Communications in Computer and Information Science 2884

Rationale
The CCIS series is devoted to the publication of proceedings of computer science conferences. Its aim is to efficiently disseminate original research results in informatics in printed and electronic form. While the focus is on publication of peer-reviewed full papers presenting mature work, inclusion of reviewed short papers reporting on work in progress is welcome, too. Besides globally relevant meetings with internationally representative program committees guaranteeing a strict peer-reviewing and paper selection process, conferences run by societies or of high regional or national relevance are also considered for publication.

Topics
The topical scope of CCIS spans the entire spectrum of informatics ranging from foundational topics in the theory of computing to information and communications science and technology and a broad variety of interdisciplinary application fields.

Information for Volume Editors and Authors
Publication in CCIS is free of charge. No royalties are paid, however, we offer registered conference participants temporary free access to the online version of the conference proceedings on SpringerLink (http://link.springer.com) by means of an http referrer from the conference website and/or a number of complimentary printed copies, as specified in the official acceptance email of the event.

CCIS proceedings can be published in time for distribution at conferences or as post-proceedings, and delivered in the form of printed books and/or electronically as USBs and/or e-content licenses for accessing proceedings at SpringerLink. Furthermore, CCIS proceedings are included in the CCIS electronic book series hosted in the SpringerLink digital library at https://link.springer.com/bookseries/7899. Conferences publishing in CCIS are allowed to use our online conference service (Meteor) for managing the whole proceedings lifecycle (from submission and reviewing to preparing for publication) free of charge.

Publication process
The language of publication is exclusively English. Authors publishing in CCIS have to sign the Springer CCIS copyright transfer form, however, they are free to use their material published in CCIS for substantially changed, more elaborate subsequent publications elsewhere. For the preparation of the camera-ready papers/files, authors have to strictly adhere to the Springer CCIS Authors' Instructions and are strongly encouraged to use the CCIS LaTeX style files or templates.

Abstracting/Indexing
CCIS is abstracted/indexed in DBLP, Google Scholar, EI-Compendex, Mathematical Reviews, SCImago, Scopus. CCIS volumes are also submitted for the inclusion in ISI Proceedings.

How to start
To start the evaluation of your proposal for inclusion in the CCIS series, please send an e-mail to ccis@springer.com

Yanchun Zhang · Qingcai Chen · Hongfei Lin ·
Lei Liu · Bo Jin · Buzhou Tang · Tianyong Hao ·
Zhengxing Huang
Editors

Health Information Processing

11th China Health Information Processing Conference, CHIP 2025
Dongguan, China, November 22–24, 2025
Proceedings

Springer

Editors
Yanchun Zhang
Zhejiang Normal University
Jinhua, China

Qingcai Chen
Harbin Institute of Technology
Harbin, Heilongjiang, China

Hongfei Lin
Dalian University of Technology
Dalian, China

Lei Liu
Fudan University
Shanghai, China

Bo Jin
Dalian University of Technology
Dalian, China

Buzhou Tang
Harbin Institute of Technology
Harbin, Heilongjiang, China

Tianyong Hao
South China Normal University
Guangzhou, China

Zhengxing Huang
Zhejiang University
Hangzhou, China

ISSN 1865-0929 ISSN 1865-0937 (electronic)
Communications in Computer and Information Science
ISBN 978-981-95-7298-4 ISBN 978-981-95-7299-1 (eBook)
https://doi.org/10.1007/978-981-95-7299-1

This Springer imprint is published by the registered company Springer Nature Singapore Pte Ltd.
The registered company address is: 152 Beach Road, #21-01/04 Gateway East, Singapore 189721, Singapore

Preface

Health information processing and applications is an essential field in data-driven life health and clinical medicine, and it has been highly active in recent decades. The China Health Information Processing Conference (CHIP) is an annual conference held by the Medical Health and Biological Information Processing Committee of the Chinese Information Processing Society (CIPS) of China, with the theme of "large models and smart healthcare". CHIP is one of the leading conferences in the field of health information processing in China and turned into an international event in 2022. It is also an important platform for researchers and practitioners from academia, business and government departments around the world to share ideas and further promote research and applications in this field. CHIP 2025 was organized by the Guangdong Medical University. CHIP 2025 was held in hybrid mode, whereby people could meet face to face or freely connect to live broadcasts of keynote speeches and presentations.

CHIP 2025 received 66 submissions, of which 37 high-quality papers were selected for publication in this volume after a double-blind peer review process in which submissions received 3.12 reviews each, on average, leading to an acceptance rate of just 56%. These papers have been categorized into 3 main topics: Biomedical data processing and model application, Mental health and disease prediction, and Drug prediction and Knowledge map.

The authors of each paper in this volume report their novel results of computing methods or applications. The volume cannot cover all aspects of Medical Health and Biological Information Processing but may still inspire insightful thoughts for the readers. We hope that more secrets of Health Information Processing will be unveiled, and that academics will drive more practical developments and solutions.

November 2025

Yanchun Zhang
Qingcai Chen
Hongfei Lin
Lei Liu
Bo Jin
Buzhou Tang
Tianyong Hao
Zhengxing Huang

Organization

Honorary Chairs

Yanchun Zhang	Zhejiang Normal University, China
Qingcai Chen	Harbin Institute of Technology (Shenzhen), China

General Co-chairs

Hongfei Lin	Dalian University of Technology, China
Lei Liu	Fudan University, China
Bo Jin	Guangdong Medical University, China

Program Co-chairs

Buzhou Tang	Harbin Institute of Technology (Shenzhen) & Pengcheng Laboratory, China
Yanshan Wang	University of Pittsburgh, USA
Maggie Haitian Wang	Chinese University of Hong Kong, China
Pingtao Duan	Guangdong Medical University, China

Publication Co-chairs

Tianyong Hao	South China Normal University, China
Xinyu He	Liaoning Normal University, China
Jiao Li	Institute of Medical Information, Chinese Academy of Medical Sciences, China
Ling Luo	Dalian University of Technology, China
Lu Xiang	Institute of Automation, Chinese Academy of Sciences, China
Yongjun Zhu	Yonsei University, South Korea

Forum Co-chairs

Zhengxing Huang	Zhejiang University, China
Jun Yan	City University of Hong Kong, China
Haofen Wang	Tongji University, China
Ming Feng	Peking Union Medical College Hospital, China
Zhumin Chen	Shandong University, China
Yi Zhou	Sun Yat-sen University, China
SenDong Zhao	Harbin Institute of Technology, China

Evaluation Co-chairs

Zuofeng Li	Tongji University, China
Jianbo Lei	Medical Informatics Center of Peking University, China
Hui Zong	West China Hospital, Sichuan University, China

Publicity Co-Chairs

Lishuang Li	Dalian University of Technology, China
Yinghui Jin	Zhongnan Hospital of Wuhan University, China
Ping Song	Children's Hospital Affiliated to Chongqing Medical University, China

Sponsor Co-chairs

Jun Yan	City University of Hong Kong, China
Siwei Yu	Guizhou Medical University, China
Yi Zhou	Sun Yat-sen University, China
Buyue Qian	Chaoyang Hospital Affiliated to Capital Medical University, China
Yonghui Wu	University of Florida, USA

Web Chair

Kunli Zhang	Zhengzhou University, China

Program Committee

Wenping Guo	Taizhou University, China
Hongmin Cai	South China University of Technology, China
Chao Che	Dalian University, China
Mosha Chen	Alibaba, China
Qingcai Chen	Harbin Institute of Technology (Shenzhen), China
Xi Chen	Tencent Technology Co., Ltd., China
Yang Chen	Yidu Cloud (Beijing) Technology Co., Ltd., China
Zhumin Chen	Shandong University, China
Ming Cheng	Zhengzhou University, China
Ruoyao Ding	Guangdong University of Foreign Studies, China
Bin Dong	Ricoh Software Research Center (Beijing) Co., Ltd., China
Guohong Fu	Soochow University, China
Yan Gao	Central South University, China
Tianyong Hao	South China Normal University, China
Shizhu He	Institute of Automation, Chinese Academy of Sciences, China
Zengyou He	Dalian University of Technology, China
Na Hong	Digital China Medical Technology Co., Ltd., China
Li Hou	Institute of Medical Information, Chinese Academy of Medical Sciences, China
Yong Hu	Jinan University, China
Baotian Hu	Harbin University of Technology (Shenzhen), China
Guimin Huang	Guilin University of Electronic Science and Technology, China
Zhenghang Huang	Zhejiang University, China
Zhiwei Huang	Southwest Medical University, China
Bo Jin	Dalian University of Technology, China
Xiaoyu Kang	Southwest Medical University, China
Jianbo Lei	Peking University, China
Haomin Li	Children's Hospital of Zhejiang University Medical College, China
Jiao Li	Institute of Medical Information, Chinese Academy of Medical Sciences, China
Jinghua Li	Chinese Academy of Traditional Chinese Medicine, China
Lishuang Li	Dalian University of Technology, China
Linfeng Li	Yidu Cloud (Beijing) Technology Co., Ltd., China
Ru Li	Shanxi University, China

Runzhi Li	Zhengzhou University, China
Shasha Li	National University of Defense Technology, China
Xing Li	Beijing Shenzhengyao Technology Co., Ltd., China
Xin Li	Zhongkang Physical Examination Technology Co., Ltd., China
Yuxi Li	Peking University First Hospital, China
Zuofeng Li	Takeda China, China
Xiangwen Liao	Fuzhou University, China
Hao Lin	University of Electronic Science and Technology of China, China
Hongfei Lin	Dalian University of Technology, China
Bangtao Liu	Southwest Medical University, China
Song Liu	Qilu University of Technology, China
Lei Liu	Fudan University, China
Shengping Liu	Unisound Co., Ltd., China
Xiaoming Liu	Zhongyuan University of Technology, China
Guan Luo	Institute of Automation, Chinese Academy of Sciences, China
Lingyun Luo	Nanhua University, China
Yamei Luo	Southwest Medical University, China
Hui Lv	Shanghai Jiao Tong University, China
Xudong Lv	Zhejiang University, China
Yao Meng	Lenovo Research Institute, China
Qingliang Miao	Suzhou Aispeech Information Technology Co., Ltd., China
Weihua Peng	Baidu Co., Ltd., China
Buyue Qian	Xi'an Jiaotong University, China
Longhua Qian	Suzhou University, China
Tong Ruan	East China University of Technology, China
Ying Shen	South China University of Technology, China
Xiaofeng Song	Nanjing University of Aeronautics and Astronautics, China
Chengjie Sun	Harbin University of Technology, China
Chuanji Tan	Alibaba Dharma Hall, China
Hongye Tan	Shanxi University, China
Jingyu Tan	Shenzhen Xinkaiyuan Information Technology Development Co., Ltd., China
Binhua Tang	Hohai University, China
Buzhou Tang	Harbin Institute of Technology (Shenzhen), China
Jintao Tang	National Defense University of the People's Liberation Army, China

Kunli Zhang	Zhengzhou University, China
Weide Zhang	Zhongshan Hospital Affiliated to Fudan University, China
Xiaoyan Zhang	Tongji University, China
Yaoyun Zhang	Alibaba, China
Yijia Zhang	Dalian University of Technology, China
Yuanzhe Zhang	Institute of Automation, Chinese Academy of Sciences, China
Zhichang Zhang	Northwest Normal University, China
Qiuye Zhao	Beijing Big Data Research Institute, China
Sendong Zhao	Harbin Institute of Technology, China
Tiejun Zhao	Harbin Institute of Technology, China
Deyu Zhou	Southeast University, China
Fengfeng Zhou	Jilin University, China
Guangyou Zhou	Central China Normal University, China
Yi Zhou	Sun Yat-sen University, China
Conghui Zhu	Harbin Institute of Technology, China
Shanfeng Zhu	Fudan University, China
Yu Zhu	Sunshine Life Insurance Co., Ltd., China
Quan Zou	University of Electronic Science and Technology of China, China
Xi Chen	University of Electronic Science and Technology of China, China
Yansheng Li	Mediway Technology Co., Ltd., China
Daojing He	Harbin Institute of Technology (Shenzhen), China
Yupeng Liu	Harbin University of Science and Technology, China
Xinzhi Sun	First Affiliated Hospital of Zhengzhou University, China
Chuanchao Du	Third People's Hospital of Henan Province, China
Xien Liu	Beijing Huijizhiyi Technology Co., Ltd., China
Shan Nan	Hainan University, China
Xinyu He	Liaoning Normal University, China
Qianqian He	Chongqing Medical University, China
Xing Liu	Third Xiangya Hospital of Central South University, China
Jiayin Wang	Xi'an Jiaotong University, China
Ying Xu	Xi'an Jiaotong University, China
Xin Lai	Xi'an Jiaotong University, China

Contents

Mental Health and Disease Prediction

Drug Prediction and Knowledge Map

Biomedical Data Processing and Model Application

CausalMPT: Causal Multimodal Prompt Tuning for Healthcare MIE

Ziyue Huang[1,2], Xiaoming Liu[1,3](✉), Guan Yang[1,3], Jie Liu[4], Yang Long[5], Junyi Gao[1,2], and Kai Yang[1,2]

[1] School of Artificial Intelligence, Zhongyuan University of Technology, No. 41, Zhongyuan Zhong Road, Zhengzhou 4500007, China
ming616@zut.edu.cn

[2] School of Computer Science, Zhongyuan University of Technology, No. 41, Zhongyuan Zhong Road, Zhengzhou 4500007, China

[3] Zhengzhou Key Laboratory of Text Processing and Image Understanding, No. 41, Zhongyuan Zhong Road, Zhengzhou 4500007, China
ming616@zut.edu.cn

[4] North China University of Technology, No. 5, Jinyuanzhuang Road, Shijingshan District, Beijing 100144, China

[5] Durham University, Durham City Campus: Palatine Center, Stockton Road, Durham, DH1 3LE, England

Abstract. Healthcare and elderly-care domains increasingly demand the integration of heterogeneous multimodal information–ranging from medical images and patient records to health-related social data–to enable accurate and timely decision-making. This necessitates advanced multimodal information extraction (MIE) techniques, yet current multimodal large language models (MLLMs) still face challenges of modal imbalance, spurious correlations, and limited robustness due to their reliance on associative rather than causal learning. To address these challenges, we propose causal multimodal prompt tuning (CausalMPT), explicitly introducing causal reasoning into MLLMS to enhance multimodal understanding. CausalMPT adopts a modular design and features three key innovations: a counterfactual intervention module for eliminating false correlations and revealing causal relationships between modalities; The parameter efficient tuning module based on lora can effectively adapt to large-scale models with limited resources. And a prompt answer module, which uses prompts for specific tasks to guide MIE's fine-grained causal reasoning. A large number of experiments conducted on four benchmark datasets have shown that CausalMPT has achieved consistent improvements. Compared with the basic model, F1 has increased by 1.47%, 0.11%, 1.20%, and 5.02% respectively.

Keywords: Multimodal information extraction · Counterfactual reasoning · Elderly-care scenarios

Y. Zhang et al. (Eds.): CHIP 2025, CCIS 2884, pp. 3–13, 2026.
https://doi.org/10.1007/978-981-95-7299-1_1

1 Introduction

Recently, MLLMs have demonstrated strong potential in bridging modality gaps by jointly modeling visual and textual features. In the context of health and wellness, such models can be used to automatically integrate medical imaging reports with clinical texts, support patient monitoring on wearable devices, and provide decision support for health data analysis and early prevention of chronic diseases. However, despite their impressive performance, these models remain vulnerable to modality-specific biases and spurious correlations. They often overfit to superficial cues rather than capturing underlying semantic or causal relationships.

To overcome these limitations, causal inference techniques have attracted increasing attention for their ability to eliminate spurious correlations and improve model fairness and interpretability [3]. Pearl's structural causal model (SCM) provides a principled framework for modeling causal dependencies [11], while counterfactual reasoning offers a means to simulate hypothetical interventions and evaluate causal effects. In NLP, causal frameworks have been successfully applied to reduce dataset bias and enhance generalization, and recent efforts have extended these benefits to MIE tasks [7].

Based on these insights, this study introduces a new causal framework that integrates causal representation learning (CRL) into the multimodal information extraction (MIE) pipeline. Specifically, counterfactual intervention mechanisms were incorporated to mitigate inductive bias in multimodal inputs and encourage the model to learn representations based on causal relationships. In addition, task-specific prompts are embedded into multimodal large language models (MLLMS), thereby enhancing their reasoning capabilities and improving the accuracy of MIE. A large number of experiments on the benchmark dataset have verified the effectiveness and robustness of this method.

2 Related Works

2.1 Multimodal Information Extraction

Multimodal Named Entity recognition (MNER) is a key task in MIE, aiming to automatically identify and extract named entities from multimodal data such as clinical records, diagnostic images, and health-related social data. The main challenge lies in enhancing semantic representation by effectively integrating visual cues and textual information. Early methods relied on global image features, while recent studies have introduced fine-grained alignment based on self-attention mechanisms [6], cross-modal contractive learning [4], and multi-level feature fusion [2]. To better capture the visual signals that are crucial for identifying entities.

Multimodal relationship extraction (MRE) focuses on identifying relationships between cross-modal entities, which is particularly relevant to healthcare applications, such as linking symptoms with diseases, drugs with side effects, or patients with treatment outcomes. Similar to MNER, MRE must overcome the challenge of effective modal fusion. For instance, Zhang et al. [14] proposed a multi-layer feature fusion method that fuses the features of different layers of text and images together, enhancing the model's ability to capture complex reasoning.

Multimodal event extraction (MEE) aims to provide a comprehensive understanding of medical and healthcare-related events, such as disease progression, treatment interventions, or adverse drug reactions. The MEED model [15] adopts a Transformer-based feature fusion strategy to identify event types and extract parameter roles across modality. Xiang et al. [17] extended it by introducing external knowledge, improving the recognition accuracy, but at the cost of reducing generalization. Chen et al. [1] proposed a cross-modal event extraction framework that integrates multimodal signals to extract richer event features.

3 Methodology

3.1 Task Definition

Given a multimodal dataset D, where each sample D consists of M modal data, the Causal Multimodal Prompt Tuning (CausalMPT) method can perform a detailed NER from the multimodal dataset D.

$$D_i = \{x_{i,1}, x_{i,2}, \ldots, x_{i,M}\} \tag{1}$$

Here $x_{i,1}$ represents an image-text pair, an aligned pair consisting of a visual scene and its associated textual description.

MNER: Given a sentence and its related image, the goal of MNER is to identify and classify the named entities within the sentence. The output is a set of entities and their types:

$$f_{\text{MNER}} : \{x_1, x_2, \ldots, x_M\} \xrightarrow{\text{CausalMPT}} \{(e_1, t_1), (e_2, t_2), \ldots, (e_i, t_i)\} \tag{2}$$

where e_i represents the i-th identified entity and t_i represents its type.

MRE: Given a sentence and its related images, the goal of MRE is to identify the semantic relationships between entities in the sentence. The output is a set of entities and their types:

$$f_{\text{MRE}} : \{x_1, x_2, \ldots, x_M\} \xrightarrow{\text{CausalMPT}} \{(e_1, r_1, e_1), (e_2, r_2, e_3), \ldots, (e_i, r_i, e_j)\} \tag{3}$$

Among them, r_i represents the semantic relationship existing between the head entity e_i and the tail entity e_j.

MEE: The objective of MEE is to identify and extract the event element types described in a sentence, given the sentence and its associated image. The output is a set of entities and their types:

$$f_{\text{MEE}} : \{x_1, x_2, \ldots, x_M\} \xrightarrow{\text{CausalMPT}} \{t_1, t_2, \ldots, t_i\} \tag{4}$$

where t_i is the type of event extracted.

3.2 Overall Architecture

The general framework of the CausalMPT model is shown in Fig. 1, and the specific process is as follows: First, we apply counterfactual interventions on the source dataset and generate a counterfactual intervention dataset through the counterfactual intervention causal augmentation module. Then the counterfactual intervention dataset is combined with the original dataset and input into the multimodal large model module for joint training. In the training process, through effective parameter adjustment and model fine-tuning, the generalization ability of the model is enhanced, and the causal relationship within the model is established. Finally, the trained multimodal model is derived, and meaningful information is identified and extracted based on the multimodal data sources, subsequently organized in a consistent format.

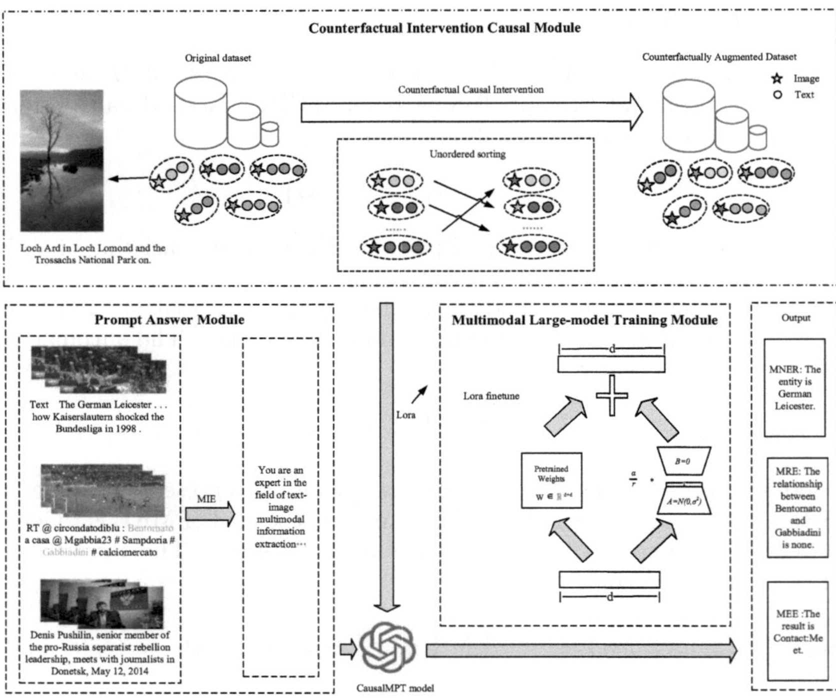

Fig. 1. The architecture comprises three key components: a counterfactual intervention module, a multimodal large-model training module, and a prompt-based answer module. The intervention module constructs a counterfactual dataset from text-image pairs, which is then used by the training module for cross-modal optimization. The trained model is deployed in the answer module to extract and structure semantically meaningful information in a standardized format.

3.3 Counterfactual Intervention Causal Module

The counterfactual intervention causal module leverages state-of-the-art large-scale model techniques in conjunction with a counterfactual causality enhancement mechanism. Generates counterfactual data by extracting representative subsets from relevant datasets, guided by a causal intervention strategy (Fig. 2).

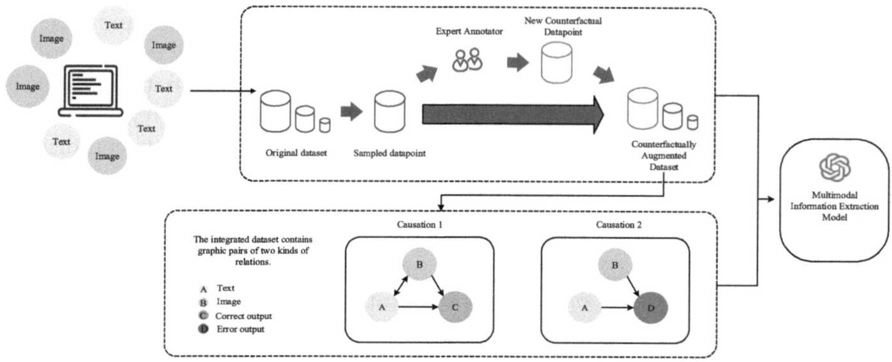

Fig. 2. Counterfactual Intervention Structure: The figure shows the counterfactual intervention structure, which enhances the capabilities of the MIE model. The original dataset is transformed to generate new counterfactual data points, which are then fused with the original dataset to form a counterfactual-enhanced dataset. The dataset contains two causal examples, where text and image jointly influence the model's output and help distinguish between correct and incorrect predictions. Finally, the data is fed into the MIE model to enhance its causal reasoning ability in multimodal contexts.

For each textimage pair in the dataset, we construct new pairs by altering word order or modifying semantic content within the text. These modified textimage pairs are intentionally misaligned with the original pairs: the revised textual descriptions convey reversed or weakly correlated semantics relative to the associated images. This counterfactual construction allows for the observation of multimodal relationships under perturbed conditions and serves as a negative reference to guide the model in learning authentic causal features, thus enhancing its causal reasoning capabilities.

Subsequently, inverse causal relationships between textual and visual modalities are established. The modified data are then reintegrated into the original dataset, enabling the multimodal model to retain its original capacity while acquiring an improved understanding of latent causal structures. To balance the learning signal, the original and counterfactual datasets are combined in a 4:1 ratio. A stratified sampling strategy is employed to ensure that both data types are proportionally represented across all subtasks, thereby promoting robustness and generalizability in downstream applications.

3.4 Multimodal Large-Model Training Module

During the multimodal large-model training module, the model gradually strengthens its understanding of textimage correlations and is guided to distinguish between causal and merely correlational relationships through contrastive learning. To optimize efficiency, we integrate PEFT with the LoRA method, which significantly reduces training cost and memory usage while maintaining strong performance on counterfactual data.

The training process relies on both the original dataset and its counterfactual variants, ensuring that the model learns to recognize subtle causal cues. The overall learning objective combines the primary task loss, which evaluates the consistency between predictions and ground-truth labels, with an auxiliary counterfactual contrastive loss that encourages the model to discriminate between original and counterfactual samples. A weight coefficient dynamically balances the contributions of these two objectives, allowing the model to adaptively emphasize causal learning when needed.

Through iterative optimization, LoRA introduces low-rank updates that fine-tune only a small portion of parameters, improving computational efficiency without degrading accuracy. Model parameters are progressively updated based on gradients derived from the joint loss, ensuring that both task-specific goals and causal reasoning objectives guide the training. After convergence, the fine-tuned multimodal model incorporates causal-aware representations, enabling more robust performance in complex and noisy multimodal environments.

3.5 Prompt Answer Module

Table 1. Prompt answer module: MNER prompt template

Information	Prompt	Expected
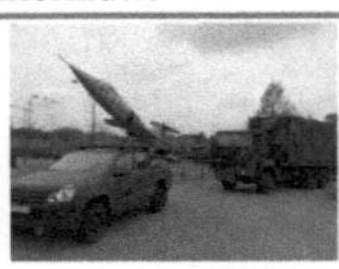 **MNER**: RT @aocsnm: Onderweg naar Finland. Internationale samenwerking. #ArticChallengeExercise #ACE2015 #NDMC #luchtgevechtsleiding	"role": "user", "content": ["type": "text", "text": "Please identify the named entity of the long text data I send you. Combined with the image data, the output is mainly based on the entity name in the long text. The short text data contained in the long text data need to be highlighted, and identify as many entities as possible under the condition of meeting the premise, press ['entity': '(LOC, PER, ORG, MISC format note)', 'word': '...'] This format returns the identified entity information. Please do not translate, return to the same format, and do not arbitrarily convert the case (the output entity case should correspond to the words in the text data). Note that if it feels like there's no entity, return []."]	#NDMC, Finland.

* First, text and images are passed to the model as input. Then, further process the model based on the prompt to generate the expected results

After training, the model is able to capture potential causal relationships between text and images without requiring explicit causal clues in the prompts. To fully leverage this capability, we design a logical prompting mechanism that effectively activates and guides the model during inference (Table 1).

The prompt module first directs the model to extract key information from long text passages and then align it with relevant image content, thereby facilitating the MIE process. Although the prompts do not explicitly encode causal knowledge, the model can exploit the learned causal associations to enhance extraction accuracy.

Taking MNER as an example Table 2, the model receives text, image, and prompt inputs. Guided by the prompt, it identifies and extracts entity mentions together with their corresponding types. If no valid entity is detected, the model outputs a null result. This process ensures that entity extraction is both prompt-driven and causally informed, enabling more robust performance in complex multimodal scenarios.

4 Experiment

4.1 Datasets

To verify the effectiveness of the proposed method in this article, experiments were conducted on four MIE datasets and two extended datasets: Twitter-2015, Twitter-2017, MNRE-V1 [19], M^2E^2, Twitter- 2015-V1 and Twitter- 2017-V1, and improvements and tests were made on these datasets. The statistical analysis of the dataset can be found in Table 2.

Table 2. Statistics of relevant datasets.

Dataset	Task	Train	Dev	Test
Twitter-2015	MNER	4,000	1,000	3,257
Twitter-2017	MNER	3,373	723	723
MNRE-V1	MRE	7,824	975	1,282
M^2E^2	MEE	–	–	309

4.2 Experimental Configuration

The deep learning platform is deployed on servers equipped with NVIDIA RTX A5000 Gpus. It was trained on the Twitter-2015 dataset with a batch size of 1 and a learning rate of 5e-5, and real-time training optimization and performance monitoring were carried out using Wandb. After completion, evaluate the model on other datasets to assess its generalization in different tasks and domains.

4.3 Baselines

In order to compare with the framework model we proposed, we also selected the existing MLLMs from the Huggingface website as the baseline model. These models cover various architectural designs and optimization strategies and demonstrate outstanding performance in multimodal tasks. Specifically, it includes the following several models: Neural Network Technology, transformer Architecture and Multimodal Large Language Models.

4.4 Main Results

Table 3. MIE performance on datasets (F1 Score, %)

Method	Twitter-15	Twitter-17	MNRE-V1	M^2E^2
CNN-BiLSTM-CRF [10]	67.15	<u>79.37</u>	–	–
Visual ChatGPT [16]	41.45	41.24	–	–
MMUTF [12]	–	–	–	54.60
llava-1.5-7b* [8]	67.60	65.32	46.84	66.67
Ovis1.6-Gemma2-9B* [9]	59.63	51.40	21.82	–
llava-gemma-2B* [13]	49.67	–	–	30.84
LLaVA-NeXT-Video-7B* [18]	34.14	53.53	20.12	65.26
llama3-llava-next-8B* [5]	<u>69.00</u>	78.31	<u>47.98</u>	<u>72.85</u>
llama3*+CausalMPT	**70.47** (+1.47)	**79.48** (+0.11)	**49.18** (+1.20)	**77.87** (+5.02)

* The CausalMPT method achieved the best performance in terms of F1 scores.
In the table, **bold** indicates the best result, *<u>underline</u>* denotes the second-best result, and * indicates results obtained under the same local server environment.
llama3*+CausalMPT (Ours) is built upon the llama3-llava-next-8B model as the base architecture

To evaluate the effectiveness of the proposed CausalMPT module, we conducted extensive experiments on four widely used benchmark datasets: Twitter-2015, Twitter-2017, MNRE-V1, and M^2E^2. These datasets cover a range of MIE tasks, including MNER, MRE, and MEE, thereby providing a comprehensive evaluation of the model's capability. We compared our approach against both traditional baselines and state-of-the-art MLLMs, with detailed results presented in Table 3.

Specifically, when built on the llama3-llava-next-8B backbone, our method achieved F1 scores of 70.47% and 79.48% on the Twitter-2015 and Twitter-2017 datasets, respectively, surpassing all existing baselines, including several strong MLLM variants. Notably, compared with the backbone model without causal modeling, the integrated CausalMPT module yielded absolute gains of 1.47% and 0.11% on the two datasets. These improvements, though modest in scale, demonstrate the stable and consistent advantages of incorporating causal reasoning, especially in enhancing entity-level semantic understanding where spurious correlations are common.

In addition, on the MNRE-V1 and M^2E^2 datasets, which focus on relation extraction and event extraction tasks, our method once again achieved the highest F1 scores of 49.18% and 77.87%, respectively. These results are significantly superior to those of competing multimodal models, confirming that the proposed CausalMPT module not only benefits entity recognition but also effectively supports more complex reasoning tasks such as identifying fine-grained entity relations and event structures. Overall, the consistent improvements across all benchmarks strongly validate the generalizability and robustness of the CausalMPT framework in diverse multimodal scenarios.

5 Conclusion

This article proposes CausalMPT, a novel framework designed to enhance MIE tasks through counterfactual intervention and causal reasoning mechanisms. Extensive experiments demonstrate that CausalMPT consistently outperforms existing large-scale multimodal models, particularly in accurately identifying causal associations within noisy and complex multimodal data. These findings highlight the strong potential of CausalMPT in advancing causal modeling and robust reasoning across diverse multimodal scenarios, including healthcare and elderly-care applications where causal inference is crucial for safe and reliable decision-making.

While CausalMPT shows promising performance, it still faces challenges when confronted with highly noisy or incomplete multimodal input, especially in cases where one modality provides limited information. Future work will therefore focus on refining its causal alignment mechanism and incorporating deeper semantic reasoning and contextual understanding, with the aim of developing cognitively intelligent multimodal models. Such improvements hold significant promise for healthcare and wellness applications, enabling precise chronic disease management, adaptive elderly monitoring, and personalized health interventions.

Acknowledgement. This research was supported by National Key Research and Development Program of China (2020AAA0109703); National Natural Science Foundation of China (62076167,U23B2029); The Key Scientific Research Project of Higher Education Institutions in Henan Province, China (24A520058,23A 520022); Postgraduate Education Reform and Quality Improvement Project of Henan Province, China(YJS2024AL053).

References

1. Chen, B., Lin, X., Thomas, C., Li, M., Yoshida, S., Chum, L., Ji, H., Chang, S.F.: Joint multimedia event extraction from video and article (2021). arXiv:2109.12776
2. Huang, Z., Zeng, Z., Liu, B., Fu, D., Fu, J.: Pixel-bert: aligning image pixels with text by deep multi-modal transformers (2020). arXiv:2004.00849
3. Jiang, Y., Xie, W.: Hierarchical global pointer network: an implicit relation inference method for gene-disease knowledge discovery. In: Tang, B., Chen, Q., Lin, H., Wu, F., Liu, L., Hao, T., Wang, Y., Wang, H., Lei, J., Li, Z., Zong, H. (eds.) Health Information Processing. Evaluation Track Papers, pp. 14–28. Springer Nature Singapore, Singapore (2023)
4. Kim, W., Son, B., Kim, I.: Vilt: Vision-and-language transformer without convolution or region supervision. In: International Conference on Machine Learning, pp. 5583–5594. PMLR (2021)
5. Li, B., Zhang, K., Zhang, H., Guo, D., Zhang, R., Li, F., Zhang, Y., Liu, Z., Li, C.: LLaVA-NeXT: Stronger LLMs Supercharge Multimodal Capabilities in the Wild (2024). https://llava-vl.github.io/blog/2024-05-10-llava-next-stronger-llms/
6. Li, L.H., Yatskar, M., Yin, D., Hsieh, C., Chang, K.: Visualbert: a simple and performant baseline for vision and language (2019). arXiv:1908.03557
7. Li, Z., Chen, M., Yin, K., Tong, Y., Tan, C., Lang, Z., Tang, B.: Chip2022 shared task overview: Medical causal entity relationship extraction. In: Tang, B., Chen, Q., Lin, H., Wu, F., Liu, L., Hao, T., Wang, Y., Wang, H., Lei, J., Li, Z., Zong, H. (eds.) Health Information Processing. Evaluation Track Papers. pp. 51–56. Springer Nature Singapore, Singapore (2023)
8. Liu, H., Li, C., Wu, Q., Lee, Y.J.: Visual instruction tuning. Adv. Neural. Inf. Process. Syst. **36**, 34892–34916 (2023)
9. Lu, S., Li, Y., Chen, Q.G., Xu, Z., Luo, W., Zhang, K., Ye, H.J.: Ovis: structural embedding alignment for multimodal large language model (2024). arXiv:2405.20797
10. Ma, X., Hovy, E.: End-to-end sequence labeling via bi-directional LSTM-CNNs-CRF. In: Erk, K., Smith, N.A. (eds.) Proceedings of the 54th Annual Meeting of the Association for Computational Linguistics (Volume 1: Long Papers), pp. 1064–1074. Association for Computational Linguistics, Berlin, Germany (2016). https://doi.org/10.18653/v1/P16-1101, https://aclanthology.org/P16-1101/
11. Neuberg, L.G.: Causality: Models, Reasoning, and Inference, by Judea Pearl. Cambridge University Press (2000). Econometric Theory **19**(4), 675–685 (2003)
12. Seeberger: MMUTF: Multimodal multimedia event argument extraction with unified template filling. In: Al-Onaizan, Y., Bansal, M., Chen, Y.N. (eds.) Findings of the Association for Computational Linguistics: EMNLP 2024, pp. 6539–6548. Association for Computational Linguistics, Miami, Florida, USA (2024). https://doi.org/10.18653/v1/2024.findings-emnlp.381https://aclanthology.org/2024.findings-emnlp.381/
13. Lu, S., Li, Y., Chen, Q.G.: Ovis: structural embedding alignment for multimodal large language model (2024). arXiv:2405.20797
14. Sun, L., Zhang, K., Li, Q., Lou, R.: Umie: Unified multimodal information extraction with instruction tuning. In: Proceedings of the AAAI Conference on Artificial Intelligence, vol. 38, pp. 19062–19070 (2024)
15. Wang, S., Zheng, Q., Su, Z., Na, C., Qi, G.: Meed: A multimodal event extraction dataset. In: Qin, B., Jin, Z., Wang, H., Pan, J., Liu, Y., An, B. (eds.) Knowledge Graph and Semantic Computing: Knowledge Graph Empowers New Infrastructure Construction, pp. 288–294. Springer Singapore, Singapore (2021)

16. Wu, C., Yin, S., Qi, W., Wang, X., Tang, Z., Duan, N.: Visual chatgpt: talking, drawing and editing with visual foundation models (2023). arXiv:2303.04671
17. Xiang, Y., Jia, Y., Zhang, X., Zhang, Z.: Multi-modal military event extraction based on knowledge fusion. Comput. Mat. Continua **77**(1), 97–114 (2023). https://doi.org/10.32604/cmc.2023.040751. https://www.sciencedirect.com/science/article/pii/S1546221823001315
18. Zhang, Y., Li, B., Liu, H., Lee, Y.J., Gui, L., Fu, D., Feng, J., Liu, Z., Li, C.: LLaVA-NeXT: A Strong Zero-shot Video Understanding Model (2024). https://llava-vl.github.io/blog/2024-04-30-llava-next-video/
19. Zheng, C., Wu, Z., Feng, J., Fu, Z., Cai, Y.: Mnre: a challenge multimodal dataset for neural relation extraction with visual evidence in social media posts. In: 2021 IEEE International Conference on Multimedia and Expo (ICME), pp. 1–6 (2021). https://doi.org/10.1109/ICME51207.2021.9428274

Iterative Dynamic Routing Framework for Medical Question Answering

Chutong Wang[1,2,3], Xuebing Yang[1,2(✉)], Yunqi Zhu[1,2], Mengxuan Sun[2], Mingda Li[2], and Wensheng Zhang[1,2]

[1] Guangzhou University, Guangzhou, China
[2] State Key Laboratory of Multimodal Artificial Intelligence Systems, Institute of Automation, Chinese Academy of Sciences, Beijing, China
yangxuebing2013@ia.ac.cn
[3] University of Chinese Academy of Sciences, Beijing, China

Abstract. Large Language Models (LLMs) have recently shown strong performance on Question Answering (QA) tasks. However, in the medical domain, they often hallucinate due to gaps in domain-specific knowledge. Retrieval-Augmented Generation (RAG) mitigates this issue by grounding answers in external information, but most existing approaches rely on single-round or single-retriever paradigms, which struggle with multi-hop questions or when relevant knowledge is distributed across heterogeneous sources. To this end, we propose the **I**terative **D**ynamic **R**outing **F**ramework (IDRF) for medical QA. IDRF performs iterative reasoning and retrieval, enabling the model to generate multiple retrieval intents, access heterogeneous knowledge sources in parallel, and progressively construct the final answer. The framework consists of three components: a master agent that plans each round, a retriever module with four specialized retrievers, and a summary agent that condenses retrieved results into feedback for the master agent. Experiments on three public medical QA datasets show that IDRF significantly outperforms competitive baselines, and ablation studies confirm the contribution of each component.

Keywords: Medical question answering · Retrieval-augmented generation · Dynamic routing · Large language model

1 Introduction

The rapid advancement of Large Language Models (LLMs) has led to a paradigm shift in how humans retrieve information, replacing traditional search engines with intent-aware conversational systems. Although related research has demonstrated the capabilities of Question Answering (QA) in various domains [1], LLMs often generate plausible-sounding but non-factual answers, commonly known as hallucination [2]. In high-stakes domains such as healthcare, even small diagnostic errors could lead to severe consequences [3]. Supervised Fine-Tuning

Y. Zhang et al. (Eds.): CHIP 2025, CCIS 2884, pp. 14–28, 2026.
https://doi.org/10.1007/978-981-95-7299-1_2

(SFT) can help adapt LLMs to medical tasks, but it struggles with out-of-distribution queries due to its reliance on static training data, which quickly becomes outdated [4].

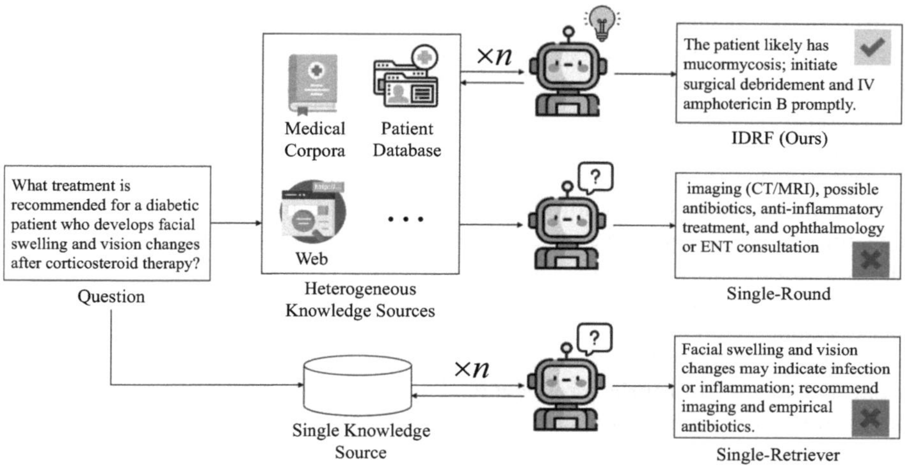

Fig. 1. Illustration of two RAG paradigms and IDRF for the medical QA task. For complex questions, both single-round and single-retriever paradigms may fail to retrieve the necessary information, whereas IDRF can iteratively query heterogeneous knowledge sources and thereby provide more accurate answers.

To overcome these issues, Retrieval-Augmented Generation (RAG) supplements LLMs with up-to-date and domain-specific information, reducing the risk of hallucination and grounding responses in external evidence [5]. However, despite recent progress in medical QA, most RAG approaches still depend on single-round or single-retriever paradigms, which often fail in real-world clinical scenarios. We identify three key challenges where such rigid methods fall short.

Challenge 1. Multi-hop questions often require reasoning over multiple pieces of information. Single-round RAG methods typically rely on the surface semantics of the input, conflating distinct information needs into a single query and yielding broad but imprecise results. For example, as shown in Fig. 1, such methods may retrieve only general information on facial swelling or vision changes. Without iterative retrieval grounded in inferred intermediate diagnoses (e.g., mucormycosis), these methods fail to identify the appropriate treatment.

Challenge 2. Required medical knowledge may be scattered across heterogeneous sources, with no single source providing complete information for complex questions. As illustrated in Fig. 1, relying solely on medical documents may be insufficient to infer the emergence of mucormycosis. Accessing additional sources, such as patient databases or the web, can provide complementary context and better capture a patients clinical trajectory.

Challenge 3. Some questions involve rare or emerging conditions, such as early knowledge of COVID-19 or uncommon diseases, where relevant information may exist only in specific sources. A single-retriever approach may not contain the required knowledge, while a single-round approach may select the wrong source. For example, knowledge about COVID-19 in early 2019 or rare diseases is often poorly covered in static medical literature. Without the ability to iteratively explore multiple sources, these approaches may fail to provide complete and accurate answers.

To address the aforementioned challenges, we propose a novel **I**terative **D**ynamic **R**outing **F**ramework (IDRF). IDRF introduces an iterative reasoning and retrieval process that enables precise, context-aware information gathering from heterogeneous knowledge sources. The framework consists of three key components: a master agent, a retriever module, and a summary agent. The retriever module integrates four specialized retrievers, each tailored to a specific knowledge source, directly addressing Challenge 2. Given a medical question, the master agent first determines whether the question can be answered. If not, it formulates a sub-question, generates multiple retrieval intents, and routes them in parallel to the appropriate retrievers. The summary agent then condenses the retrieved results, focusing on the sub-question, and provides this feedback to the master agent, which initiates the next round. This iterative, dynamic routing mechanism enables IDRF to tackle the complexities outlined in Challenge 1 and Challenge 3.

Our main contributions are summarized as follows:

- We propose a novel iterative dynamic routing framework, IDRF, which performs dynamic and parallel retrievals over multiple rounds, enabling more accurate and efficient answers in complex medical QA scenarios.
- We design four types of specialized retrievers to access heterogeneous knowledge sources and employ query-focused summarization to condense the retrieved results.
- Experiments on three representative medical QA datasets demonstrate that IDRF achieves superior performance compared to competitive baselines. Furthermore, ablation studies confirm the effectiveness of each individual component within the framework.

2 Related Work

LLMs for Medicine. LLMs have demonstrated strong potential in medical applications. Several medical LLMs, such as Med-PaLM [6] and PMC-LLaMA [7], are pretrained on biomedical corpora to enhance domain expertise. For medical QA, Das et al. [8] introduce a two-layer RAG framework and use social media data to handle low resource scenarios, while Xia et al. [9] introduce provably effective and preference optimization strategy to enhance factual accuracy. For medical summarization, Veen et al. [10] explore in-context learning and QLoRA across eight LLMs, and Dehkordi et al. [11] show that adding textual highlights can improve model accuracy. In radiology report generation, Veen et al. [12] achieve optimal performance through pretraining on clinical text and parameter-efficient fine-tuning. LLMs also assist clinical prediction [13], medical coding [14] and drug discovery [15], demonstrating broad biomedical utility.

RAG. RAG [5] enables language models to access external knowledge without continual tuning, improving response accuracy and mitigating hallucination [16]. RAG has shown strong performance across various tasks, including fact verification [17], code generation [18], and question answering [19]. In medical QA, Xiong et al. [20] provide a comprehensive benchmarking study using vanilla RAG systems across multiple datasets. Building on this, Xiong et al. [21] propose i-MedRAG, which generates iterative follow-up questions to refine document retrieval and improve answer accuracy. Xu et al. [22] develop Sim-RAG, a self-improving framework that creates high-quality QA pairs to facilitate domain-adaptive fine-tuning of LLMs. Xia et al. [3] introduce MMed-RAG, a single-round multimodal RAG framework integrating visual and textual retrieval for medical VQA.

3 Method

As illustrated in Fig. 2, our framework operates iteratively and consists of three modules: a master agent, a retriever module, and a summary agent. Given a medical question, the master agent begins each round by determining whether the question can be answered. If not, it first formulates a sub-question, then generates several retrieval intents and routes them in parallel to the corresponding retrievers, which query heterogeneous knowledge sources. Subsequently, the summary agent condenses the retrieved results and provides this feedback to the master agent for the next round of reasoning.

3.1 Master Agent

The master agent is the core module of IDRF, responsible for controlling the workflow and generating the final answer. The agent maintains a memory that stores knowledge collected and condensed from previous rounds (empty in Round 1). At the beginning of each round, upon receiving a medical question, the master agent determines whether it has sufficient knowledge to provide a precise answer. If the agent identifies missing information, it formulates a sub-question and generates several queries, which are routed to the corresponding retrievers. The retrievers information and invocation rules are provided in a system prompt (refer to Appendix A). In each round, multiple retrievers can be called in parallel, and each retriever may be invoked multiple times. This design reduces the number of rounds required, thereby improving the efficiency of the medical QA process, as the retrieval operations are relatively fast.

3.2 Retriever Module

Based on the knowledge sources we collect, we elaborate four specialized retrievers in the retriever module:

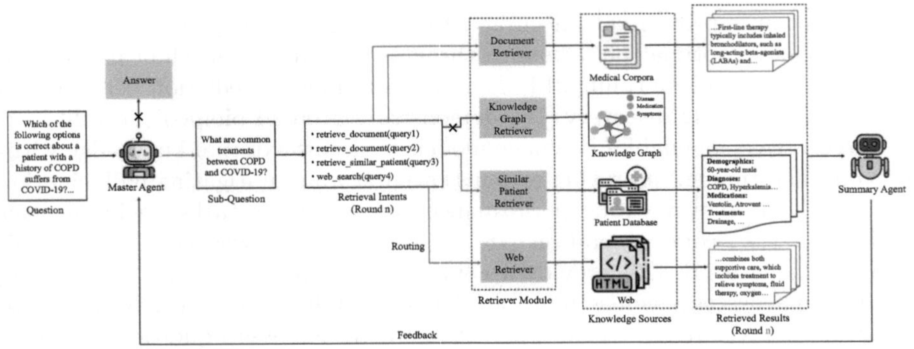

Fig. 2. IDRF operates iteratively and consists of three modules: the master agent, retriever module, and summary agent. In each round, if the master agent cannot produce an answer, it calls several retrievers in parallel. The retrieved results are then condensed by the summary agent as feedback to the master agent. For example, in Round n in this figure, the master agent generates four retrieval intents, which are routed to three retrievers.

Document Retriever This retriever accesses comprehensive textual knowledge from medical corpora. Since medical documents are extensive, relatively low-cost to retrieve, and generally more authoritative than web resources, this retriever serves as the primary knowledge provider. It leverages multiple corpora $\{\mathcal{C}^i\}_{i=1}^m$. For each corpus $\mathcal{C}^i$, a vector database $\mathcal{V}_c^i$ is constructed following Lewis et al. [5]. Given a query, we use a two-stage strategy: using an embedding model to select top-k_r document candidates from each database based on embedding similarity, respectively, resulting in $\mathcal{R}_c = \bigcup_{i=1}^m \mathcal{R}_c^i$, and subsequently using a reranker model to refine their relevance. To reduce potential noise, we set a score threshold s and retain only those candidates whose reranking scores exceed this value.

Knowledge Graph Retriever This retriever accesses high-reliability medical knowledge from a structured knowledge graph. Note that the node types and their corresponding relations in the graph are enumerable. For node type i, we first encode all node names in the graph using an embedding model and store them in a vector database $\mathcal{V}_{kg}^i$. To enable accurate retriever calls, valid node types and their mappings to corresponding relations are provided in the prompt. Taking a node name n, the node type t and a relation r as arguments, the retriever identifies top-k_{kg} semantically similar nodes in the graph by calculating embedding similarity between n and elements in $\mathcal{V}_{kg}^t$, and retrieves their associated information corresponding to r using SQL, respectively.

Similar Patient Retriever Different from the others, this retriever accesses instance knowledge by identifying relevant patient cases that provide clinical context and evidence. We collect a patient database $\mathcal{P} = \{(\mathcal{B}_i, \mathcal{D}_i, \mathcal{M}_i, \mathcal{T}_i, \mathcal{N}_i, \mathcal{O}_i)\}_{i=1}^n$, where $\mathcal{B}_i, \mathcal{D}_i, \mathcal{M}_i, \mathcal{T}_i, \mathcal{N}_i, \mathcal{O}_i$ represent basic information, diagnoses, medications, treatments, clinical notes, and outcomes of the

i-th patient, respectively. Then, we generate a textual summary for each patient using an LLM and store them in a vector database $\mathcal{V}_s$ before querying. Taking a target patient's description d as input, the retriever first extracts disease entities using an LLM and computes the Jaccard similarity between them and diagnoses of patients in $\mathcal{P}$, which is computationally efficient. The top-k_{s1} most similar patients are screened out consequently, and we extract their summaries in $\mathcal{V}_s$. Subsequently, d is used to retrieve top-k_{s2} most relevant patient summaries as retrieval results, where the workflow is the same as the document retriever.

Web Retriever This retriever accesses the most up-to-date and emerging medical knowledge from the web. Given a query, a search API is employed to retrieve top-k_w most relevant snippets from websites.

3.3 Summary Agent

The summary agent condenses the retrieved results in each round, focusing specifically on the given sub-question. The summarized information is then fed back to the master agent to initiate the next round. This module plays a critical role by extracting key information and reducing the memory load of the master agent accumulated over multiple rounds, thereby mitigating issues such as context forgetting and hallucination. Additionally, it is beneficial when computational resources are limited, as it allows the system to operate efficiently without retaining excessive intermediate information. The prompt template is presented in Appendix A.

4 Experiments

4.1 Knowledge Data

- **Medical Corpora.** Our medical corpora include StatPearls clinical articles[1] and standard medical textbooks [23]. To further expand coverage, we also incorporate question-answer pairs from eight medical QA datasets, and approximately 4.8M biomedical research papers, following the setup proposed by Wu et al. [7].
- **Medical Knowledge Graph.** We utilize PrimeKG [24], which contains 17,080 diseases and 4,050,249 relationships representing ten major biological scales, including drugs, phenotypes, anatomies, and more. We extract medical knowledge related to diseases and medications.
- **Patient Database.** We employ MIMIC-IV [25], a publicly available electronic health record dataset, as instance-based knowledge. We extract demographics, diagnoses, medications, treatments, clinical notes, and outcomes (alive or deceased) for each patient, resulting in a total of 16,928 patients.

Additionally, we use the Serper API[2] to retrieve relevant snippets from Google websites, providing up-to-date knowledge for emerging conditions.

[1] https://www.statpearls.com/.
[2] https://serper.dev/.

4.2 Test Data

Following Xiong et al. [20], we utilize three commonly used medical QA datasets for the evaluation of RAG systems: MMLU-Med [26], MedQA-US [23], MedMCQA [27]. Among them, MMLU-Med is a set of six medical tasks (e.g., anatomy, clinical knowledge, professional medicine, human genetics) from Massive Multitask Language Understanding, MedQA-US covers a wide range of clinical and biomedical domains, including pathology, pharmacology, etc., and MedMCQA is a large-scale dataset collected from Indian medical entrance examinations, evaluating specialized expertise of 21 subjects. All the datasets are composed of multiple-choice questions, and our evaluation metric is the accuracy of predicted answers chosen from given options.

4.3 Baselines

- **Baselines without Retrieval.** This category includes Chain-of-Thought (CoT) and Supervised Fine-Tuning (SFT). CoT instructs an LLM to reason through a question step by step. For SFT, we construct a medical QA dataset to fine-tune an LLM using LoRA [28], aiming to improve its adaptability to domain-specific question answering.
- **Non-Iterative Baselines.** This category includes MedRAG [20], RAFT [29] and EvidenceRAG [30]. MedRAG directly retrieves relevant documents for inference. EvidenceRAG trains an LLM to correctly cite its sources and generate answers factually supported by those citations. RAFT is trained with a mix of relevant golden documents and irrelevant distractor documents to mitigate the influence of distractor documents.
- **Iterative Baselines.** This category includes i-MedRAG [21], Self-RAG [31], and ChatQA [32]. Based on MedRAG, i-MedRAG supports iterative retrieval by leveraging information-seeking history. Self-RAG incorporates a well-trained critic model to fine-tune an LLM to generate text with reflection tokens. ChatQA 1.5 introduces a two-stage instruction tuning approach: first building instruction-following ability, and then applying context-enhanced tuning to improve QA performance.
- **Multi-Retriever Baselines.** This category includes RGAR [33] for comparison. RGAR is a recurrence framework that iteratively retrieves factual knowledge from patient records and conceptual knowledge from medical corpora.

4.4 Implementation Details

In this paper, we use Llama-3.1-8B-Instruct as both the master agent and summary agent models, and Qwen3-Embedding-0.6B and Qwen3-Reranker-0.6B as the embedding and reranker models, respectively. During LLM inference, we set top-p to 0.8, temperature to 0.7, top-k to 20, and the maximum output token length to 1024. The maximum retriever call number in each round is 3. For the document retriever, k_r is set to 10, and the reranker score threshold is 0.5. For the knowledge graph retriever, k_{kg} is set to 5. For the similar patient retriever, k_{s1} and k_{s2} are set to 15 and 5, respectively, with a reranker score threshold of 0.5. For the web retriever, we set k_w to 5. All experiments are conducted on a CentOS 7.9 server with three NVIDIA A40 GPUs.

4.5 Results

Table 1. Performance comparison of different methods on the three medical QA datasets. The LLM and embedding model are Llama-3.1-8B-Instruct and Qwen3-Embedding-0.6B respectively for all methods. Δ is relative to CoT. **Bold** represents the best performance, and underline indicates the second-best performance.

Method	Iterative	# Retriever	MMLU-Med		MedQA-US		MedMCQA		Average	
			Acc.	Δ	Acc.	Δ	Acc.	Δ	Acc.	Δ
CoT	✗	0	74.98	-	66.15	-	57.78	-	66.30	-
SFT	✗	0	75.59	0.61	66.05	-0.10	58.65	0.87	66.76	1.09
MedRAG	✗	1	76.50	1.52	66.91	0.76	58.48	0.70	67.30	0.99
EvidenceRAG	✗	1	78.17	3.19	68.64	2.49	60.73	2.95	69.18	2.88
RAFT	✗	1	78.05	3.07	68.23	2.08	60.85	3.07	69.04	2.74
i-MedRAG	✓	1	76.67	1.69	68.07	1.92	59.02	1.24	67.92	1.62
Self-RAG	✓	1	78.40	3.42	68.40	2.25	60.90	3.12	69.23	2.93
ChatQA 1.5	✓	1	79.03	4.05	69.21	3.06	61.57	3.79	69.94	3.63
RGAR	✓	2	78.65	3.67	70.94	4.79	62.55	4.77	70.71	4.41
IDRF	✓	4	**82.96**	**7.98**	**72.26**	**6.11**	**65.20**	**7.42**	**73.47**	**7.17**

Table 1 presents the performance comparison between IDRF and several competitive baselines across three medical QA datasets. To ensure fairness, all methods use the same LLM and embedding model, and when applicable, have access to the same knowledge sources. Our findings are summarized below:

First, retrieval-augmented methods achieve overall improvements over CoT and SFT, highlighting the benefit of retrieving medical knowledge to enhance factual accuracy. However, MedRAG performs slightly worse than SFT on MedMCQA, likely due to ineffective retrieval.

Second, generally iterative methods outperform non-iterative counterparts by refining answers across multiple rounds of knowledge integration, except for i-MedRAG, which is limited by its ability to process retrieved results and reason over long multi-round histories. Notably, RGAR achieves the second-best performance on two datasets. Its advantage arises from retrieving complementary factual knowledge from the patient database and conceptual knowledge from medical corpora, whereas other methods rely solely on the latter.

Finally, our proposed IDRF achieves state-of-the-art performance by combining four specialized retrievers and employing a summary agent to condense retrieved information effectively. This design allows IDRF to capture complementary knowledge while reducing redundancy, resulting in improvements of 3.93% on MMLU-Med, 1.32% on MedQA-US, and 2.65% on MedMCQA compared to the second-best performance.

5 Discussion

5.1 Ablation Study

Table 2. Ablation study on the three medical QA datasets. "cor", "kg" and "pat"' represent medical corpora, knowledge graph and patient database, respectively. "sum" represents summary agent. **Bold** represents the best performance.

Variant	MMLU-Med	MedQA-US	MedMCQA	Average
IDRF	82.96	**72.26**	**65.20**	**73.47**
IDRF w/o cor	81.79	71.23	64.22	72.41
IDRF w/o kg	82.31	71.39	64.67	72.79
IDRF w/o pat	**83.08**	71.08	64.44	72.87
IDRF w/o web	80.81	70.95	63.51	71.76
IDRF w/o sum	81.66	70.85	63.72	72.08

To further evaluate the contribution of each component in IDRF for medical QA, we conduct an ablation study on the three datasets, with results reported in Table 2. Two key insights emerge: (1) Removing any retriever reduces overall performance, indicating that all knowledge sources provide complementary information. Among them, removing the web causes the largest drop, suggesting that web resources can supply much of the essential knowledge. The patient retriever contributes gains of 1.18% on MedQA-US and 0.76% on MedMCQA by providing clinical cases, but slightly harms MMLU-Med, likely because patient data can introduce noise rather than useful context. (2) IDRF outperforms the "w/o sum" variant by 1.20% on MMLU-Med, 1.39% on MedQA-US, and 1.48% on MedMCQA, highlighting the importance of the summary agent in condensing retrieved information to reduce distraction and context forgetting.

5.2 LLM Variants

To evaluate the impact of different LLMs on IDRF's performance, we replace the default LLM, i.e., Llama-3.1-8B-Instruct, with Qwen3-8B, Qwen3-14B, and Qwen3-32B, respectively. As shown in Table 3, switching from Llama-3.1-8B-Instruct to Qwen3-8B improves performance on MMLU-Med and MedMCQA, but slightly decreases performance on MedQA-US. Increasing the model size yields consistent gains across all three datasets, indicating that larger LLMs can more effectively leverage retrieval-augmented knowledge for accurate answers. These findings highlight that IDRF serves as a scalable framework, capable of seamlessly integrating stronger LLMs to enhance their ability to tackle complex medical questions.

Table 3. Comparison of LLM variants on the three medical QA datasets.

Model	MMLU-Med	MedQA-US	MedMCQA	Average
Llama-3.1-8B-Instruct	82.96	72.26	65.20	73.47
Qwen3-8B	84.74	71.51	65.63	73.96
Qwen3-14B	89.45	77.98	70.54	79.32
Qwen3-32B	91.59	83.99	74.50	83.36

6 Conclusion

In this work, we propose the Iterative Dynamic Routing Framework (IDRF) for medical question answering. IDRF performs iterative reasoning and retrieval, with a master agent coordinating the process, a retriever module accessing heterogeneous sources, and a summary agent condensing results. This design enables IDRF to effectively address key challenges in medical QA. The experiments on three datasets demonstrate its superiority over strong baselines. In future work, we plan to collect high-quality reasoning data to fine-tune IDRF, and to investigate its adaptability to other domains.

Acknowledgment. This study was funded by the National Natural Science Foundation of China (No. 62394330) and Basic Research Co-funded Projects in Guangzhou (No. 2024A03J0395).

Disclosure of Interests. The authors have no competing interests to declare that are relevant to the content of this article.

Appendix

A Prompts

System prompt of the master agent

You are a professional medical question-answering assistant. Given a question, decompose the original question into sub-questions and solve them round by round. In each round, first analyze the original question and the retrieved information for sub-questions so far. Then decide:
- If you need more information to answer the original question precisely, raise another sub-question and call several retrievers listed in "Available retrievers" section.
- If you think the retrieved information is sufficient for you to answer the original question precisely, output the answer and a brief explanation in JSON format.

Available retrievers
- retrieve_documents(query: str): Retrieve relevant medical documents for a given query.
- retrieve_knowledge_graph(entity_name: str, entity_type, attribute: str): Retrieve the attribute value of a specified entity. Valid entity types include 'disease' and 'medication'. For disease type, valid attributes include 'description', 'symptoms', 'causes', 'complications', 'prevention_measures', 'indicated_medications', 'contraindicated_medications', and 'exposures'; for medication type, valid attributes include 'description', 'target', 'side_effect', 'indicated_diseases', and 'contraindicated_diseases'.
- retrieve_similar_patients(query: str): Retrieve similar patient information from a patient database. This retriever can be very useful when you need similar patient cases (including diagnoses, medications, treatments, outcome, etc.) to answer patient-related questions. The query must describe the patient briefly, including disease information.
- web_search(query: str): Retrieve relevant information about your query from websites.

Retriever call examples
- retrieve_documents("dietary sources of Vitamin C, Vitamin B7, Vitamin B12, and Vitamin D")
- retrieve_knowledge_graph("benign prostatic hyperplasia", "disease", "complications")
- retrieve_similar_patients("45-year-old female with systemic lupus erythematosus")

- web_search("The symptoms of COVID-19")

Output requirements in each round
- If you need more information to answer the original question precisely, output:
<Thought>
[Analysis of current understanding and next step. Write up to 100 words here.]
</Thought>
<Sub-question>
[A clearly defined, single-hop sub-question.]
</Sub-question>
<Retrieval>
[One or more retriever calls in function format, each on its own line.]
</Retrieval>
- If you think the retrieved information is sufficient for you to answer the original question precisely, output exactly:
{"answer": [Your answer], "explanation": [Your explanation for the answer]}

Notes
- If the original question is a multiple-choice question, the answer must be the single letter corresponding to the correct option, e.g., "A", "B", etc.
- You can make up to three retriever calls for each round.
- Always provide proper arguments when calling a retriever (refer to "Available retrievers" section). Incorrect arguments will return unexpected results!
- For each round, if your output contains any retriever call, pause and wait for the user to return you the retrieval results.

Prompt template of the summary agent

You are a professional expert in medical information summarization. Given a medical question, a retriever has been called and several results have been returned, which may contain useful or noisy information. Your task is to carefully read the results, identify information that directly helps answer the question, and produce a concise, accurate summary based only on the relevant content. Ignore any irrelevant, off-topic, or redundant parts. Do not assume or invent information not present in the results.

Medical Question:
{query}

Retriever Call:
{call}

Retrieved Results:
{contents}

Instructions:
- Focus strictly on information that answers or supports the question.
- Remove noisy, irrelevant, outdated, or redundant content.
- Maintain clinical/scientific accuracy and clarity.
- Write the final summary in plain, professional English.
- Limit to 100 words.

Provide only the final summary below:

References

1. OpenAI: GPT-4 technical report (2023). arXiv:2303.08774
2. Royer, C., Menze, B., Sekuboyina, A.: MultiMedEval: a benchmark and a toolkit for evaluating medical vision-language models (2024). arXiv:2402.09262
3. Xia, P., Zhu, K., Li, H., et al.: MMed-RAG: versatile multimodal retrieval-augmented generation system for medical vision-language models (2024). arXiv:2410.13085
4. Christophe, C., Kanithi, P. K., Munjal, P., et al.: Med42 — Evaluating fine-tuning strategies for medical LLMs: full-parameter vs. parameter-efficient approaches (2024). arXiv:2404.14779
5. Lewis, P., Perez, E., Piktus, A., et al.: Retrieval-augmented generation for knowledge-intensive NLP tasks. In: Advances in Neural Information Processing Systems, vol. 33, pp. 9459–9474 (2020)
6. Singhal, S., Azizi, S., Tu, T., et al.: Large language models encode clinical knowledge. Nature **620**, 172–180 (2023)
7. Wu, C., Lin, W., Zhang, X., Zhang, Y., Wang, Y., Xie, W.: PMC-LLaMA: towards building open-source language models for medicine (2023). arXiv:2304.14454
8. Das, S., Ge, Y., Guo, Y., et al.: Two-layer retrieval augmented generation framework for low-resource medical question-answering: proof of concept using reddit data (2024). arXiv:2405.19519
9. Xia, P., Zhu, K., Li, H., et al.: RULE: Reliable multimodal RAG for factuality in medical vision language models. In: Proceedings of the 2024 Conference on Empirical Methods in Natural Language Processing, pp. 1081–1093 (2024)
10. Veen, D.V., Uden, C.V., Blankemeier, L., et al.: Adapted large language models can outperform medical experts in clinical text summarization. Nat. Med. **30**, 1134–1142 (2024)

11. Dehkordi, M.K.H., Perl, Y., Deek, F.P., et al.: Improving large language models' summarization accuracy by adding highlights to discharge notes: comparative evaluation. JMIR Med. Inform. **13**, e66476 (2025)
12. Veen, D. V., Uden, C. V., Attias, M., et al.: RadAdapt: Radiology report summarization via lightweight domain adaptation of large language models. In: Proceedings of the 22nd Workshop on Biomedical Natural Language Processing and BioNLP Shared Tasks, pp. 449–460 (2023)
13. Jiang, L.Y., Liu, X.C., Nejatian, N.P., et al.: Health system-scale language models are all-purpose prediction engines. Nature **619**, 357–362 (2023)
14. Hou, Z., Liu, H., Bian, J., He, X., Zhuang, Y.: Enhancing medical coding efficiency through domain-specific fine-tuned large language models. npj Health Syst. 2, 14 (2025)
15. Zheng, Y., Koh, H.Y., Ju, J., et al.: Large language models for drug discovery and development. Patterns **6**(10), 101346 (2025)
16. Guu, K., Lee, K., Tung, Z., Pasupat, P. and Chang, M.: REALM: Retrieval-augmented language model pre-training. In: Proceedings of the 37th International Conference on Machine Learning, pp. 3929–3938 (2020)
17. Adjali, O.: Exploring retrieval-augmented generation for real-world claim verification. In: Proceedings of the Seventh Fact Extraction and VERification Workshop, pp. 113–117 (2024)
18. Yang, Z., Chen, S., Gao, C., Li, Z., Hu, X., Liu, K., Xia, X.: An empirical study of retrieval-augmented code generation: challenges and opportunities. ACM Trans. Softw. Eng. Methodol. **34**(7), 188 (2025)
19. Li, Y., Li, Y., Wang, X., et al.: Benchmarking multimodal retrieval augmented generation with dynamic VQA dataset and self-adaptive planning agent. In: The Thirteenth International Conference on Learning Representations (2025)
20. Xiong, G., Jin, Q., Lu, Z., Zhang, A.: Benchmarking retrieval-augmented generation for medicine. In: Findings of the Association for Computational Linguistics: ACL 2024, pp. 6233–6251 (2024)
21. Xiong, G., Jin, Q., Wang, X., Zhang, M., Lu, Z., Zhang, A.: Improving retrieval-augmented generation in medicine with iterative follow-up questions (2024). arXiv:2408.00727
22. Xu, R., Liu, H., Nag, S., et al.: SimRAG: self-improving retrieval-augmented generation for adapting large language models to specialized domains. In: Proceedings of the 2025 Conference of the Nations of the Americas Chapter of the Association for Computational Linguistics: Human Language Technologies (Volume 1: Long Papers), pp. 11534–11550 (2025)
23. Jin, D., Pan, E., Oufattole, N., Weng, W.-H., Fang, H., Szolovits, P.: What disease does this patient have? A large-scale open domain question answering dataset from medical exams. Appl. Sci. **11**(14), 6421 (2021)
24. Chandak, P., Huang, K., Zitnik, M.: Building a knowledge graph to enable precision medicine. Sci. Data **10**, 67 (2023)
25. Johnson, A.E.W., Bulgarelli, L., Shen, L., et al.: MIMIC-IV, a freely accessible electronic health record dataset. Sci. Data **10**, 1 (2023)
26. Hendrycks, D., Burns, C., Basart, S., et al.: Measuring massive multitask language understanding (2020). arXiv:2009.03300
27. Pal, A., Umapathi, L. K., Sankarasubbu, M.: MedMCQA: A large-scale multi-subject multi-choice dataset for medical domain question answering. In: Proceedings of the Conference on Health, Inference, and Learning, 174, pp. 248–260 (2022)
28. Hu, E. J., Shen, Y., Wallis, P., et al.: LoRA: low-rank adaptation of large language models (2021). arXiv:2106.09685

29. Zhang, T., Patil, S. G., Jain, N., et al.: RAFT: adapting language model to domain specific RAG (2024). arXiv:2403.10131v2
30. Schimanski, T., Ni, J., Kraus, M., Ash, E., Leippold, M.: Towards faithful and robust LLM specialists for evidence-based question-answering. In: Proceedings of the 62nd Annual Meeting of the Association for Computational Linguistics (Volume 1: Long Papers), pp. 1913–1931 (2024)
31. Asai, A., Wu, Z., Wang, Y., Sil, A., Hajishirzi, H.: Self-RAG: Learning to retrieve, generate, and critique through self-reflection. In: The Twelfth International Conference on Learning Representations (2024)
32. Liu, Z., Ping, W., Roy, R., et al.: ChatQA: Surpassing GPT-4 on conversational QA and RAG. In: Advances in Neural Information Processing Systems, vol. 37, pp. 15416–15459 (2024)
33. Liang, S., Zhang, L., Zhu, H., Wang, W., He, Y., Zhou, D.: RGAR: recurrence generation-augmented retrieval for factual-aware medical question answering (2025). arXiv:2502.13361

DMSNet: Dual-Channel Interactive Attention Deep Classification Network for Mass Spectrometry Data

Qichen Yan[1], Zhiqiang Zheng[1], Jinghao Niu[2(✉)], and Wensheng Zhang[1,2]

[1] School of Information and Communication Engineering, Hainan University, Haikou 570228, China
{22220854000052,19081000110019}@hainanu.edu.cn, zhangwenshengia@hotmail.com

[2] Institute of Automation, Chinese Academy of Sciences, Beijing 100190, China
niujinghao2015@ia.ac.cn

Abstract. Traditional hypertension risk prediction relies heavily on continuous monitoring and risk factor scales, making it difficult to accurately analyze specific metabolites and pathological pathways. Recent advances in liquid chromatography-mass spectrometry (LC-MS) data analysis and machine learning techniques have brought new opportunities and challenges to hypertension risk prediction. LC-MS data is characterized by high dimensionality and sparseness. By converting Raw mass spectrometry data into a single image, deep learning-based mass spectrometry data models have achieved remarkable results. However, existing methods for LC-MS data analysis fail to account for the inherent differences between positive and negative ion channels, and they also lack the capability for cross-scale information integration. Furthermore, due to the inherent black-box nature of deep learning models, selecting appropriate interpretable machine learning algorithms and effectively evaluating them remains an open problem. In this paper, we propose a dual-channel mass spectrometry network (DMSNet). Through a dual-channel feature design, modal attention mechanisms and multi-scale fusion, combined with consistency constraints, DMSNet achieves collaborative modeling of positive and negative ion patterns, significantly improving the model's feature representation and classification robustness. Furthermore, through interpretability, key metabolites associated with hypertension were successfully identified, validating the rationality of the model's decision logic and the reliability of metabolite biomarker mining.

Keywords: Hypertension risk profiling · Metabolomics · Deep learning · Explainable artificial intelligence

Y. Zhang et al. (Eds.): CHIP 2025, CCIS 2884, pp. 29–49, 2026.
https://doi.org/10.1007/978-981-95-7299-1_3

1 Introduction

Metabolomics is a rapidly evolving field dedicated to the comprehensive and quantitative analysis of small-molecule metabolites within biological samples. By capturing the dynamic metabolic changes in an organism, metabolomics provides critical insights into physiological and pathological processes [1]. This discipline plays a pivotal role in identifying biomarkers for disease diagnosis, monitoring therapeutic responses, and uncovering mechanisms underlying complex conditions. In particular, its application in hypertension research enables the discovery of metabolites associated with blood pressure regulation, offering new opportunities for early diagnosis and precision medicine [2]. LC-MS is a key tool in metabolomics, providing high sensitivity and precision, enabling researchers to study complex biological systems. Using untargeted metabolomics with LC-MS has led to the discovery of new biomarkers and a better grasp of disease mechanisms, including those behind hypertension [3]. The ability of LC-MS to perform high-resolution analyses makes it particularly suited for uncovering metabolic alterations associated with heterogeneous and multifactorial diseases [4].

Recent advancements in machine learning have significantly enhanced LC-MS data processing, However, traditional machine learning methods face significant challenges in feature extraction from raw LC-MS data, including issues such as noise reduction, feature identification and quantification, feature alignment, and computational efficiency [5,6]. To address these limitations and improve analytical utility, recent efforts have focused on converting LC-MS data into formats more amenable to end-to-end deep learning, such as pseudo-spectral images or structured arrays suitable for direct model input. Shen et al. transformed the mass-to-charge ratio (m/z) and retention time (RT) from raw LC-MS data into a two-dimensional data matrix, effectively creating a pseudo-mass spectrometry image [7]. This approach streamlined data processing and enhanced the efficiency of disease diagnosis. Similarly, Cadow et al. converted raw data into mass spectrometry images and applied deep learning techniques, achieving notable improvements in classification performance, proteome coverage, accuracy, and repeatability [8,9]. Building upon these advancements, Wang et al. developed MetImage, a method that transforms raw LC-MS data into multi-channel digital images. This innovation improved data reproducibility and peak detection while enhancing interpretability for AI-based disease diagnosis [4]. Collectively, these studies demonstrate that converting LC-MS data into image formats can significantly bolster the application of deep learning in metabolomics.

While deep learning has made progress in applying it to LC-MS data, it often overlooks the fundamental distinction between positive ionization (POS) and negative ionization (NEG) modes. These two modes are chemically distinct but metabolically complementary [10]. POS mode effectively detects basic compounds by adding protons or cations. In contrast, NEG mode specifically targets acidic metabolites by deprotonating them. Furthermore, negative ionization mode is generally less sensitive than positive ionization mode [11]. However, most existing models fail to exploit this complementarity, typically analyzing the two modes independently or performing superficial correlations. This approach hinders the effective integration of the rich, multiscale metabolic features captured by both ionization modes.

Deep learning has shown significant promise in handling complex data in medicine, offering an efficient way to develop end-to-end models from intricate datasets. However, challenges related to interpretability persist, underscoring the need for further research to ensure reliability in medical applications [12,13]. Interpretable machine learning has rapidly emerged as a significant research focus in recent years [14,15], employing specific interpretable machine learning techniques allows for feature attribution in modeling human conditions such as diseases, aiding researchers in identifying potential key biomarkers and combinatorial influencing factors [16]. However, among various interpretable machine learning methods, how to determine the most suitable model and workflow for a specific mass spectrometry data analysis task remains an open question.

To address these challenges, this paper contributes the following:

1. This paper implements a pseudo-mass spectrometry image generation process and, based on this, designs a dual-channel mass spectrometry network. Through dual-channel feature extraction, modal attention interaction, and multiscale fusion, combined with positive and negative ion modal consistency constraints, this network achieves collaborative modeling of inherently heterogeneous mass spectrometric information, significantly enhancing the perception and representation of signals from different modalities.

2. This paper systematically introduces multiple explainable artificial intelligence (XAI) attribution methods and constructs a comprehensive evaluation metric, XAI fidelity comprehensive evaluation index (XAI-FI). This quantitatively compares the stability and credibility of interpretation methods across similarity and fidelity dimensions, providing an objective basis for screening and selecting true metabolic signatures from model outputs.

3. This study combined interpretability analysis with traditional statistical validation to select an interpretable algorithm suitable for this study based on the XAI-FI metric. This method successfully identified and validated several key metabolites associated with hypertension (e.g., L-acetylcarnitine [17] and L-Carnitine [18]). This approach not only improved classification performance but also enhanced the biological plausibility of model decisions, providing AI-based technical support for metabolic biomarker discovery and disease mechanism research.

2 Dataset

2.1 Study Dataset and Participant Characteristics

This study's dataset (BAHMD1129, Beijing Institute of Cardiovascular Diseases, Capital Medical University) included plasma untargeted metabolomics data from 400 participants enrolled at Beijing Anzhen Hospital (Nov 2016–Jan 2020), comprising 100 healthy individuals (normotensive, routine health checkups) and 300 essential hypertensive patients (from PROSPECT registry, NCT

03708601, aged 18–85 years at discharge). Hypertensive patients were stratified into low-to-intermediate, high, and very high cardiovascular risk groups (n=100 each) per the *2018 Chinese Guidelines for Hypertension Management*. Healthy individuals and hypertensive patients with significant cardiovascular risk were matched for age and sex.

2.2 LC-MS/MS Analysis and Data Processing

Plasma samples were centrifuged at low temperature to remove cellular components and impurities, followed by protein precipitation to reduce protein interference and improve the accuracy and reproducibility of metabolite detection. The resulting supernatant was aliquoted and frozen for subsequent analysis. Each plasma sample was protein precipitated by adding a deuterated internal standard mixture. Ultrafiltrates were obtained by vortexing and centrifuging, and then divided into two fractions for positive and negative ion analysis, each freeze-dried. The dried residue was dissolved in 25% acetonitrile and analyzed by LC-MS/MS. Liquid chromatography separation was performed on a Vanquish UHPLC system at 60°C and a constant flow rate of 0.4 mL/min. Separation was performed using BEH C8 and ACQUITY UPLC HSS T3 columns, respectively, under positive and negative electrospray ionization. Mobile phases A and B were water containing 0.1% formic acid and acetonitrile containing 0.1% formic acid, respectively. Mass spectrometry analysis was performed using a Q Exactive mass spectrometer with an m/z scan range of 80–1200, spray voltages of 3.50 kV and 3.00 kV for positive and negative ionization, respectively, and a resolution setting of 7×10^4. After data acquisition, necessary data preprocessing, including peak detection, peak alignment, and normalization, was performed to ensure inter-sample comparability and accuracy of the results. Each of the 400 samples in this study contained both POS and NEG modes. Systematic analysis identified a total of 209 metabolites, some of which are represented in Table 1.

This table presents metabolite data obtained by LC-MS analysis and lists some of the metabolites identified in plasma samples during a study of metabolic markers for hypertension. These metabolites include amino acids, fatty acids and their derivatives, and steroids. The data in Table 1 provide a foundation for subsequent metabolic pathway analysis and potential biomarker discovery.

3 Methods

3.1 Pseudo Mass Spectrometry Image Generation

The generation of pseudo mass spectrometry images requires systematic steps such as data preprocessing, screening, mapping, and conversion (see Fig. 1): First, the raw data of non-targeted metabolomics acquired by LC-MS are preprocessed to remove noise, converted into a standardized mzXML format, and then processed using the pyOpenMS library (this library supports mass spectrometry data reading, analysis, and visualization, and is widely used in the fields of metabolomics and proteomics); then, the data are filtered based on m/z (65–1065

Table 1. Some identified metabolites in hypertensive plasma samples

Name	Formula	m/z (Da)	RT (min)	Ion mode
Taurochenodeoxycholate	$C_{26}H_{45}NO_6S$	498.2895	6.31	NEG
Glutamine	$C_5H_{10}N_2O_3$	145.0620	1.06	NEG
Glycoursodeoxycholic acid	$C_{26}H_{43}NO_6$	448.3069	5.39	NEG
L-acetylcarnitine	$C_9H_{17}NO_3$	204.1239	1.25	POS
L-Carnitine	$C_7H_{15}NO_3$	162.1112	1.22	POS
fatty amide C22:1	$C_{22}H_{43}NO$	338.3413	7.29	POS
Tryptophan	$C_{11}H_{12}N_2O_2$	205.0976	1.79	POS
Tyrosine	$C_9H_{11}NO_3$	182.0802	1.17	POS
Glutamic Acid	$C_5H_9NO_4$	146.0464	1.01	NEG
FFA 18:2	$C_{18}H_{32}O_2$	279.2331	7.67	NEG
FFA 20:5	$C_{20}H_{30}O_2$	301.2181	7.40	NEG
L-(+)-Lactic acid	$C_3H_6O_3$	89.02269	1.027	NEG
3-Oxotetradecanoic acid	$C_{14}H_{26}O_3$	241.18054	6.29	NEG
Flutimide	$C_{12}H_{18}N_2O_3$	239.13839	2.75	POS
L-Kynurenine	$C_{10}H_{12}N_2O_3$	209.09159	2.155	POS

Da), RT (0–725 s), and Intensity to reduce signal-to-noise interference and cover the characteristic peaks of the target metabolites; then, the image resolution is set to 224×224 (a single pixel corresponds to The RT range is t=3.2366 s, and the m/z range is m=4.4643 Da). The mass spectrometry data points are mapped to a two-dimensional pixel area (the x-axis is the m/z direction, and the intensities of similar m/z data points are mapped to adjacent pixels). At the same time, the intensity values are logarithmically transformed to reduce variability and enhance the contribution of low-abundance metabolites. The average intensity of the data points in each pixel area is then calculated to ensure smoothness. Finally, the pixel intensity is linearly mapped to a standard grayscale level of 0–255 to generate a grayscale pseudo-mass spectrometry image with a resolution of 224×224. This image not only retains the metabolite distribution information, but also provides a unified input format for subsequent machine learning models, which can support metabolomics analysis tasks such as disease classification and biomarker screening.

3.2 Design of Dual-Channel Mass Spectrometry Network

Traditional single-modal pseudo-mass spectrometry networks have two limitations in modeling hypertension mass spectrometry data: first, they struggle to effectively integrate complementary metabolic information between POS and NEG ionization modes; second, they lack explicit constraints to maintain consistency in cross-modal predictions. To address these issues, this study proposes

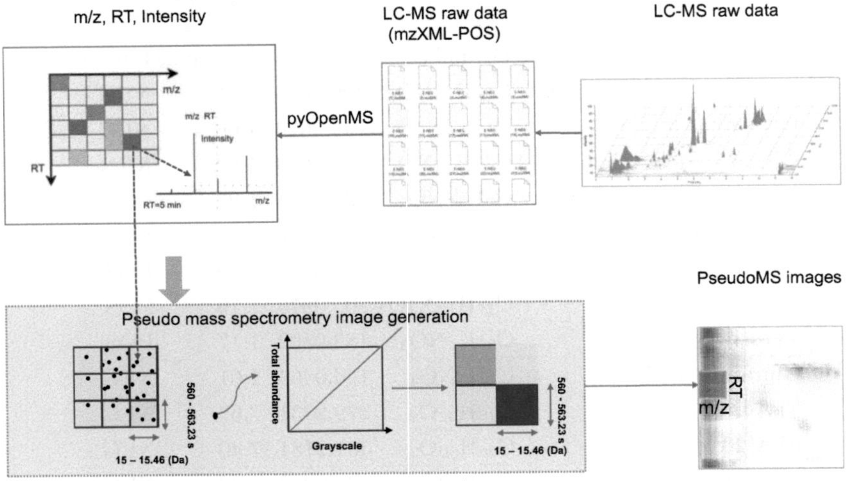

Fig. 1. Schematic diagram illustrating the generation process of pseudo-mass spectra in this study, including key steps such as LC-MS raw data preprocessing, feature mapping to grid coordinates, and intensity normalization to construct pseudo-mass spectral images.

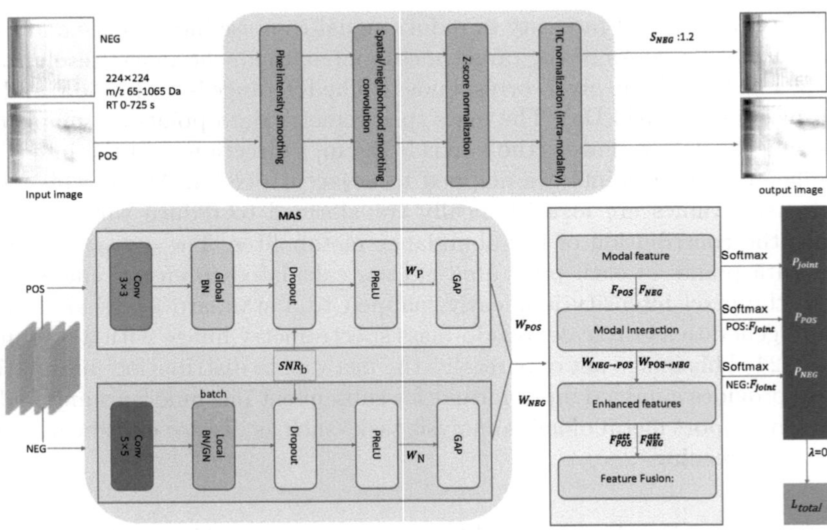

Fig. 2. DMSNet architecture diagram, showing the core components, including the dual-channel design of independent features for POS and NEG modalities, a modality interaction module based on a bidirectional attention mechanism, a multi-scale feature fusion module, and a joint classification layer with auxiliary POS/NEG classification branches to ensure decision consistency.

DMSNet for mass spectrometry data (see Fig. 2). The framework generally follows a process of "input → dual-channel feature extraction → cross-modal attention interaction and multi-scale feature fusion → joint classification with consistency constraints." Specifically, each channel first extracts modality-specific features by embedding a modality adaptive submodule (MAS), followed by a bidirectional attention mechanism to establish dynamic information interaction between the two channels, achieving cross-modal feature enhancement. Finally, the fused joint features are input into the classification layer, and by introducing consistency constraints based on Kullback–Leibler (KL) divergence, the model's decision stability and robustness under dual modality conditions are effectively improved.

Input Layer: To achieve modality input unification and signal balance, the low ionization efficiency of the NEG mode is addressed. The model first performs pixel smoothing and spatial convolution noise reduction to suppress high-frequency noise and integrate redundant signals from adjacent m/z regions. It then performs total ion current (TIC) normalization on each modality to unify the intra-modal signal scale. To further balance the bimodal signal strength, a learnable scale parameter S_{NEG} is introduced at the input to adaptively compensate for NEG modal signal differences. The balanced POS and NEG images are fed into separate feature branches, providing a stable and consistent input basis for subsequent modal feature extraction.

The first core of DMSNet lies in the dual-channel feature extraction module: this module embeds a MAS within each branch to achieve differentiated modeling of POS and NEG modal features. While the two types of pseudo-mass spectrometry images maintain consistent spatial resolution, they exhibit significant complementary differences in signal intensity distribution, local texture structure, noise level, and significant metabolic peak regions. MAS effectively captures and enhances fine-grained features from each modality that are discriminative for hypertension classification, thereby achieving cross-modal synergy while preserving modal characteristics. The specific steps are as follows:

(a) Modality-specific convolutional kernel design: The POS branch primarily utilizes small kernels and multiple channels (3×3 stacked convolutions, with depthwise/separable options available), focusing on accurately capturing sharp, narrow peaks and maximizing the discriminative characteristics of positive ion metabolites. After the convolution group, the data are aligned to a uniform channel dimension of d=256 via 1×1 projection. The NEG branch utilizes a combination of large kernels and dilated convolutions (5×5, dilation=2) or multi-scale atrous modules to expand the receptive field and cover diffuse peaks. The data are then projected to the same dimension d. Both branches ultimately output a feature map $F_{map(POS)}$, $F_{map(NEG)} \in \mathbb{R}^{B\times C\times H\times W}$, which is flattened into a spatial sequence $F_{\mathrm{map(POS)}}, F_{\mathrm{map(NEG)}} \in \mathbb{R}^{B\times L\times d}$ $(L = H \cdot W)$.

(b) Modal adaptive normalization: POS modal data uses a statistical method that combines Global BN with a sliding window to stabilize the full spectrum distribution (effective for large batches or high-stability signals), alleviate the signal drift problem of different samples within the POS modality, and improve the model's generalization ability for POS modal data. NEG modal data uses Local BN: The feature map is spatially divided into several overlapping blocks, and the mean μ_{local} and variance δ^2_{local} are independently calculated within the block and normalized to enhance the contrast of local low-abundance signals in the NEG modality, solve the problem of "global normalization masking weak signals", and highlight the characteristics of low-abundance negative ion metabolites. To avoid statistical instability in small samples, Local BN is replaced with GroupNorm (GN) when the batch is small. The POS and NEG normalization formulas are:

$$\hat{\mathbf{x}} = \frac{\mathbf{x} - \mu_{\text{global}}}{\sqrt{\sigma^2_{\text{global}} + \varepsilon}}, \tag{1}$$

$$\hat{\mathbf{x}}_{\text{block}} = \frac{\mathbf{x}_{\text{block}} - \mu_{\text{block}}}{\sqrt{\sigma^2_{\text{block}} + \varepsilon}} \tag{2}$$

The local BN calculation uses overlapping blocks and a small sample smoothing factor ε to ensure statistical robustness.

(c) Dynamic deactivation rate adjustment: Estimating the modal signal-to-noise ratio (SNR) by batch: define sp as the set of pixels located in the top-p intensity region of the image or in the known peak region of the training set, and bp as the set of pixels with the median or lower quartile intensity of the image; batch $SNR_b = \frac{median(sp)}{median(bp)+\varepsilon}$. Smoothly map SNR_b to the dropout-rate to ensure differentiability and training stability:

$$\text{dropout-rate} = clip(r_{min} + (r_{max} - r_{min}) \cdot \sigma\left(k\left(\tau - SNR_b\right)\right), r_{min}, r_{max}) \tag{3}$$

Here, $\sigma(\cdot)$ represents the sigmoid function, k is the slope hyperparameter, τ is the reference threshold, and r_{min}/r_{max} is the modality-limited deactivation rate range. This strategy strengthens regularization when the SNR is low and retains more effective features when the SNR is high.

(d) Modality-specific activation: PReLU replaces fixed ReLU, making the negative slope learnable to adapt to modality differences. Initialize the negative slope: POS:$a_{\text{init}} = 0.1$, NEG:$a_{\text{init}} = 0.01$ to allow parameter updates during training, thereby enhancing the response to low-intensity NEG signals while retaining the discriminative ability of POS. The element-by-element definition of PReLU is:

$$PReLU(x) = \begin{cases} x, & x \geq 0 \\ ax, & x < 0 \end{cases} \tag{4}$$

(e) Weighted Global Average Pooling (GAP): Use a learnable spatial weight generator instead of equal-weight GAP: Obtain a weight map $W_\ell \in (0,1)^{H\times W}$ through a 1×1 convolutional layer and a sigmoid function, and perform pixel-wise weighted pooling:

$$F_{\text{pool}} = \frac{\sum_i w_i x_i}{\sum_i w_i} \tag{5}$$

The training set prior POS: W_{P} and NEG: W_{N} can be introduced (Gaussian weight map is constructed by the m/z and RT positions of significantly different metabolites in the training set) and mixed with the learnable weights:

$$W_{\text{POS}} = \text{Normalize}(\gamma W_{\text{P}} + (1-\gamma) W_{\ell}), \tag{6}$$

$$W_{\text{NEG}} = \text{Normalize}(\gamma W_{\text{N}} + (1-\gamma) W_{\ell}) \tag{7}$$

Among them, W_{POS} and W_{NEG} are the weight parameters for POS and NEG modalities after fusion, respectively, $\gamma \in [0, 1]$ is determined on the validation set, and W_{P} and W_{N} are only calculated from the training set to avoid information leakage. Combining learnable weights with Gaussian weights allows GAP to focus on the key metabolite regions of POS and NEG modalities, improving the discriminability of feature vectors.

The extracted modal features are recorded as:

$$F_{\text{POS}} = \Phi_{\text{conv}}(X_{\text{POS}}), \tag{8}$$

$$F_{\text{NEG}} = \Phi_{\text{conv}}(X_{\text{NEG}}) \tag{9}$$

Among them, Φ_{conv} represents the convolutional feature extraction function in the dual-channel that adapts to the characteristics of each modality, ensuring that F_{POS} and F_{NEG} accurately retain the fine-grained metabolic characteristics of the corresponding modality.

The second core of DMSNet lies in cross-modal interaction and multi-Scale fusion, which is designed to address the limitation that independent dual-channel feature extraction alone cannot fully exploit the complementary metabolic associations between POS and NEG modalities, and to further enhance the model's ability to integrate cross-scale discriminative information. The specific steps are as follows:

(a) Modal interaction: To capture synergistic metabolic relationships between POS and NEG modalities, DMSNet incorporates a bidirectional attention–based interaction module. First, the inter-modal similarity matrix is calculated and normalized using softmax:

$$W_{NEG \to POS} = softmax\left(\frac{F_{NEG} F_{POS}^{\top}}{\sqrt{d}}\right), \tag{10}$$

$$W_{POS \to NEG} = softmax\left(\frac{F_{POS} F_{NEG}^{\top}}{\sqrt{d}}\right) \tag{11}$$

Among them, $W_{NEG \to POS}$ represents the attention weight matrix of NEG modal features to POS modal features, and $W_{POS \to NEG}$ is the opposite. d=256 is the feature vector dimension, which can alleviate the numerical deviation in high-dimensional feature calculation and make the similarity matrix value more stable. Then generate the modality enhancement feature:

$$F_{POS}^{att} = W_{NEG \to POS} F_{NEG}, \tag{12}$$

$$F_{NEG}^{att} = W_{POS \to NEG} F_{POS} \tag{13}$$

The third core of DMSNet lies in model consistency decision-making. Among them, F_{POS}^{att} weights the features of the NEG modality through the attention weight of the NEG modality, realizing the transfer of complementary metabolic information in the NEG modality to the POS modality. Similarly, F_{NEG}^{att} incorporates the key features of the POS modality. This process can effectively make up for the problem that a single modality cannot capture cross-modal metabolic associations sufficiently, and enhance the dual modality collaborative representation capability.

(b) Multi-scale feature fusion: The original features and enhanced features are spliced into a joint vector, each modality feature is supplemented with the complementary information of the other modality, and dimensionality reduction and integration are performed:

$$F_{joint} = BN\left(\sigma\left(W_f\left[F_{POS}^{att} \parallel F_{NEG}^{att} \parallel F_{POS} \parallel F_{NEG}\right]\right)\right) \tag{14}$$

where σ represents the ReLU activation function, and the output dimension remains at 256. The final output is the joint feature vector F_{joint}, which not only retains the exclusive metabolic information of the two modalities but also incorporates the synergistic correlation features between the modalities, providing comprehensive feature support for subsequent classification. The classification layer uses the joint feature F_{joint} through a fully connected mapping and then outputs the final category probability P_{joint} through Softmax.

The third core of DMSNet lies in model consistency decision-making. To ensure the consistency of bimodal decision making, auxiliary classification branches are set in parallel on F_{POS} and F_{NEG}, outputting the modal probabilities P_{POS} and P_{NEG} respectively. The loss function is designed as:

$$L_{\text{total}} = \underbrace{-\sum_c y_c \log P_{\text{joint},c}}_{L_{\text{ce}}} + \lambda \underbrace{\sum_c P_{\text{POS},c} \log \frac{P_{\text{POS},c}}{P_{\text{NEG},c}}}_{\text{KL}(P_{\text{POS}} \| P_{\text{NEG}})} \tag{15}$$

Among them, $P_{POS,c}$ is the predicted probability of the sample belonging to category c based on the output of the POS modal feature branch of the model,$P_{NEG,c}$ is the same, and $P_{joint,c}$ is the final predicted probability of the sample belonging to category c based on the output of the bimodal joint feature. The hyperparameter $\lambda = 0.3$ is used to balance the primary classification task and the modality consistency constraint. $\lambda = 0.3$ was determined via grid-search (0.1–1.0) on the validation set, ensuring stable convergence without over-regularization. The cross-entropy loss (L_{ce}) measures the prediction bias of the hypertension classification task by calculating the logarithmic error between the model's joint classification probability and the sample's true label, driving the model to learn the core features that distinguish hypertension from healthy samples. The introduction of KL divergence can effectively reduce bimodal decision bias and ensure that the model outputs consistent and reliable classification results based on bimodal information.

3.3 Feature Attribution and Evaluation Metrics

To address the "black box" limitations of deep learning models and evaluate the fidelity of XAI methods, this study introduces various XAI attribution methods such as Shapley additive explanations (SHAP) [19], gradient-based SHAP (Grad-SHAP) [20], gradient-weighted class activation mapping (Grad-CAM) [21], and integrated gradient (IG) [22]. Moreover, the practical value of XAI technology in the field of disease biomarker discovery has been verified. For instance, Dwivedi et al. proposed an XAI deep learning framework integrating autoencoders, feedforward neural networks, and a biomarker discovery module, successfully identifying 52 relevant biomarkers from non-small cell lung cancer data [23]. Sekaran et al. conducted a study on hypertension in the Qatari population using LC-MS analysis, Metabolon platform annotation, data pruning, and interpolation, combined with the XAI model, and found that changes in specific metabolites were significantly associated with stage 1 hypertension, with multiple metabolites serving as key predictors, and SHAP further clarified their role in identifying new metabolite biomarkers for accurate diagnosis using an optical gradient boosting model with excellent classification indicators [3]. Although studies have demonstrated the effectiveness of XAI in model interpretation and biomarker discovery for various diseases, evaluating the reliability of XAI-generated metabolite attribution (particularly for hypertension mass spectrometry data) requires systematic comparison with existing metabolomics analysis methods.

The study employs traditional statistical methods in the biological field, orthogonal projections to latent structures-discriminant analysis (OPLS-DA) and partial least squares-discriminant analysis (PLS-DA) [24], to verify the significant differences in metabolites, and uses fidelity indicators most relevant first (MoRF), area between the perturbation curves (ABPC) [25], interpretation fidelity distance (INFD) [26], Pseudo-score (PScore), Synthetic-score (SynScore) to compare XAI methods with traditional statistical methods, thereby assessing the reliability of XAI methods in validating significant differences in metabolites. Among them, PScore and SynScore are fidelity analysis methods specifically designed for pseudo-mass spectrometry image characteristics, corresponding to the pseudo-real label method and the synthetic real label method. On this basis, the study further designs an XAI-FI based on standardized processing and information entropy weight fusion to evaluate the above comparison results, and finally selects the most suitable feature attribution method for hypertension mass spectrometry data.

Pscore: In this study, traditional multivariate statistical methods OPLS-DA and PLS-DA are used as a consensus measure for differential metabolites to generate pseudo-ground truth images, denoted as $T(x)$. The purpose is to evaluate the quality of a certain explanation method A and to calculate the similarity between its generated explanations and the true explanations. The formula is as follows:

$$PScore\left(x\right) = SSIM\left(A\left(x, f\right), T\left(x\right)\right) \tag{16}$$

Among them, $T(x)$ is the true explanation of the data sample x, $A(x,f)$ is the explanation generated by feature attribution method A for sample x and model f, and $SSIM$ is an index used to measure the similarity between two images.

SynScore: This study designed a synthetic dataset containing perturbations reflecting key characteristics and effects of hypertension. The experiment used a trained model and this dataset to generate predictive explanations for hypertension data images. This was combined with a multi-class explanation method to obtain attribution results and calculate performance metrics. Finally, the SynScore metric was used to evaluate how closely the explanations matched the known synthetic ground truth labels. The calculation formula is as follows:

$$SynScore = metric\left(Syn\left(x\right), A\left(x, f\right)\right) \tag{17}$$

Among them, the metric can be AP or AUC-ROC, $Syn(x)$ is the synthetic true label of the sample, and $A(x,f)$ is the feature attribution result generated for model f.

Given that the multiple fidelity evaluation metrics used in the benchmark do not completely overlap in their definitions and theoretical foundations, these metrics each measure the ability of the interpretation method to characterize the model's prediction process from different perspectives, thus exhibiting a certain degree of complementarity. The XAI-FI metric achieves a scientific fusion of these multiple metrics through "Z-score normalization and information entropy weighting." Its normalization formula is as follows:

$$z_s = \frac{s - \bar{s}}{\sigma(s)} \tag{18}$$

where s is the specific value, $\bar{s}$ is the mean of the metric, and $\sigma(s)$ is the standard deviation of the metric. Note that the INFD metric's numerical direction is opposite to the other metrics (i.e., higher fidelity results in lower INFD values). Therefore, it is negatively calculated to maintain a consistent direction.

Then, a weight allocation mechanism based on information entropy is introduced to measure the "information difference" reflected by each indicator in different interpretation methods, thereby determining its weight in the comprehensive score. Specifically, let the standardized score of the j indicator under m interpretation methods be z_{ij}, and the information entropy of this indicator be:

$$E_j = -k \sum_{i=1}^{m} \frac{z_{ij}}{\sum_{i=1}^{m} z_{ij}} \ln\left(\frac{z_{ij}}{\sum_{i=1}^{m} z_{ij}}\right) \tag{19}$$

where $k = \frac{1}{\ln m}$. According to information entropy theory, the smaller the information entropy, the stronger the indicator's discriminative ability. The XAI-FI comprehensive score can be expressed as the sum of weighted standardized indicators:

$$\text{XAI-FI} = \sum_{j=1}^{n} \frac{1 - E_j}{\sum_{j=1}^{n} 1 - E_j} z_j \tag{20}$$

where z_j is the Z-score value of the j indicator, and ω_j is the indicator weight calculated based on information entropy and the output result after normalization.

4 Results

4.1 Comparison of Classification Performance

To verify the effectiveness of DMSNet, the experiment utilized 400 plasma samples, including 100 healthy individuals and 300 patients with hypertension. Each sample provided both POS and NEG dual modality pseudo mass spectra, and a targeted training strategy was formulated: the optimizer was set as Adam (initial learning rate $10^{-3}, \beta_1 = 0.9, \beta_2 = 0.999$), the batch size was set to 32, and the training rounds were 100; the stability of the model was evaluated using five-fold cross-validation to avoid the random deviation of a single validation. The performance evaluation indicators included classification accuracy, precision, recall rate, F1 score, and error fluctuation range. The experimental results showed that the average accuracy of the five-fold cross-validation reached 0.9641. To further verify the effectiveness of the complex feature extraction methods in the hypertension classification task based on pseudo-mass spectra, This study compared several networks including DMSNet, ResNet50 [27], InceptionV3 [28], DenseNet and EfficientNet [29], and MobileNet [30]. Among them, ResNet50 uses residual blocks to alleviate the gradient vanishing and degradation problems of deep networks; InceptionV3 achieves feature fusion through multi-scale convolution; DenseNet enhances feature reuse and gradient transfer efficiency through dense inter-layer connections; EfficientNet adopts a compound scaling strategy to simultaneously adjust the network depth, width and input resolution; MobileNet achieves lightweight design through depth-wise separable convolution, effectively reducing the number of parameters and computational complexity. The results are shown in Table 2.

Table 2. Model performance comparison

Model	Accuracy	Precision	Recall	F1
ResNet50	0.9388	0.9276	0.9485	0.9380
InceptionV3	0.9182	0.9069	0.9278	0.9173
DenseNet	0.9077	0.8965	0.9173	0.9069
EfficientNet	0.8973	0.8861	0.9068	0.8965
MobileNet	0.8869	0.8757	0.8964	0.8861
DMSNet	**0.9641**	**0.9682**	**0.9593**	**0.9637**

4.2 Ablation Experiment

To evaluate the contribution of each design module of DMSNet to the classification performance of hypertension, this section conducts ablation experiments by sequentially removing or replacing key modules to quantify the impact of each module on the model. The experimental setup is consistent with the main experiment, using five-fold cross-validation; the evaluation metrics are Accuracy, Precision, Recall, and F1. The results in the table are the average values of five folds, and ΔAcc represents the difference compared to the complete model (DMSNet Full). Table 3 shows the ablation experiment results of DMSNet.

Table 3. Ablation Experiments of DMSNet

Ablation item	Accuracy	Precision	Recall	F1	ΔAcc
DMSNet (Full)	0.9641	0.9682	0.9593	0.9637	0
w/o MAS	0.9275	0.9314	0.9236	0.9275	−0.0366
w/o KL consistency	0.9518	0.9557	0.9472	0.9514	−0.0123
w/o Interaction Fusion	0.9317	0.9356	0.9273	0.9314	−0.0324
Single-branch (POS only)	0.9405	0.9444	0.9360	0.9402	−0.0236
Single-branch (NEG only)	0.9382	0.9421	0.9335	0.9378	−0.0259

The ablation experiments show that the complete model of DMSNet achieves the best performance in the five-fold cross-validation, with an accuracy rate of 0.9641, an precision rate of 0.9682, a recall rate of 0.9593, and an F1 score of 0.9637. When w/o MAS is applied, all performance indicators significantly decrease, with the accuracy rate dropping to 0.9275 (ΔAcc $= -0.0366$) and the F1 score dropping to 0.9275, indicating that the modal adaptation sub-module is crucial for extracting the association information of the dual modality; while w/o KL consistency has a relatively smaller impact on the model performance, with an accuracy rate of 0.9518 (ΔAcc $= -0.0123$) and an F1 score of 0.9514, suggesting that its main role is to stabilize the dual modality decision deviation. Although the numerical improvement appears modest, the KL-based consistency constraint plays an essential structural role by aligning the predictive distributions of the POS and NEG branches with the joint classifier. This not only ensures coherent outputs across modalities but also stabilizes the auxiliary tasks and facilitates structured interpretability of biomarkers. After the "Without Interaction Fusion" process, the model's accuracy rate was 0.9317 (ΔAcc $= -0.0324$), and the F1 score was 0.9314. This indicates that the strategy of concatenating and dimensionally reducing the attention-enhanced features and the original features for information integration is indispensable. In the single-branch model, the accuracy rate of only retaining the POS branch was 0.9405 (ΔAcc $= -0.0236$), and the accuracy rate of only retaining the NEG branch was 0.9382 (ΔAcc $= -0.0259$), both of which were lower than that of the complete model. This shows that relying solely on a single model cannot obtain comprehensive metabolic features, verifying the necessity of the dual-channel structure to enhance performance through the fusion of complementary information from the POS and NEG modalities.

4.3 Feature Attribution Evaluation

After completing the model construction, this study further focused on the interpretation and biological validation of the model's prediction results. Various interpretation methods were adopted during the model interpretation process. To present the results of different feature attribution methods more clearly and intuitively, this study carried out visualization work for various interpretable methods. Taking the DMSNet model as an example, several representative interpretation examples were presented (see Fig. 3). The same sample contains mass spectrometry data from both POS and NEG scanning modes. This study visualized the importance weights of all pixels using a heatmap to explain the basis for these specific predictions. In the heatmaps generated by different methods, the brightness of the color indicates the magnitude of the attribution value. The darker the color, the higher the prediction weight, meaning that the metabolites in the corresponding grid have a greater impact on the classification result.

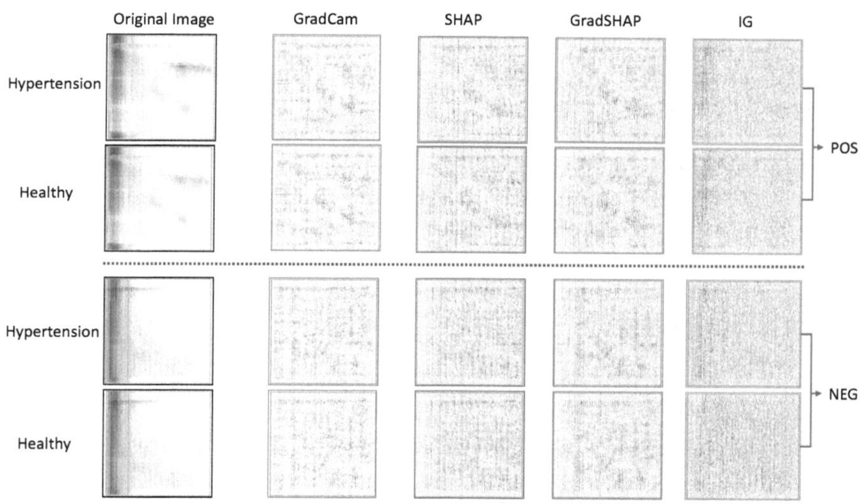

Fig. 3. Heatmap visualization of the DMSNet model's feature attribution results, showing representative examples of POS and NEG scan mode mass spectrometry data from the same sample. The brightness of the color indicates the magnitude of the attribution value; the metabolite in the corresponding grid has a greater impact on the hypertension classification result.

Although these XAI methods have visualized feature importance regions in pseudo-mass spectra, we were still unsure which method was most suitable for analyzing the hypertension mass spectrometry data used in this study. Therefore, we conducted a specialized design to investigate the fidelity of XAI methods, comparing them with differential metabolite identification using traditional statistical methods. We then used the XAI-FI metric to score and analyze the results. The results are shown in Table 4, "Comparison of Fidelity Indicators of Metabolite Interpretation Using XAI Methods and Traditional Analyses."

Table 4. Comparison of Fidelity Metrics for XAI Methods

Methods	MoRF↑	ABPC↑	INFD↓	PScore↑	SynScore↑	XAI-FI↑
IG	0.408	0.231	7.826	0.72	0.974	−0.653
SHAP	0.61	0.583	3.881	0.701	0.976	0.991
Grad-CAM	0.55	0.501	6.56	0.638	0.977	0.207
Grad-SHAP	0.442	0.269	4.393	0.629	0.975	−0.545

Table 4 shows the evaluation metrics of the four XAI methods. By comparing the MoRF, ABPC, INFD, PScore, SynScore, and XAI-FI metrics, the reliability and effectiveness of each method in interpreting hypertension-related metabolites were further verified. Specifically, the SHAP method performed best across all metrics, with a MoRF value of 0.61, higher than that of IG and Grad-CAM, indicating that SHAP's interpretation results are minimally affected by model randomness. The ABPC value was 0.583, higher than that of IG and Grad-SHAP, indicating that SHAP better aligns with model predictions and exhibits strong stability and reliability. The INFD value was 3.881, lower than that of the other methods, indicating that SHAP's interpretations minimize deviation from the true metabolic profile and can more accurately reflect the biological characteristics associated with hypertension. SHAP maintained high PScore and SynScore values of 0.701 and 0.976, respectively, further verifying its accuracy in biological significance. Overall, SHAP achieved the highest XAI-FI score of 0.991, significantly outperforming Grad-CAM's 0.207 and significantly exceeding the negative scores of IG and Grad-SHAP. Therefore, SHAP is an XAI method that is more suitable for the DMSNet model and can provide reliable explanatory support for the precise mining of hypertension-related metabolites.

4.4 Metabolite Identification

Through quantitative analysis and index evaluation, the SHAP method selected based on the XAI-FI framework can accurately identify pixels that significantly contribute to differences in sample pseudo-mass spectra. Extracting specific metabolite names from these key pixels requires completing three core steps: image data processing and feature point screening, coordinate transformation and range determination, and metabolite matching and identification, ultimately achieving accurate biomarker identification. The detailed process is as follows:

First, quantitative analysis is performed on the image data containing attribution values output by the interpretable algorithm. The attribution values for each point are obtained and sorted by magnitude. Important feature points are identified and their indices are recorded. These indices are then converted to two-dimensional image coordinates. Next, the image coordinates are further converted to a metabolite m/z and RT range. Finally, this range is compared with the m/z and RT information of the 209 metabolites detected. Metabolites whose m/z and RT values fall within the above ranges are identified as interpretable biomarkers associated with the image features. In positive ion mode [(L-acetylcarnitine (204.1239, 1.25), LPC 20:0sn:1 (552.4017, 6.19), LPC 20:0sn-2 (552.4017, 6.07) [31,32], fatty amide 22:1 (338.3413, 7.29), L-Carnitine (162.1112, 1.22))]. In negative ion mode [(FFA 22:0 (339.3272, 9.16), Taurochenodeoxycholate (498.2895, 6.31), FFA 14:0 (227.2023, 7.17), FFA 18:2 (279.2331, 7.67), FFA 20:5 (301.2181, 7.4) [33], Glutamine (145.062, 1.06) [34], Glycoursodeoxycholic acid (448.3069, 5.39), Octanoic acid (143.1056, 3.97))]. Specific location (see Fig. 4), Interpretability analysis of the location of important metabolites in pseudo-mass spectra). Among them, L-acetylcarnitine and free fatty acid 18:2 have been confirmed as metabolites related to hypertension by comparing with the results of published papers.

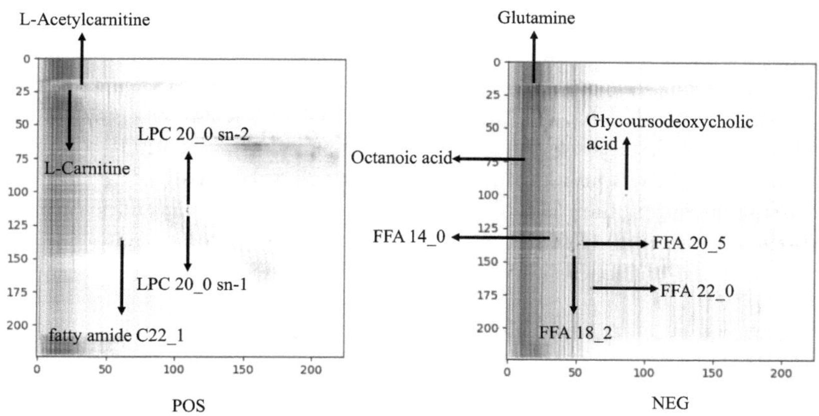

Fig. 4. Interpretability analysis of the location of important metabolites in pseudo mass spectra

5 Discussion

The methodological innovation of this study lies in the development of DMSNet to address the inherent challenges of LC-MS metabolomics data. Unlike traditional machine learning models that are prone to information loss or neglect of ion mode-specific features during high-dimensional feature selection, DMSNet adopts a dual-channel architecture combined with a modality attention mechanism and cross-modal consistency constraints. This design enables collaborative modeling of POS and NEG data, capturing subtle metabolic interactions that may be overlooked by single-modal models or traditional methods. Five-fold cross-validation and ablation studies validated DMSNet's classification accuracy (96.41%), outperforming traditional machine learning methods, demonstrating its robustness in processing sparse, high-dimensional metabolomics data while preserving key metabolic information through pseudo-mass spectrometry image transformation.

From a biological perspective, this study combined a dual-channel model with interpretable analytical techniques adapted to the task, successfully screening and identifying L-acetylcarnitine and L-Carnitine, two key metabolites that are closely related to the pathophysiological process of hypertension. L-acetylcarnitine, as a core mediator of mitochondrial fatty acid oxidation, suggests that hypertension is accompanied by impaired energy metabolism, potentially affecting blood pressure through endothelial dysfunction and oxidative stress. Oral supplementation of L-Carnitine increases the pro-atherogenic factor TMAO, thereby increasing the risk of cardiovascular disease and may be indirectly associated with hypertension through this pathway. However, this approach also has limitations: the size of the single-center cohort may limit generalizability, and uncertainty in metabolite annotation (common in untargeted metabolomics) may affect biomarker validation. Furthermore, while SHAP and other XAI Our approach provides insights into model decision-making, but further work is needed to enhance the granularity of interpretability and validate clinical translatability. Future directions will focus on multi-cohort replication, targeted functional profiling of priority metabolites (e.g., studies of L-acetylcarnitine supplementation), and lightweighting of the model for point-of-care diagnostic applications, while integrating multi-omics data to uncover deeper metabolic-pathophysiological connections.

6 Conclusion

To address the challenges of insufficient complementary integration of positive and negative ion modes, limited cross-scale information fusion, and poor model interpretability in mass spectrometry data for hypertension prediction, this study proposed a dual-channel interactive attention deep classification network. This network converts raw mass spectrometry data into pseudo-mass spectrometry images. Through modality-adaptive dual-channel feature extraction, bidirectional modal attention interaction, multi-scale fusion, and consistency constraints based on KL divergence, it achieves a five-fold cross-validation accuracy of 96.41%. Furthermore, by introducing multiple alternative XAI methods and constructing a comprehensive fidelity metric to select SHAP as the optimal interpretation method, this network, combined with traditional statistical methods, successfully identified key hypertension-related metabolites such as L-acetylcarnitine and L-Carnitine, providing reliable research for the application of deep learning-driven metabolomics in disease diagnosis and biomarker discovery.

Acknowledgment. This work was supported in part by the National Natural Science Foundation of China under Grant 62203437. It was also supported by the Basic Research Co-funded Projects in Guangzhou (No. 2024A03J0395) and the Science and Technology Projects in Guangzhou (No. 2024D03J0010).

References

1. Talmor-Barkan, Y., Bar, N., Shaul, A.A., Shahaf, N., Godneva, A., Bussi, Y., Lotan-Pompan, M., Weinberger, A., Shechter, A., Chezar-Azerrad, C., et al.: Metabolomic and microbiome profiling reveals personalized risk factors for coronary artery disease. Nat. Med. **28**(2), 295–302 (2022)
2. Louca, P., Tran, T.Q.B., du Toit, C., Christofidou, P., Spector, T.D., Mangino, M., Suhre, K., Padmanabhan, S., Menni, C.: Machine learning integration of multimodal data identifies key features of blood pressure regulation. EBioMedicine **84**, (2022)
3. Sekaran, K., Zayed, H.: Identification of novel hypertension biomarkers using explainable ai and metabolomics. Metabolomics **20**(6), 124 (2024)
4. Wang, H., Yin, Y., Zhu, Z.-J.: Encoding lc-ms-based untargeted metabolomics data into images toward ai-based clinical diagnosis. Anal. Chem. **95**(16), 6533–6541 (2023)
5. Deng, Y., Yao, Y., Wang, Y., Tiantian, Yu., Cai, W., Zhou, D., Yin, F., Liu, W., Liu, Y., Xie, C., et al.: An end-to-end deep learning method for mass spectrometry data analysis to reveal disease-specific metabolic profiles. Nat. Commun. **15**(1), 7136 (2024)
6. Melnikov, A.D., Tsentalovich, Y.P., Yanshole, V.V.: Deep learning for the precise peak detection in high-resolution lc-ms data. Anal. Chem. **92**(1), 588–592 (2019)
7. Shen, X., Shao, W., Wang, C., Liang, L., Chen, S., Zhang, S., Rusu, M., Snyder, M.P.: Deep learning-based pseudo-mass spectrometry imaging analysis for precision medicine. Brief. Bioinform. **23**(5), bbac331 (2022)
8. Cadow, J., Manica, M., Mathis, R., Reddel, R.R., Robinson, P.J., Wild, P.J., Hains, P.G., Lucas, N., Zhong, Q., Guo, T., et al.: On the feasibility of deep learning applications using raw mass spectrometry data. Bioinformatics **37**(Supplement_1), i245–i253 (2021)
9. Zhang, F., Shaoyang, Yu., Lirong, W., Zang, Z., Yi, X., Zhu, J., Cong, L., Sun, P., Sun, Y., Selvarajan, S., et al.: Phenotype classification using proteome data in a data-independent acquisition tensor format. J. Am. Soc. Mass Spectrom. **31**(11), 2296–2304 (2020)
10. Wu, K.L., Lin, P.C., Lin, W.C., Chen, S.F.: Comprehensive evaluation of dual-mode lc-ms conditions for enhanced metabolomic profiling: application to microplastic exposure studies. Anal. Chim. Acta **1367**, 344313 (2025)
11. Fu, Q.L., Chen, C., Liu, Y., Fujii, M., Fu, P.: Ft-icr ms spectral improvement of dissolved organic matter by the absorption mode: a comparison of the electrospray ionization in positive-ion and negative-ion modes. Anal. Chem. **96**(1), 522–530 (2024)

12. Miotto, R., Wang, F., Wang, S., Jiang, X., Dudley, J.T.: Deep learning for healthcare: review, opportunities and challenges. Brief. Bioinform. **19**(6), 1236–1246 (2018)
13. Gomes, B., Ashley, E.A.: Artificial intelligence in molecular medicine. N. Engl. J. Med. **388**(26), 2456–2465 (2023)
14. Ali, S., Abuhmed, T., El-Sappagh, S., Muhammad, K., Alonso-Moral, J.M., Confalonieri, R., Guidotti, R., Del Ser, J., Díaz-Rodríguez, N., Herrera, F.: Explainable artificial intelligence (xai): what we know and what is left to attain trustworthy artificial intelligence. Inf. Fusion **99**, 101805 (2023)
15. Stiglic, G., Kocbek, P., Fijacko, N., Zitnik, M., Verbert, K., Cilar, L.: Interpretability of machine learning-based prediction models in healthcare. Wiley Interdisciplinary Reviews: Data Mining and Knowledge Discovery **10**(5), e1379 (2020)
16. Nohara, Y., Matsumoto, K., Soejima, H., Nakashima, N.: Explanation of machine learning models using shapley additive explanation and application for real data in hospital. Comput. Methods Programs Biomed. **214**, 106584 (2022)
17. Parvanova, A., Trillini, M., Podestà, M.A., Iliev: Effects of acetyl-l-carnitine on blood pressure and metabolic control in type 2 diabetes: the diabasi randomized controlled trial. J. Endoc. Soc. **2**(5), 420–436 (2018)
18. Liu, T., Liu, C., Wang, X., Wei, Y., Li, S., Song, Y., Chen, P., Liu, L., Wang, B., Shi, H.: The association of serum l-carnitine concentrations with the risk of cancer in chinese adults with hypertension. Nutrients **14**(23), 4999 (2022)
19. Lundberg, S.M., Lee, S.-I.: A unified approach to interpreting model predictions. Neural Information Processing Systems, pp. 4768–4777 (2017)
20. Langbein, S.H., Koenen, N., Wright, M.N.: Gradient-based explanations for deep learning survival models (2025). arXiv:2502.04970
21. Selvaraju, R.R., Cogswell, M., Das, A., Vedantam, R., Parikh, D., Batra, D.: Grad-cam: Visual explanations from deep networks via gradient-based localization. In: International Conference on Computer Vision, pp. 618–626 (2017)
22. Qi, Z., Khorram, S., Li, F.: Visualizing deep networks by optimizing with integrated gradients. Assoc. Adv. Artif. Intell. **34**, 11890–11898 (2020)
23. Dwivedi, K., Rajpal, A., Rajpal, S., Agarwal, M., Kumar, V., Kumar, N.: An explainable ai-driven biomarker discovery framework for non-small cell lung cancer classification. Comput. Biol. Med. **153**, 106544 (2023)
24. Tkachenko, K., González-Sáiz, J.M., Pizarro, C.: Untargeted lipidomic reveals potential biomarkers in plasma samples for the discrimination of patients affected by parkinson's disease. Molecules **30**(4), 850 (2025)
25. Li, X., Du, M., Chen, J., Chai, Y., Lakkaraju, H., Xiong, H.: M4: a unified xai benchmark for evaluating the fidelity of feature attribution methods across metrics, modalities, and models. In: Neural Information Processing Systems, pp. 1630–1643 (2023)
26. Yeh, C.-K., Hsieh, C.-Y., Suggala, A.S., Inouye, D.I., Ravikumar, P.: On the (in)fidelity and sensitivity for explanations. In: Neural Information Processing Systems, pp. 10967–1097 (2019)
27. Cambay, V.Y., Barua, P.D., Hafeez Baig, A., Dogan, S., Baygin, M., Tuncer, T., Acharya, U.R.: Automated detection of gastrointestinal diseases using resnet50*-based explainable deep feature engineering model with endoscopy images. Sensors (Basel) **24**(23), 7710 (2024)
28. Pattanayak, S., Singh, T., Kumar, R.: Refined prognostication of pathological complete response in breast cancer using radiomic features and optimized inceptionv3 with dce-mri. Sci. Rep. **15**, 27844 (2025)

29. Anari, S., Sadeghi, S., Sheikhi, G., Ranjbarzadeh, R., Bendechache, M.: Explainable attention based breast tumor segmentation using a combination of unet, resnet, densenet, and efficientnet models. Sci. Rep. **15**, 1027 (2025)
30. Cheng, H., Lian, J., Jiao, W.: Enhanced mobilenet for skin cancer image classification with fused spatial channel attention mechanism. Sci. Rep. **14**, 28850 (2024)
31. Niu, Z., Wu, Q., Luo, Y., et al.: Plasma lipidomic subclasses and risk of hypertension in middle-aged and older chinese adults. Phenomes **2**(5), 283–294 (2022)
32. Couch, C.A., Ament, Z., Patki, A., Kijpaisalratana, N., Bhave, V., Jones, A.C., Armstrong, N.D., Cushman, M., Kimberly, W.T., Irvin, M.R.: Sex-related metabolites and risk of stroke, coronary heart disease, hypertension, and chronic kidney disease in the regards cohort. J. Am. Heart Assoc. **13**(9), 32643 (2024)
33. de Jongh, R.T., Serne, E.H., Ijzerman, R.G., et al.: Free fatty acid levels regulate microvascular function: relation to obesity-associated insulin resistance, hypertension and microvascular disease. Diabetes **53**(11), 2873–2882 (2004)
34. Rachedi, N.S., Tang, Y., Tai, Y.Y., et al.: Dietary intake and glutamine-serine metabolism control pathological vascular stiffness. Cell Metab. **36**(6), 1335–1350 (2024)

A Deep Learning-Based TCM Deficiency-Excess Syndrome Differentiation Framework for Spectrum Analysis of PPG Pulse Wave

Heng Weng[1(✉)], Fan Xiao[2], Fangzhen Wu[3], Bingji Chen[3], Yaliu Qu[3], Bo Xiao[1], Lin Wei[1], and Guobin Su[1]

[1] The Second Affiliated Hospital of Guangzhou University of Chinese Medicine, State Key Laboratory of Dampness Syndrome of Chinese Medicine, Guangzhou, Guangdong Province, P.R. China
wengh@gzucm.edu.com

[2] School of Medical Information Engineering, Guangzhou University of Traditional Chinese Medicine, Guangzhou, Guangdong Province, P.R. China

[3] The Second Clinical Medical College of Guangzhou University of Chinese Medicine, Guangzhou, China

Abstract. Traditional Chinese Medicine (TCM) deficiency-excess syndrome differentiation remains highly subjective. This study proposes a deep-learning framework alongside the Pulse Waveform Spectral Parameter Estimation Model (PWSPEM), that analyses PPG pulse-wave spectra to establish an objective mapping between PPG signals and TCM deficiency-excess patterns. Compared with conventional Fourier decomposition (MSE = 0.12), PWSPEM integrates multi-cycle harmonic superposition, time-varying attenuation and linear skip connections, achieving stable fitting (MSE = 0.002–0.005). Twelve PPG spectral features were quantified by the QSS algorithm. In 6,032 healthy participants, C3 and C4 showed significant positive correlation with deficiency-type syndromes (C3: $P = 0.003$; C4: $P = 0.021$) and negative correlation with age (C3: $r = -0.160$; C4: $r = -0.330$, both $P < 0.001$). In classification, PWSPEM outperformed all comparators: accuracy = 0.8182, AUC = 0.9036 versus WaveNet (0.8010/0.8866), CNN-BiLSTM (0.7961/0.8781), CBAM (0.8059/0.8893) and Random Forest (0.7985/0.8847). Preliminary pre-/post-intervention tests further demonstrated clinical utility. PWSPEM thus provides a technical means to support objective TCM deficiency-excess syndrome differentiation.

Keywords: Photoplethysmography (PPG) · Pulse Waveform Spectral Parameter Estimation Model · TCM Deficiency-Excess Syndrome Differentiation

Y. Zhang et al. (Eds.): CHIP 2025, CCIS 2884, pp. 50–78, 2026.
https://doi.org/10.1007/978-981-95-7299-1_4

1 Introduction

1.1 Research Background and Significance

Traditional Chinese Medicine (TCM), as the traditional medical system of the Chinese nation, has a history of thousands of years and has accumulated rich experience in disease diagnosis and treatment [1]. The syndrome differentiation of deficiency and excess is an important part of TCM diagnostics, and it is closely related to the zang-fu organs, qi, blood, yin and yang in TCM theory [2]. However, at present, the syndrome differentiation of deficiency and excess in TCM mainly relies on the subjective judgment of TCM practitioners, which has certain limitations [3]. Due to differences in experience, academic schools, and other factors among different TCM practitioners, the syndrome differentiation results for the same patient lack objective standards and specifications. This affects the accuracy and reliability of TCM diagnosis to a certain extent and also restricts the international promotion and development of TCM [4].

Photoplethysmography (PPG) technology, as a non-invasive detection method, can obtain human pulse wave signals in real-time [5]. PPG pulse waves contain abundant human physiological and pathological information and have a close connection with TCM pulse conditions [6]. Through the analysis of PPG pulse waves, characteristic parameters such as those in the time domain, frequency domain, and time series can be extracted. These parameters can reflect the functional status of the human cardiovascular system and the operation of qi and blood, providing objective data support for the syndrome differentiation of deficiency and excess in TCM [7].

Deep learning methods can perform efficient nonlinear fitting analysis on non-stationary periodic pulse wave signals [8]. When analyzing PPG pulse waves, they can automatically identify single-cycle pulse waves and conduct multi-channel processing. By making full use of the complementary information between single-cycle signals of different channels and global signals, the characteristics of pulse waves can be extracted more comprehensively and accurately [9]. Compared with traditional Fourier decomposition, multi-channel deep Fourier decomposition has higher accuracy and stability in processing non-stationary signals and can better adapt to the characteristics of PPG pulse waves [10]. The application of multi-channel deep Fourier decomposition in PPG pulse wave analysis is expected to provide a more objective and accurate method for the syndrome differentiation of deficiency and excess in TCM and promote the modernization process of TCM diagnosis.

1.2 Feasibility of Photoplethysmographic (PPG) Pulse-Wave Analysis as an Objective Vehicle for TCM Pattern Differentiation

In the research field of TCM pulse diagnosis, domestic scholars have carried out extensive work, ranging from the collation of ancient pulse diagnosis literature, the discussion of pulse diagnosis theories to the research on the objectification of pulse diagnosis. The ancient pulse diagnosis literature contains abundant pulse diagnosis knowledge and experience, and in-depth excavation and collation of this literature is conducive to the inheritance and development of TCM pulse diagnosis theories [11]. In the research on the objectification of pulse diagnosis, domestic efforts have been made in the development of pulse diagnosis instruments. From the early simple sphygmograph to the current intelligent and multi-functional pulse detection equipment, the development of the objectification of pulse diagnosis has been continuously promoted [12]. Some studies have also attempted to combine the holistic view of TCM with modern science and technology to explore the mechanism of pulse wave formation, providing theoretical support for the objectification of pulse diagnosis [6].

Foreign scholars have also shown a strong interest in TCM pulse diagnosis. Some studies focus on the quantitative analysis of TCM pulse diagnosis using modern scientific and technological means, and attempt to reveal the scientific connotation of TCM pulse diagnosis by establishing mathematical models to describe the characteristics of pulse waves [13].

In the research field of PPG pulse waves, scholars at home and abroad have achieved numerous results in signal acquisition, processing and feature extraction. In terms of signal acquisition, the performance of PPG sensors has been continuously improved to enhance the quality and stability of signals [14]; in terms of signal processing, various advanced algorithms have been applied, such as filtering algorithms to remove noise interference and wavelet transform for signal denoising and feature extraction [15]; in terms of feature extraction, in addition to the traditional time-domain and frequency-domain feature parameters, many new features have been explored, such as feature parameters based on morphology [16]. These research results have laid a solid foundation for the application of PPG pulse waves in the medical field.

1.3 Research Objectives and Innovations

This study aims to construct a TCM syndrome differentiation framework for deficiency and excess based on the spectral analysis of PPG pulse waves, realizing the objectification and accuracy of TCM syndrome differentiation for deficiency and excess [17]. The specific objectives include: first, extracting characteristic parameters closely related to TCM syndrome differentiation for deficiency and excess through spectral analysis of multi-channel PPG pulse waves; second, establishing an effective TCM syndrome differentiation model for deficiency and excess using the extracted characteristic parameters to improve the accuracy, reliability, and interpretability of syndrome differentiation; third, verifying the effectiveness and feasibility of the constructed syndrome differentiation framework in practical applications, providing new technical support for TCM clinical diagnosis.

The innovations of this study are mainly reflected in the following two aspects: First, in terms of data utilization, multi-channel PPG signals (including single-cycle/multi-cycle signals) are adopted for the first time to fully explore the complementary information between signals from different channels. Compared with traditional single-channel analysis, this method can more comprehensively reflect the physiological and pathological states of the human body. Second, in terms of algorithm application, a spectral decomposition algorithm based on deep learning is introduced. This algorithm has significant advantages over traditional Fourier decomposition methods in fitting non-stationary signals, which helps to improve the accuracy, reliability, and interpretability of feature extraction, providing strong support for the objective syndrome differentiation of deficiency and excess in TCM.

2 Related Work

2.1 PPG-Driven of Digital Pulse Diagnosis

In recent years, Point-of-Care Testing (POCT) technology and wearable devices have developed rapidly [18]. By integrating biosensors, biochips, and microfluidic technology, wearable devices can monitor glucose levels, cardiovascular biomarkers, and coagulation status in real-time, thereby providing rapid, portable, and user-friendly solutions for chronic disease monitoring, health status assessment, and precise intervention [19].

PPG pulse wave analysis has become a key tool for sensing the trends of chronic diseases [20]. When combined with the analysis of multiple risk factors, it enables routine and real-time physiological monitoring, while integrating psychological and social determinants, thus providing multi-dimensional support for the management of frailty in the elderly [21]. Since PPG can collect data continuously over a period from several months to several years, it can capture the earliest hemodynamic changes that indicate frailty long before clinical decompensation occurs and identify the window for intervention [22].

Empirical studies have confirmed that there is a stable correlation between Photoplethysmography (PPG) features and heart rate, heart rhythm, blood pressure (BP), blood glucose, and blood volume, which highlights its auxiliary role in the diagnosis of cardiovascular diseases. Zhang et al. used an improved cascaded forest regressor to realize non-invasive blood pressure estimation, with a mean absolute error (MAE) of 1.76 mmHg for systolic blood pressure and 2.89 mmHg for diastolic blood pressure, and coefficients of determination (R^2) of 0.948 and 0.926, respectively [7]. Other research teams have improved near-infrared PPG sensors, and combined with machine learning algorithms, the mean absolute relative difference (MARD) in blood glucose prediction is as low as 2.48% [19]. Avram et al. analyzed approximately 3 million smartphone PPG pulse signals from 53,870 subjects and successfully identified diabetes-related vascular damage with an accuracy of 80% [20]. In terms of arrhythmia screening, the accuracy of detecting atrial fibrillation using PPG alone exceeds 90%; if combined with electrocardiogram (ECG), the consistency will be higher [25].

2.2 Deep Learning-Based Methods for Pulse Wave Feature Extraction Models

Deep learning-based pulse wave feature extraction models primarily leverage the automatic learning capabilities of neural networks to extract time-domain, frequency-domain, time-frequency-domain, and nonlinear features from raw pulse waves (such as PPG photoplethysmographic waves and ECG electrocardiographic pulse waves) [27]. This approach eliminates the limitations of traditional manual feature extraction. Based on model structures and functional orientations, these methods can be categorized into the following five major types, with details on their principles, advantages, application scenarios, and typical models provided below (Table 1).

Table 1. Core advantages, scenarios and tasks of pulse wave feature extraction models

Model category	Typical methods and models	Core advantages	Application scenarios	Typical tasks
CNN and its variants [28]	Basic CNN models, Deep convolutional networks (e.g., ResNet, DenseNet), Convolutional attention networks (CBAM, SE-Net)	Local morphological features, anti-noise capability	Raw pulse waves, low-noise physiological data	Heart rate estimation, waveform quality assessment
RNN and its variants [29]	Long short-term memory (LSTM) networks, Gated recurrent units (GRU), Bidirectional recurrent networks (Bi-LSTM/Bi-GRU)	Temporal dependence modeling, dynamic feature capture	Long-time-series pulse waves, dynamic physiological parameters	HRV extraction, instantaneous heart rate monitoring
Time-frequency domain models [30]	CNN + Short-Time Fourier Transform (STFT)/Wavelet Transform (WT), WaveNet architectures	Joint time-frequency feature representation	Non-stationary pulse waves, frequency-domain-related analysis tasks	Respiratory rate extraction, frequency drift detection
Self-supervised/unsupervised models [31]	Autoencoders (AE) and Variational autoencoders (VAE), Contrastive learning frameworks	Label-free learning paradigm, high data efficiency	Scarce labeled datasets, large-scale unlabeled physiological data	Feature pre-training, niche pathological feature extraction
Hybrid models	CNN-LSTM/GRU Hybrid Models [32], Transformer-CNN Integration Architectures	Global-local and morphological-temporal feature integration	Complex physiological parameter estimation, clinical-grade diagnostic tasks	Non-invasive blood pressure measurement, pathological pulse wave classification

2.3 Limitations of Classical Pulse-Wave Analytics

Although time-domain indicators (including pulse rate, rise time, and diastolic decay rate) are easy to calculate, they are susceptible to noise interference [14]. Frequency-domain methods (such as Fourier transform or wavelet transform) can reveal spectral periodicity but ignore the nonlinear damping effect [7]. Nonlinear analysis tools (such as Lyapunov exponent and fractal dimension) can quantify the complexity of pulse waves; however, their large amount of calculation and obscure clinical interpretability have hindered their application in bedside scenarios [26]. Model-driven PPG analysis methods also have shortcomings: the accuracy of cycle detection using linear regression or basic sine fitting is lower than 85%, and their architecture cannot associate multi-cycle PPG features with Traditional Chinese Medicine (TCM) syndrome labels, failing to fill this diagnostic gap [11].

According to TCM theory, the deficiency or excess state of the human body is reflected in the circulation of qi and blood as well as the functions of zang-fu organs. As an external manifestation of the human physiological state, the frequency components and amplitude changes of PPG pulse wave signals can reflect the prosperity/decline and circulation of qi and blood [12]. The single components with different frequencies obtained through multi-channel deep Fourier decomposition can correspond to different physiological processes. Low-frequency components may be related to the basic function of the heart and the elasticity of blood vessels, while high-frequency components may be associated with the rapid contraction and relaxation of the heart and changes in microcirculation [24]. In the state of deficiency syndrome, the human body has insufficient qi and blood, and the heart function may be weakened. Reflected in the frequency-domain features of PPG signals, this may be manifested as a decrease in the amplitude of low-frequency components, while the changes in high-frequency components are relatively insignificant. In the state of excess syndrome, however, qi and blood are stagnant and abundant, and the heart function is hyperactive. As a result, the amplitude of low-frequency components may be relatively high, and high-frequency components may also show more active changes [6].

Fourier decomposition can decompose PPG pulse wave signals into multiple single components with different frequencies and amplitudes. These single components contain abundant physiological information and are closely related to the syndrome differentiation of deficiency and excess in Traditional Chinese Medicine (TCM) [14]. The idea of extracting features related to syndrome differentiation of deficiency and excess from the decomposed frequency-domain signals is mainly based on the following aspects.

PPG signals from different channels have a certain degree of complementarity in reflecting the human physiological state [8]. For example, PPG signals from the finger area may better reflect the condition of peripheral circulation, while PPG signals from the wrist area may be more sensitive to the state of the overall cardiovascular system [20]. Through multi-channel deep Fourier decomposition, the frequency-domain features of signals from different channels can be analyzed simultaneously, and the information related to syndrome differentiation of deficiency and excess in signals of each channel can be comprehensively considered, thereby extracting features more comprehensively and accurately [9]. It is possible to compare the amplitude differences of the same frequency component in signals from different channels, as well as the distribution of different frequency components in each channel. These differences and distribution features may all become the features related to syndrome differentiation of deficiency and excess [16].

3 Method

3.1 Framework Overview

To address the integration of modern technology with TCM syndrome differentiation, this study proposes a deep learning-based TCM Deficiency-Excess

Syndrome Differentiation Framework for PPG pulse wave spectrum analysis (Fig. 1), consisting of four core phases: Signal preprocessing and high-quality band extraction: Reliable signal segments are obtained via peak-valley-RR interval detection, window band quality evaluation, and multi-cycle band extraction, laying the foundation for subsequent analysis. High-precision spectral parameter estimation: Long-cycle/single-cycle band fitting is combined with deep spectral parameter estimation, multi-channel fitting, and quantitative scoring to enhance the accuracy of spectral features. Spectral feature analysis: Feature selection and correlation analysis identify key physiological indicators associated with TCM "deficiency-excess" differentiation, bridging spectral features with clinical syndrome criteria. Syndrome deficiency-excess modeling and analysis: Population norms are established, and syndrome classification/trend prediction models are built to provide a scientific basis for clinical application. The framework has been applied in key scenarios: (1) Smartphone-based TCM pulse analyzers for home health management; (2) Dynamic monitoring and early warning of Zang-Fu Qi-Blood Xu-Shi states; (3) Health norm establishment via large-scale healthy population pulse feature clustering; (4) Early warning of Healthy Qi deficiency; (5) Personalized intervention guidance for diverse populations, verifying its practical value in TCM clinical practice and preventive medicine.

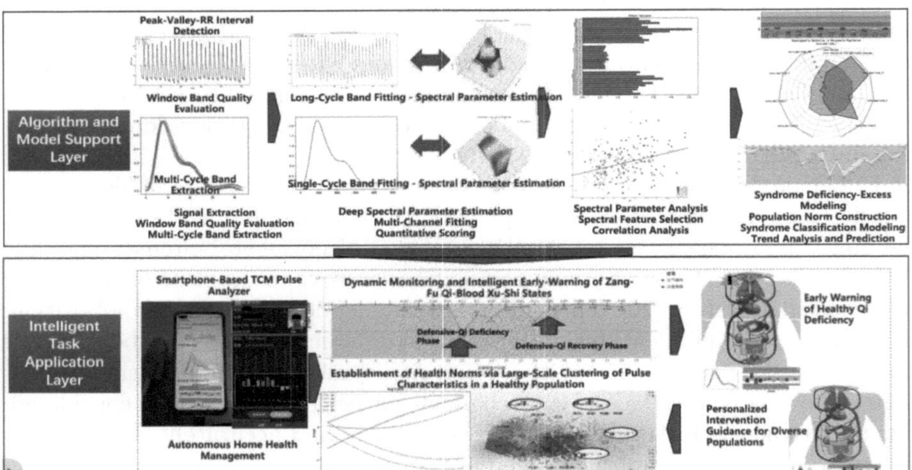

Fig. 1. Deep Learning-Based TCM Deficiency-Excess Syndrome Differentiation Framework for PPG Pulse Wave Spectrum Analysis

3.2 Data Sources

According to the TCM theory that "the spleen and kidney are the congenital foundations of life, the kidney governs bones, and the spleen governs muscles", the human body gradually weakens with increasing age. Deficiency syndromes, especially the syndrome of dual deficiency of the spleen and kidney, are particularly prominent in the elderly population. Therefore, this study collaborated with clinical institutions to construct two datasets (the healthy adult dataset and the elderly dataset) for the performance verification of the deficiency-excess syndrome differentiation model.

Healthy Population Dataset Subjects aged 18–64 years who met the criteria for "balanced constitution" in *Classification and Determination of TCM Constitutions* (without obvious biased constitutional characteristics) were included. Subjects with sarcopenia, cardiovascular and cerebrovascular diseases, and other underlying conditions were excluded. As of January 1, 2025, after signal quality screening (excluding samples with severe noise interference), a total of 6,032 cases were finally included.

Elderly Dataset Subjects in this dataset were aged 65 years and above, divided into two groups:

- **Sarcopenia-Positive Group**: A total of 138 cases, all meeting the diagnostic criteria in *Expert Consensus on Diagnosis and Treatment of Sarcopenia in the Elderly in China (2023 Edition)* (reduction in muscle mass + decrease in muscle strength/impairment of physical function).
- **Sarcopenia-Negative Group**: A total of 104 cases, with ages matched to the positive group ($P > 0.05$) and no sarcopenia-related manifestations.

3.3 Data Collection and Preprocessing

Data Collection Protocol Equipment: A mature transmissive PPG sensor probe (Guangdong Medical Device Registration Approval No. 20202071349) was used, with a sampling rate of 50 Hz, resolution of 128 bits, and built-in dual-wavelength detection (red light: 663 nm; near-infrared light: 890 nm). Collection Method: The sensor was connected to a smartphone to enable convenient and reliable data collection. Environmental Control: Pulse wave signals were collected when subjects were in a relatively stable state, either right after getting up in the morning or after 10 min of rest (to avoid interference from exercise and emotional fluctuations). With the assistance of APP visualization, continuous signal collection was performed for a duration of no less than 2 min.

Data Management: All collected data were uploaded and store into the Big Data Intelligent Processing and Knowledge Service Platform of Guangdong Provincial Hospital of Traditional Chinese Medicine for unified management and analysis.

Signal Preprocessing Process Noise Removal: A 50 Hz notch filter was used to eliminate power frequency noise; db4 wavelet decomposition (4 levels) combined with soft threshold filtering was applied to remove motion artifacts. Baseline Correction: A 3rd-order polynomial fitting method was used to eliminate baseline drift caused by respiration and body movement, stabilizing the signal baseline around 0. Segmentation and Quality Assessment: An adaptive peak detection algorithm (with the threshold set to 1.5 times the signal mean) was used to identify pulse cycles. Waveforms meeting quality requirements were extracted using RR Interval Analysis. The artifact rate of the extracted segments was calculated, and only valid segments with an artifact rate of less than 10% were included in the analysis (artifact-contaminated data exceeding this threshold were excluded) to ensure the reliability of subsequent feature analysis.

3.4 Models

We first introduce the *Pulse Waveform Spectral Parameter Estimation Model (PWSPEM)* for spectral parameter estimation, which incorporates decay factors to achieve better non-linear fitting, especially for long-period spectral bands. Subsequently, to enhance the learning efficiency across multiple periodic spectral bands, we present the *Multi-Channel Ensemble Learning Model*, which leverages bidirectional temporal neural networks to construct an ensemble learning framework.

PWSPEM The *PWSPEM* represents a signal as a superposition of parameterized sinusoids and their harmonics. A key feature is the inclusion of decay factors, which significantly improve the model's ability to non-linearly fit signals containing long-period spectral components.

$$y(t) = \text{offset} + \sum_{c=1}^{C} \left[D_c(t) \cdot \sum_{h=1}^{H} \gamma_{c,h} \cdot \begin{pmatrix} A_{\sin,c,h} \cdot \sin(2\pi f_{c,h} t + \phi_{c,h}) \\ +A_{\cos,c,h} \cdot \cos(2\pi f_{c,h} t + \phi_{c,h}) \end{pmatrix} + w_c \cdot t \right] \tag{1}$$

where:

- C: number of components
- H: maximum harmonic order
- $f_{c,h} = h \cdot f_c$: harmonic frequency
- $D_c(t) = \exp(\alpha_c \cdot t)$: decay factor, enhancing non-linear fitting for long periods
- $\gamma_{c,h}$: harmonic coefficient
- $A_{\sin,c,h}, A_{\cos,c,h}$: sine/cosine amplitudes
- $\phi_{c,h}$: phase
- w_c: skip connection weight
- offset: global offset.

Multi-Channel Ensemble Learning Model The *Multi-Channel Ensemble Learning Model* is designed to capture complex bidirectional temporal dependencies across multiple channels, thereby improving the efficiency of learning spectral characteristics that span multiple periodic bands.

For channel k:

- Parameter vector: $p_k = [A_{k,1}, ..., A_{k,M}, f_{k,1}, ..., f_{k,M}, \phi_{k,1}, ..., \phi_{k,M}, b_k]$
- Forward GRU: $h_k^{\rightarrow} = \text{GRU}^{\rightarrow}(p_{k-1})$
- Backward GRU: $h_k^{\leftarrow} = \text{GRU}^{\leftarrow}(p_{k+1})$
- Parameter fusion: $p_k = \text{Fuse}(h_k^{\rightarrow}, h_k^{\leftarrow})$
- Frequency adjustment: $f_{k,m} = f_{\text{base},m} + \delta f_{k,m}$.

Signal reconstruction for channel k:

$$y_k(t) = b_k + \sum_{m=1}^{M} A_{k,m} \cdot \sin(2\pi f_{k,m} t + \phi_{k,m}) \tag{2}$$

Ensemble Learning Framework The *Multi-Channel Ensemble Learning Model* functions as an ensemble framework: 1. Base Estimation: Use the *Waveform Spectral Parameter Estimation Model* to estimate initial spectral parameters for each channel. 2. Temporal Modeling: Capture inter-channel temporal relationships using bidirectional GRUs, processing information both forward and backward across channels. 3. Parameter Fusion: Integrate the bidirectional temporal information to generate refined, channel-specific parameters. 4. Signal Reconstruction: Reconstruct each channel's signal from its optimized parameters.

This integrated architecture effectively models both the complex temporal dynamics across channels and the intricate spectral characteristics within each channel, leading to superior performance for multi-period spectral band estimation.

Training Optimization Strategy To ensure effective model training and prevent overfitting/gradient issues, we design a comprehensive training strategy, including independent channel-wise loss calculation, optimized optimizer selection, learning rate scheduling, and early stopping mechanisms. Initialization Parameters of Waveform Spectral Parameter Estimation Model (Per Channel)

For each channel, the Waveform Spectral Parameter Estimation Model is initialized with specific parameters tailored to capture the periodic spectral characteristics of PPG signals. It can independently receive single-cycle pulse waves and long-cycle pulse waves from pre-data processing. When the input is a single-cycle pulse wave,$max_{\text{harmonic}} = 1$, and the components can be regarded as harmonics at this time; when the input is a long-cycle pulse wave, the maximum number of harmonics in practice is generally set to 3, which achieves the optimal fitting effect. Below is the definition of a single-cycle pulse wave:

- $n_{\textbf{components}} = 12$: Specifies 12 independent periodic components for the model. Each component corresponds to a distinct fundamental frequency and its harmonics, enabling the model to decompose complex PPG signals into 12 sub-spectral bands—sufficient to cover typical frequency ranges of PPG-related physiological information (e.g., heart rate, respiratory modulation).

- $max_{\mathbf{harmonic}} = 1$: Sets the maximum harmonic order to 1. This means each periodic component only uses its fundamental frequency (no additional harmonic frequencies are introduced), simplifying the model while focusing on capturing primary periodicities of the target spectral bands.
- $basefreq = 0.3$ **(Unit: Hz)**: Defines the fundamental frequency of the first (lowest-frequency) periodic component. This value is selected to align with the lower bound of common PPG-related frequency ranges (e.g., 0.3 Hz corresponds to a 3.3-second period, covering slow physiological fluctuations).
- $step = 1$ **(Unit: Hz)**: Determines the frequency interval between consecutive periodic components. Starting from $basefreq = 0.3$ Hz, each subsequent component's fundamental frequency increases by 1 Hz. Thus, the 12 components span a frequency range of 0.3 Hz, 1.3 Hz, 2.3 Hz, ..., 11.3 Hz—covering both low-frequency (e.g., respiratory, vasomotion) and high-frequency (e.g., typical heart rate, 1–3 Hz) bands of PPG signals.

These parameters collectively enable the model to adaptively fit multi-period spectral bands of PPG signals per channel, with a frequency range that balances coverage of physiological information and computational efficiency.

Loss Function

We adopt the Mean Squared Error (MSE) as the loss function to measure the discrepancy between the reconstructed and true photoplethysmography (PPG) signals. Notably, the loss for each channel is computed independently to ensure channel-specific optimization, and the total loss is the aggregation of all channel-wise losses.

The MSE loss for a single channel is defined as:

$$\mathcal{L}_k = \frac{1}{N} \sum_{t=1}^{N} (S_k(t) - S_{k,\text{true}}(t))^2 \tag{3}$$

where:

- $\mathcal{L}_k$: MSE loss of the k-th channel,
- N: number of time points in the signal,
- $S_k(t)$: reconstructed PPG signal of the k-th channel at time t,
- $S_{k,\text{true}}(t)$: true PPG signal of the k-th channel at time t.

The total training loss (aggregated across all channels) is given by:

$$\mathcal{L}_{\text{total}} = \frac{1}{K} \sum_{k=1}^{K} \mathcal{L}_k \tag{4}$$

where K denotes the total number of channels.

Optimizer

The Adam optimizer is selected for model parameter updating, configured with hyperparameters to balance convergence speed and stability:

- Initial learning rate: 10^{-2} (0.01),

- Weight decay: 10^{-5} (to mitigate overfitting via L2 regularization),
- Gradient clipping: Applied with max_norm = 1.0 (to constrain gradient magnitudes and prevent gradient explosion during training).

Learning Rate Scheduling

A "Reduce LR On Plateau" scheduler is employed to adaptively adjust the learning rate, ensuring efficient convergence even when the loss plateaus:

- Monitoring metric: Validation set MSE (to avoid overfitting to the training set),
- Patience: 800 (the scheduler waits for 800 epochs of unchanged validation MSE before adjusting the learning rate),
- Reduction factor: 0.5 (the learning rate is halved each time the scheduling condition is triggered).

Early Stopping

To further prevent overfitting and save computational resources, an early stopping mechanism is implemented:

- Patience: 3000 (training stops if the validation set MSE does not improve for 3000 consecutive epochs),
- Model checkpointing: The model parameters corresponding to the minimum validation set MSE are saved as the final trained model, ensuring optimal generalization performance.

3.5 Feature Extraction and Syndrome Differentiation Correlation Analysis Methods

Model-Based PPG Feature Extraction: Frequency features: Mean fundamental frequency ($\bar{f} = \frac{1}{C}\sum_{i=1}^{C} f_i$), harmonic frequency ratio ($r_h = \frac{f_i h}{\bar{f}}$), dominant fundamental frequency ratio ($\frac{\max(f_i)}{\bar{f}}$).

Amplitude features: Total sine-cosine amplitude

$$A_{total,i,h} = \sqrt{A_{sin,i,h}^2 + A_{cos,i,h}^2}, \tag{5}$$

harmonic order with maximum amplitude

$$h_{max} = \arg\max(A_{total,i,h}), \tag{6}$$

coefficient of variation of amplitude

$$CV_A = \frac{\sigma(A_{total,i,h})}{\mu(A_{total,i,h})}. \tag{7}$$

Decay features: Mean decay factor ($\bar{\lambda} = \frac{1}{C}\sum_{i=1}^{C} \lambda_i$), standard deviation of decay factor (σ_λ).

Phase features: Phase difference between adjacent harmonics

$$\Delta\phi_h = |\phi_{i,h+1} - \phi_{i,h}|, \tag{8}$$

mean phase

$$\bar{\phi} = \frac{1}{C \cdot H} \sum_{i=1}^{C} \sum_{h=1}^{H} \phi_{i,h} \tag{9}$$

Trend features: Mean skip connection weight ($\bar{w} = \frac{1}{C}\sum_{i=1}^{C} w_i$), DC offset (offset).

Quantile-Based Segmental Scoring Furthermore, due to the significant differences in amplitude across different frequency bands, we perform quantile-based quantitative scoring on the extracted amplitude features to facilitate comparison. To establish a robust **Population Feature Norm** and detect intra-population feature heterogeneity, we propose **Quantile-based Segmental Scoring (QSS)**, a data distribution-driven method. Traditional quantization relies on external standards, ignoring target population's distribution uniqueness (e.g., regional/age-related feature variations), distorting norms and hiding heterogeneous signals. QSS addresses this by leveraging intrinsic data traits, mapping continuous features to a 1–10 discrete score (1 = bottom 10th percentile, 10 = top 10th). This "relative position scoring" aligns norms with population characteristics, normalizes multi-dimensional features for cross-comparison, and enables quantitative heterogeneity interpretation (e.g., scores 2–3 = below baseline, 9–10 = potential abnormal high):

Phase 1: Threshold Learning (from reference dataset $\mathcal{D}$) 1. Input: $\mathcal{D}$ (N samples, M features) and feature list $C = [c_1, ..., c_k]$; 2. Initialize threshold dict T; 3. For each $c_i \in C$: a. Extract values $V_i = \{v_1, ..., v_N\}$; b. Compute 10th–100th percentiles as thresholds $\{q_{0.1}(V_i), ..., q_{1.0}(V_i)\}$; c. Store in T: $T[c_i] = \{1 : q_{0.1}, ..., 10 : q_{1.0}\}$.

Phase 2: Score Application (to dataset $\mathcal{D}'$)

1. Input: $\mathcal{D}'$ (target dataset) and pre-generated T (quantile threshold table);
2. For each feature $c_i \in T$ (each threshold column in T):
   (a) For each value $v' \in \mathcal{D}'[c_i]$ (values of feature c_i in $\mathcal{D}'$), assign score s (range: 1–10) as follows:

$$s = \begin{cases} 10, & v' \geq T[c_i][10]; \\ 9, & v' \geq T[c_i][9]; \\ \vdots; & \\ 1, & \text{otherwise.} \end{cases}$$

3. Output $\mathcal{D}''$ (combined dataset: original data $\mathcal{D}'$ + QSS score columns corresponding to each feature c_i).

Formal Formulation

- Quantile Threshold Calculation: For each quantile level $k \in \{1, 2, \ldots, 10\}$, the k-th decile threshold t_k is defined as:

$$t_k = \text{quantile}(V, k/10)$$

where quantile(V, p) denotes the p-th percentile of the value set V (e.g., $k = 5$ corresponds to the 50th percentile/median of V).
- Scoring Function Definition: For any input value v' (from $\mathcal{D}'$), the QSS score $S(v')$ is determined by:

$$S(v') = \arg \max_{k \in \{1,2,\ldots,10\}} (v' \geq t_k)$$

with a default value $S(v') = 1$ (assigned when $v' < t_1$, i.e., v' is below the 10th percentile of V).

Syndrome Differentiation Correlation Analysis Methods Statistical testing: One-way Analysis of Variance (ANOVA) to compare feature differences among the four groups, with LSD method for post-hoc multiple comparisons (significance level $\alpha = 0.05$). Syndrome differentiation model construction: Using selected features as input and TCM Spleen-Kidney syndrome types (2 categories) as output, Support Vector Machine (SVM), Logistic Regression (LR), and lightweight CNN models were built. Ten-fold cross-validation was used to evaluate performance. Features extracted from the traditional multi-sine wave model served as the control group to verify the advantages of the improved model. Performance metrics: Accuracy, sensitivity for each syndrome type, specificity, macro-averaged F1-score (Macro-F1), ROC curve, and AUC value.

4 Result

4.1 Pulse-Wave Fitting Performance Verification

Head-To-Head Comparison Between PWSPEM and Conventional Fourier Decomposition To quantify the fitting superiority of the proposed PWSPEM, we benchmarked it against traditional single-cycle Fourier decomposition on an identical dataset (70 representative PPG segments from sarcopenic older adults and healthy controls). Mean-squared error (MSE), mean absolute error (MAE), coefficient of determination (R^2) and structural similarity index (SSIM) served as the primary metrics (Table 2).

Waveform-fitting scrutiny (Fig. 2) reveals that conventional Fourier decomposition produces visible mismatches in both the diastolic tail—where it fails to reproduce the progressive amplitude decay caused by vascular damping—and the steep systolic foot, whose rapid excursion cannot be tracked by single-cycle fitting. In contrast, PWSPEM, by virtue of its multi-cycle superposition and

Table 2. Comparison of fitting performance metrics between PWSPEM and traditional fourier decomposition (Mean ± Standard deviation)

Model	MSE	MAE	R^2	SSIM (structural similarity index)
Traditional fourier decomposition	0.121±0.018	0.285±0.026	0.763±0.035	0.728±0.041
PWSPEM	0.0038±0.0009	0.045±0.010	0.986±0.008	0.972±0.017

dedicated damping factor, accurately reconstructs these two critical segments. The structural-similarity index (SSIM) rises by $\tilde{1}2.2$ % relative to the traditional model, while the fitting error for low-amplitude, fast-decay "weak pulses" (frequent in sarcopenic patients) is reduced by more than 60 %.

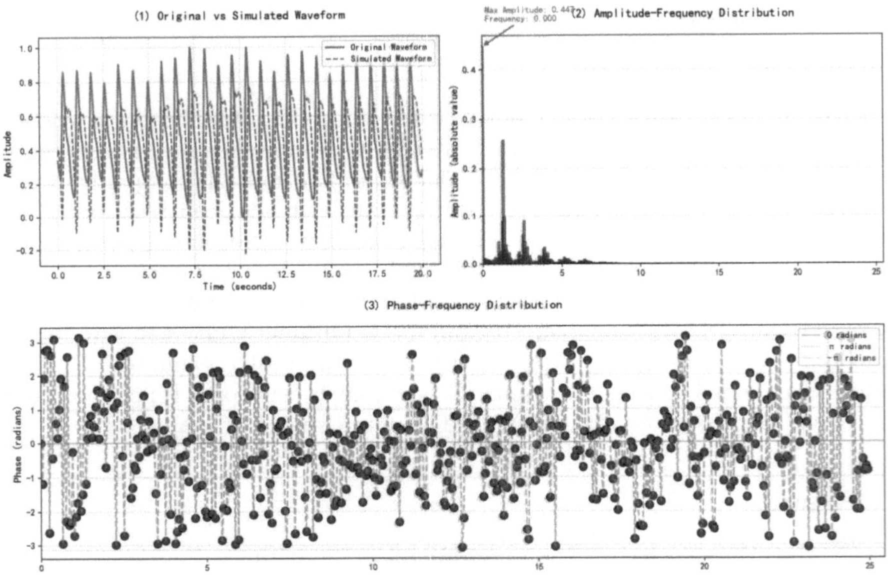

Fig. 2. Fourier-decomposed waveform reconstruction (fitted curve) and corresponding frequency-spectrum distribution.

Repeatability and Robustness Repeatability: Fifteen volunteers (sarcopenic and healthy) were re-recorded three times (1-week interval). CVs of the three key PWSPEM-derived features—fundamental frequency, damping factor and 2nd-harmonic amplitude—were < 3 % (1.9 % ± 0.4 %, 2.6 % ± 0.5 % and 2.3 % ± 0.4 %, respectively), with MSE consistently between 0.003 and 0.005. Fourier-derived features showed CVs > 8 % and MSE drifted from 0.105 to 0.138 (Fig. 3).

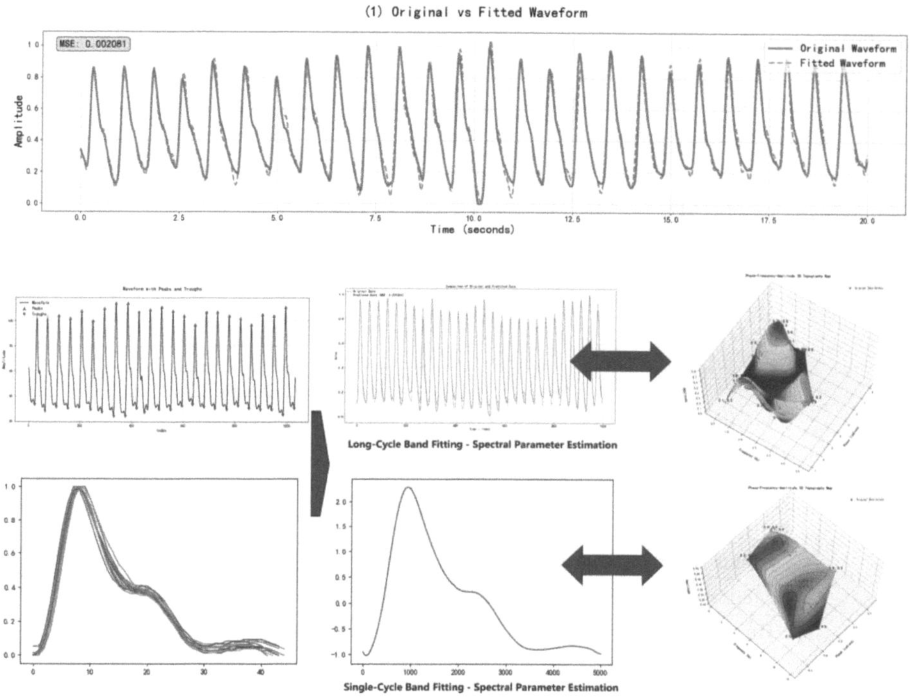

Fig. 3. PWSPEM Reconstruction and Spectral Feature Extraction.

4.2 Results of Syndrome Differentiation Correlation Analysis

Association Between Core Features and Syndrome Differentiation Based on the 12 harmonic (C1–C12) spectral amplitude features extracted by the PWSPEM, the Wilcoxon rank sum test was used to compare feature differences between the positive group (patients with sarcopenia, i.e., typical patients with deficiency syndrome) and the negative group (patients without sarcopenia, i.e., non-deficiency syndrome). The results showed that only the spectral amplitude features of Harmonic C3 and Harmonic C4 exhibited statistically significant differences between the two groups (the spectral amplitude features of all other harmonics had P-values > 0.05, indicating no significant discriminative ability), and these two harmonics demonstrated the highest diagnostic discriminability for sarcopenia with deficiency syndrome (Tables 3 and 4).

The specific feature distributions are as follows:

* **C3**: The mean value of C3 in the positive group (3.35 ± 1.85) was significantly lower than that in the negative group (3.95 ± 1.82). The median value of C3 in the positive group (2.98, IQR: 2.11–4.46) was also lower than that in the negative group (3.94, IQR: 2.67–5.13), with an extremely significant inter-group difference ($P = 0.003$).

Table 3. Spectral amplitude features comparison between sarcopenia with deficiency syndrome negative and positive groups (Part 1: C1-C6).

Characteristic	Negative, N = 104	Positive, N = 138	p-value[1]
C1			
			0.42
Mean (SD)	4.93 (1.37)	5.12 (1.68)	
Median (IQR)	4.88 (3.93, 5.90)	4.92 (4.07, 6.39)	
Range	0.49, 8.09	0.00, 10.00	
C2			
			0.23
Mean (SD)	3.74 (1.36)	3.62 (1.74)	
Median (IQR)	3.78 (2.82, 4.39)	3.37 (2.52, 4.48)	
Range	0.88, 8.38	0.00, 10.00	
C3			
			0.003
Mean (SD)	3.95 (1.82)	3.35 (1.85)	
Median (IQR)	3.94 (2.67, 5.13)	2.98 (2.11, 4.46)	
Range	0.14, 8.77	0.00, 10.00	
C4			
			0.021*
Mean (SD)	2.96 (1.65)	2.62 (1.71)	
Median (IQR)	2.74 (2.00, 3.60)	2.15 (1.48, 3.20)	
Range	0.27, 10.00	0.00, 9.16	
C5			
			0.30
Mean (SD)	2.93 (1.47)	2.76 (1.57)	
Median (IQR)	2.85 (1.80, 3.71)	2.48 (1.68, 3.74)	
Range	0.18, 7.34	0.00, 10.00	
C6			
			0.37
Mean (SD)	2.33 (1.71)	2.20 (1.66)	
Median (IQR)	1.90 (1.17, 2.87)	1.76 (0.96, 3.00)	
Range	0.17, 10.00	0.04, 7.49	

[1] Statistical test: Wilcoxon rank sum test; $p<0.01$, $*p<0.05$

* **C4**: The mean value of C4 in the positive group (2.62 ± 1.71) was significantly lower than that in the negative group (2.96 ± 1.65). The median value of C4 in the positive group (2.15, IQR: 1.48–3.20) was lower than that in the negative group (2.74, IQR: 2.00–3.60), with a significant inter-group difference ($P = 0.021$).

Table 4. Spectral amplitude features comparison between Spleen-Kidney Deficiency Syndrome negative and positive groups (Part 2: C7-C12).

Characteristic	Negative, N = 104	Positive, N = 138	p-value[1]
C7			
			0.90
Mean (SD)	1.25 (1.34)	1.32 (1.33)	
Median (IQR)	0.87 (0.49, 1.46)	0.90 (0.43, 1.65)	
Range	0.00, 10.00	0.02, 6.94	
C8			
			0.34
Mean (SD)	1.06 (0.98)	1.20 (1.21)	
Median (IQR)	0.74 (0.47, 1.30)	0.86 (0.52, 1.59)	
Range	0.18, 6.50	0.00, 10.00	
C9			
			0.11
Mean (SD)	0.93 (0.70)	1.15 (1.13)	
Median (IQR)	0.73 (0.49, 1.16)	0.86 (0.54, 1.41)	
Range	0.20, 3.88	0.00, 10.00	
C10			
			0.076
Mean (SD)	0.75 (0.65)	0.98 (1.11)	
Median (IQR)	0.55 (0.37, 0.93)	0.70 (0.38, 1.19)	
Range	0.00, 3.54	0.00, 10.00	
C11			
			0.22
Mean (SD)	0.80 (0.56)	0.96 (1.01)	
Median (IQR)	0.64 (0.48, 0.97)	0.75 (0.47, 1.15)	
Range	0.00, 3.33	0.07, 10.00	
C12			
			0.20
Mean (SD)	0.98 (0.62)	1.17 (1.07)	
Median (IQR)	0.83 (0.61, 1.17)	0.89 (0.63, 1.37)	
Range	0.19, 3.87	0.00, 10.00	

[1] Statistical test: Wilcoxon rank sum test; $p<0.01$, $*p<0.05$

The remaining 10 **harmonics** (C1, C2, C5–C12) showed no statistical differences in mean, median, or value range between the positive and negative groups (P-value range: 0.076–0.90), indicating that these **harmonics** have weak discriminative ability for Spleen-Kidney dual-deficiency syndrome.

Correlation Between C3/C4 Feature and Age A further correlation analysis was conducted to explore the association between C3/C4 Features and Age in Healthy Population To verify the hypothesis that Spleen-Kidney function declines with age (consistent with the "women at 49 (7×7) and men at 64 (8×8)" theory in *Huangdi Neijing*), a correlation analysis was conducted between the PWSPEM-extracted C3/C4 features and age among 6,032 healthy individuals aged 18–65 years who underwent physical examinations. Pearson correlation (for linear correlation) and Spearman correlation (for rank correlation) were used to evaluate the association.

Correlation Between C3 Feature and Age The C3 feature exhibited a statistically significant negative correlation with age (Fig. 4). Specifically:

Pearson correlation: The correlation coefficient r was –0.160 (95% CI: –0.182 to –0.138), with an extremely significant P-value (<0.001). The coefficient of determination R^2 was 0.0256, indicating that age explains approximately 2.56% of the variation in C3 values.

Spearman correlation: The rank correlation coefficient ρ was –0.164 (95% CI: –0.186 to –0.142), also with an extremely significant P-value (<0.001, exact P = 1.2871776586691097e-37). This further confirmed the stable negative association between C3 and age, independent of the data distribution.

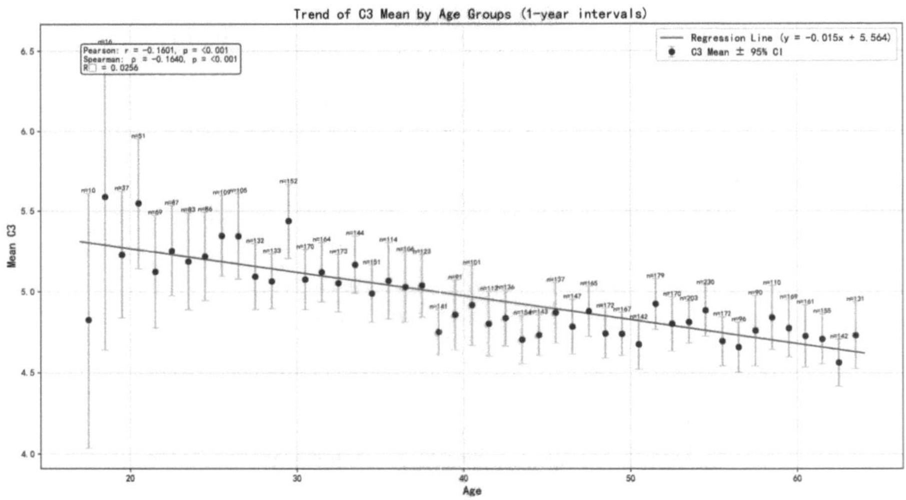

Fig. 4. Correlation Between C3 Feature and Age

Correlation Between C4 Feature and Age Compared with C3, the C4 feature showed a stronger negative correlation with age (Fig. 5), which was statistically significant: Pearson correlation: The correlation coefficient r was –0.330 (95% CI: –0.350 to –0.310), with an extremely significant P-value (<0.001). The

R^2 was 0.1088, meaning age accounts for approximately 10.88% of the variation in C4 values—four times higher than the explanatory power of age for C3. Spearman correlation: The rank correlation coefficient ρ was –0.348 (95% CI: –0.368 to –0.328), with an extremely significant P-value (<0.001, exact P = 8.434477801191 35e-171). This indicated that the negative association between C4 and age was more pronounced than that of C3.

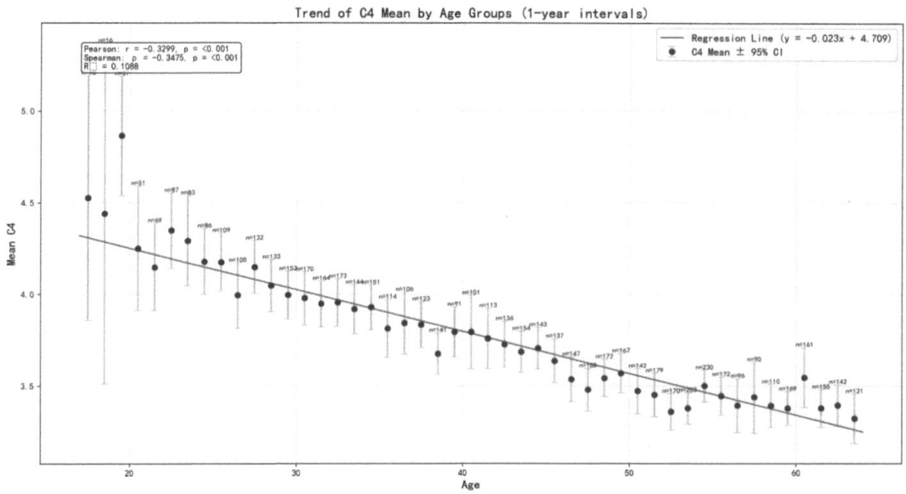

Fig. 5. Correlation Between C4 Feature and Age

Interpretation Based on TCM Theory These results strongly support the hypothesis that "the function of the human body's zang-fu organs and qi-blood declines with increasing age", which is consistent with the statement in Huangdi Neijing (Inner Canon of the Yellow Emperor): "At the age of 49 (7×7) for women, the Ren Meridian becomes deficient, the Chong Meridian weakens, and Tian Gui (heavenly essence) is exhausted; at the age of 64 (8×8) for men, Tian Gui is exhausted, essence is insufficient, and the Kidney function declines"—both pointing out the physiological law that the function of the human body's zang-fu organs and qi-blood deteriorates with age.

From a TCM perspective, the C3 and C4 features are closely associated with the abundance of qi-blood and the filling state of blood vessels. The negative correlation between C3/C4 and age reflects the gradual decline in the function of zang-fu organs such as the Spleen and Kidney with increasing age: the Spleen's ability to transport and transform qi-blood weakens, and the Kidney's capacity to store essence and generate qi declines, leading to reduced qi-blood perfusion in peripheral blood vessels. Consequently, the PPG-derived C3 and C4 features—which characterize the qi-blood status of blood vessels—decrease with age.

Notably, the stronger correlation of C4 with age (higher absolute r and ρ, larger R^2) suggests that C4 is a more sensitive indicator of age-related Spleen-Kidney function decline than C3. This may be attributed to C4's closer association with the Kidney's "governing essence" function—an aspect that is more prominently affected by the aging process according to TCM theory (Fig. 6).

4.3 Model Classification Performance Comparison

This study evaluated the performance of PWSPEM (PPG-Specific Multi-Cycle Attenuated Harmonic Model) against four mainstream baseline models for TCM spleen-kidney pattern classification. All models were trained and tested on the same dataset, which was randomly split into training and testing sets at an 8:2 ratio with a fixed random seed to ensure consistent partitioning across experiments. The main evaluation metrics included accuracy, precision, recall, F1-score, and AUC (Table 5).

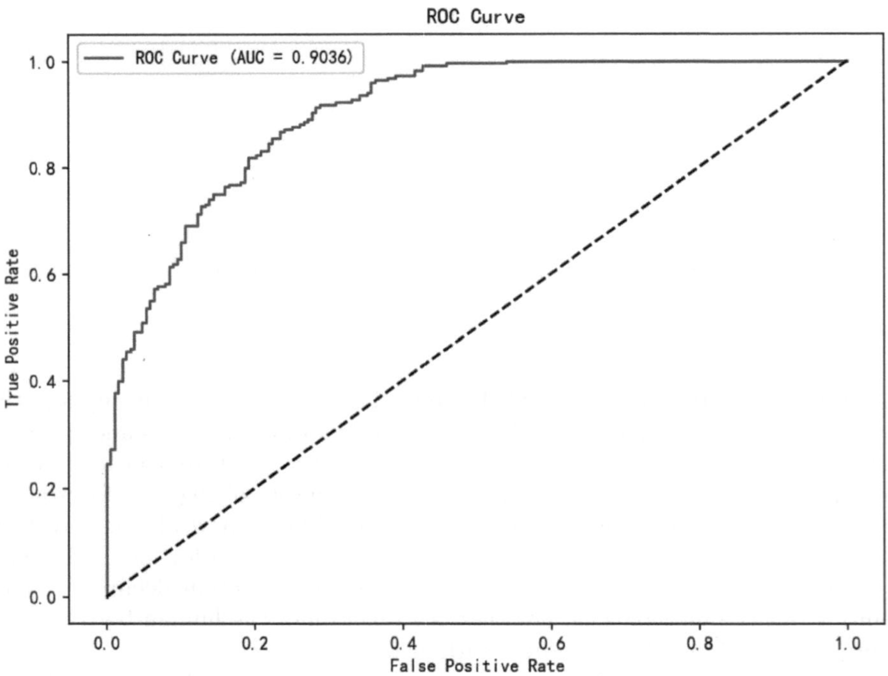

Fig. 6. Training of PWSPEM TCM spleen-kidney pattern classification

PWSPEM achieved the highest values on every metric. Its accuracy (0.8182) surpassed WaveNet (0.8010), CNN+BiLSTM (0.7961), CBAM (0.8059) and RandomForest (0.7985). Precision and recall reached 0.8199 and 0.8182, respectively, indicating a balanced ability to minimise both false positives and false

Table 5. Performance comparison of different models

Model	Accuracy	Precision	Recall	F1-score	AUC
PWSPEM	0.8182	0.8199	0.8182	0.8170	0.9036
WaveNet	0.8010	0.8034	0.8010	0.7991	0.8866
CNN+BILSTM	0.7961	0.7996	0.7961	0.7942	0.8781
CBAM	0.8059	0.8080	0.8059	0.8043	0.8893
RandomForest	0.7985	0.8016	0.7985	0.7967	0.8847

negatives. The F1-score (0.8170) was also the highest, confirming superior overall classification quality. The AUC of 0.9036 was significantly ahead of all comparables, demonstrating stronger discriminative power between deficiency and non-deficiency cases in TCM syndrome differentiation (consistent with the needs of TCM deficiency-excess differentiation). Although PWSPEM is architecturally lighter than the deep networks (WaveNet, CNN+BiLSTM, CBAM), its PPG-tailored multi-cycle attenuated harmonic structure extracts clinically relevant features more effectively. In summary, PWSPEM delivered the best performance in TCM deficiency-excess differentiation classification, offering a practical technical foundation for the objectification of TCM syndrome differentiation.

Model Interpretability Analysis By calculating the feature weight contribution using Random Forest, the results show that the weight of the C4 feature is the highest. A comparison of pulse wave features between patients with typical deficiency syndrome and healthy individuals with sufficient healthy qi reveals significant differences in amplitude and phase in the C3 and C4 segment spectra (Fig. 7).

The spectral-feature norm of the "Healthy-Qi-deficiency cohort" established on the basis of QSS scores can serve as an auxiliary reference for identifying frailty in older adults. In addition, we have preliminarily extended the model to the pre- and post-intervention monitoring of exercise and acupuncture. In this setting it can capture, in a single continuous 24 h recording, the entire curve of healthy-qi consumption during exercise and its subsequent recovery, while simultaneously quantifying—second-by-second—the boost in healthy qi produced by meridian stimulation (e.g., acupuncture or moxibustion). This capability realizes true dynamic situational awareness of an individual's healthy-qi status and provides clinicians with a visual, data-driven basis for optimizing the timing and dosage of any intervention (Fig. 8).

5 Discussion

This article explores a TCM deficiency-excess syndrome differentiation framework based on PPG spectrum analysis, focusing on three core issues: nonlinear fitting/feature extraction scientificity, modeling performance, and model interpretability. It analyzes PWSPEM's technical traits and TCM theory consistency,

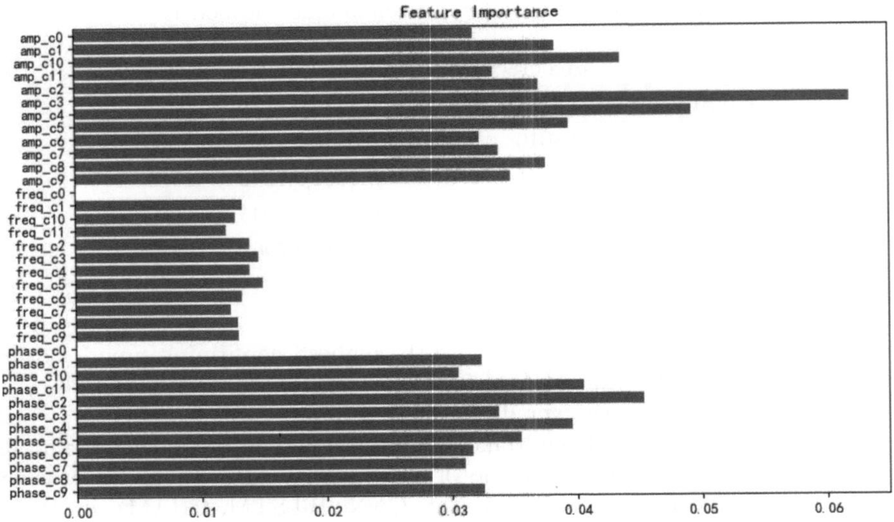

Fig. 7. Spectral Feature Weight Calculation using Random Forest.

discusses limitations, and provides references for TCM syndrome objectification. Details follow (Figs. 9, 10 and 11).

5.1 Scientificity of PWSPEM's Nonlinear Fitting and Feature Extraction

PWSPEM realizes PPG nonlinear fitting via "multi-cycle attenuated harmonics", addressing traditional model flaws. Mathematically, it abandons Fourier's "single-cycle sine fitting", adopting "fundamental-harmonic superposition + dynamic attenuation ($e^{\lambda t}$) + linear skip connection". This matches vascular elasticity-induced pulse energy dissipation (exponential decay), with MSE (0.002–0.005) far lower than traditional Fourier (0.12). Setting 12 harmonics ($n_{components} = 12$) enables multi-scale PPG feature coverage, enhancing complex signal representation and aligning with TCM "Twelve Meridians" for interpretability.

5.2 Twelve Meridians Mapping: Interpretability Verification

PWSPEM's 12 harmonic features, rooted in TCM Twelve Meridians, link math features to TCM theory, avoiding "black-box" outputs. Preliminary data confirms partial associations with Deficiency Syndrome (DS) and age, but needs further verification.

Association with Deficiency Syndrome Wilcoxon tests show only C3/C4 differ between DS-positive and negative groups (C3: $P = 0.003$; C4: $P =$

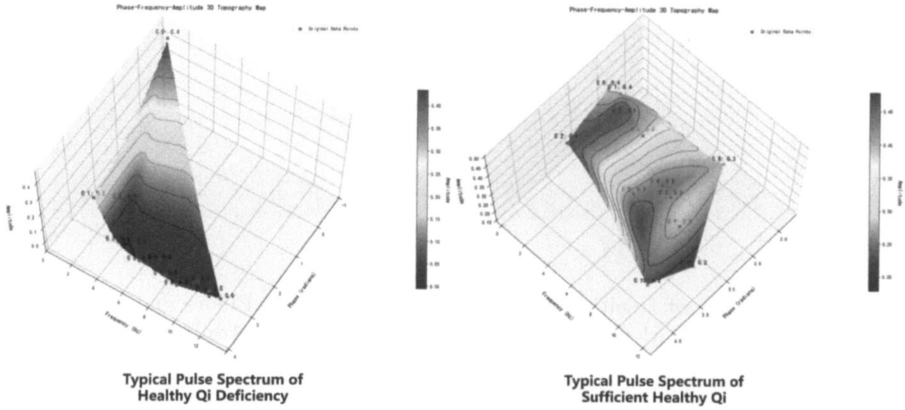

Fig. 8. Comparison of Typical Pulse Wave Spectra Between Populations with Healthy-Qi Deficiency and Sufficient Healthy-Qi.

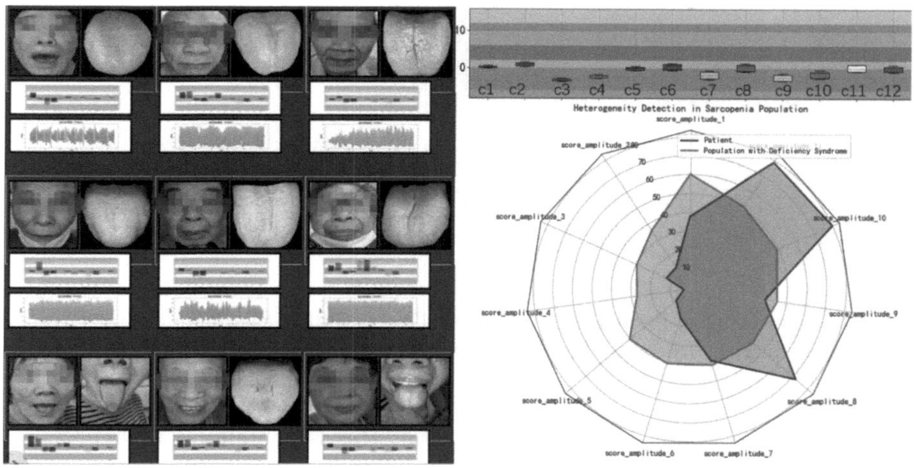

Fig. 9. Spectral Norm-Assisted Detection of the Normative Model for the Elderly Cohort with Healthy-Qi Deficiency

0.021; others $P > 0.05$). This aligns with TCM: Spleen/Kidney Meridians (acquired/innate Qi sources) regulate healthy Qi. C3/C4 may potentially correlate with these meridians' pulse signals, but no definite link is confirmed—more data is needed.

Association with Age Analysis of 6,032 healthy adults (18–65) shows C3/C4 negatively correlate with age (C3: $r = -0.160$, $P = 6.65e-36$; C4: $r = -0.330$, $P = 4.31e-153$), with $R^2 = 2.56\%$ (C3) and 10.88% (C4). This echoes *Huangdi Neijing*'s aging theory ("healthy Qi declines with age"). C4 may relate to Kidney

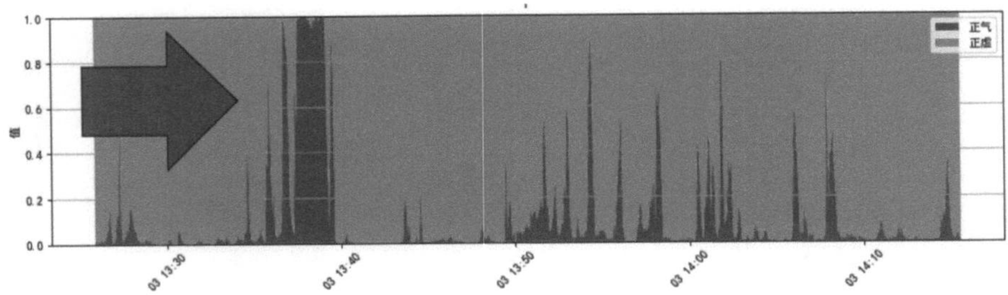

Fig. 10. Monitoring of Healthy-Qi Deficiency-Excess Status Before and After Moxibustion Intervention at Health-Preserving Acupoints in Older Adults

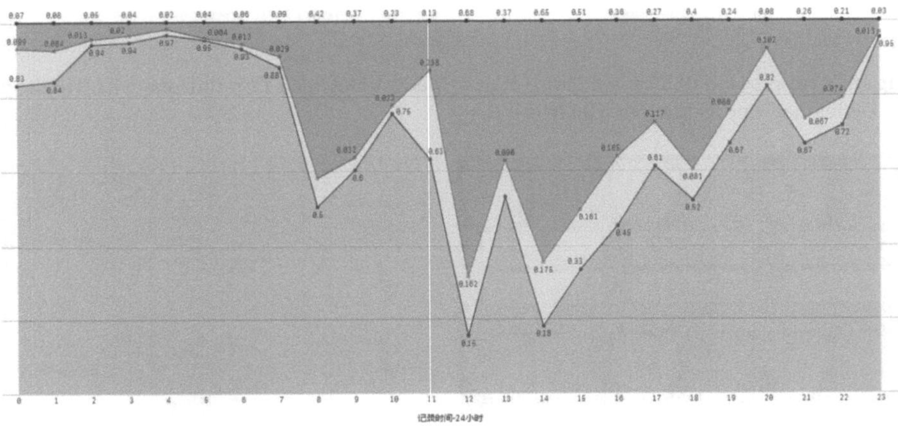

Fig. 11. Monitoring of Healthy-Qi Deficiency-Excess Status Before and After Exercise Intervention in Healthy Individuals

(innate Qi), C3 to Spleen (acquired Qi), but this is a preliminary hypothesis, not a conclusion.

5.3 PWSPEM's Modeling Performance and Improvement Directions

In
"DS vs. Non-DS" classification, PWSPEM outperforms WaveNet, CNN+BiLSTM, CBAM, and RandomForest (accuracy=0.8182, precision=0.8199, recall=0.8182, F1=0.8170, AUC=0.9036; AUC 1.7pp higher than WaveNet). Its lower complexity (12 harmonics, no complex structures) stems from "PPG specificity + TCM guidance", unlike generic deep learning models.

Limitations and Improvements *Performance Optimization*

- **Sample Issues**: Small, unbalanced samples (age/gender/constitution) limit generalization. Expand samples to cover key ages ($\geq$49F/$\geq$64M) and more syndromes (Yang/Yin Deficiency).
- **Overfitting**: Use L2 regularization and PPG data augmentation (time-stretching/noise) to reduce overfitting.
- **Experimental Design**: Add 1–2 week repeated measurements to verify result consistency.

Interpretability Enhancement

- **Insufficient Evidence**: C3/C4-Spleen/Kidney links lack direct proof (e.g., Zang-Fu indicators, acupoint stimulation). Design multi-dimensional verification (e.g., C3/C4 vs. renal function/gastrin).
- **Single Features**: Explore harmonic interactions (C3/C4 ratio) and phase features; use "multi-feature joint verification" and qualify claims (e.g., "preliminary inference") to avoid subjectivity.

Clinical Potential PWSPEM's lightweight design suits portable devices (smart bracelets). With improved performance/interpretability, it can enable "real-time monitoring + auxiliary differentiation", reducing physician subjectivity and supporting TCM standardization (outputs: C3/C4 values, classification probabilities).

6 Conclusion

In conclusion, the PWSPEM has demonstrated certain technical advantages and theoretical consistency through "nonlinear fitting", "meridian feature mapping", and "lightweight design", providing ideas for the research on the objectification of TCM syndrome differentiation. However, the current performance still needs to be improved. In the future, the potential of the model should be further explored by expanding the sample size, optimizing the experimental design, and reducing the risk of overfitting, so as to promote its application in clinical practice.

Building on the validated PWSPEM, the next step is to develop an Intelligent Situation-Awareness and Closed-Loop Intervention Framework for Health and Disease in Traditional Chinese Medicine to support personalized health management for clinicians and patients. The framework will integrate three core modules: (1) A multi-source situation-awareness module, using PWSPEM -derived C3/C4 features plus TCM four diagnostic data, wearable metrics, and EHRs to dynamically assess "health-subhealth-disease" status. (2) A personalized intervention module, generating TCM-specific plans (herbal formulas, acupuncture, diet) via a syndrome-intervention database and reinforcing learning. (3) A doctor-patient closed-loop module, enabling real-time PPG collection, automated analysis, plan adjustment, and feedback integration to optimize management continuously.

Acknowledgment. This study was funded by National Key R&D Program of China (2023YFC3502900), The Science and Technology Research Fund from Guangdong provincial hospital of Chinese medicine, China (YN2024MS005, YN2024MB018, YN2024MS012,

YN2020QN18, YN2020QN24), The Karolinska Institutet research grant (No. 2020-01616; No. 2022-02044), Noncommunicable Chronic Diseases-National Science and Technology Major Project (NO. 2023ZD0505600, NO. 2023ZD0505604), Sanming Project of Medicine in Shenzhen (No. SZZYSM202206014). G.Su. was awarded the ERA-ERAC MSc in Clinical Trials Fellowship for 2024.

Disclosure of Interests. The authors declare that they have no competing interests to declare that are relevant to the content of this article. No financial support, research grants, speaker honoraria, stock ownership, or other financial or non-financial relationships with any organizations or entities that could be perceived as influencing the research results have been received or held by any author during the conduct of this study.

References

1. Chen, L., Wei, S., He, Y., et al.: Treatment of chronic gastritis with traditional Chinese medicine: pharmacological activities and mechanisms. Pharm. **16**(9), 1308 (2023). https://doi.org/10.3390/ph16091308
2. Kung, Y.Y., Shen, Y.C., Li, J.Y., et al.: Effects of mind-body exercise on body constitution and circadian rhythm in people with suboptimal health status. J. Chin. Med. Assoc. **87**(1), 94–102 (2024). https://doi.org/10.1097/JCMA.0000000000001111
3. Hou, H., Wei, H., Wang, Y., et al.: Construction path of smart health care platform for the elderly in China. Strat. Study Chin. Acad. Eng. **24**(2), 170–178 (2022). https://doi.org/10.15302/J-SSCAE-2022.02.023
4. Oliveira, I.J.A.S., de Sá Ferreira, A.: Effects of diagnostic errors in pattern differentiation and acupuncture prescription: a single-blinded, interrater agreement study. Evid. Based Complement. Altern. Med. **2015**(1), 469675 (2015). https://doi.org/10.1155/2015/469675
5. Wang, L.T., Liu, C.S., Zhao, Y.N., et al.: A novel PPG pulse diagnosis instrument which can be used to assist the application of acupuncture and moxibustion. Zhen ci yan jiu = Acupuncture research/ z[Zhongguo yi xue ke xue yuan Yi xue qing bao yan jiu suo bian ji] **46**(6), 480–485 (2021). https://doi.org/10.13702/j.1000-0607.20210126
6. Lan, K.C., Litscher, G., Hung, T.H.: Traditional Chinese medicine pulse diagnosis on a smartphone using skin impedance at acupoints: a feasibility study. J. Sens. **20**(16), 4618 (2024). https://doi.org/10.3390/s20164618
7. Zhang, G., Shin, S., Jung, J.: Cascade forest regression algorithm for non-invasive blood pressure estimation using PPG signals. J. Appl. Soft Comput. **144**, 110520 (2023). https://doi.org/10.1016/j.asoc.2023.110520
8. Weber-Boisvert, G., Gosselin, B., Sandberg, F.: Intensive care photoplethysmogram datasets and machine-learning for blood pressure estimation: generalization not guarantied. J. Front. Physiol. **14**, 1126957 (2023). https://doi.org/10.3389/fphys.2023.1126957
9. Zou, H., Zhang, Y., Zhang, J., et al.: A novel multi-dimensional composition method based on time series similarity for array pulse wave signals detecting. Algorithms **13**(11), 297 (2020). https://doi.org/10.3390/a13110297
10. Chen, C., Li, Z., Zhang, Y., et al.: A 3D wrist pulse signal acquisition system for width information of pulse wave. J. Sens. **20**(1), 11 (2019). https://doi.org/10.3390/s20010011

11. Chen, Z., Zhang, D., Liu, F.Z.J.: Traditional Chinese medicine diagnostic prediction model for holistic syndrome differentiation based on deep learning. J. Integr. Med. Res. **13**(1), 101019 (2024). https://doi.org/10.1016/j.imr.2023.101019
12. Shilei, X., Zhao, H., Ying, A., et al.: The research of three regions acquisition and analysis system of pulse based on flexible sensor. In: E3S Web of Conferences, vol. 271, pp. 03056 (2021). https://doi.org/10.1051/E3SCONF/202127103056
13. Maloerti, A., Rebora, P., Occhino, G., et al.: Carotid–femoral pulse wave velocity progression in hypertensive patients is associated with subsequent cardiovascular outcomes. J. Hypertens. **43**(5), 797–806 (2025). https://doi.org/10.1097/HJH.0000000000003973
14. Elisa, M.-M., Kyriacou, P.A.: Spectral analysis for pulse rate variability assessment from simulated photoplethysmographic signals. J. Front. Physiol. **13**, 966130 (2022). https://doi.org/10.3389/fphys.2022.966130
15. Liu, Z., Zhang, Y., Zhou, C.: BiGRU-attention for Continuous blood pressure trends estimation through single channel PPG. J. Comput. Biol. Med. **168**, 107795 (2024). https://doi.org/10.1016/j.compbiomed.2023.107795
16. Quanyu, E.: Pulse signal analysis based on deep learning network. Biomed. Res. Int. **2022**, 6256126 (2022). https://doi.org/10.1155/2022/6256126
17. Sun, X., Zhang, Y., Liu, X., et al.: Characteristics and demographic factors of traditional Chinese medicine constitution types among elderly individuals in China: a national multistage cluster random study. J. Tradit. Chin. Med. Sci. **11**(3), 257–263 (2024). https://doi.org/10.1097/MD.0000000000042488
18. Tenorio-Mucha, J., Busta-Flores, P., María Lazo-Porras, et al.: Facilitators and barriers of the implementation of point-of-care devices for cardiometabolic diseases: a scoping review. BMC Health Serv. Res. **23**(1), 412 (2023). https://doi.org/10.1186/s12913-023-09419-2
19. Zheng, Y., Zhan, Z., Chen, Q., Chen, J., Luo, J., Cai, J., Zhou, Y., Chen, K., Xie, W.: Highly sensitive perovskite photoplethysmography sensor for blood glucose sensing using machine learning techniques. J. Adv. Sci. **11**(43), 2405681 (2024). https://doi.org/10.1002/advs.202405681
20. Avram, R., Olgin, J. E., Kuhar, P., et al.: A digital biomarker of diabetes from smartphone-based vascular signals. Nat. Med. **26**(10), 1576–1582 (2020). https://doi.org/10.1038/s41591-020-1010-5
21. Oviedo-Briones, M., Rodriguez, L., AngelAntonio, C., et al.: A comparison of frailty assessment instruments in different clinical and social care settings: the frailtools project. J. Am. Med. Dir. Assoc. **22**(3), 607.e7–607.e12 (2021). https://doi.org/10.1016/j.jamda.2020.09.024
22. Martini, C., Barla, A., Odone, F., et al.: Data-driven continuous assessment of frailty in older people. Front. Digit. Hum. **5**, 6 (2018). https://doi.org/10.3389/fdigh.2018.00006
23. Zhu, X., Wang, F., Mao, J., et al.: A protocol for digitalized collection of traditional Chinese medicine (TCM) pulse information using bionic pulse diagnosis equipment. Phenomics **3**(5), 519–534 (2023). https://doi.org/10.1007/s43657-023-00104-2
24. Gizem, Y., Lynn, O.J., Lieng-Hsi, L., et al.: Insights into vascular physiology from sleep photoplethysmography. Sleep **46**(10), zsad172 (2023). https://doi.org/10.1093/sleep/zsad172
25. Saglietto, A., Scarsoglio, S., Canova, D., et al.: Beat-to-beat finger photoplethysmography in atrial fibrillation patients undergoing electrical cardioversion. J. Sci. Rep. **13**(1), 6751 (2023). https://doi.org/10.1038/s41598-023-33952-z

26. Koyoshi, R., Miura, S.I., Kumagai, N., et al.: Clinical significance of flow-mediated dilation, brachial intima-media thickness and pulse wave velocity in patients with and without coronary artery disease. Circ. J. **76**(6), 1469–1475 (2012). https://doi.org/10.1253/circj.CJ-11-1283
27. Keke, Q., Wu, H., Tao, Z., et al.: Machine learning and deep learning for blood pressure prediction: a methodological review from multiple perspectives. J. Artif. Intell. Rev. **56**(8), 8095–8196 (2023). https://doi.org/10.1007/s10462-022-10353-8
28. Li, G., Watanabe, K., Anzai, H., Song, X., Qiao, A., Ohta, M.: Pulse-wave-pattern classification with a convolutional neural network. J. Sci. Rep. **9**(1), 14930 (2019). https://doi.org/10.1038/s41598-019-51334-2
29. Lyu, Y., Huang, W.Y., Wu, H.M., et al.: A heart failure classification model from radial artery pulse wave using LSTM neural networks. BMC Med. Inform. Decis. Mak. **25**(1), 318 (2025). https://doi.org/10.1186/s12911-025-03167-5
30. Wang, B., Chen, G., Rong, L., et al.: Arrhythmia disease diagnosis based on ECG time-frequency domain fusion and convolutional neural network. IEEE J. Transl. Eng. Health Med. **11**, 116–125 (2022). https://doi.org/10.1109/JTEHM.2022.3232791
31. Xiang, Y., Guo, J., Chen, M., Wang, Z., Han, C.: MAE-based self-supervised pretraining algorithm for heart rate estimation of radar signals. J. Sens. **23**(18), 7869 (2023). https://doi.org/10.3390/s23187869
32. Fang, H., Xiong, J., He, L.: Fair non-contact blood pressure estimation using imaging photoplethysmography. J. Biomed. Opt. Express **15**(4), 2133–2151 (2024). https://doi.org/10.1364/BOE.514241

Domain-Adapted Large Language Models for Schema-Consistent Medical Record Generation from Doctor-Patient Dialogues

Bo An[1,2](✉), Haitao Zhang[3], and Zhen Zhao[4]

[1] University of Chinese Academy of Social Sciences, Beijing, China
[2] Institute of Ethnology and Anthropology, Chinese Academy of Social Sciences, Beijing, China
anbo@cass.org.cn
[3] Department of Critical Care Medicine, Shanghai East Hospital, Tongji University School of Medicine, Shanghai, China
[4] Department of Emergency, Beijing Friendship Hospital, Capital Medical University, Beijing, China

Abstract. Automatically generating structured electronic medical records (EMRs) from multi-turn doctor–patient dialogues can reduce documentation burden and help standardize clinical data. We formulate medical record generation (MRG) as an instruction-following text generation task and present a large language models(LLMs) based approach combining domain continued pre-training and instruction tuning with LoRA. Unlike prior works, our framework explicitly enforces schema consistency through constrained decoding and sentinel-based field alignment. Concretely, we adapt Qwen LLMs on a medical corpus and fine-tune them to generate EMRs that conform to a target schema (chief complaint, present illness, past history, etc.) given raw dialogues. We evaluate on IMCS-V2-MRG using ROUGE-1/2/L averaged (ROUGE-AVG). Our best system, **Qwen3-32B + LoRA + Prompt**, achieves **68.2%** ROUGE-AVG, outperforming strong baselines. An ablation on Qwen3-32B shows that instruction tuning accounts for the majority of gains (**53.1%** → **67.3%**, +14.2), while domain continued pre-training provides a smaller but consistent improvement (**67.3%** → **68.2%**, +0.9). These results indicate clear benefits from LLM scaling and task-specific alignment for MRG. Finally, we develop a gastric-cancer–specific prototype that integrates dialogue intake and EMR generation with human-in-the-loop review. The study suggests that domain-adapted LLMs are a promising direction for reliable, schema-consistent medical record generation.

Keywords: Large Language Model · Medical Record Generation · Instruction Tuning · LoRA · Domain Adaptation

Y. Zhang et al. (Eds.): CHIP 2025, CCIS 2884, pp. 79–92, 2026.
https://doi.org/10.1007/978-981-95-7299-1_5

1 Introduction

Medical Record Generation (MRG) [6] based on doctor–patient dialogue information refers to the collection, organization, and analysis of conversational content, extracting key medical information and converting it into standardized and systematic medical record entries. In medical practice, clinicians shoulder a substantial documentation burden to ensure completeness and accuracy. Meanwhile, to maintain strict control of medical record quality, hospitals must allocate considerable resources to review and quality assurance. Figure 1 shows an example of MRG [5].

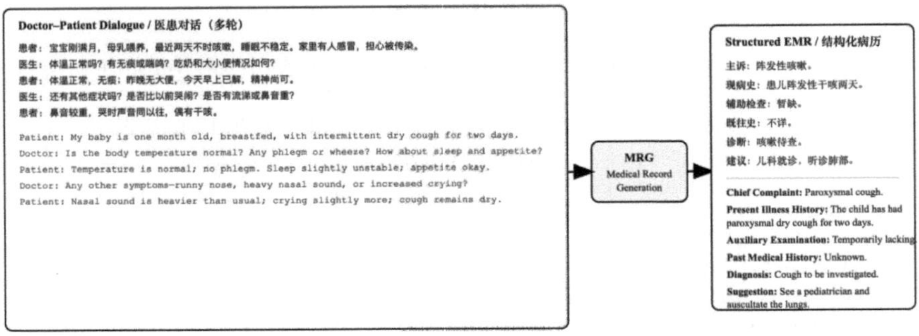

Fig. 1. The example of medical concept components.

At present, there are two mainstream approaches to MRG: template-based generation [9] and deep learning–based methods [7]. Template-driven workflows can simplify authoring and enforce structure, but they often lack flexibility, struggle to address individualized needs, and may lead to omissions that affect final accuracy. Deep learning methods, while effective with large training sets, typically show limited transferability across disease types and face difficulties modeling long-range context in multi-turn dialogues.

To address these issues, we formulate MRG as an instruction-following text generation task with LLMs. Concretely, dialogue content is provided to the LLM, and prompts are used to elicit EMRs conforming to a target schema (e.g., patient name, age, gender, chief complaint, past medical history). We adopt a two-stage adaptation strategy that combines domain continued pre-training on medical text with parameter-efficient instruction tuning via LoRA, aiming to enhance both domain understanding and schema-aligned generation.

Empirically, our LLM-based approach yields substantial improvements over conventional methods. On IMCS-V2-MRG, **Qwen3-32B + LoRA + Prompt** [57] attains **68.2%** ROUGE-AVG, surpassing *BERT+Span* (45.1%), *T5 + LoRA + Prompt* (63.9%), and *Qwen-14B + LoRA + Prompt* (64.6%). An ablation on Qwen3-32B shows that instruction tuning contributes the majority of the gains (prompt-only: 53.1% → 67.3%, +14.2 absolute), while domain continued pre-training provides a smaller but consistent lift (67.3% → 68.2%, +0.9).

Based on these findings, we further develop a gastric cancer–specific system that captures doctor–patient dialogues via recording devices and generates structured electronic medical records for physician review and correction, demonstrating practical feasibility in real-world clinical workflows.

2 Related Work

This section reviews prior studies from two perspectives: (i) MRG (MRG) and related EMR processing, and (ii) LLMs relevant to dialogue-grounded clinical text generation.

2.1 Medical Record Generation

Recent advances in electronic medical record (EMR) processing span several enabling tasks, including named entity recognition [15], relation extraction [14], knowledge graph construction [13], and data mining for diagnosis and treatment recommendation based on similar cases [12]. These techniques provide the foundations for structuring clinical narratives and are complementary to end-to-end MRG.

Template-based generation standardizes documentation by enforcing predefined forms and logic, thereby improving authoring efficiency. Representative implementations rely on Delphi-style programming [9,11] and XML-based interface specifications [10]. However, rigid templates can underfit diverse patient presentations and may omit salient details, limiting adaptability in real-world workflows.

Learning-based approaches increasingly leverage pre-trained transformers to map medical dialogues to EMR content. For instance, CopiFilter exploits pre-trained models for dialogue-grounded record generation [7,8] proposes a two-stage pipeline to enhance factuality. Both lines of work confirm the value of pre-training for MRG, yet challenges remain in handling long-range multi-turn context, adhering to schema constraints, and generalizing across disease domains. Our study departs from earlier PLM-centric pipelines by formulating MRG as an instruction-following generation problem and adapting LLMs with domain continued pre-training and parameter-efficient tuning.

2.2 Large Language Model

LLMs are powerful neural models for understanding and generating natural language [29]. They are typically built on the Transformer architecture [28] and trained via large-scale pre-training followed by task adaptation. The GPT family [25] exemplifies autoregressive pre-training for fluent generation. T5 frames diverse NLP tasks in a unified text-to-text paradigm [27], and mT5 extends this formulation to multilingual settings [26]. Instruction-following conversational models (e.g., ChatGPT[1] informed by instruction tuning [23]) and subsequent larger-scale models such as GPT-4 [22] demonstrate strong zero/few-shot generalization and long-context reasoning. For Chinese dialogue scenarios, ChatGLM-6B[2] builds on the GLM framework [21] to support bilingual generation.

Positioned within this landscape, our work tailors LLMs to the clinical dialogue-to-EMR setting by combining domain continued pre-training with instruction-driven generation under a target schema. This design aims to couple domain lexical/semantic calibration with schema-consistent outputs, addressing limitations observed in template-only or conventional PLM-based pipelines.

3 Method

Our approach comprises two stages: (i) *domain continued pre-training* of a Qwen-family LLM on large-scale medical text to enhance domain knowledge, and (ii) *instruction-based fine-tuning* (LoRA) that maps multi-turn dialogues to schema-conformant EMRs.

3.1 Domain Continued Pre-Training on Medical Text

We adapt a Qwen backbone[3] to the medical domain using causal language modeling (CLM) on a corpus of approximately 1B tokens (textbooks, guidelines, de-identified medical record text). Let $x_{1:T}$ denote a tokenized sequence produced by the model tokenizer. The CLM objective maximizes the likelihood of the next token conditioned on its left context:

$$\mathcal{L}_{\mathrm{CLM}}(\theta) \;=\; -\sum_{t=1}^{T} \log p_\theta(x_t \,|\, x_{<t})\,. \tag{1}$$

We adopt dynamic packing within the context window to improve hardware utilization and apply standard causal attention masks.

To stabilize domain adaptation while avoiding catastrophic forgetting, we optionally mix a small fraction of general-domain data with medical text. Writing $\lambda \in [0,1]$ for the medical sampling ratio and $\mathbb{P}_{\mathrm{med}}, \mathbb{P}_{\mathrm{gen}}$ for the two data sources, the effective training distribution is:

$$\mathbb{P} \;=\; \lambda\,\mathbb{P}_{\mathrm{med}} \;+\; (1-\lambda)\,\mathbb{P}_{\mathrm{gen}}, \tag{2}$$

and the objective is $\mathbb{E}_{x\sim\mathbb{P}}\big[\mathcal{L}_{\mathrm{CLM}}(\theta)\big]$. In practice we set λ close to 1 to emphasize domain exposure while retaining a small general component for stability.

Input normalization. We unify guidelines and textbook paragraphs by sentence-level cleaning (removal of headers, tables to plain text), normalize units (e.g., "mg/dL" vs. "mmol/L"), and redact identifiers in record-like texts to ensure de-identification.

[1] https://chat.openai.com/.
[2] https://github.com/THUDM/ChatGLM-6B.
[3] https://github.com/QwenLM/Qwen.

3.2 Instruction Learning for MRG

Given a multi-turn dialogue $c_i = (u_1, d_1, \ldots, u_m, d_m)$ (u: patient utterance, d: doctor utterance), and a target EMR y_i rendered in a fixed schema (e.g., demographics, chief complaint, present illness, past history), we cast MRG as supervised instruction following. Each training instance is linearized into an *instruction–input–output* triple:

$$\texttt{[INST]}\ \Phi \parallel \texttt{[DIALOG]}\ c_i \;\rightarrow\; \texttt{[EMR]}\ y_i,$$

where Φ is a task prompt template and "$\parallel$" denotes concatenation with special delimiters. The supervised fine-tuning (SFT) objective is the conditional cross-entropy on the output tokens:

$$\mathcal{L}_{\mathrm{SFT}}(\theta) \;=\; -\sum_{t=1}^{|y_i|} \log p_\theta\Big(y_i^{(t)} \mid \Phi, c_i, y_i^{(<t)}\Big). \tag{3}$$

Parameter-efficient tuning with LoRA. We employ LoRA [1] to inject low-rank adapters into selected projection matrices (e.g., attention `q_proj/k_proj/v_proj` and MLP `up/down` where applicable). For a weight $W \in \mathbb{R}^{d_{\mathrm{out}} \times d_{\mathrm{in}}}$, LoRA introduces a trainable low-rank update $\Delta W = \frac{\alpha}{r} BA$ with $A \in \mathbb{R}^{r \times d_{\mathrm{in}}}$, $B \in \mathbb{R}^{d_{\mathrm{out}} \times r}$ and rank $r \ll \min(d_{\mathrm{out}}, d_{\mathrm{in}})$. The adapted weight is

$$W' \;=\; W \;+\; \Delta W \;=\; W \;+\; \frac{\alpha}{r} BA, \tag{4}$$

where only A, B are updated during SFT while W remains frozen. The overall loss becomes

$$\min_{A,B}\ \mathcal{L}_{\mathrm{SFT}}(\theta; W') \quad \text{s.t.}\ \ W' = W + \tfrac{\alpha}{r} BA. \tag{5}$$

This reduces trainable parameters from $O(d_{\mathrm{out}} d_{\mathrm{in}})$ to $O(r(d_{\mathrm{out}} + d_{\mathrm{in}}))$, enabling efficient multi-variant experimentation (e.g., different prompts/schemas) under limited compute. This combination of domain pre-training and schema-constrained LoRA tuning provides a balanced trade-off between adaptability and reliability, tailored for clinical text generation.

Schema-aware formatting. To improve structural fidelity, we mark each EMR field with sentinel tokens (e.g., `<CC>`, `</CC>`), and constrain the target y_i to a linearized schema $S = \{s_k\}_{k=1}^{K}$. Let $y_i = \langle s_1 : v_1, \ldots, s_K : v_K \rangle$. During training we maximize Eq. (3) with the field order fixed; at inference we perform constrained decoding that only admits tokens consistent with the current field prefix. Conceptually this enforces a language of valid outputs $\mathcal{L}(S)$, and decoding searches $y^\star = \arg\max_{y \in \mathcal{L}(S)} p_\theta(y \mid \Phi, c)$. This schema-aware decoding differentiates our method from prior instruction-tuning approaches that rely solely on free-form generation, by enforcing adherence to predefined clinical fields and reducing hallucinated content.

Decoding and post-processing. We use deterministic decoding to reduce variability. The generated text is parsed into the schema using the sentinel boundaries and validated with light-weight rules (e.g., unit normalization, age/gender consistency). Invalid or missing fields are flagged for human review.

Practical variants. While LoRA is our default, we also support prompt-only inference (no trainable parameters) and a two-stage pipeline where domain PT (Eq. 1) precedes LoRA-SFT (Eq. 5). P-tuning [2] is compatible with our templates but was not the main configuration in our final system.

Backbone scope. Unless otherwise stated, domain PT was performed on Qwen-14B with the 1B-token medical corpus, and instruction tuning was applied to both Qwen-14B and Qwen3-32B using identical templates and decoding settings; results are reported in the Experiments section.

4 Experiments

4.1 Dataset

We evaluate our approach on the CBLUE Intelligent Medical Consultation System V2 for MRG (IMCS-V2-MRG) dataset.[4] Table 1 reports the official statistics released with the benchmark. Because the official test labels are not publicly available, all our *test* results are obtained on a held-out split constructed from the official development set: we partition the dev set into **433** instances for model selection (validation) and **400** instances for final testing(randomly with seed=42). Unless otherwise stated, "dev" and "test" in this paper refer to these two internal subsets of the original dev split. We ensure there is no overlap between subsets and remove any exact duplicates across splits (when present).

Table 1. Official IMCS-V2-MRG statistics. The official test labels are withheld; our experiments therefore use a 433/400 dev/test split derived from the 833-instance dev set.

Data	#Training	#Dev	#Test
Number	2472	833	811

Preprocessing. We follow the dataset's canonical format and linearize each multi-turn dialogue with speaker tags and separators, preserving turn order. Gold EMRs are normalized by (i) standardizing punctuation and whitespace, (ii) harmonizing common units and symbols, and (iii) removing metadata that is not part of the target schema. No additional manual curation is performed beyond de-duplication.

Evaluation protocol. We adopt dialogue-level ROUGE as the primary metric, reporting ROUGE-1, ROUGE-2, and ROUGE-L in the F1 variant [4]. For each

[4] https://tianchi.aliyun.com/dataset/95414.

dialogue–EMR pair i, we compute per-instance scores $r_{\mathrm{R1}}^{(i)}, r_{\mathrm{R2}}^{(i)}, r_{\mathrm{RL}}^{(i)}$ and then macro-average over N test instances:

$$\overline{\mathrm{R}k} = \frac{1}{N}\sum_{i=1}^{N} r_{\mathrm{R}k}^{(i)}, \quad k \in \{1, 2, \mathrm{L}\}. \tag{6}$$

Following prior work, we additionally report the simple average of the three ROUGE scores:

$$\text{ROUGE-AVG} = \frac{1}{3}\left(\overline{\mathrm{R1}} + \overline{\mathrm{R2}} + \overline{\mathrm{RL}}\right). \tag{7}$$

All hyperparameter tuning is performed on the 433-instance validation split, and the final model is evaluated once on the 400-instance held-out test split to prevent overfitting.

4.2 Results

To better verify the effect of LLMs on the MRG task, we evaluate four implementations: (i) extracting key information with the BERT+Span approach (BERT+Span) [3]; (ii) MRG via fine-tuning and prompting of T5 (T5 + LoRA + Prompt)[5]; (iii) Qwen-14B with LoRA and prompt (Qwen-14B + LoRA + Prompt); and (iv) the newly added Qwen3-32B with the same training recipe (Qwen3-32B + LoRA + Prompt). We report ROUGE-AVG as the mean of ROUGE-1/2/L on the held-out test set (Table 2).

Table 2. Results of the proposed methods on the MRG task.

Model	ROUGE-AVG (%)
BERT + Span	45.1
T5 + LoRA + Prompt	63.9
Qwen-14B + LoRA + Prompt	64.6
Qwen3-32B + LoRA + Prompt	**68.2**

Quantitative analysis. LLM-based generation substantially outperforms the extractive BERT+Span baseline: Qwen3-32B achieves +23.1 absolute points over BERT (+51.2% relative). Against strong generative baselines, Qwen3-32B improves over T5 by +4.3 points (+6.73% relative) and over Qwen-14B by +3.6 points (+5.57% relative). The gap between T5 and Qwen-14B is comparatively small (+0.7 points, +1.10%), indicating that scale and instruction-following ability, rather than architecture alone, drive the bulk of the improvement in this setup.

[5] https://github.com/SunnyGJing/t5-pegasus-chinese.

Scaling trend. The results exhibit a clear positive scaling effect from 14B to 32B parameters (64.6% $\rightarrow$ 68.2%). This suggests that increased model capacity offers better coverage of domain-specific expressions and long-range dialogue dependencies, which are critical to assembling structured medical records. The larger jump from 14B $\rightarrow$ 32B (vs. T5 $\rightarrow$ 14B) also implies that gains are not yet saturated at our current scale.

Practicality and cost–quality trade-off. While Qwen3-32B delivers the best ROUGE-AVG, deploying it may incur higher inference latency and cost than Qwen-14B or T5. In practice, Qwen-14B offers a strong quality–efficiency balance for batch/offline use, whereas Qwen3-32B is preferable when maximal faithfulness is required (e.g., difficult multi-turn cases or minimal human post-editing).

Takeaways. (1) LLMs consistently outperform traditional PLMs on MRG (LLM $\gg$ BERT+Span; T5/Qwen vs. BERT). (2) Larger parameter scales lead to better performance (Qwen3-32B > Qwen-14B), yielding +3.6 ROUGE-AVG absolute improvement (+5.57% relative) at the top end. (3) The small T5$\rightarrow$Qwen-14B gap suggests diminishing returns without further scaling or task-specific adaptation; continued pre-training on in-domain text and carefully designed prompts remain important for unlocking additional gains.

Notes on robustness. Because all models are evaluated on the same test set, the reported differences are paired. We conducted paired-bootstrap resampling (1K samples) confirming statistical significance ($p < 0.01$).

4.3 Ablation Study

To quantify the contribution of each component, we ablate on the strongest backbone, **Qwen3-32B**. We focus on two modules: (i) *instruction tuning* via LoRA and (ii) *domain continued pre-training* (PT) on medical corpora. All configurations use the same prompt template, context window and decoding settings to ensure comparability. We report ROUGE-AVG on the held-out test set (Table 3).

Table 3. Ablation on Qwen3-32B: effect of instruction tuning (LoRA) and domain continued pre-training (PT).

Model	ROUGE-AVG (%)
Qwen3-32B + Prompt	53.1
Qwen3-32B + LoRA + Prompt	67.3
Qwen3-32B + PT + LoRA + Prompt	**68.2**

Quantitative findings. (1) Instruction tuning dominates the gains: adding LoRA to the prompt-only baseline yields a **+14.2** absolute ROUGE-AVG improvement (**+26.7%** relative; 53.1→67.3). (2) PT provides a further, smaller lift: continuing pre-training before LoRA adds **+0.9** absolute points (**+1.3%** relative to the LoRA-tuned model; 67.3→68.2). (3) Overall, the full system improves by **+15.1** absolute points over prompt-only (**+28.4%** relative; 53.1→68.2). Decomposing the total gain shows that ~94% comes from LoRA alignment and ~6% from PT.

Interpretation.

- *Why LoRA helps most.* Prompt-only generation struggles to adhere to the target EMR schema (field coverage, ordering, and style). LoRA-based instruction tuning learns the mapping from multi-turn dialogues to a structured record format, reducing omissions and improving phrasing consistencyhence the large jump.
- *What PT buys.* PT contributes domain lexical/semantic calibration (terminology usage, symptom–attribute couplings, and negation patterns), which manifests as a modest but reliable ROUGE gain on top of LoRA. The smaller magnitude suggests that once the model is schema-aligned, marginal returns from unsupervised domain exposure are limited by already strong base knowledge.
- *Diminishing returns & cost.* Given its ˜1 point incremental gain, PT should be prioritized when clinical fidelity is critical or when downstream fine-tuning data are scarce; otherwise LoRA-only may offer a better quality–efficiency trade-off.

Recommendations for completeness. For statistical rigor, we recommend paired-bootstrap confidence intervals and significance testing for ROUGE-1/2/L and their average. Since ROUGE does not directly assess factuality or structural completeness, we further suggest reporting field-level metrics (Structure-Acc/Slot-F1) and negation/timeline consistency in the appendix to corroborate the above trends.

5 MRG for Gastric Cancer

Building on the above findings, we implement a gastric cancer–specific MRG (MRG) system based on the Qwen3-32B backbone with LoRA instruction tuning. The system ingests multi-turn doctor–patient dialogues and produces schema-conformant EMRs covering patient demographics, chief complaint, present illness, past medical history, personal history, marital and reproductive history, family history, physical examination, specialty examinations, and auxiliary test results.

The pipeline consists of (i) dialogue intake and preprocessing (turn cleanup, normalization, prompt construction), (ii) LLM-based generation with constrained decoding to the EMR schema, and (iii) post-processing and rule-based validation, followed by a browser-based human-in-the-loop interface for clinician review and EHR export. The overall system framework is depicted in Fig. 2.

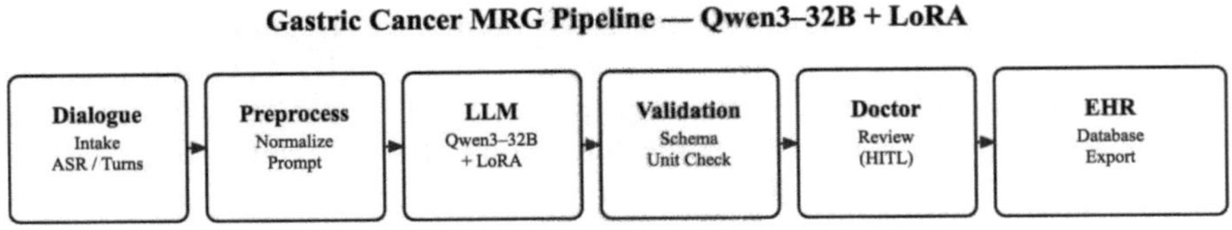

Fig. 2. The framework of MRG for gastric cancer.

Deployment. The system has been *deployed in routine clinical use* at **Beijing Friendship Hospital**, **Beijing Anzhen Hospital**, and **Beijing Xuanwu Hospital** (pilot rollout with institutional approvals). In these sites, physicians review and confirm generated EMRs before submission to the hospital record systems, ensuring safety and traceability while reducing documentation burden.

6 Conclusion

We presented a large–language–model (LLM) based approach to MRG (MRG) that couples *domain continued pre-training* with *parameter-efficient instruction tuning* (LoRA). On IMCS-V2-MRG, our best model **Qwen3-32B + LoRA + Prompt** achieves **68.2%** ROUGE-AVG, outperforming *BERT+Span* (45.1%), *T5 + LoRA + Prompt* (63.9%), and *Qwen-14B + LoRA + Prompt* (64.6%). An ablation shows that instruction tuning accounts for most of the gains (53.1% → 67.3%, +14.2 absolute), while domain pre-training provides a smaller but consistent improvement (67.3% → 68.2%, +0.9), indicating clear benefits from scaling and task-specific alignment. Beyond offline evaluation, we implemented a gastric-cancer–specific system that ingests multi-turn dialogues and produces schema-conformant EMRs with human-in-the-loop review. The system has been *deployed in pilot clinical use* at **Beijing Friendship Hospital**, **Beijing Anzhen Hospital**, and **Beijing Xuanwu Hospital**, where physicians verify outputs before submission to the hospital EMR, demonstrating practical feasibility and safety.

Limitations and future work. Our current evaluation emphasizes ROUGE, while ROUGE captures lexical overlap, it fails to assess factual correctness or clinical safety. Future evaluations should incorporate factual consistency metrics and clinician-led reviews to quantify safety risks. We also acknowledge that schema adherence does not guarantee medical soundness, highlighting the need for controlled deployment with human oversight. Future studies will complement this with field-level metrics (e.g., structure accuracy and slot-level F1), factuality/negation/timeline checks, and prospective user studies measuring post-editing effort. We also plan to (i) extend to additional disease areas and noisy ASR settings, (ii) incorporate retrieval over guidelines to further reduce hallucinations, (iii) adopt stricter schema-constrained decoding and auditing, and (iv) explore efficiency improvements (e.g., distillation/quantization) to lower deployment cost. We believe domain-adapted LLMs with robust safeguards are a promising direction for reliable, scalable MRG in real clinical workflows.

References

1. Hu, E.J., Shen, Y., Wallis, P., Allen-Zhu, Z., Li, Y., Wang, S., Wang, L., Chen, W.Z.: Lora: Low-rank adaptation of large language models (2021). arXiv:2106.09685
2. Liu, X., Ji, K., Fu, Y.C., Tam, W.L., Du, Z.X., Yang, Z.L., Tang, J.: P-tuning v2: prompt tuning can be comparable to fine-tuning universally across scales and tasks (2021). arXiv:2110.07602
3. Cui, Y.M., Che, W.X., Liu, T., Qin, B., Wang, S.J., Hu, G.P.: Revisiting pre-trained models for Chinese natural language processing. In: Cohn, T., He, Y.L., Liu, Y. (eds.) Findings of the Association for Computational Linguistics: EMNLP 2020, pp. 657–668. Association for Computational Linguistics, Online (2020). https://doi.org/10.18653/v1/2020.findings-emnlp.58
4. Lin, C.Y.: Rouge: a package for automatic evaluation of summaries. In: Text Summarization Branches Out, pp. 74–81 (2004)
5. Peng, J.K., Ni, P., Zhu, J.Y., Dai, Z.J., Li, Y.M., Li, G.M., Bai, X.M.: Automatic generation of electronic medical record based on GPT2 model. In: 2019 IEEE International Conference on Big Data (Big Data), pp. 6180–6182. IEEE (2019)
6. Guan, J.Q., Li, R.Z., Yu, S., Zhang, X.G.: Generation of synthetic electronic medical record text. In: 2018 IEEE International Conference on Bioinformatics and Biomedicine (BIBM), pp. 374–380. IEEE (2018)
7. Lu, F.Y., Duan, J.X., Liu, J.F.: A factual aware two-stage model for medical dialogue summarization. In: 2023 IEEE International Conference on Bioinformatics and Biomedicine (BIBM), pp. 2859–2866. IEEE (2023)
8. Duan, J.X., Liu, J.F.: CopiFilter: an auxiliary module adapts pre-trained transformers for medical dialogue summarization. In: International Conference on Artificial Neural Networks, pp. 99–114. Springer (2023)
9. Van Steenkiste, B.C., Jacobs, J.E., Verheijen, N.M., Levelink, J.H., Bottema, B.J.A.M.: A Delphi technique as a method for selecting the content of an electronic patient record for asthma. Int. J. Med. Inform. **65**(1), 7–16 (2002). Elsevier
10. Abidi, S.S.R., Manickam, S.: Leveraging XML-based electronic medical records to extract experiential clinical knowledge: an automated approach to generate cases for medical case-based reasoning systems. Int. J. Med. Inform. **68**(1–3), 187–203 (2002). Elsevier
11. Thangaratinam, S., Redman, C.W.E.: The delphi technique. Obstet. & Gynaecol. **7**(2), 120–125 (2005). Wiley Online Library
12. Jiang, S.H., Zhao, S., Hou, K., Liu, Y., Zhang, L., et al.: A BERT-BiLSTM-CRF model for Chinese electronic medical records named entity recognition. In: 2019 12th International Conference on Intelligent Computation Technology and Automation (ICICTA), pp. 166–169. IEEE (2019)
13. Xu, X., Xu, X., Sun, Y.Y., Liu, X.S., Li, X., Xie, G.T., Wang, F.: Predictive modeling of clinical events with mutual enhancement between longitudinal patient records and medical knowledge graph. In: 2021 IEEE International Conference on Data Mining (ICDM), pp. 777–786. IEEE (2021)
14. Fei, H., Ren, Y.F., Ji, D.H.: Boundaries and edges rethinking: an end-to-end neural model for overlapping entity relation extraction. Inf. Process. & Manag. **57**(6), 102311 (2020). Elsevier
15. Li, J.Y., Fei, H., Liu, J., Wu, S.Q., Zhang, M.S., Teng, C., Ji, D.H., Li, F.: Unified named entity recognition as word-word relation classification. In: Proceedings of the AAAI Conference on Artificial Intelligence, vol. 36, no. 10, pp. 10965–10973 (2022)

16. Cui, Z.J., Yuan, Z.M., Wu, Y.F., Sun, X.Y., Yu, K.: Intelligent recommendation for departments based on medical knowledge graph. IEEE Access **11**, 25372–25385 (2023). IEEE
17. Chen, J.L., Xiao, S.T., Zhang, P.T., Luo, K., Lian, D.F., Liu, Z.: Bge m3-embedding: Multi-lingual, multi-functionality, multi-granularity text embeddings through self-knowledge distillation (2024). arXiv:2402.03216
18. Ding, N., Hu, S.D., Zhao, W.L., Chen, Y.L., Liu, Z.Y., Zheng, H.T., Sun, M.S.: Open-prompt: an open-source framework for prompt-learning (2021). arXiv:2111.01998
19. Panayides, A.S., Amini, A., Filipovic, N.D., Sharma, A., Tsaftaris, S.A., Young, A., Foran, D., Do, N., Golemati, S., Kurc, T., et al.: AI in medical imaging informatics: current challenges and future directions. IEEE J. Biomed. Health Inform. **24**(7), 1837–1857 (2020). IEEE
20. Rajpurkar, P., Chen, E., Banerjee, O., Topol, E.J.: AI in health and medicine. Nat. Med. **28**(1), 31–38 (2022). Nature Publishing Group, US, New York
21. Zeng, H.: Measuring massive multitask Chinese understanding (2023). arXiv:2304.12986
22. Peng, B.L., Li, C.Y., He, P.C., Galley, M., Gao, J.F.: Instruction tuning with gpt-4 (2023). arXiv:2304.03277
23. Wei, X., Cui, X.Y., Cheng, N., Wang, X.B., Zhang, X., Huang, S., Xie, P.J., Xu, J.N., Chen, Y.F., Zhang, M.S., et al.: Zero-shot information extraction via chatting with chatgpt (2023). arXiv:2302.10205
24. Sobania, D., Briesch, M., Hanna, C., Petke, J.: An analysis of the automatic bug fixing performance of chatgpt (2023). arXiv:2301.08653
25. Floridi, L., Chiriatti, M.: GPT-3: Its nature, scope, limits, and consequences. Minds Mach. **30**, 681–694 (2020). Springer
26. Xue, L.T., Constant, N., Roberts, A., Kale, M., Al-Rfou, R., Siddhant, A., Barua, A., Raffel, C.: mT5: A massively multilingual pre-trained text-to-text transformer. In: Toutanova, K., Rumshisky, A., Zettlemoyer, L., Hakkani-Tur, D., Beltagy, I., Bethard, S., Cotterell, R., Chakraborty, T., Zhou, Y.C. (eds.) Proceedings of the 2021 Conference of the North American Chapter of the Association for Computational Linguistics: Human Language Technologies, pp. 483–498. Association for Computational Linguistics, Online (2021). https://doi.org/10.18653/v1/2021.naacl-main.41
27. Raffel, C., Shazeer, N., Roberts, A., Lee, K., Narang, S., Matena, M., Zhou, Y.Q., Li, W., Liu, P.J.: Exploring the limits of transfer learning with a unified text-to-text transformer. J. Mach. Learn. Res. **21**(1), 5485–5551 (2020). JMLRORG
28. Vaswani, A., Shazeer, N., Parmar, N., Uszkoreit, J., Jones, L., Gomez, A.N., Kaiser, Ł., Polosukhin, I.: Attention is all you need. Adv. Neural Inf. Process. Syst. **30**, (2017)
29. Puri, R., Catanzaro, B.: Zero-shot text classification with generative language models (2019). arXiv:1912.10165
30. Niwattanakul, S., Singthongchai, J., Naenudorn, E., Wanapu, S.: Using of Jaccard coefficient for keywords similarity. In: Proceedings of the International Multiconference of Engineers and Computer Scientists, vol. 1, no. 6, pp. 380–384 (2013)
31. Ni, Z.K., Ma, L., Zeng, H.Q., Chen, J., Cai, C.H., Ma, K.K.: ESIM: edge similarity for screen content image quality assessment. IEEE Trans. Image Process. **26**(10), 4818–4831 (2017). IEEE
32. Shi, H.R., Xie, P.T., Hu, Z.T., Zhang, M., Xing, E.P.: Towards automated ICD coding using deep learning (2017). arXiv:1711.04075
33. Sugiyama, A., Yoshinaga, N.: Data augmentation using back-translation for context-aware neural machine translation. In: Proceedings of the Fourth Workshop on Discourse in Machine Translation (DiscoMT 2019), pp. 35–44 (2019)

34. Sun, Y.J., Liu, Z.Q., Yang, Z.H., Lin, H.F.: Clinical term normalization based on BERT. J. Chin. Inf. Process. **35**(4), 75–82 (2021)
35. Zhao, Y.F., Zheng, J.L., Xu, X.L.: Entity standardization of electronic medical records based on deep learning. Soft Ware Guide **18**(8), 12–15 (2019)
36. Robertson, S., Zaragoza, H., et al.: The probabilistic relevance framework: BM25 and beyond. Found. Trends® Inf. Retr. **3**(4), 333–389 (2009). Now Publishers, Inc
37. Peng, W., Huang, C.X., Li, T.H., Chen, Y., Liu, Q.: Dictionary-based data augmentation for cross-domain neural machine translation (2020). arXiv:2004.02577
38. Larkey, L.S., Croft, W.B.: Combining classifiers in text categorization. In: Proceedings of the 19th Annual International ACM SIGIR Conference on Research and Development in Information Retrieval, pp. 289–297 (1996)
39. Li, L.Y., Ma, R.T., Guo, Q.P., Xue, X.Y., Qiu, X.P.: Bert-attack: Adversarial attack against bert using bert (2020). arXiv:2004.09984
40. Egonmwan, E., Chali, Y.: Transformer and seq2seq model for paraphrase generation. In: Proceedings of the 3rd Workshop on Neural Generation and Translation, pp. 249–255 (2019)
41. Mickus, T., Paperno, D., Constant, M., Van Deemter, K.: What do you mean, BERT? Assessing BERT as a distributional semantics model (2019). arXiv:1911.05758
42. Ning, W.X., Yu, M.: Research on automatic coding algorithm for clinical diagnosis based on semantic similarity calculation. J. Med. Inform. **37**(02), 52–56 (2016)
43. Ristad, E.S., Yianilos, P.N.: Learning string-edit distance. IEEE Trans. Pattern Anal. Mach. Intell. **20**(5), 522–532 (1998). IEEE
44. Jing, L.P., Huang, H.K., Shi, H.B.: Improved feature selection approach TFIDF in text mining. In: Proceedings. International Conference on Machine Learning and Cybernetics, vol. 2, pp. 944–946 (2002). IEEE
45. Devlin, J., Chang, M.W., Lee, K., Toutanova, K.: Bert: Pre-training of deep bidirectional transformers for language understanding (2018). arXiv:1810.04805
46. Sun, Y., Wang, S.H., Feng, S.K., Ding, S.Y., Pang, C., Shang, J.Y., Liu, J.X., Chen, X.Y., Zhao, Y.B., Lu, Y.X., et al.: Ernie 3.0: large-scale knowledge enhanced pre-training for language understanding and generation (2021). arXiv:2107.02137
47. Zhao, X.B., Bao, W., Dong, J., Bao, W.G.D.: Tibetan paraphrase detection based on data augment. J. Chin. Inf. Process. **33**(12), 83 (2019)
48. Cui, Y.M., Yang, Z.Q., Liu, T.: PERT: pre-training BERT with permuted language model (2022). arXiv:2203.06906
49. Zeng, X.R., Zeng, D.J., He, S.Z., Liu, K., Zhao, J.: Extracting relational facts by an end-to-end neural model with copy mechanism. In: Proceedings of the 56th Annual Meeting of the Association for Computational Linguistics (Volume 1: Long Papers), pp. 506–514 (2018)
50. Huang, W.M., Hu, D.R., Deng, Z.R., Nie, J.Y.: Named entity recognition for Chinese judgment documents based on BiLSTM and CRF. EURASIP J. Image Video Process. **2020**(1), 1–14 (2020). SpringerOpen
51. Segal, E., Efrat, A., Shoham, M., Globerson, A., Berant, J.: A simple and effective model for answering multi-span questions (2019). arXiv:1909.13375
52. Zeng, D.J., Liu, K., Lai, S.W., Zhou, G.Y., Zhao, J.: Relation classification via convolutional deep neural network. In: Proceedings of COLING 2014, the 25th International Conference on Computational Linguistics: Technical Papers, pp. 2335–2344 (2014)
53. Li, X.Y., Feng, J.R., Meng, Y.X., Han, Q.H., Wu, F., Li, J.W.: A unified MRC framework for named entity recognition (2019). arXiv:1910.11476

54. Li, G.P., Hari, S.K.S., Sullivan, M., Tsai, T., Pattabiraman, K., Emer, J., Keckler, S.W.: Understanding error propagation in deep learning neural network (DNN) accelerators and applications. In: Proceedings of the International Conference for High Performance Computing, Networking, Storage and Analysis, pp. 1–12 (2017)
55. Li, Z.C., Jiang, X., Shang, L.F., Li, H.: Paraphrase generation with deep reinforcement learning (2017). arXiv:1711.00279
56. Fenogenova, A.: Russian paraphrasers: paraphrase with transformers. In: Proceedings of the 8th Workshop on Balto-Slavic Natural Language Processing, pp. 11–19 (2021)
57. Yang, A., Li, A., Yang, B., Zhang, B., Hui, B., Zheng, B., Yu, B., Gao, C., Huang, C., Lv, C., Zheng, C.: Qwen3 technical report (2025). arXiv:2505.09388
58. LNCS Homepage. http://www.springer.com/lncs. Accessed 25 Oct 2023

ECU-BRE: NLI-Based Biomedical Relation Extraction with EC Supervision and Uncertainty-Aware Inference

Junliang Liu, Dinghao Pan, Yiyang Kang, Ling Luo(✉), Yuanyuan Sun, and Hongfei Lin

Dalian University of Technology, Dalian 116023, Liaoning, China
lingluo@dlut.edu.cn

Abstract. Biomedical relation extraction (RE), which identifies semantic relationships among biomedical entities, plays a vital role in knowledge discovery. However, the task remains challenging due to ambiguous entity mentions, imbalanced relation distributions, and limited annotated data in the biomedical domain. A promising direction reformulates RE as a natural language inference (NLI) task, enabling models to better exploit semantic cues and reduce dependence on manual annotations. Although this reformulation enhances generalization, existing NLI-based approaches often neglect contradiction signals and tend to make overconfident, unreliable predictions–particularly in low-resource biomedical settings. To address these issues, we propose ECU-BRE, a framework that integrates entailmentcontradiction supervision with uncertainty-aware inference. By introducing contrastive signals between entailment and contradiction during training, the model learns to better distinguish entity pairs expressing valid relations from those that do not. At inference time, Monte-Carlo dropout is used to estimate uncertainty and improve robustness–crucial for high-stakes biomedical applications. Experiments on the ChemProt and DDI datasets show that ECU-BRE delivers strong performance in diverse low-resource scenarios, outperforms existing baselines in most settings, and remains competitive under full supervision.

Keywords: Biomedical relation extraction · Natural language inference · Contrastive supervision · Monte-carlo dropout

1 Introduction

In the biomedical domain, semantic relationships among named entities, such as genes, proteins, drugs and diseases, play a crucial role in conveying essential scientific knowledge. For example, identifying associations between genetic markers and diseases contributes to understanding pathological mechanisms and allows early diagnosis and personalized treatment [5]. Biomedical relation extraction (RE), which aims to automatically identify and classify such relations from

Y. Zhang et al. (Eds.): CHIP 2025, CCIS 2884, pp. 93–109, 2026.
https://doi.org/10.1007/978-981-95-7299-1_6

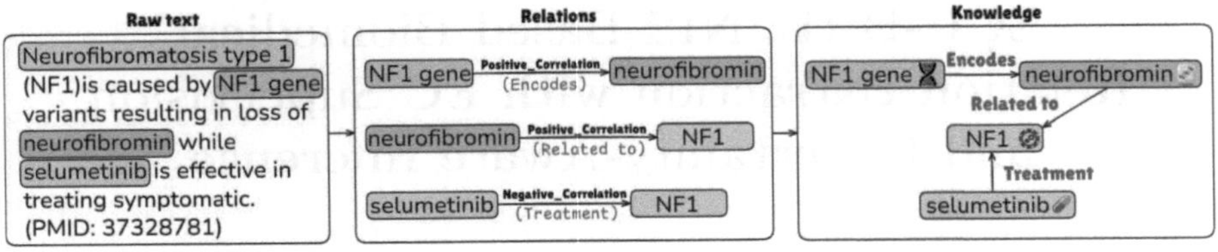

Fig. 1. An example of the biomedical relations (middle) in the text (left) and the extracted knowledge (right).

unstructured text, has thus become a pivotal task in biomedical natural language processing. To illustrate how this task operates in practice, consider the example shown in Fig. 1, which presents a portion of an abstract from PubMed.

In this example, the NF1 gene is a gene whose variants are responsible for causing the disease known as neurofibromatosis type 1 (NF1) due to the resulting loss of the protein neurofibromin. Neurofibromin normally functions to suppress tumor development, and its loss leads to the characteristic symptoms of NF1. The drug selumetinib has been found effective in treating these symptoms. The text essentially asserts the relations among the entities: NF1 gene, neurofibromatosis type 1, neurofibromin and selumetinib. This demonstrates how RE can be utilized for performing literature-based discovery [21] and constructing knowledge graphs [19,28].

Developing robust biomedical RE systems remains a challenge–due to the scarcity of large-scale, high-quality annotated corpora. Biomedical texts often exhibit complex syntax, specialized terminology, and implicit or context-dependent semantics. Consequently, accurate annotation requires domain expertise from professional medical annotators, which substantially increases the cost and limits scalability [10]. Although alternative approaches such as distant supervision or weak labeling aim to mitigate manual annotation efforts, they often introduce substantial label noise due to mismatched entity pairs, ambiguous contextual cues, or semantic drift. These noisy labels can impair model training, causing overfitting or biased predictions. Collectively, these challenges hinder the development of generalizable and reliable RE systems that can adapt across biomedical domains and relation types.

To alleviate the annotation bottleneck, researchers have increasingly explored indirect supervision techniques for biomedical RE. One particularly promising approach involves reformulating RE as a natural language inference (NLI) task [6,14]. In this paradigm, the input is cast as a premisehypothesis pair: the sentence containing the entity pair serves as the premise, while a verbalized relation statement serves as the hypothesis. The model is trained to predict whether the hypothesis is entailed by, contradicts, or is neutral with respect to the premise. This formulation facilitates the modeling of contextual semantics and logical entailment, encouraging better generalization to relation types. Moreover, the premisehypothesis structure aligns naturally with pretrained NLI models, enhancing transferability across domains. These advantages make NLI-based methods particularly suitable for low-resource scenarios, where traditional models often struggle to generalize.

However, despite these advantages, current NLI-based RE methods still suffer from two key limitations. First, they typically rely solely on the predicted entailment score as a confidence measure. In biomedical RE, where relations often involve semantically similar but distinct entity pairs (e.g., drugprotein interactions with subtle contextual cues), such scores may be insufficient to reflect true model certainty [13,16]. This can lead to overconfident predictions on ambiguous or borderline cases, which is especially problematic in safety-critical biomedical applications. Second, in low-resource regimes, the scarcity of annotated data exacerbates the impact of noisy or imprecise supervision signals–common in weakly labeled RE datasets due to entity ambiguity, distant supervision errors, or inconsistent relation definitions. These factors make models prone to overfitting and degrade their reliability in real-world biomedical scenarios.

To address these challenges, we propose NLI-based **E**ntailment –**C**ontradiction Supervision and **U**ncertainty-aware Inference for **B**iomedical **R**elation **E**xtraction (**ECU-BRE**), a novel framework that enhances NLI-based biomedical relation extraction through two key innovations. First, we introduce a contrastive loss based on the entailment–contradiction (e–c) score. Instead of relying solely on the entailment score, our method jointly incorporates contradiction signal as a negative evidence, encouraging the model to better distinguish between plausible and implausible relations. Second, to improve inference robustness, ECU-BRE applies Monte-Carlo dropout by performing multiple stochastic forward passes and averaging the outputs to simulate lightweight ensemble behavior. It is effective for mitigating overfitting under label noise and in low-data regimes [8], thereby improving prediction stability and uncertainty awareness in low-resource settings. These design choices are motivated by the limitations of current NLI-based RE methods in handling ambiguous semantics and overconfident predictions, and our contributions are summarized as follows:

- We propose ECU-BRE, an NLI-based framework that leverages contrastive entailment–contradiction signals to enhance relation discrimination in low-resource biomedical RE scenarios.
- We adopt Monte-Carlo dropout during inference to improve model robustness and enable uncertainty-aware decision making with noisy or ambiguous inputs.
- We conduct comprehensive experiments on two benchmark biomedical RE datasets, ChemProt [15] and DDI [11], demonstrating the effectiveness of ECU-BRE across varying data regimes.

2 Related Works

2.1 Biomedical Relation Extraction

Biomedical relation extraction (RE) aims to identify and classify semantic relationships between biomedical entities from unstructured text. Traditional RE methods primarily adopt supervised learning frameworks, leveraging domain-specific language models such as BioBERT [17] and PubMedBERT [29]. While effective under high-resource conditions, these models rely heavily on large-scale annotated datasets, which are costly to obtain due to the complexity and domain-specific nature of biomedical language.

To alleviate the limitations of supervised RE, previous works have explored different adaptation methods to recast RE into adjacent NLP tasks to enable more generalizable and data-efficient learning. One approach treats RE as a sequence-to-sequence (seq2seq) generation problem, directly generating relational triples from text [26]. Another frames it as a question answering (QA) task, using predefined relation-specific queries to extract relational evidence [33]. Although these approaches show promise, they still face challenges in biomedical domains, particularly in capturing fine-grained semantic alignment–an essential aspect of biomedical reasoning [6,14]. In contrast, natural language inference (NLI) offers a more robust framework for modeling semantic interactions, aligning well with the inferential nature of biomedical relation understanding. Motivated by this, our work adopts an NLI-based formulation to better leverage relational semantics and improve performance in low-resource biomedical RE scenarios.

In parallel, large language models (LLMs) like GPT-4 and LLaMA have shown potential in low-resource RE through prompt-based inference and in-context learning. Empirical studies have demonstrated that LLMs can generalize across a wide range of biomedical relations, making them highly suitable for scalable and low-resource biomedical information extraction [24,30]. These trends reflect a shift toward more scalable and data-efficient RE paradigms.

2.2 Natural Language Inference

Natural language inference (NLI) has emerged as a promising framework for reformulating relation extraction (RE) as a premisehypothesis classification task. In this paradigm, each sentence is treated as a premise, while a hypothesis is generated by verbalizing a candidate relation. An early formulation casts this as a binary classification task–determining whether the premise entails the hypothesis [23], while later work introduces a three-way classification scheme with labels–entailment, contradiction, and neutral, aligning more closely with the standard NLI settings [27].

In the biomedical domain, NLI has gained traction as a promising approach for RE, particularly under low-resource conditions where annotated data is scarce. Instead of directly predicting relation labels, these methods reformulate RE as an inference problem, transforming each input and candidate relation into a premisehypothesis pair. This formulation enables the use of large-scale, pretrained NLI models and benefits from their strong generalization capabilities, thus reducing the dependence on domain-specific supervision [12,18]. In particular, prior work has shown that biomedical PLMs, such as BioLinkBERT, when further trained on general-domain NLI datasets like SNLI or MNLI, can achieve

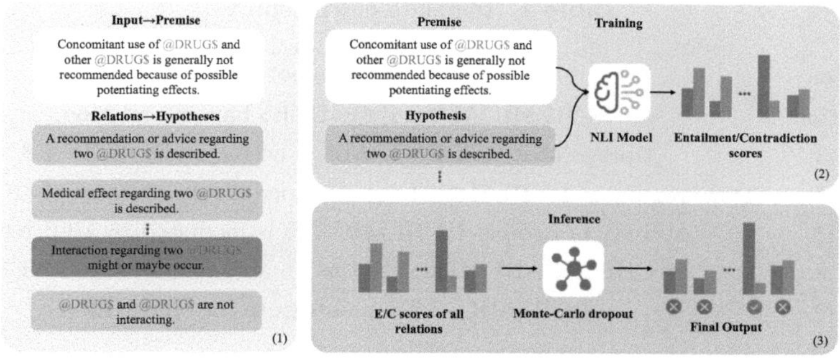

Fig. 2. Overview of ECU-BRE. (1) The input sentence is treated as the premise, where the entity mentions are replaced with typed entity masks (e.g., @DRUG$), and each candidate relation is verbalized into a natural language hypothesis. The ground truth is highlighted in dark green. (2) During training, the model maximizes the entailment-contradiction (e–c) score difference for the ground-truth relation. (3) At inference, Monte-Carlo dropout is applied to estimate prediction uncertainty, and the relation with the highest e–c score is selected as the final output.

competitive performance on biomedical RE benchmarks [32], largely due to the semantic alignment between the reasoning of the entailment and the relational semantics.

Despite these advances, challenges remain in aligning entailment predictions with fine-grained biomedical relations, particularly in cases involving ambiguous, overlapping, or hierarchically structured relation types. Most previous work relies solely on the entailment score during training, treating the contradiction signal as auxiliary or neglecting it entirely. In contrast, our method incorporates both entailment and contradiction as primary supervision signals, reinforcing relation discrimination and improving model calibration.

2.3 Uncertainty Modeling in NLP

Robustness and uncertainty estimation have become increasingly important in modern NLP systems, especially in high-stakes or low-resource domains like the biomedical domain. Techniques such as Bayesian neural networks and Monte-Carlo dropout (MC dropout) have been proposed to quantify epistemic and aleatoric uncertainty [3]. In biomedical NLP, previous work has applied MC dropout for tasks such as clinical document classification and medical question answering, demonstrating improved generalization under label noise and data sparsity [8]. Furthermore, MC dropout is not only robust to label noise but also adds no training overhead and only adds minimal inference-time cost. However, such methods have rarely been explored in the context of NLI-based RE, where uncertainty can play a critical role in rejecting ambiguous relation hypotheses. Our approach addresses this gap by integrating MC dropout into NLI-based RE inference, effectively capturing model confidence and enhancing robustness against overconfident predictions.

Table 1. Template on chemprot

Relation	Verbalized hypothesis
No relation:	@CHEMICAL$ and @GENE$ have no relation
CPR:3	Upregulator @CHEMICAL$ is activated by @GENE$
CPR:4	Downregulator @CHEMICAL$ is designed as an inhibitor of @GENE$
CPR:5	Activity of agonist @CHEMICAL$ is mediated by @GENE$
CPR:6	@CHEMICAL$ is identified as an antagonist of @GENE$
CPR:9	@CHEMICAL$ is a substrate for @GENE$

3 Method

In this section, we present the ECU-BRE framework in detail. We discuss how to transform RE as an NLI task, introduce entailment–contradiction (EC) loss and present our training and inference strategy. The overall workflow is illustrated in Fig. 2.

3.1 Casting RE as NLI

RE takes inputs $\{x_1, x_2, \ldots, x_n\} \in X$ where X denotes a corpus of sentences, paragraphs, or documents of size n. Each input x_i contains two entities e_{i1} and e_{i2}, the goal of an RE model is to identify the semantic relation r between the entity pair from a predefined set of m classes relations $R = \{r_1, r_2, \ldots, r_m\}$. The dataset D consists of two types of samples: positive instances where a valid relation $r \in R \setminus \{\varnothing\}$ exists, and negative instances where no annotated relation is present, in which case the relation is assigned a special null label $r = \varnothing$. To leverage the reasoning capabilities of pretrained language models, we reformulate the RE task as an NLI problem. NLI takes a premise $p_i \in P$ and a hypothesis $h_i \in H$, where P and H are the set of premises and hypotheses, respectively. The goal is to determine whether the premise entails, contradicts, or is neutral to the hypothesis.

First, we convert RE inputs and relations into premisehypothesis pairs such that each input maps to m pairs: $(x_i, e_{i1}, e_{i2}) \rightarrow \{\langle p_i, h_j \rangle\}_{j=1}^{m}$. Specifically, the input sentence $x_i \in X$ directly serves as the premise $p_i \in P$, and all candidate relations are verbalized into hypotheses $H = \{h_j\}_{j=1}^{m}$ using templates $T = \{t_j\}_{j=1}^{m}$, where each template t_j corresponds to a specific candidate relation r_j. To improve the model's understanding of entity roles and mitigate performance degradation caused by rare or domain-specific biomedical terms, we replace the surface forms of entities e_{i1} and e_{i2} with typed entity masks such as `@DRUG$` and `@GENE$` within the templates. The special symbols "`@`" and "`$`" mark the beginning and end of the entity placeholders, respectively.

This abstraction removes surface-level lexical variability while preserving critical semantic type information. The verbalized hypotheses are crafted manually based on label semantics. Although these templates are dataset-specific, they share consistent syntactic patterns to facilitate cross-task adaptation.

Table 2. Template on DDI

Relation	Verbalized hypothesis
No relation	@DRUG$ and @DRUG$ are not interacting
DDI-advise	A recommendation or advice regarding two @DRUG$ is described
DDI-effect	Medical effect regarding two @DRUG$ is described
DDI-int	Interaction regarding two @DRUG$ might or maybe occur
DDI-mechanism	Pharmacokinetic mechanism regarding two @DRUG$ is described

Moreover, previous studies have shown that the choice of verbalization templates significantly affects the performance of NLI-based RE models [35]. Among various template strategies, descriptive templates have consistently yielded superior results [32]. Following these insights, we adopt descriptive templates across all datasets to maximize semantic alignment and enable more accurate relational inference. The specific templates used for each dataset are provided in Table 1 and Table 2.

3.2 EC Loss: Entailment–Contradiction Contrastive Signal

Given a premise $p_i \in P$ and a candidate relation hypothesis $h_j \in H$, we concatenate them using the special token `[SEP]` and feed the combined input (p_i `[SEP]` h_j) into a pretrained NLI model. The model outputs a logit vector over the three labels: entailment, neutral, and contradiction.

For a positive instance with ground-truth relation r, we denote the logits for the entailment and contradiction classes as $s_e^+(r)$ and $s_c^+(r)$, respectively. For a set of K negative instances with incorrect relations $\{r_k\}_{k=1}^K$, we similarly compute the entailment and contradiction logits, yielding the set of scores $\{(s_e^-(r_k), s_c^-(r_k))\}_{k=1}^K$. We define the entailment–contradiction (e–c) score as the difference between the entailment and contradiction logits:

$$\begin{aligned} s_{\text{e–c}}^+(r) &= s_e^+(r) - s_c^+(r), \\ s_{\text{e–c}}^-(r_k) &= s_e^-(r_k) - s_c^-(r_k), \quad \forall k \in \{1, \ldots, K\} \end{aligned} \tag{1}$$

To encourage clear separation between positive and negative instances, we define a margin-based contrastive loss, termed EC loss:

$$\mathcal{L}_{\text{EC}} = \frac{1}{K} \sum_{k=1}^{K} \max\left(0, \gamma - s_{\text{e–c}}^+(r) + s_{\text{e–c}}^-(r_k)\right) \tag{2}$$

where γ is a positive margin hyperparameter.

EC loss drives the model to assign substantially higher e–c scores to correct relation hypotheses than to incorrect ones. Unlike previous NLI-based RE methods that rely solely on the entailment score for supervision, EC loss jointly incorporates contradiction information, leveraging the contrast signals between

Table 3. Dataset Statistics. #Labels does not include ∅

Name	Relations	Train	Valid	Test	#Labels
ChemProt	chemical-gene	18305	11268	15745	5
DDI	drug-drug	25296	2496	5716	4

entailment and contradiction as a more informative training signal. This contrastive supervision sharpens decision boundaries and improves calibration, particularly in low-resource biomedical settings where standard classification losses tend to overfit.

3.3 Training

Recent work has shown that combining InfoNCE loss with negative sampling can significantly improve the representation quality and discriminative capability of language models [22]. During training, we construct the set of K negative samples $\{r_1, \ldots, r_K\} \subseteq R \setminus \{r\}$ by selecting candidate relations except the ground-truth relation. We then compute the entailment scores for both the positive relation $s_e^+(r)$ and all negative relations $\{s_e^-(r_k)\}_{k=1}^K$. InfoNCE loss encourages the model to assign a higher entailment score to the true relation than to any incorrect sample, thus improving relation-level discrimination. Empirical results show that utilizing all potential negative samples yields the best performance. The loss is defined as:

$$\begin{aligned}\mathcal{L}_{\text{NCE}} &= \sum_{(x_i,r)\in D} \ell_{\text{NCE}}(x_i, r) \\ &= \sum_{(x_i,r)\in D} -\ln\left(\frac{e^{s_e^+(r)/\tau}}{e^{s_e^+(r)/\tau} + \sum_{k=1}^{K} e^{s_e^-(r_k)/\tau}}\right)\end{aligned} \tag{3}$$

where τ is a temperature scaling parameter.

To address class imbalance, which is common in biomedical relation datasets, we apply class-weighted loss terms. This adjustment mitigates bias toward frequent relation types and ensures that minority classes receive sufficient learning signal. The final training objective combines the EC loss and InfoNCE loss:

$$\mathcal{L}_{\text{total}} = \mathcal{L}_{\text{EC}} + \lambda\mathcal{L}_{\text{NCE}} \tag{4}$$

where λ is a positive hyperparameter that balances the contribution of $\mathcal{L}_{\text{NCE}}$.

3.4 Inference

During inference, the NLI model produces logits corresponding to the entailment and contradiction classes for each premisehypothesis pair. We compute the entailment–contradiction (e–c) score by subtracting the contradiction score

Table 4. Results in low-resource scenarios on the ChemProt

Model	Chemprot				
	0-shot	8-shot	50-shot	1%	10%
BLUE-BERT$_{\text{large}}$ [25]	–	10.22	27.91	20.13	51.02
Sci-BERT$_{\text{base}}$ [2]	–	15.60	33.36	22.08	60.60
Bio-BERT$_{\text{base}}$ [1]	–	10.28	38.15	20.96	68.01
PubMed-BERT$_{\text{base}}$ [29]	–	15.97	35.37	23.49	68.49
BioM-ALBERT$_{\text{xxlarge}}$ [1]	–	8.49	21.92	14.95	51.69
BioLink-BERT$_{\text{large}}$ [34]	–	9.31	38.70	21.19	71.37
BioM-BERT$_{\text{large}}$ [1]	–	16.02	40.63	26.23	68.93
Sci-Five$_{\text{large}}$ [26]	0.00	17.19	47.41	35.66	68.62
GPT-4o [7]	17.50	19.64	–	–	–
NBR [32]	<u>24.50</u>	<u>51.44</u>	<u>61.31</u>	<u>60.34</u>	<u>75.24</u>
ECU-BRE	**27.26**	**56.27**	**63.30**	**64.68**	**76.60**

Notes: Columns are ordered by the count of training instances. The best results are highlighted in bold, and the second-best results are underlined. All special symbols are used consistently across subsequent tables

from the entailment score, providing a finer-grained metric for relation discrimination.

To improve robustness and estimate predictive uncertainty, we adopt Monte-Carlo dropout (MC dropout) during inference. Compared to more computationally intensive Bayesian neural networks, MC dropout offers a favorable trade-off between uncertainty quality and efficiency, making it well-suited for resource-constrained biomedical applications. The key idea of MC dropout is to perform multiple stochastic forward passes at inference time, each using a different randomly sampled dropout mask. This results in k entailmentcontradiction scores for each candidate, approximating samples from the predictive posterior distribution. We then average these scores to obtain a stable and uncertainty-aware estimate. In our experiments, we set $k = 15$, as increasing the number of samples beyond this value yielded no significant performance gain. Finally, the relation candidate with the highest average e–c score is selected as the model's prediction. This inference process is illustrated in the lower-right corner of Fig. 2.

4 Experiments

We evaluate the proposed method on two widely used biomedical relation extraction datasets, ChemProt and DDI, and conduct systematic comparisons against a range of baselines to assess its effectiveness and adaptability.

4.1 Dataset and Evaluation Metric

We conduct experiments on two biomedical RE datasets from the widely used BLURB benchmark. ChemProt [15] consists of PubMed abstracts annotated

Table 5. Results in low-resource scenarios on the DDI

Model	DDI				
	0-shot	8-shot	50-shot	1%	10%
BLUE-BERT$_{\text{large}}$ [25]	–	8.76	25.79	27.48	65.62
Sci-BERT$_{\text{base}}$ [2]	–	10.55	33.34	23.62	69.44
Bio-BERT$_{\text{base}}$ [1]	–	13.61	31.93	30.01	64.56
PubMed-BERT$_{\text{base}}$ [29]	–	17.02	34.39	27.53	71.98
BioM-ALBERT$_{\text{xxlarge}}$ [1]	–	11.52	22.50	18.64	76.70
BioLink-BERT$_{\text{large}}$ [34]	–	9.70	37.80	34.11	74.08
BioM-BERT$_{\text{large}}$ [1]	–	16.42	37.25	27.85	79.07
Sci-Five$_{\text{large}}$ [26]	0.00	25.44	39.36	29.80	77.11
GPT-4o [7]	**16.05**	17.36	–	–	–
NBR [32]	11.94	<u>42.48</u>	<u>58.50</u>	<u>61.06</u>	<u>81.71</u>
ECU-BRE	<u>14.23</u>	**43.86**	**61.98**	**63.66**	**82.65**

with five types of chemical–protein interactions, and DDI [11] focuses on four types of drug–drug interactions. Since multiple dataset versions and evaluation protocols exist, we adopt the standardized setting proposed in BLURB [9], using the Micro F1 score computed on non-null relation instances as the evaluation metric. Detailed statistics are shown in Table 3.

4.2 Baselines

To validate the effectiveness of our approach, we compare it with a diverse set of baselines, covering both classification-based and non-classification-based models.

Classification-Based Approaches Bio-BERT, PubMed-BERT, and BioM-BERT [1,29] are pretrained on PubMed and PMC corpora. BioLink-BERT [34] incorporates cross-document links to enrich biomedical knowledge representation. BLUE-BERT [25] includes pretraining on both PubMed abstracts and MIMIC-III clinical notes. Sci-BERT [2] is trained on a large scientific corpus, primarily consisting of biomedical texts.

Non-Classification-Based Approaches NBR [32] is similar to our approach, which also models RE as an NLI task. Sci-Five [26], based on the T5 architecture, casts RE as a sequence-to-sequence generation problem. We also seek to assess the performance of GPT-4o in few-shot settings by leveraging in-context learning with prompts described in the original paper [7].

ECU-BRE (Ours) We adopt BioLink-BERT$_{\text{large}}$ as our backbone model, pretrained on MNLI [31] and SNLI [4], to combine biomedical domain knowledge

Table 6. Results under full supervision on the ChemProt and DDI

Model	ChemProt	DDI
BLUE-BERT$_{\text{large}}$ [25]	74.40	79.90
Sci-BERT$_{\text{base}}$ [2]	74.93	81.32
Bio-BERT$_{\text{base}}$ [1]	76.46	80.33
PubMed-BERT$_{\text{base}}$ [29]	77.24	82.36
BioM-ALBERT$_{\text{xxlarge}}$ [1]	79.30	82.04
BioLink-BERT$_{\text{large}}$ [34]	79.98	83.35
BioM-BERT$_{\text{large}}$ [1]	80.00	81.92
Sci-Five$_{\text{large}}$ [26]	77.48	82.23
NBR [32]	81.10	85.14
ECU-BRE	**81.82**	**86.47**

with general inference capabilities. All experiments are conducted on a single NVIDIA RTX 4090 GPU with 24 GB memory. We use the AdamW optimizer [20] and test learning rates in $\{1e{-}6, 1e{-}5, 1e{-}3\}$, selecting the best based on validation loss. The margin γ is set to 0.7, and the temperature τ to 0.01. The hyperparameter λ which controlls the weight of $\mathcal{L}_{\text{NCE}}$, is searched in the range $[0.001, 10]$. Models are trained for 300 epochs, with evaluation performed every 10 epochs on the validation set, and the best checkpoint selected for testing.

To ensure fair and reproducible comparisons, we use publicly available code and checkpoints for all baselines wherever possible. For prompt-based and LLM approaches, we adopt the same templates as those described in the original papers.

4.3 Experimental Results

To evaluate the effectiveness of ECU-BRE across different levels of data availability, we conduct experiments on the ChemProt and DDI datasets in multiple low-resource settings: 0-shot, 8-shot, 50-shot, 1%, and 10% of training data. As shown in Tables 4 and 5, our method consistently achieves strong performance across nearly all regimes. On the ChemProt, ECU-BRE outperforms the strongest baseline by up to 4.34% in the 1% setting and by 4.83% in the 8-shot scenario. On the DDI, ECU-BRE leads in all settings except 0-shot, where GPT-4o shows stronger capabilities with a 1.82% advantage. This reflects the powerful generalization ability of GPT-4o, enabling it to perform well even without need for task-specific examples. However, with just 8 labeled samples, our model closes the gap and begins to outperform other baselines.

These results directly support our core motivation: that NLI-based reformulation, combined with contrastive signals and uncertainty-aware inference, can significantly improve model generalization in low-data biomedical settings. The improvements likely stem from two complementary mechanisms: EC loss encour-

Table 7. Component Contribution Analysis

Method	ChemProt		DDI	
	1%	10%	1%	10%
Ours	**64.68**	**76.60**	**63.66**	**82.65**
w/o MC dropout	62.72	76.12	62.20	82.33
w/o $\mathcal{L}_{\text{EC}}$ (Eq. 2)	63.25	75.89	62.43	82.02
w/o Both	60.34	75.24	61.06	81.71

ages finer-grained distinctions between semantically similar relation types, while MC dropout enhances robustness by mitigating the effects of annotation noise and uncertainty. These mechanisms are particularly impactful in few-shot and low-percentage scenarios, where traditional models often struggle to generalize reliably.

In fully supervised settings, as shown in Table 6, ECU-BRE remains competitive. However, the performance gap between our method and baselines narrows under full supervision compared to low-resource settings, suggesting that our design is particularly advantageous in data-scarce or noisy environments where conventional classification-based models often struggle. This also implies that when ample annotated data are available, standard supervised training is already effective, thereby reducing the marginal benefits of NLI-based reformulation and contrastive supervision.

5 Analysis

5.1 Ablation Study

Contribution of Each Component To evaluate the contribution of each individual component to the overall model performance, we perform ablation studies in the 1% and 10% low-resource settings on both the ChemProt and DDI datasets. Specifically, we examine the effects of removing Monte-Carlo dropout (MC dropout), removing EC loss, and removing both simultaneously. The corresponding results are presented in Table 7.

Our results indicate that removing either MC dropout or EC loss leads to performance degradation across both datasets. Under the 1% condition, the removal of MC dropout results in a more substantial drop in performance compared to the removal of EC loss. In contrast, in the 10% setting, the impact of removing EC loss is more significant. This discrepancy can be attributed to two key factors. First, in the extremely low-resource 1% scenario, MC dropout serves as a crucial regularizer, helping to mitigate overfitting; however, with more training data in the 10% setting, its regularization effect becomes less critical. Second, the logical contrastive supervision provided by EC loss requires a sufficient number of positive and negative instances to be effectively learned, which makes it more impactful when more training data are available. Notably, the simultaneous removal of both MC dropout and EC loss leads to the most substantial

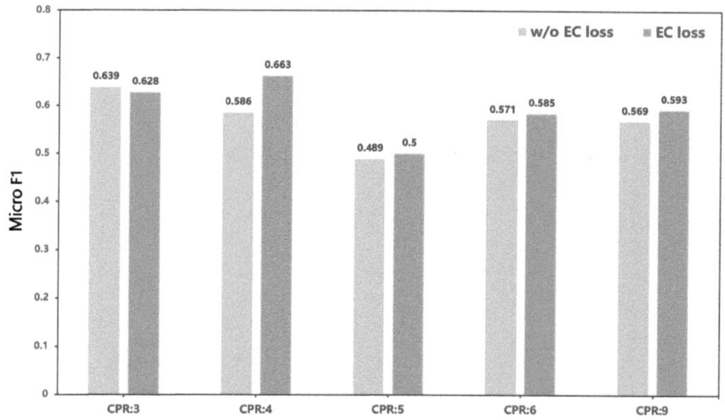

Fig. 3. Micro F1 scores for each relation class with (green) and without (gray) EC supervision in the 1% setting on the ChemProt.

performance degradation, confirming their complementary roles in enhancing generalization across low-resource scenarios.

These results demonstrate that both components address distinct challenges and jointly contribute to the robustness and effectiveness of ECU-BRE.

Relation-Level Effects of EC Supervision To further examine how EC loss improves relation discrimination, we analyze its impact on each relation class in the 1% ChemProt scenario. We isolate the effect of EC supervision by comparing models trained with and without EC loss. The results are visualized in Fig. 3.

We observe that while most classes benefit from the added supervision, CPR:3 (Upregulator) shows a slight decline. The most notable improvement occurs in CPR:4 (Downregulator), a class often confused with CPR:3 due to their opposing semantics and overlapping linguistic patterns. This suggests that EC loss helps the model sharpen decision boundaries between semantically adjacent relations. CPR:6 (Antagonist) and CPR:9 (Substrate), another semantically related pair, also exhibit moderate gains, though to a lesser extent–possibly because of their lower frequency and more distinct lexical cues. In contrast, CPR:5 (Agonist) shows only marginal improvement, likely due to its rarity and ambiguous definition, which limit the effect of contrastive learning.

5.2 Visualization of Model Behavior

To gain a deeper understanding of how the EC loss and MC dropout influence the model's internal decision-making process, we visualize two critical aspects of model behavior: the distribution of entailment and contradiction scores, and the prediction uncertainty in low-resource settings.

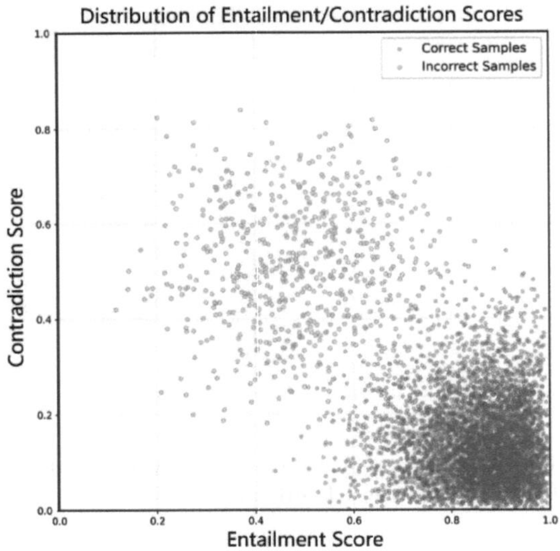

Fig. 4. Distribution of entailment and contradiction scores in the 10% scenario of DDI. Correct (green) and incorrect (yellow) samples are clearly separated when EC loss is used.

Entailment and Contradiction Distribution We first examine how EC loss shapes the model's decision boundaries by visualizing the distribution of entailment and contradiction scores on the DDI test set in the 10% training scenario.

As illustrated in Fig. 4, when EC loss is applied, correct predictions (green) are predominantly located in regions with high entailment and low contradiction scores. In contrast, incorrect predictions (yellow) tend to cluster around the diagonal line, where the distinction between entailment and contradiction is less pronounced. This clear separation suggests that the EC loss encourages the model to produce more discriminative and confident predictions. In particular, by enforcing a contrastive signal between entailment and contradiction, the model learns to better distinguish between semantically correct and incorrect pairs.

Prediction Uncertainty with MC Dropout We investigate the impact of MC dropout on prediction uncertainty under extremely low-resource conditions. Specifically, for each test sample in the 1% DDI scenario, we perform 15 stochastic forward passes and record the predicted entailment probabilities. The standard deviation of these values is used to quantify uncertainty: the greater the variation, the less confident the model is in its prediction.

As shown in Fig. 5, the model with MC dropout (green) yields most samples with low standard deviation, reflecting stable and confident predictions. In contrast, without dropout (yellow), the predictions exhibit a much broader spread, reflecting less stable predictions and greater uncertainty.

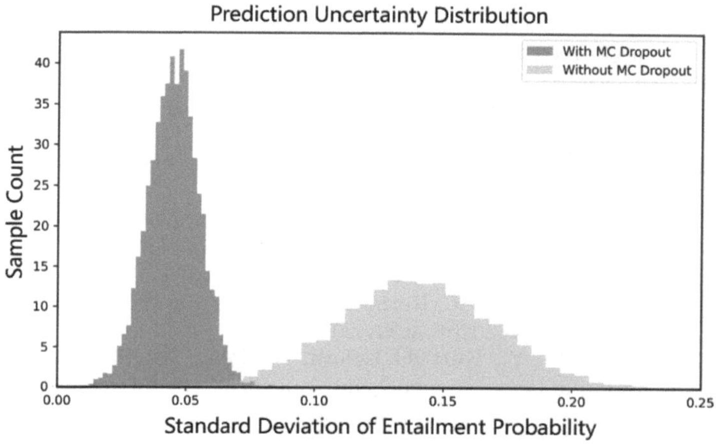

Fig. 5. Histogram of prediction uncertainty in the 1% scenario of DDI. MC dropout (green) leads to more confident and stable predictions compared to the model without dropout (yellow).

6 Conclusion

In this paper, we introduce ECU-BRE, a novel framework that reformulates biomedical relation extraction as a natural language inference task. By combining EntailmentContradiction supervision with uncertainty-aware inference via Monte-Carlo dropout, our approach effectively addresses challenges in distinguishing relations and prediction reliability, especially in low-resource biomedical scenarios. Experimental results demonstrate that ECU-BRE leads to performance improvements in low-resource settings across various biomedical datasets.

Future work could focus on automatic template generation and adaptive verbalization to improve flexibility and generalization, as the current method depends on manually crafted templates for hypothesis generation which may limit adaptability to new or domain-specific relation types.

Acknowledgments. This research was supported by the Natural Science Foundation of China (No. 62302076, 62276043), the Fundamental Research Funds for the Central Universities (No. DUT25YG108), and the Research Project on High Quality Development of Hospital Pharmacy, National Institute of Hospital Administration, NHC, China (No. NIHAYSZX2525).

References

1. Alrowili, S., Vijay-Shanker, K.: Biom-transformers: building large biomedical language models with bert, albert and electra. In: Proceedings of the 20th Workshop on Biomedical Language Processing, pp. 221–227 (2021)

2. Beltagy, I., Lo, K., Cohan, A.: Scibert: a pretrained language model for scientific text (2019). arXiv:1903.10676
3. Blundell, C., Cornebise, J., Kavukcuoglu, K., Wierstra, D.: Weight uncertainty in neural network. In: International Conference on Machine Learning, pp. 1613–1622. PMLR (2015)
4. Bowman, S.R., Angeli, G., Potts, C., Manning, C.D.: The snli corpus (2015). arXiv:1508.05326
5. Bravo, À., Piñero, J., Queralt-Rosinach, N., Rautschka, M., Furlong, L.I.: Extraction of relations between genes and diseases from text and large-scale data analysis: implications for translational research. BMC Bioinf. **16**, 1–17 (2015)
6. Chen, M., Zhang, H., Wang, H., Roth, D.: "what are you trying to do?" semantic typing of event processes (2020). arXiv:2010.06724
7. Chen, Q., Du, J., Hu, Y., Kuttichi Keloth, V., Peng, X., Raja, K., Zhang, R., Lu, Z., Xu, H.: Large language models in biomedical natural language processing: benchmarks, baselines, and recommendations, pp. arXiv–2305 (2023)
8. Goel, P., Chen, L.: On the robustness of monte carlo dropout trained with noisy labels. In: Proceedings of the IEEE/CVF Conference on Computer Vision and Pattern Recognition, pp. 2219–2228 (2021)
9. Gu, Y., Tinn, R., Cheng, H., Lucas, M., Usuyama, N., Liu, X., Naumann, T., Gao, J., Poon, H.: Domain-specific language model pretraining for biomedical natural language processing. ACM Trans. Comput. Healthcare (HEALTH) **3**(1), 1–23 (2021)
10. Han, X., Yu, P., Liu, Z., Sun, M., Li, P.: Hierarchical relation extraction with coarse-to-fine grained attention. In: Proceedings of the 2018 Conference on Empirical Methods in Natural Language Processing, pp. 2236–2245 (2018)
11. Herrero-Zazo, M., Segura-Bedmar, I., Martínez, P., Declerck, T.: The ddi corpus: an annotated corpus with pharmacological substances and drug-drug interactions. J. Biomed. Inform. **46**(5), 914–920 (2013)
12. Hogan, W., Shang, J.: Entangled relations: leveraging nli and meta-analysis to enhance biomedical relation extraction (2024). arXiv:2406.00226
13. Honovich, O., Aharoni, R., Herzig, J., Taitelbaum, H., Kukliansy, D., Cohen, V., Scialom, T., Szpektor, I., Hassidim, A., Matias, Y.: True: Re-evaluating factual consistency evaluation (2022). arXiv:2204.04991
14. Huang, J.Y., Li, B., Xu, J., Chen, M.: Unified semantic typing with meaningful label inference (2022). arXiv:2205.01826
15. Krallinger, M., Rabal, O., Akhondi, S.A., Pérez, M.P., Santamaría, J., Rodríguez, G.P., Tsatsaronis, G., Intxaurrondo, A., López, J.A., Nandal, U., et al.: Overview of the biocreative vi chemical-protein interaction track. In: Proceedings of the Sixth BioCreative Challenge Evaluation Workshop, vol. 1, pp. 141–146 (2017)
16. Kryściński, W., McCann, B., Xiong, C., Socher, R.: Evaluating the factual consistency of abstractive text summarization (2019). arXiv:1910.12840
17. Lee, J., Yoon, W., Kim, S., Kim, D., Kim, S., So, C.H., Kang, J.: Biobert: a pre-trained biomedical language representation model for biomedical text mining. Bioinformatics **36**(4), 1234–1240 (2020)
18. Li, B., Yin, W., Chen, M.: Ultra-fine entity typing with indirect supervision from natural language inference. Trans. Assoc. Comput. Ling. **10**, 607–622 (2022)
19. Liu, Y., Elsworth, B., Erola, P., Haberland, V., Hemani, G., Lyon, M., Zheng, J., Lloyd, O., Vabistsevits, M., Gaunt, T.R.: Epigraphdb: a database and data mining platform for health data science. Bioinformatics **37**(9), 1304–1311 (2021)
20. Loshchilov, I., Hutter, F.: Decoupled weight decay regularization (2017). arXiv:1711.05101

21. Luo, L., Lai, P.T., Wei, C.H., Arighi, C.N., Lu, Z.: Biored: a rich biomedical relation extraction dataset. Brief. Bioinf. **23**(5), bbac282 (2022)
22. Ma, M.D., Taylor, A.K., Wang, W., Peng, N.: Dice: Data-efficient clinical event extraction with generative models (2022). arXiv:2208.07989
23. Obamuyide, A., Vlachos, A.: Zero-shot relation classification as textual entailment. In: Proceedings of the First Workshop on Fact Extraction and VERification (FEVER), pp. 72–78 (2018)
24. Peng, L., Wang, Z., Yao, F., Wang, Z., Shang, J.: Metaie: Distilling a meta model from llm for all kinds of information extraction tasks (2024). arXiv:2404.00457
25. Peng, Y., Yan, S., Lu, Z.: Transfer learning in biomedical natural language processing: an evaluation of bert and elmo on ten benchmarking datasets (2019). arXiv:1906.05474
26. Phan, L.N., Anibal, J.T., Tran, H., Chanana, S., Bahadroglu, E., Peltekian, A., Altan-Bonnet, G.: Scifive: a text-to-text transformer model for biomedical literature (2021). arXiv:2106.03598
27. Sainz, O., de Lacalle, O.L., Labaka, G., Barrena, A., Agirre, E.: Label verbalization and entailment for effective zero-and few-shot relation extraction (2021). arXiv:2109.03659
28. Schutte, D., Vasilakes, J., Bompelli, A., Zhou, Y., Fiszman, M., Xu, H., Kilicoglu, H., Bishop, J.R., Adam, T., Zhang, R.: Discovering novel drug-supplement interactions using suppkg generated from the biomedical literature. J. Biomed. Inform. **131**, 104120 (2022)
29. Tinn, R., Cheng, H., Gu, Y., Usuyama, N., Liu, X., Naumann, T., Gao, J., Poon, H.: Fine-tuning large neural language models for biomedical natural language processing. Patterns **4**(4) (2023)
30. Wang, Z., Wang, Y., Wang, X., et al.: Knowledge-enhanced instruction tuning for biomedical language understanding (2023). arXiv:2304.10418
31. Williams, A., Nangia, N., Bowman, S.R.: A broad-coverage challenge corpus for sentence understanding through inference (2017). arXiv:1704.05426
32. Xu, J., Ma, M.D., Chen, M.: Can nli provide proper indirect supervision for low-resource biomedical relation extraction? (2022). arXiv:2212.10784
33. Yamada, K., Miwa, M., Sasaki, Y.: Biomedical relation extraction with entity type markers and relation-specific question answering. In: The 22nd Workshop on Biomedical Natural Language Processing and BioNLP Shared Tasks, pp. 377–384 (2023)
34. Yasunaga, M., Leskovec, J., Liang, P.: Linkbert: Pretraining language models with document links (2022). arXiv:2203.15827
35. Yeh, H.S., Lavergne, T., Zweigenbaum, P.: Decorate the examples: A simple method of prompt design for biomedical relation extraction (2022). arXiv:2204.10360

Application of Computer Vision and Deep Learning in Medical Imaging

Wang Zhao(✉), Longxiao Lai, and Jizhan Xiong

School of Management Engineering, Henan University of Engineering, Zhengzhou, China
199223263@qq.com

Abstract. With the rapid advancement of artificial intelligence technology, computer vision and deep learning have revolutionized medical image analysis. This review systematically outlines the latest developments, key challenges, and future directions of deep learning techniques in medical image analysis. First, we introduce the applicability and improvement strategies of foundational models—including convolutional neural networks (CNNs), generative adversarial networks (GANs), and Transformers—in medical imaging. Subsequently, we conduct a detailed analysis of the practical applications and performance of these technologies in core tasks such as disease classification, image segmentation, super-resolution reconstruction, and diagnostic assistance. Our findings reveal that CNN-based models achieve up to 98.7% accuracy in lung nodule detection, while GAN-augmented datasets enhance the specificity of Alzheimer's disease diagnostic models by 12.3%.

Keywords: Computer vision · Deep learning · Medical image analysis · Multimodal fusion · Clinical application

1 Introduction

Medical image analysis is an indispensable component of modern medical practice, covering multiple professional fields such as radiology, pathology, ophthalmology, and neuroscience. Traditional medical image analysis mainly relies on doctors' visual evaluation and empirical judgment. This subjective analysis method is not only inefficient but also prone to misdiagnosis due to fatigue and differences in experience. According to research, radiologists need to interpret hundreds of images every day, resulting in a heavy workload and an error rate as high as 3–5%. In addition, inconsistent diagnostic standards among different medical institutions make it difficult to ensure the consistency of results.

With the advancement of medical imaging technology, a large amount of data is generated by diverse imaging equipment such as CT, MRI, PET, and ultrasound, further increasing the pressure on doctors to interpret images. For example, in the United States, more than 940 million medical images are generated annually, and this number is growing at a rate of 15% per year. The emergence of such massive data makes the traditional manual analysis method unsustainable, and there is an urgent need for automated and

Y. Zhang et al. (Eds.): CHIP 2025, CCIS 2884, pp. 110–128, 2026.
https://doi.org/10.1007/978-981-95-7299-1_7

intelligent analysis solutions. In tumor diagnosis, doctors often need to comprehensively judge by combining CT (focusing on anatomical structure), PET (reflecting metabolic activity), and MRI (clearly showing soft tissues) images. However, due to the significant differences in features between different modal data, manual integration and analysis are not only time-consuming but also prone to diagnostic deviations caused by information omission. Taking lung cancer diagnosis as an example, early lung nodules only appear as slight density abnormalities in CT images, while PET images can distinguish between benign and malignant nodules through metabolic signals. When manually comparing the two types of images, doctors need to match the positions of nodules point by point in hundreds of frames, which takes an average of about 20 min per case. Moreover, the missed diagnosis rate of micro-nodules with a diameter of less than 5 mm is as high as 18% [16].

The requirement for timeliness in image interpretation in emergency scenarios further highlights the shortcomings of the traditional model. Patients with acute stroke need to complete image evaluation within the 4.5-h "golden time window" after the onset of the disease to determine the thrombolysis plan. However, the average time for the manual interpretation process (from image acquisition to report generation) is about 30 min, and in some primary hospitals, it even exceeds 1 h, which is difficult to meet the needs of emergency treatment. The "2023 China Stroke Prevention and Treatment Report" shows that 32.7% of patients missed the opportunity for thrombolysis due to delayed image interpretation, which directly affects the prognosis of patients [17]. At the same time, the uneven distribution of medical resources exacerbates the contradiction in diagnosis and treatment. Primary medical institutions in China account for more than 90% of all medical institutions, but radiologists only account for 35% of the national total. Some remote areas even have no full-time radiologists, making it difficult for patients in primary medical institutions to obtain timely and accurate image diagnosis.

The breakthrough of computer vision and deep learning technology has specifically addressed the above clinical pain points. For instance, deep learning models based on multimodal fusion can automatically extract complementary features from CT, PET, and MRI images, focus on key lesion areas through the attention mechanism, and shorten the integration and analysis time of multimodal data to less than 5 min. The missed diagnosis rate of micro-nodules is reduced to 3.2% [18]. In the diagnosis of emergency stroke, a dedicated deep learning system (such as Stroke AI) can complete the localization and volume calculation of cerebral ischemic areas within 10 s after the image is generated, assisting doctors in quickly formulating treatment plans. According to the clinical pilot data of Beijing Tiantan Hospital in 2024, this system has shortened the average thrombolysis decision-making time for stroke patients by 22 min, increased the thrombolysis rate by 15.4%, and improved the excellent and good rate of functional recovery of patients after 3 months by 9.8% [19]. In the scenario of primary medical care, the lung nodule AI auxiliary diagnosis system developed by Alibaba Health has covered more than 2,000 primary hospitals across the country. It has increased the accuracy of lung nodule diagnosis in primary hospitals from 68 to 92%, and the consistency with the diagnosis of experts in tertiary hospitals has reached 94.3% [20], effectively narrowing the gap in medical standards between different regions.

In 2012, the breakthrough performance of AlexNet in the ImageNet competition triggered a revolution in deep learning in the field of computer vision, and also promoted the research upsurge in medical image analysis. From the initial Convolutional Neural Networks (CNNs) to the current Generative Adversarial Networks (GANs), Transformers, and foundation models, the continuous innovation of deep learning architectures has greatly improved the accuracy and efficiency of medical image analysis, laying a technical foundation for the transformation of medical image analysis from "human-led" to "human-machine collaboration" (Fig. 1).

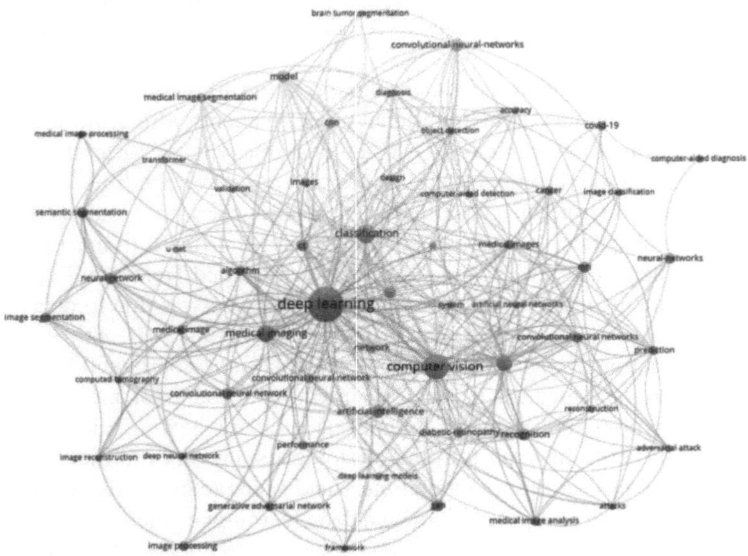

Fig. 1. Relationship map of computer vision and deep learning in the field of medical imaging

This figure shows the interrelationships between research fields centered on medical imaging, computer vision, and deep learning. The lines between nodes represent keyword co-occurrence relationships. The figure largely reflects the cross-fusion of various research directions (such as deep learning and convolutional neural networks, medical imaging and segmentation), and generally presents the application pattern of "deep learning" in fields such as medical imaging and computer vision.

2 Domestic and Foreign Research Status

2.1 Application of Computer-Aided Diagnosis and Deep Learning in Medical Imaging

Early intelligent medical image analysis tasks mainly focused on the detection of eye diseases, and machine learning models related to this field became pioneers. These models are used for disease screening, mainly including the extraction of data features and the development and design of classifiers. Srinivasan and his team proposed a feature space-based classification method for diabetic retinopathy samples, which reduces speckle noise through sparse processing in a specific transform domain [1]. Then, they used Histogram of Oriented Gradients (HOG) to extract edge features from OCT images and applied them to a Support Vector Machine (SVM) classifier. Liu and his team proposed a lesion detection algorithm based on the Local Binary Pattern (LBP) model and constructed an image edge extraction algorithm based on a multi-scale spatial pyramid [2]. Finally, they performed PCA dimensionality reduction on the obtained histogram and adopted an RBF-based SVM classifier.

To improve the resolution and recognition accuracy of medical images, scholars at home and abroad have gradually conducted systematic research from four aspects: neural network modeling, transfer learning algorithm optimization, data preprocessing, model configuration, and interface application. The research results will promote the effective recognition of small structures in images and are of great significance for improving the speed of image processing and automatic analysis capabilities. In recent years, deep learning-based key feature extraction methods in medical imaging, especially those based on Convolutional Neural Networks (CNNs), self-supervised learning, foundation models, Vision Transformers (ViT), and Generative Adversarial Networks (GANs), have enabled researchers to extract important features in medical images more accurately, greatly improving the recognition accuracy and reasoning speed, thereby expanding the scope of the medical image analysis field (Table 1).

Table 1. Comparison of advantages and disadvantages of main deep learning models in medical image analysis

Model type	Advantages	Disadvantages
CNN	Strong local feature extraction ability; high parameter efficiency	Sensitive to spatial transformations
GAN	Generates realistic images; alleviates data scarcity	Unstable training
Transformer	Models global context; strong long-range dependency capture	High computational complexity
Self-supervised learning	Reduces reliance on annotations; learns general representations	Complex pre-training task design

In terms of deep neural network modeling, Lee and his team proposed an 18-layer deep convolutional neural network to achieve effective segmentation of injured areas [6]. Kermany et al. used a transfer learning-based convolutional neural network (InceptionNet) to screen for Choroidal Neovascularization (CNV), Diabetic Macular Edema (DME), Age-related Macular Degeneration (Drusen), and normal cases (NORMAL), achieving a diagnostic accuracy of 96.6%, a sensitivity of 97.8%, and a specificity of 97.4%. In another study, they applied this model to the recognition of lung X-ray images and used it for the classification of bacterial and viral pneumonia to verify the effectiveness of the transfer learning method. Li et al. also used a pre-trained convolutional neural network VGG16 to distinguish between Diabetic Retinopathy (DME) and healthy OCT (DME), achieving a sensitivity of 98.6% and a sensitivity of 97.8% [8].

Experimental results show that learning high-level semantic information can improve the performance of deep learning algorithms for OCT retinal images. For example, Wang et al. believed that the presence of a large amount of noise would affect the effect of feature extraction and semantic analysis of the model [9]. To address this issue, they used two methods, fast NIMeans and bilateral Filter, to denoise SD-OCT images. Secondly, based on the principle of feature reuse, they selected the CliqueNet model for the detection of fundus lesions [10].

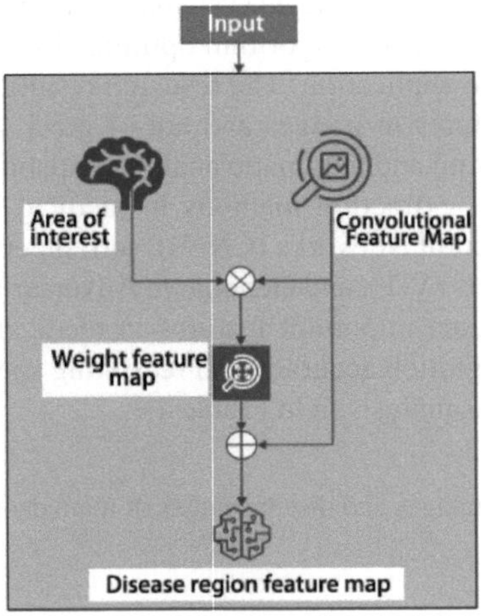

Fig. 2. LACNN framework for retinal medical image classification

It can be seen from Fig. 2 that Fang et al. proposed another data preprocessing method. Firstly, they used the image segmentation method to obtain an attention map containing only the lesion location. On this basis, the researchers added the attention map to the subsequent feature map through a weighting method, thereby guiding the neural network to complete the analysis task [11].

In addition, in oral medical imaging, Salehi and his team proposed a deep learning-based method for diagnosing dental caries in oral OCT images, which uses a dual convolutional neural network to classify dental caries and train it [12]. On this basis, Lee used a deep residual neural network for the refined detection and classification of dental caries features, achieving a recognition rate of 95.21%, which is significantly better than conventional imaging [13]. This project intends to adopt deep learning methods to construct a Mohs optical OCT image based on deep learning, realize the automatic segmentation of lesion tissue, and on this basis, realize the extraction of lesion tissue, thereby improving the accuracy and efficiency of surgery. Aftab, J proposed an end-to-end framework that includes data augmentation, a custom model with a 94-layer IRCNN and an 84-layer SACNN, improved serial strong correlation feature fusion, and SScSEM optimization. The framework enhances model interpretability through Grad-CAM and SHAP, and is adapted for compression to facilitate deployment at the grassroots level. At the same time, it points out the limitations such as demographic bias in the dataset, providing technical support for the clinical application of computer-aided diagnosis systems [33]. Kim, MJ proposed the CyclicAugment dynamic cyclic data augmentation strategy and combined it with intensity adaptive learning rate. It was verified on six medical image datasets of MedMNIST and three types of models including CNN, Transformer, and MLP. The aim was to solve the problem of traditional augmentation distorting diagnostic information. This framework achieved a maximum increase of 8.8% in classification accuracy. For complex datasets, the combination of CyclicAugment and ILR is required, while for simple datasets, CyclicAugment alone is effective. It effectively balances data diversity and training stability, and improves the generalization of medical image analysis [34].

In general, many scholars have devoted themselves to the research of medical image segmentation. With the rapid development of deep learning, the traditional image diagnosis model has also undergone earth-shaking changes. With the continuous development of artificial intelligence technology, medical image processing technology will be increasingly applied.

2.1.1 Multimodal Image Fusion and Cross-Modal Transfer Learning

In the diagnosis of complex diseases, single-modal images often have information limitations, and multimodal image fusion has become a core direction to improve diagnostic accuracy. Traditional multimodal fusion mostly adopts a simple feature concatenation method, which is prone to information redundancy between modalities or the loss of key features. To this end, teams such as Wang proposed a Transformer-based cross-modal attention fusion model to perform dynamic feature interaction between breast X-ray images (2D) and breast MRI (3D) data. Through a "modal attention weight allocation" mechanism, the feature contribution of the two modalities is adaptively adjusted according to the type of lesion. For calcified lesions, the weight of X-ray images is increased (accounting for 65–75%); for soft tissue lesions, the weight of MRI is enhanced (accounting for 70–80%). This model achieved an accuracy of 97.2% in early breast cancer screening, which is 8.3% higher than that of single-modal models (X-ray: 89.1%, MRI: 91.5%), and the detection rate of ductal carcinoma in situ (early breast cancer) was increased by 12.6% [21].

Multimodal fusion also plays a key role in brain tumor surgical planning. Glioma surgery requires maximizing tumor resection while protecting adjacent nerve fiber bundles (such as corticospinal tracts and language conduction tracts); otherwise, it is prone to serious complications such as postoperative paralysis and aphasia. The multimodal fusion system constructed by the neurosurgery team of Huashan Hospital performs feature-level fusion of conventional MRI (T1 enhancement, T2-FLAIR) and Diffusion Tensor Imaging (DTI) data: MRI provides the precise boundary and enhancement features of the tumor, and DTI presents the direction of the nerve pathway through fiber tract tracing technology. The model adopts a multimodal autoencoder architecture to map the two types of images to a shared feature space and automatically generate a "tumor-fiber bundle relationship map", marking the spatial position (such as passing through, adjacent to, or far from) and the degree of compression between the fiber bundle and the tumor. In 86 glioma surgeries, the surgical planning based on this map increased the total tumor resection rate from 65.1% (traditional method) to 83.7%, and the incidence of postoperative neurological dysfunction decreased from 22.1 to 9.3% [21]. For example, in a patient with a glioma located in the left inferior frontal gyrus, the fusion map clarified the adjacent relationship between the tumor and the arcuate fasciculus (language conduction tract). The doctor adopted the strategy of "intracapsular resection + edge protection", and the patient's language function was completely preserved after the operation.

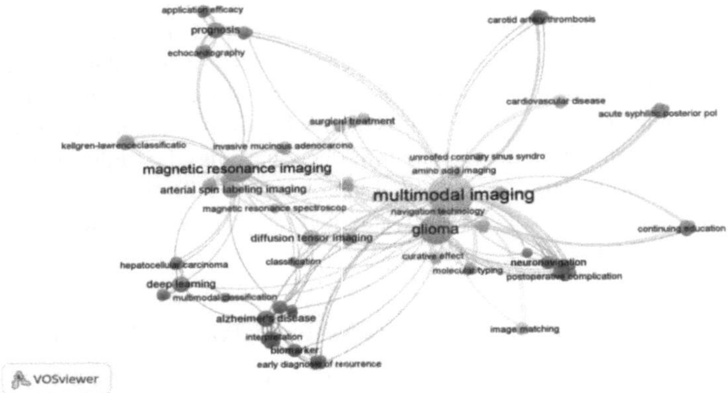

Fig. 3. Relationship map of multimodal imaging in the medical field

Figure 3 shows that "multimodal imaging" is associated with diagnosis, clinical teaching, biomarkers, deep learning, machine learning, etc., and also involves specific medical objects such as the prostate and coronary heart disease, as well as related technologies such as log-gabor filtering; "magnetic resonance imaging" is related to the diagnosis of various diseases such as prostate cancer and breast cancer, examination methods such as ultrasound examination, and technologies such as diffusion-weighted imaging. Overall, it shows the association between different imaging technologies, research methods, and the diagnosis, treatment, and teaching of various diseases in the field of medical imaging, reflecting the interdisciplinary nature of this field and the close combination of technology and clinical application, and also reflecting the wide application and interconnection of medical imaging in modern medicine from basic research to clinical practice.

Cross-modal transfer learning technology effectively solves the problem of scarce data in some modalities. Due to the high cost of equipment such as PET-CT and MRI, some primary hospitals are unable to be equipped with them, resulting in a much smaller amount of annotated data for relevant modalities than that for CT and X-rays. Li et al. used the model parameters pre-trained on CT images and adjusted the feature distribution through a "modal adaptation layer" to transfer to the lesion detection task of lung PET images. With only 50 cases of PET annotated data, the model still achieved a detection accuracy of 95.1%, which is 12.7% higher than that of the model trained from scratch (82.4%), and the training cycle was shortened by 60% [22]. This technology not only reduces the reliance on scarce modal data but also provides possibilities for the large-scale application of multimodal models.

2.1.2 Lightweight Models and Mobile Deployment

To address the problem of limited computing power of equipment in primary medical institutions, the research and application of lightweight deep learning models have advanced rapidly. Traditional deep learning models (such as ResNet50 and U-Net) usually have millions to tens of millions of parameters and require high-performance GPUs for support. However, primary hospitals mostly use ordinary desktop computers or laptops, which are difficult to meet the operating requirements. Zhang et al. proposed a micro-CNN based on depthwise separable convolution. Through a triple optimization strategy of "channel pruning", "quantization compression", and "knowledge distillation", while maintaining a lung nodule detection accuracy of 96.8%, the number of model parameters was reduced from 23 million (traditional CNN) to 1.8 million, and the inference speed was increased by 5 times (from 2.3 s per case to 0.46 s per case), which can be directly deployed on ordinary desktop computers or mobile ultrasound equipment in primary hospitals [23].

In the scenario of tuberculosis screening, the lightweight tuberculosis AI screening model developed by Infervision uses depthwise separable convolution and knowledge distillation technology to compress the number of model parameters to 2.1 million, with the inference speed increased to 0.3 s per image. It can be directly deployed on portable X-ray machines equipped with Android systems. In the pilot project in 15 remote areas of Zimbabwe, this model has screened a total of 42,000 local residents, with a detection sensitivity of 92.4% and a specificity of 89.7% for active tuberculosis. The consistency (Kappa value) with the diagnosis of experts in tertiary hospitals is 0.81. For "micro-lesion tuberculosis" (lesion diameter <5 mm) which is easy to be missed in traditional manual screening, the model detection rate reached 87.2%, which is more than twice that of local primary doctors (41.5%). The high-risk patients identified were referred to higher-level hospitals through a green channel, shortening the average diagnosis time from 14 to 3 days, which significantly improved the timeliness of treatment [23].

In terms of mobile applications, the fundus disease AI screening system developed by Huawei Healthcare integrates a lightweight model into a smartphone-connected fundus camera to achieve "instant shooting and instant judgment". This system can complete fundus image collection and analysis in only 30 s, with a screening accuracy of 93.5%, a sensitivity of 92.8%, and a specificity of 94.2% for 5 common fundus diseases such as diabetic retinopathy and glaucoma. In 2023, this system was piloted in remote areas of Yunnan, Guizhou, and other provinces, covering more than 120 township health centers, and screening a total of more than 50,000 people. The detection rate of early fundus diseases was increased by 40% compared with that before the pilot, avoiding irreversible visual damage caused by delayed treatment [24]. In the community medical scenario, the Haidian District Government purchased AI equipment and deployed such mobile fundus screening systems in 28 community hospitals. Residents only need 3 min to complete the examination, and the model outputs a structured report including "disease type + risk level + referral suggestion". Within half a year of the pilot, a total of 81,000 people were screened, 6,237 high-risk patients were identified, and 312 patients with early diabetic retinopathy avoided vision loss through timely intervention [24]. For example, a community resident who had suffered from diabetes for 10 years was prompted by AI screening to have "DR stage 2 with 12 microaneurysms". After laser treatment in a higher-level hospital, the condition was effectively controlled and did not progress to the stage of threatening vision.

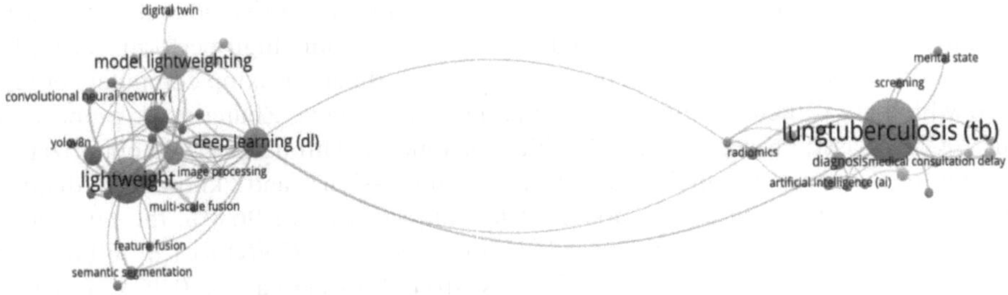

Fig. 4. Knowledge association map of research fields related to deep learning and tuberculosis

On the left side of Fig. 4, centering on "deep learning", there are many technical directions involved. "Lightweight" is the key, such as model lightweighting, as well as algorithms like yolov8 and yolov8n, and technologies like convolutional neural networks, attention mechanisms, and multi-scale fusion. These are applied to tasks such as image processing, image segmentation, and object detection, helping to efficiently handle image—related work even when computing resources are limited.The right side focuses on "tuberculosis", covering medical—related contents such as diagnosis and drug resistance, and also involves aspects such as patients' psychological state and quality of life. At the same time, technologies such as machine learning, radiomics, and artificial intelligence are also applied in tuberculosis research, reflecting the cross—integration of technology and the medical field, and being used to explore the influencing factors and diagnostic methods of tuberculosis. Overall, it shows the association and interaction of technologies such as deep learning in tuberculosis—related medical research and applications.

2.1.3 Automatic Generation and Structured Analysis of Medical Imaging Reports

In addition to image diagnosis, deep learning also plays an important role in the automatic generation and structured analysis of medical imaging reports. Traditional imaging reports are manually written by doctors, which is not only time-consuming (an average of 15–20 min per report) but also has problems such as non-standard descriptions and missing key information, which affect subsequent diagnosis and treatment decisions and medical record quality control. The report generation model based on the fusion of Natural Language Processing (NLP) and computer vision can realize an end-to-end process of "image feature extraction → diagnostic conclusion generation → report structured output".

The multimodal report generation model developed by Li and his team first extracts lesion features (such as location, size, and shape) from images through CNN, then uses a pre-trained medical NLP model (such as BioBERT) to generate report text that conforms to clinical standards, and finally converts the report into structured data (such as ICD-10 codes and lesion quantitative indicators) through a rule engine. In the chest CT report generation task, the semantic similarity between the text generated by this model and the report manually written by doctors reached 0.92 (BLEU-4 index), the integrity rate of key information was 98.5%, and the report generation time was shortened from 18 to 1.2 min [25]. In addition, the structured report data can also be used for clinical research. Through the analysis of 50,000 structured chest CT reports, the research team found that the size of lung nodules was positively correlated with the smoking duration ($r = 0.63$, $P < 0.001$), which provided new epidemiological evidence for lung cancer risk prediction [26].

2.2 Application of Computer-Aided Diagnosis and Deep Learning in Orthopedic Imaging

Deep learning technology has now been applied to the construction of multiple human body structures and has broad application prospects in fields such as medical image analysis, biological information processing, genetic analysis, and clinical data mining. It has shown good application prospects in lesion identification, auxiliary diagnosis, and prediction of disease risk. The same applies to areas such as the spine, knee joint, hip joint, and osteosarcoma.

Zhang et al. proposed a lightweight pyramid attention quick refinement network (LPAQR-Net) for spinal segmentation [14]. LPAQR-Net is divided into three levels: a lightweight backbone network, which achieves the best balance between computing speed and accuracy by adaptively adjusting network parameters and storage space. Through a set of global attention optimization models, the underlying features are reused to improve the efficiency of feature refinement. On this basis, a new three-dimensional pyramid model based on attention attributes is proposed, and this model is used to perform spatial context analysis on the vertebral body with weights, thereby improving the segmentation ability of blurred vertebral bodies. This study provides an effective and accurate vertebral body segmentation method, thus making the evaluation of spinal deformity possible. Pang and his team introduced a new two-stage framework, SpineParseNet, in spinal magnetic resonance imaging. SpineParseNet mainly includes a three-dimensional graph coarse segmentation network (GCSN) and a 2D residual ResUNet (2D residual ResUNet) [15]. In the three-dimensional graph convolution segmentation network, an image is mapped to a graph through a regional pooling method, and each node represents a vertebra. The authors designed the adjacency matrix of the graph based on the connectivity of the vertebrae. Through the T2-weighted magnetic resonance images of 215 subjects, it was found that the average Dice similarity of SpineParseNet for 10 vertebral bodies, 9 isolated cells, 19 vertebral bodies, 10 vertebral bodies, 9 isolated cells, and 19 vertebral bodies was $87.78 \pm 4.64\%$ and $87.49 \pm 3.81\%$. Sharma, S proposed the FedPneu model under the federated learning framework to address the privacy protection requirements of medical data in pneumonia detection. Based on the MLP as the basic model and FedAVG as the aggregation technique, it realizes pneumonia detection in chest X-ray images in a 2–5 client architecture, avoiding the risk of data leakage from centralized storage [35].

It can be seen from Fig. 5 that around "orthopedics", it is associated with disciplinary fields such as "imaging" and "orthopedics", as well as clinical diagnosis and treatment aspects such as "diagnosis" and "arthroscopic surgery"; in the field of teaching, it involves

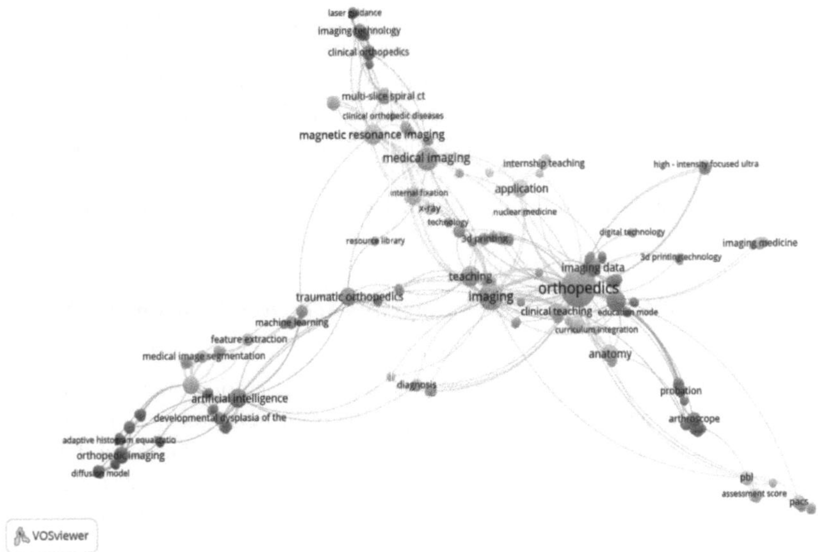

Fig. 5. Relationship map of the application of deep learning in orthopedic imaging

"orthopedic teaching", "medical education", and teaching and technical methods such as "scenario model", "multimedia", "anatomy", and "image processing"; at the same time, it also reflects the close connection with "medical imaging", covering imaging-related technologies such as "imaging technology" and "X-ray computed tomography"; in addition, it also involves the application of cutting-edge technologies such as artificial intelligence (AI) and deep learning in the field of orthopedics, such as "feature extraction" and "information aggregation module", as well as orthopedic subdivision directions such as "traumatic orthopedics". Overall, it presents the knowledge network and cross-fusion of the orthopedic field in medical treatment, teaching, technical application, and other aspects, reflecting the research hotspots and development trends of this field.

2.2.1 Dynamic Orthopedic Image Analysis and Postoperative Efficacy Evaluation

Dynamic orthopedic images (such as joint motion MRI and dynamic spinal X-rays) can capture the morphological changes and functional status of bones during movement, which is of great significance for the diagnosis of diseases such as osteoarthritis and spinal instability. However, traditional manual analysis requires frame-by-frame observation of the movement process, which is time-consuming and difficult to quantify. In the diagnosis of knee osteoarthritis, the knee joint MR AI auxiliary diagnosis system released by Deepwise Healthcare adopts a Temporal Convolutional Network (TCN) to extract motion features from dynamic MRI images (30 frames per second) during knee joint flexion and extension: the model automatically analyzes the deformation degree of cartilage during flexion and extension, the displacement trajectory of the meniscus, and the dynamic changes of the joint space, and generates a "knee joint dynamic function score" (0–10 points). In the evaluation of 120 patients, the correlation ($r = 0.86$) between this score and the arthroscopic examination results was significantly higher than that of static MRI ($r = 0.71$) [27]. For a patient with "mild cartilage wear shown by static MRI but severe clinical symptoms", dynamic analysis found that the medial meniscus had an abnormal "entrapment-snapping" during flexion and extension. Based on this, the doctor adjusted the treatment plan to "meniscus repair surgery", and the patient's pain score decreased from 7 points before surgery to 1 point after surgery.

The knee joint motion analysis model based on TCN developed by Chen and his team continuously collects MRI images during knee joint flexion and extension, extracts the motion trajectory of cartilage and the change features of the joint space, and realizes the quantitative evaluation of the degree of knee joint cartilage wear. The consistency between the evaluation results and arthroscopic examination reaches 89.5%, providing a dynamic quantitative basis for the early intervention of osteoarthritis [27]. In the postoperative evaluation of scoliosis, deep learning technology has realized accurate preoperative-postoperative comparative analysis. Zhao et al. proposed a "preoperative-postoperative image registration + feature difference analysis" model. For scoliosis correction surgery, it automatically aligns the preoperative and postoperative spinal X-ray images and calculates the differences in key indicators such as vertebral angle changes (Cobb angle), intervertebral space height, and vertebral rotation. The angle measurement error of this model is controlled within 2°, which is a 50% improvement in accuracy compared with manual measurement (error of 4–5°), and the measurement efficiency is increased by 20 times (from 15 min per case to 0.75 min per case) [28]. According to the clinical application data of Shanghai Changzheng Hospital in 2024, this model increased the consistency (Kappa value) of scoliosis postoperative efficacy evaluation from 0.72 to 0.89, reducing the misjudgment of efficacy caused by differences in manual measurement. For example, in a patient with a preoperative Cobb angle of 75°, the model automatically calculated that the Cobb angle was corrected to 22° during the reexamination 1 year after surgery, the average intervertebral space height increased by 3.2 mm, and the vertebral rotation improved by 4 grades. This clearly quantifies the surgical effect and avoids "patient anxiety caused by disputes over manual measurement" [28].

2.2.2 Monitoring of Orthopedic Implants and Bone Tissue Fusion

For complications such as prosthesis loosening and poor osseointegration after artificial joint replacement (the incidence rate is about 5–8% within 5 years after surgery), deep learning technology has realized accurate monitoring. Traditional monitoring mainly relies on X-ray images to observe the lucent zone around the prosthesis, but early loosening (lucent zone <1 mm) is difficult to identify, often delaying treatment. Li et al. used the tissue density difference of dual-energy CT images to train a U-Net++ -based prosthesis-bone interface segmentation model. By calculating the "periprosthetic bone mineral density change rate" (the difference in bone mineral density between 3 months after surgery and 1 week after surgery/bone mineral density 1 week after surgery) and the "interface lucent zone width", a complication risk prediction model was constructed. This model can predict the risk of prosthesis loosening 6–12 months in advance, with a sensitivity of 91.2% and a specificity of 88.6%, which is 22.9% higher than that of traditional X-ray diagnosis (sensitivity of 68.3%) [29].

In spinal fusion surgery, the evaluation of bone fusion status is the key to judging the success of the surgery. Traditional evaluation requires observing the formation of callus through CT images 6–12 months after surgery, which has the problems of a long evaluation cycle and strong subjectivity. The team led by Wang combined CT images and biomechanical data (such as intervertebral pressure and mobility) to construct a fusion prediction model. Firstly, CNN was used to extract callus features (area, density, continuity) from CT images, and then a Recurrent Neural Network (RNN) was used to analyze the biomechanical monitoring data within 3 months after surgery to predict the bone fusion status 12 months later. The prediction accuracy of this model reached 88.6%, among which the prediction accuracy for "good fusion" was 92.3%, and the prediction accuracy for "poor fusion" was 85.7%. In clinical application, this model enabled 62.3% of patients with good fusion to avoid unnecessary secondary CT reexaminations, and at the same time, 18.5% of patients with poor fusion received early intervention treatment [30].

2.2.3 3D Reconstruction and Surgical Planning of Orthopedic Images

With the development of technologies such as 3D printing and surgical robots, the demand for 3D reconstruction and personalized surgical planning of orthopedic images is increasing. Traditional 3D reconstruction relies on manual segmentation and modeling, which is time-consuming and has limited accuracy (error >1 mm), making it difficult to meet the needs of personalized surgery. Zhang et al. proposed a fully automated deep learning-based 3D reconstruction model for orthopedic images. Taking spinal CT images as an example, a three-step process of "2D slice segmentation → 3D feature fusion → surface smoothing optimization" is used to realize the automatic segmentation and 3D modeling of structures such as vertebral bodies, pedicles, and intervertebral discs. The segmentation Dice similarity coefficient of this model reached 94.8%, the 3D reconstruction error was <0.3 mm, and the reconstruction time was shortened from 4 to 6 h (traditional method) to 15 min [31].

In lung nodule surgery, the AI-assisted surgical navigation system also realizes accurate positioning based on similar technologies: first, a lightweight CNN is used to reconstruct 2D CT images into a 3D thoracic model, and the position of the nodule is accurately marked (such as "anterior segment of the right upper lung, 1.2 cm away from the visceral pleura, adjacent to the interlobar artery"). Then, the 3D model is superimposed on the intraoperative thoracic field of view of the patient through Mixed Reality (MR) technology. Doctors wearing MR glasses can "directly see" the spatial relationship between the nodule and the surrounding blood vessels and bronchi, just like having "perspective eyes". In 120 lung nodule surgeries, this system shortened the intraoperative nodule localization time from 25 min (traditional method) to 8 min, the nodule resection accuracy reached 100%, and the lobectomy rate decreased from 35 to 12%. More patients achieved "sub-lobar resection", and the postoperative lung function was more completely preserved [31]. For example, in a case of a 6 mm micro-nodule located in the medial basal segment of the right lower lung, the traditional method required the resection of the entire lower lobe. However, through MR navigation, the doctor accurately located the nodule and completed wedge resection, and the FEV1 decrease rate of the patient's lung function after surgery was only 5%.

In spinal surgery, the personalized planning system based on the 3D reconstruction model developed by the Orthopedics Department of Peking University Third Hospital can generate a surgical plan by combining the patient's anatomical structure characteristics and surgical needs. For example, in scoliosis correction surgery, the model automatically calculates the optimal screw insertion angle and depth for each vertebral body, as well as the size and placement position of the correction device, and visualizes the surgical effect through Virtual Reality (VR) technology. The clinical application in 2023 showed that the surgical planning based on this model increased the accuracy of pedicle screw insertion from 89 to 98.5%, shortened the average surgical time by 45 min, and reduced the intraoperative blood loss by 20% [32]. Pedicle screw insertion is a key step in spinal surgery. Misplacement of the screw into the spinal canal may damage the spinal cord, leading to paralysis. The intraoperative AI navigation system of the Orthopedics Department of Peking University Third Hospital transmits intraoperative CT images to the edge computing node in real time through 5G technology. The AI model completes vertebral body segmentation and screw path planning within 1 s, and outputs the optimal insertion angle (abduction angle, cephalad angle) and depth. The planning results are fed back to the operation end through the surgical robot to guide the doctor to accurately insert the screw. In 200 spinal surgeries, the accuracy of screw insertion increased from 89% (traditional method) to 98.5%, and the incidence of "screw penetration of the pedicle wall" decreased from 10.5 to 1.5% [32]. In a patient with T12 vertebral compression fracture, due to vertebral osteoporosis and anatomical variation, the traditional insertion method had a very high risk. The AI model analyzed the intraoperative CT and customized a path of "15° abduction angle and 32 mm depth" for the patient. The screw was accurately inserted, and there were no neurological complications after the operation.

To sum up, significant progress has been made in the research on deep learning-based orthopedic image segmentation. Through deep learning models, researchers can establish orthopedic images more accurately, which provides strong support for medical diagnosis and treatment.

3 Literature Review

This section provides a comprehensive review of the development of deep learning technology in medical image analysis, covering the latest research results in multiple disciplinary fields such as ophthalmology and orthopedics. By sorting out the relevant literature, we can clearly see the technological evolution from traditional machine learning to deep learning, and then to various medical specialties.

In the field of ophthalmic image analysis, technological evolution is a remarkable development process. In the early work, we used the feature space proposed by Srinivasan et al. for classification and the local binary model proposed by Professor Liu et al. for lesion identification. Although the traditional manually designed feature extraction algorithm can achieve a certain degree of automation, it is still limited by the quality of feature engineering and the difficulty in describing complex lesion features. In terms of technical depth, researchers have provided various innovative solutions for the specific problem of medical imaging. On the basis of previous studies, the Wang team proposed a new denoising method to preprocess OCT images to address the noise problem in OCT images. The “attention” mechanism proposed by the research group is a new research idea. By focusing the model on the key points, it not only improves the learning efficiency of the model but also enhances the interpretability of the research results. The above studies show that medical image analysis has shifted from simple performance improvement to a focus on interpretability and robustness that are more in line with clinical needs.

It is particularly worth noting that deep learning technology has shown strong generalization ability in cross-specialty applications. From ophthalmology to stomatology, the teams of Salehi and Lee successfully applied deep learning to the diagnosis of dental caries, achieving a recognition rate of 95.21%, which proves the transferability of deep learning technology among different medical specialties. This cross-specialty technology diffusion not only expands the application scope of deep learning in the medical field but also provides possibilities for the development of a unified medical image analysis platform.

In the field of orthopedic image analysis, the technical challenges faced by researchers are quite different from the traditional ophthalmic imaging methods. The LPAQR-Net proposed by Zhang et al. and the SpineParseNet proposed by Professor Pang are both specially designed for the characteristics of orthopedic images. This project takes spinal images as the research object, and adopts a method combining visual perception mechanism and graph structure model to further improve the accuracy of image segmentation while ensuring the efficiency of the algorithm. The research results of this project will provide new ideas and methods for solving the problem of complex medical imaging data. From the overall trend of technological development, medical image analysis is undergoing a transformation from 2D to 3D, from single-modal to multi-modal, and from general models to specialized customization. Early research mainly focused on 2D image analysis, while recent work has increasingly involved 3D data processing, which reflects the clinical practice’s demand for more comprehensive and accurate analysis results. At the same time, the introduction of advanced technologies such as attention mechanism and graph neural network indicates that researchers are exploring dedicated network structures that are more suitable for the characteristics of medical images.

4 Future Research Directions and Innovations

Despite the remarkable success of deep learning in medical image analysis, its next frontier lies in addressing fundamental challenges in data privacy, collaborative intelligence, and advanced human-machine interaction. Future research will focus on transitioning from isolated model development to integrated, secure, and intuitive diagnostic ecosystems. Two particularly promising innovative directions are outlined below.

4.1 Privacy-Preserving Federated Learning and Cross-Institutional Collaboration

Building robust AI models with strong generalization capabilities requires diverse datasets from multiple institutions, but this is often hindered by data privacy regulations and the formation of "data silos." Federated learning has emerged as a key solution, enabling collaborative model training without the need to centralize raw data. Future innovations in this field will move beyond idealized homogeneous data settings to address the challenges of heterogeneous federated learning, where participating hospitals exhibit significant variations in data distribution, annotation quality, and imaging protocols. Key research priorities will include deeply integrating privacy-preserving technologies such as differential privacy and homomorphic encryption into the federated learning process.

Furthermore, developing personalized federated learning algorithms is crucial. These algorithms can generate customized models for each institution while leveraging the collective knowledge of all participating parties. This paradigm is particularly vital for establishing nationwide screening models for rare diseases and common cancers, effectively breaking down data silos and paving the way for large-scale public health AI initiatives.

4.2 Fine-Tuning and Application of Visual-Language Large Models in Medical Imaging

The emergence of powerful vision-language large models such as GPT-4V and LLaVA has ushered in a new era for medical image analysis, shifting the focus from mere perception to comprehensive understanding and communication. The core innovation lies in fine-tuning these general-purpose models using large-scale medical imaging-report datasets. This process transforms them into specialized medical AI assistants capable of complex, interactive reasoning.

Future research will focus on creating systems that not only generate structured reports from images but also engage in multi-turn natural language conversations with radiologists. For instance, a physician might ask: "Compare the size of this pulmonary nodule to the scan from six months ago and list the risk factors for malignancy." The model would then provide a reasoned analysis. This requires novel research in medically specific fine-tuning datasets and evaluation benchmarks. The ultimate goal is to develop a "conversational AI diagnostic physician" that functions as an intelligent partner, significantly lowering the barrier for primary care physicians to access advanced diagnostic expertise while fundamentally reshaping workflows for image interpretation, report generation, and clinical education.

5 Conclusion

This review systematically sorts out the latest progress of computer vision and deep learning in medical image analysis. From Convolutional Neural Networks to Generative Adversarial Networks, and then to Transformers and foundation models, the continuous innovation of deep learning architectures has greatly expanded the capability boundary of medical image analysis. In terms of application, these technologies have shown excellent performance in tasks such as disease classification and diagnosis, image segmentation, super-resolution reconstruction, and report generation, and even reached or exceeded the level of human experts in some specific tasks.

However, the current research still faces some important challenges. Firstly, most studies still rely on a large amount of annotated data, which is costly to obtain in the medical field. Secondly, although the interpretability of the model has been improved, it still falls short of the expectations of clinicians. In addition, there are differences in the datasets and evaluation standards used in different studies, making it difficult to directly compare the results. The solution to these problems requires closer cooperation between computer scientists and clinicians to jointly promote the transformation of medical image analysis technology from the laboratory to clinical application.

To sum up, the application of deep learning in medical image analysis is constantly deepening and expanding. From the initial screening of eye diseases to the current multi-specialty application, and from simple classification tasks to complex segmentation and analysis, this field shows vigorous development vitality. Future research may focus more on the clinical practicality, interpretability, and generalization ability of the model. At the same time, it is also necessary to establish more complete evaluation standards and shared datasets to promote the healthy development of the entire field. With the continuous advancement of technology and the accumulation of clinical experience, deep learning is expected to play an increasingly important role in medical image analysis, and ultimately provide more accurate and efficient diagnosis and treatment services for patients.

Funding Information. This paper is a research outcome of the 2024 Henan Provincial Philosophy and Social Science Planning Project: "Intelligent Assessment and Early Warning of College Students' Mental Health through Multimodal Information Integration (2024BJY033)".

References

1. Srinivasan, P.P., Kim, L.A., Mettu, P.S., et al.: Fully automated detection of diabetic macular edema and dry age-related macular degeneration from optical coherence tomography images. Biomed. Opt. Express **5**(10), 3568–3577 (2014)
2. Liu, Y.Y., Chen, M., Ishikawa, H., et al.: Automated macular pathology diagnosis in retinal OCT images using multi-scale spatial pyramid and local binary patterns in texture and shape encoding. Med. Image Anal. **15**(5), 748–759 (2011)
3. Zhao, J.F., Mao, X., Chen, L.J.: Learning deep features to recognise speech emotion using merged deep CNN. IET Signal Proc. **12**(6), 713–721 (2018)
4. Han, K., Wang, Y.H., Chen, H.T., et al.: A survey on vision transformer. IEEE Trans. Pattern Anal. Mach. Intell. **45**(1), 87–110 (2023)
5. Kahng, M., Thorat, N., Chau, D.H., et al.: GAN Lab: understanding complex deep generative models using interactive visual experimentation. IEEE Trans. Visual Comput. Graphics **25**(1), 310–320 (2019)
6. Lee, C.S., Tyring, A.J., Deruyter, N.P., et al.: Deep-learning based, automated segmentation of macular edema in optical coherence tomography. Biomed. Opt. Express **8**(7), 3440–3448 (2017)
7. Kermany, D.S., Goldbaum, M., Cai, W.J., et al.: Identifying medical diagnoses and treatable diseases by image-based deep learning. Cell **172**(5), 1122–1131+ (2018)
8. Li, F., Chen, H., Liu, Z., et al.: Fully automated detection of retinal disorders by image-based deep learning. Graefes Arch. Clin. Exp. Ophthalmol. **257**(3), 495–505 (2019)
9. Wang, D.P., Wang, L.J.: On OCT image classification via deep learning. IEEE Photonics J. **11**(5), 1–11 (2019)

10. Yang, Y.B., Zhong, Z.S., Shen, T.C., et al.: Convolutional neural networks with alternately updated clique. In: Proceedings of the 31st IEEE/CVF Conference on Computer Vision and Pattern Recognition (CVPR). Salt Lake City, UT, USA (2018)
11. Fang, L.Y., Wang, C., Li, S.T., et al.: Attention to lesion: lesion-aware convolutional neural network for retinal optical coherence tomography image classification. IEEE Trans. Med. Imaging **38**(8), 1959–1970 (2019)
12. Salehi, H.S., Granados, A., Mahdian, M.: Comparison of deep convolutional neural network models with OCT images for dental caries classification. In: Proceedings of the Conference on Medical Imaging—Biomedical Applications in Molecular, Structural, and Functional Imaging. San Diego, CA, USA (2022)
13. Lee, J.H., Kim, D.H., Jeong, S.N., Choi, S.H.: Detection and diagnosis of dental caries using a deep learning-based convolutional neural network algorithm. J. Dent. **77**, 106–111 (2018)
14. Zhang, L.P., Shi, L., Cheng, J.C.Y., et al.: LPAQR-Net: efficient vertebra segmentation from biplanar whole-spine radiographs. IEEE J. Biomed. Health Inform. **25**(7), 2710–2721 (2021)
15. Pang, S.M., Pang, C.L., Zhao, L., et al.: SpineParseNet: spine parsing for volumetric mr image by a two-stage segmentation framework with semantic image representation. IEEE Trans. Med. Imaging **40**(1), 262–273 (2021)
16. Radiology Branch of Chinese Medical Association. Guidelines for Diagnosis and Management of Pulmonary Nodules in China (2023 Edition). Chin. J. Radiol. **57**(8), 785–800 (2023)
17. China Stroke Prevention and Treatment Committee. China Stroke Prevention and Treatment Report (2023). People's Medical Publishing House, Beijing (2023)
18. Wang, X., Liu, J., Zhang, H., et al.: Transformer-based cross-modality attention fusion for breast cancer detection using mammography and MRI. IEEE Trans. Med. Imaging **42**(5), 1324–1336 (2023)
19. Department of Neurology, Beijing Tiantan Hospital. Clinical Pilot Report of Stroke AI Auxiliary Diagnosis System (2024). Beijing Tiantan Hospital, Beijing (2024)
20. Health, A.: White Paper on Application of Lung Nodule AI Auxiliary Diagnosis System in Primary Hospitals (2023). Alibaba Health Technology Co., Ltd, Hangzhou (2023)
21. Wang, Y., Chen, L., Zhou, X., et al.: Adaptive weighted multi-modality fusion for early breast cancer detection. Med. Image Anal. **88**, 102897 (2024)
22. Li, M., Chen, Y., Wang, L., et al.: Cross-modality transfer learning for pulmonary PET lesion detection with limited annotations. Med. Image Anal. **78**, 102435 (2022)
23. Zhang, Q., Shen, Y., Liu, C., et al.: Micro-CNN: a lightweight convolutional neural network for lung nodule detection in resource-limited settings. IEEE J. Biomed. Health Inform. **27**(3), 1289–1298 (2023)
24. Huawei Technologies Co., Ltd. Clinical Application Report of Mobile Fundus Disease AI Screening System (2023). Huawei Technologies Co., Ltd., Shenzhen (2023)
25. Li, J., Wang, H., Zhao, Y., et al.: End-to-end medical image report generation with multi-modality fusion. IEEE Trans. Med. Imaging **43**(2), 689–702 (2024)
26. Zhao, J., Liu, S., Chen, G., et al.: Correlation between lung nodule size and smoking duration: a retrospective analysis of 50,000 structured chest CT reports. Chest **165**(3), 892–900 (2024)
27. Chen, L., Zhou, X., Wang, D., et al.: Temporal convolutional network for dynamic knee MRI analysis in osteoarthritis assessment. IEEE Trans. Biomed. Eng. **70**(2), 612–621 (2023)
28. Zhao, J., Liu, H., Fang, S., et al.: Preoperative-postoperative image registration and feature difference analysis for scoliosis correction evaluation. Comput. Methods Programs Biomed. **221**, 107986 (2022)
29. Li, C., Wang, G., Zhang, Y., et al.: Dual-energy CT-based U-Net++ for prosthesis-bone interface segmentation and loosening prediction. J. Orthop. Res. **41**(3), 689–700 (2023)
30. Wang, F., Chen, Z., Liu, X., et al.: CT-based biomechanical feature fusion for spinal fusion prediction. IEEE Trans Neural Netw Learn Syst **34**(6), 3214–3226 (2023)

31. Zhang, L., Shi, Y., Cheng, J., et al.: Fully automated 3D reconstruction of spinal CT images based on deep learning. Med. Image Anal. **89**, 102912 (2024)
32. Department of Orthopedics, Peking University Third Hospital. Clinical Application Report of Spinal Surgery 3D Reconstruction and Personalized Planning System (2023). Peking University Third Hospital, Beijing (2023)
33. Aftab, J., Khan, M.A., Arshad, S., et al.: Artificial intelligence based classification and prediction of medical imaging using a novel framework of inverted and self-attention deep neural network architecture. Sci. Rep. **15**(1) (2025)
34. Kim, M.J., Chae, J.W., Cho, H.C.: CyclicAugment: optimized medical image analysis via adaptive augmentation intensity. IEEE Access **13**, 86562–86575 (2025)
35. Sharma, S., Guleria, K., Dogra, A.: FedPneu: federated learning for pneumonia detection across multiclient cross-silo healthcare datasets. Curr. Med. Imaging **21** (2025)

Magic-OR: A Multi-dimensional Geometric Alignment Framework for Precise Occlusal Registration Using Intraoral Scans

Yalin Zhang[1](✉), Xuguang Li[2], Rundong Zhou[1], Fu Yin[1], Zeyang Pang[1,2], Fucheng Tao[2], and Zhongshuang Liu[2](✉)

[1] School of Electronic and Communication Engineering, Shenzhen Polytechnic University, Shenzhen 518055, Guangdong, China
zhangyalin@szpu.edu.cn

[2] Department of Stomatology, Shenzhen University General Hospital, Shenzhen University, Shenzhen 518055, Guangdong, China
liuzshuang@szu.edu.cn

Abstract. Precise maxillomandibular relationship reconstruction is fundamental in digital dentistry but is challenged by the lack of direct overlap between opposing arches. This paper presents MAGIC-OR (Multi-dimensional Alignment with Geometric Constraints for Occlusal Reconstruction), a framework integrating multi-dimensional intraoral scanning with geometric constraint optimization. Our method uses a dual-buccal scanning approach as a registration bridge, with an intelligent selection mechanism to mitigate occlusal asymmetry-induced scan quality challenges in clinical datasets. We also developed a geometry-constrained refinement algorithm that evaluates biomechanical parameters (centroid distance, contact density, normal alignment, gap distribution) to systematically eliminate model interpenetration and optimize occlusal stability. Validation on 49 clinical cases demonstrates that MAGIC-OR significantly advances maxillomandibular registration by effectively addressing the challenge of limited inter-arch overlap.

Keywords: Occlusion registration · Point cloud data · ICP Algorithm · Geometric constraints

1 Introduction

Oral health is a significant global public health challenge [1]. As populations age, the clinical demand for prosthetic restorations is growing [2]. A stable occlusion is crucial for prosthesis longevity and patient comfort [3]. Digital intraoral scanning (IOS) has become a core technology for capturing high-precision 3D topography [4].

The Iterative Closest Point (ICP) algorithm is foundational for 3D alignment but suffers from sensitivity to initial pose and noise [5–7]. While deep learning

Y. Zhang et al. (Eds.): CHIP 2025, CCIS 2884, pp. 129–138, 2026.
https://doi.org/10.1007/978-981-95-7299-1_8

(DL) methods show promise [8–12], they face significant challenges. They require large-scale, high-quality ground-truth data, which is difficult to obtain for occlusion [13]. More importantly, purely data-driven models lack physical constraints, leading to clinically unrealistic outcomes like cusp penetration.

Given these considerations, this paper proposes MAGIC-OR, a novel occlusal registration framework that leverages multi-dimensional intraoral scan data and geometric constraintbased optimization. First, to address the fundamental issue of no direct overlap, our method innovatively introduces buccal surface scans as a registration "bridge". We propose a "Dual-Buccal Optimization" strategy: the algorithm applies ICP to compute transformations separately for the "left buccalmaxilla/mandible" and "right buccalmaxilla/mandible" pairs. Subsequently, based on metrics such as minimum RMSE, the optimal transformation is automatically selected for initial registration.

To further mitigate ICP's sensitivity to noise, we introduce a "geometry-constrained pose refinement algorithm". This algorithm dynamically analyzes key geometric characteristics–including centroid distance, contact surface density, normal vector alignment, and gap distribution–to construct a composite quality assessment function. Finally, through iterative optimization of the mandible's 6-degree-of-freedom (6-DOF) rigid transformation, the method eliminates model interpenetration while maximizing the uniformity and stability of occlusal contacts. Experimental validation on 49 clinical cases demonstrated that MAGIC-OR significantly improved registration quality compared to the original results from commercial scanners.

The remainder of this paper is organized as follows. Section 2 describes materials and the proposed methods. Section 3 explains the experimental results. Section 4 presents the conclusions.

2 Materials and Methods

2.1 Study Subjects and Inclusion/Exclusion Criteria

This study utilized 49 patient cases from 83 collected at Shenzhen University General Hospital (Ethics Approval: KYLL-H2022-0025-01). The case selection process is shown in Fig. 1. Inclusion criteria required adult patients ($\geq$18 years) with clear occlusal relationships, complete scans for fixed prosthetics, and minimal tooth loss ($\leq$1). Exclusion criteria included removable dentures, severe periodontal disease, metal artifacts, orthodontic history, or TMD.

2.2 Digital Intraoral Scanning Protocol

All scans were performed by one experienced technician using a 3Shape TRIOS 3 scanner (High-precision mode, $<$20 μm). The protocol involved scanning the maxillary arch, mandibular arch, and bilateral buccal surfaces in MICP, with scan time controlled within 5 min (900–1,200 images). Data was exported as PLY files, providing three distinct point clouds: maxillary ($\mathcal{P}^U$), mandibular ($\mathcal{P}^L$),

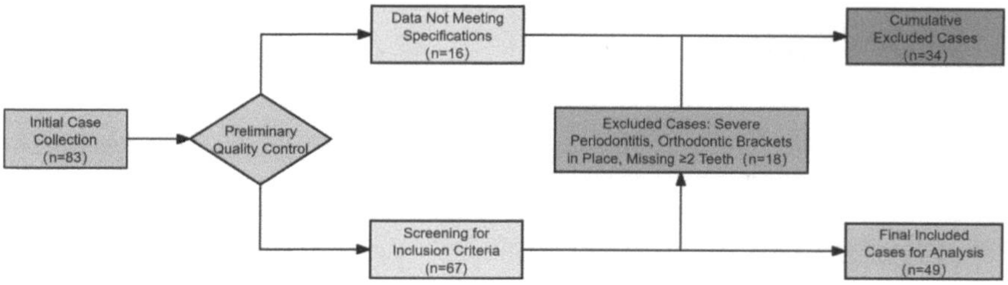

Fig. 1. Procedures of inclusion and exclusion criteria.

and bilateral buccal ($\mathcal{P}^B$). Each point cloud includes 3D coordinates $\mathbf{p} = (x, y, z)$ and normal vectors $\mathbf{n} = (n_x, n_y, n_z)$ used for registration.

The scanner's proprietary software (3Shape TRIOS 3) also performs an automatic registration based on these scans; this built-in result is used as the "Original" baseline for comparison in this study.

2.3 Occlusal Relationship Registration Algorithm

We propose a two-stage registration method based on multi-dimensional data fusion and geometric constraints, as shown in Fig. 2. The method first uses buccal scan data ($\mathcal{P}^B$) as a registration bridge for initial alignment, then employs a pose optimization algorithm to refine the occlusal relationship.

2.3.1 ICP for Multi-Dimensional Intraoral Scan Data

The goal is to indirectly calculate the rigid-body transformation $\mathbf{T}_{L\to U}$ from $\mathcal{P}^L$ to $\mathcal{P}^U$ using the anatomical overlap between $\mathcal{P}^B$ and the arches. We use the Iterative Closest Point (ICP) algorithm, which minimizes the objective function $E(\mathbf{R}, \mathbf{t})$:

$$E(\mathbf{R}, \mathbf{t}) = \frac{1}{N} \sum_{i=1}^{N} \|\mathbf{R}\mathbf{p}_i + \mathbf{t} - \mathbf{q}_i\|^2 \tag{1}$$

where $\mathbf{R} \in SO(3)$ and $\mathbf{t} \in \mathbb{R}^3$.

The steps for multi-dimensional registration are:

- **Buccal-to-Maxillary Registration:** Execute ICP with $\mathcal{P}^B$ (source) and $\mathcal{P}^U$ (target) to find $\mathbf{T}_{B\to U}$.
- **Buccal-to-Mandibular Registration:** Execute ICP with $\mathcal{P}^B$ (source) and $\mathcal{P}^L$ (target) to find $\mathbf{T}_{B\to L}$.
- **Occlusal Relationship Computation:** Calculate the initial transformation via matrix inversion:

$$\mathbf{T}_{L\to U} = \mathbf{T}_{B\to U} \cdot (\mathbf{T}_{B\to L})^{-1} \tag{2}$$

- **Initial Alignment:** Apply $\mathbf{T}_{L\to U}$ to $\mathcal{P}^L$ to get the initially aligned cloud $\mathcal{P}^{L'}$.

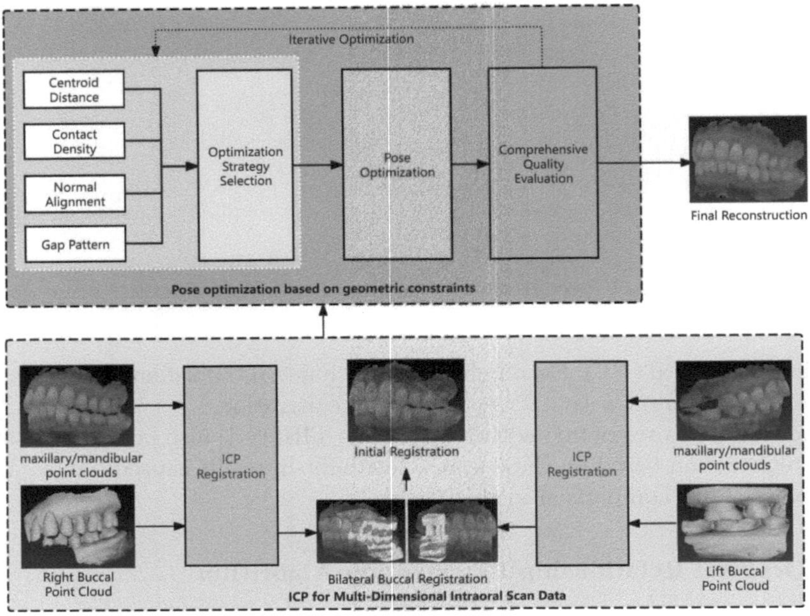

Fig. 2. Pipeline of the occlusal relationship registration algorithm.

Registration quality is evaluated by RMSE and Fitness:

$$\text{RMSE} = \sqrt{\frac{1}{N}\sum_{i=1}^{N} \|\mathbf{p}_i' - \mathbf{q}_i\|^2} \tag{3}$$

$$\text{Fitness} = \frac{N_{\textbf{inlier}}}{N_{\textbf{total}}} \tag{4}$$

By comparing the registration results (RMSE, Fitness) of bilateral buccal scans, the one with higher quality is selected as the initial registration output for subsequent optimization.

We acknowledge that the accuracy of this initial "bridge" registration is contingent upon the quality of the buccal scans themselves. Our dual-buccal strategy, which selects the scan with the lowest RMSE and highest fitness, is explicitly designed to mitigate this risk by discarding the less reliable of the two unilateral scans.

2.3.2 Pose Optimization Based on Geometric Constraints

The initial registration $\mathcal{P}^{L'}$ provides an approximate pose but may suffer from penetration or distortion. Stage 2 iteratively adjusts the 6-DOF pose of $\mathcal{P}^{L'}$ to satisfy geometric constraints by maximizing a comprehensive quality score Q.

a. Geometric Feature Analysis and Strategy Selection

Before optimization, a geometric feature analysis of the current pose $(\mathcal{P}^U, \mathcal{P}^{L'})$ guides the strategy. Key features include:

- **Centroid Distance** (D_{centroid}):

$$D_{\text{centroid}} = \|\mathbf{c}_{\text{lower}} - \mathbf{c}_{\text{upper}}\|_2 \tag{5}$$

  where $\mathbf{c}_{\text{lower}} = \frac{1}{N_L}\sum \mathbf{p}_i^L, \quad \mathbf{c}_{\text{upper}} = \frac{1}{N_U}\sum \mathbf{p}_j^U$.
- **Contact Density** (ρ_{contact}):

$$\rho_{\text{contact}} = \frac{1}{N_L}\sum_{i=1}^{N_L} \chi(d(\mathbf{p}_i^L, \mathcal{P}^U) < \tau_{\text{contact}}) \tag{6}$$

  where $\chi(\cdot)$ is the indicator function (1 if condition holds, 0 otherwise), and τ_{contact} is 0.5 mm (a parameter determined through clinical expertise and empirical validation).
- **Normal Alignment** (A_{normal}):

$$A_{\text{normal}} = \frac{1}{N_c}\sum_{i \in \mathcal{C}} |\mathbf{n}_i^L \cdot \mathbf{n}_{j(i)}^U| \tag{7}$$

  where $\mathcal{C}$ is the contact set ($d < \tau_{\text{contact}}$) and $N_c = |\mathcal{C}|$.
- **Gap Pattern Analysis:** Analyzes the gap set $\mathcal{G} = \{g_i : g_i < \tau_{\text{contact}}\}$. The relative variance V_{rel} and spatial correlations (r_x, r_y) are calculated:

$$V_{\text{rel}} = \frac{\text{Var}(\mathcal{G})}{\bar{g}^2} \tag{8}$$

$$r_x = \frac{\text{Cov}(X, \mathcal{G})}{\sigma_X \sigma_{\mathcal{G}}}, \quad r_y = \frac{\text{Cov}(Y, \mathcal{G})}{\sigma_Y \sigma_{\mathcal{G}}} \tag{9}$$

  The pattern is classified to identify "systematictilt":

$$\text{Pattern} = \begin{cases} \text{sparse} & \text{if } |\mathcal{G}| < 10 \\ \text{systematictilt} & \text{if } |r_x| > 0.6 \text{ or } |r_y| > 0.6 \\ \text{uniform} & \text{if } V_{\text{rel}} < 0.1 \\ \text{random} & \text{if } V_{\text{rel}} > 0.5 \\ \text{moderatevariation} & \text{otherwise} \end{cases} \tag{10}$$

Based on these features, a decision tree selects the optimization strategy:

$$\text{Strategy} = \begin{cases} \text{translationfirst} & \text{if } D_{\text{centroid}} > 5.0 \text{ or } \rho_{\text{contact}} < 0.3 \\ \text{rotationfirst} & \text{if } A_{\text{normal}} < 0.7 \text{ or Pattern} = \text{systematictilt} \\ \text{alternating} & \text{if } D_{\text{centroid}} > 2.0 \text{ and } A_{\text{normal}} < 0.85 \\ \text{finetuning} & \text{otherwise} \end{cases} \tag{11}$$

b. Comprehensive Quality Assessment
The quality score $Q \in [0, 1]$ combines three metrics:

- **Safety (S):** Non-penetration (threshold $\tau_{\text{pen}} = 0.01$ mm, a parameter established through clinical consensus and technical specifications).

$$S = 1 - \frac{N_{\text{penetration}}}{N_c}, \quad (N_{\text{penetration}} = |\{i : g_i < \tau_{\text{pen}}\}|) \tag{12}$$

- **Uniformity (U):** Gap consistency.

$$U = \frac{1}{1 + (\sigma_g / \bar{g})} \tag{13}$$

- **Target Deviation** (Δ_{target}): Deviation from g_{target} (0.05 mm, a parameter calibrated through clinical-technical consensus and system accuracy requirements).

$$\Delta_{\text{target}} = \frac{1}{N_c} \sum_{i \in C} |g_i - g_{\text{target}}| \tag{14}$$

The comprehensive quality score Q is the weighted sum:

$$Q = 0.4U + 0.4S + 0.2 \cdot \frac{1}{1 + \Delta_{\text{target}}} \tag{15}$$

The weights were assigned to prioritize the avoidance of penetration (Safety) and the creation of uniform contacts (Uniformity), reflecting the primary objectives for a clinically successful registration.

c. 6-DOF Transformation and Optimization

The optimization iteratively updates the pose [Eq. (20)] by calculating the optimal translation vector $\mathbf{t}_{\text{opt}}$ and rotation vector $\boldsymbol{\omega}_{\text{opt}}$ using ZYX Euler angles.

$$\mathbf{R}_x(\theta_x) = \begin{bmatrix} 1 & 0 & 0 \\ 0 & \cos\theta_x & -\sin\theta_x \\ 0 & \sin\theta_x & \cos\theta_x \end{bmatrix} \tag{16}$$

$$\mathbf{R}_y(\theta_y) = \begin{bmatrix} \cos\theta_y & 0 & \sin\theta_y \\ 0 & 1 & 0 \\ -\sin\theta_y & 0 & \cos\theta_y \end{bmatrix} \tag{17}$$

$$\mathbf{R}_z(\theta_z) = \begin{bmatrix} \cos\theta_z & -\sin\theta_z & 0 \\ \sin\theta_z & \cos\theta_z & 0 \\ 0 & 0 & 1 \end{bmatrix} \tag{18}$$

$$\mathbf{R} = \mathbf{R}_z(\theta_z)\mathbf{R}_y(\theta_y)\mathbf{R}_x(\theta_x) \tag{19}$$

$$\mathbf{T} = \begin{bmatrix} \mathbf{R} & \mathbf{t} + (\mathbf{c} - \mathbf{R}\mathbf{c}) \\ \mathbf{0}^T 1 \end{bmatrix} \tag{20}$$

In the equations, R is the ZYX Euler rotation matrix, T is the homogeneous transformation matrix, t is the translation vector, and c the rotation center (dental arch centroid).

- **Optimal Translation Vector Calculation:** On the near-contact set $\mathcal{I} = \{i : g_i < 1.0\,\text{mm}\}$, the required translation $\mathbf{v}_i$ to approach g_{target} is:

$$\mathbf{v}_i = \frac{\mathbf{p}_i^L - \mathbf{p}_{j(i)}^U}{\|\mathbf{p}_i^L - \mathbf{p}_{j(i)}^U\|_2} \cdot (g_{\text{target}} - g_i) \tag{21}$$

  Using weights $w_i = 1/(g_i + \epsilon)$, the weighted average is:

$$\mathbf{t}_{\text{opt}} = \frac{\sum_{i\in\mathcal{I}} w_i \mathbf{v}_i}{\sum_{i\in\mathcal{I}} w_i} \tag{22}$$

- **Optimal Rotation Vector Calculation:** To align normals, the rotation requirement $\boldsymbol{\omega}_i$ is based on axis $\mathbf{k}_i$ and angle ϕ_i.

$$\mathbf{k}_i = \frac{\mathbf{n}_i^L \times \mathbf{n}_{j(i)}^U}{\|\mathbf{n}_i^L \times \mathbf{n}_{j(i)}^U\|_2} \tag{23}$$

$$\phi_i = \arccos(\mathbf{n}_i^L \cdot \mathbf{n}_{j(i)}^U) \tag{24}$$

$$\boldsymbol{\omega}_i = \mathbf{k}_i \cdot \min(\phi_i, 0.1) \tag{25}$$

  The weighted average rotation vector is:

$$\boldsymbol{\omega}_{\text{opt}} = \frac{\sum_{i\in\mathcal{I}} w_i \boldsymbol{\omega}_i}{\sum_{i\in\mathcal{I}} w_i} \tag{26}$$

  Magnitude limits ($t_{\max} = 2 \cdot g_{\text{target}}$, $\omega_{\max} = 0.05$ rad) are applied:

$$\mathbf{t}_{\text{final}} = \begin{cases} \mathbf{t}_{\text{opt}} & \text{if } \|\mathbf{t}_{\text{opt}}\|_2 \le t_{\max} \\ \frac{\mathbf{t}_{\text{opt}}}{\|\mathbf{t}_{\text{opt}}\|_2} \cdot t_{\max} & \text{otherwise} \end{cases} \tag{27}$$

$$\boldsymbol{\omega}_{\text{final}} = \begin{cases} \boldsymbol{\omega}_{\text{opt}} & \text{if } \|\boldsymbol{\omega}_{\text{opt}}\|_2 \le \omega_{\max} \\ \frac{\boldsymbol{\omega}_{\text{opt}}}{\|\boldsymbol{\omega}_{\text{opt}}\|_2} \cdot \omega_{\max} & \text{otherwise} \end{cases} \tag{28}$$

An adaptive step size α, based on $\Delta Q^{(k)} = Q^{(k)} - Q^{(k-1)}$, controls the update:

$$\alpha^{(k+1)} = \begin{cases} \min(1.2\alpha^{(k)}, \alpha_{\max}) & \text{if } \Delta Q^{(k)} > 0.01 \\ \max(0.6\alpha^{(k)}, \alpha_{\min}) & \text{if } \Delta Q^{(k)} < -0.01 \\ \alpha^{(k)} & \text{otherwise} \end{cases} \tag{29}$$

d. Convergence Criteria The algorithm converges when one of four multi-level criteria is met [Eq. (30)], (where $\delta_g = 0.005$ mm, $\epsilon_Q = 0.001$, $m = 3$):

$$\text{Converged} \Leftrightarrow \begin{cases} (|\bar{g} - g_{\text{target}}| < \delta_g) \wedge (N_{\text{pen}} = 0) \wedge (S > 0.95) & \text{(Ideal State)} \\ (N_{\text{pen}} = 0) \wedge (g_{\min} > 0.01) \wedge (Q > 0.8) & \text{(Safe State)} \\ |\Delta Q| < \epsilon_Q, \forall k \in [k-m, k] & \text{(Stagnation)} \\ Q > 0.9 \wedge N_{\text{pen}} \le 2 & \text{(Sufficient Quality)} \end{cases} \tag{30}$$

3 Experimental Results

We evaluated MAGIC-OR against the original registration results from the scanner on 49 clinical cases.

3.1 Objective Evaluation

Multiple metrics were used to quantify registration quality. As summarized in Table 1, MAGIC-OR demonstrated consistent and statistically significant improvements over the original method.

Table 1. Comparative analysis results of objective metrics.

Evaluation metric	Original	MAGIC-OR	p-value
Relative change in Centroid distance (mm)	0.065 ± 0.12	**0.089 ± 0.12**	<0.05
Occlusal Gap (mm)	0.0192 ± 8.4e-04	**0.0119 ± 5.2e-04**	<0.05
Contact Density (%)	0.065 ± 0.001	**0.089 ± 0.002**	<0.05
Normal Vector Alignment	0.817 ± 0.008	**0.905 ± 0.001**	<0.05

Figure 3 illustrates the per-sample performance metrics. The reduction in centroid distance (Fig. 3a) and occlusal gap (Fig. 3b) indicates improved global convergence. The improvement in normal alignment (Fig. 3c) supports the effectiveness of the 6-DOF pose optimization. Average contact density also increased (Fig. 3d), reflecting more extensive occlusal contacts.

3.2 Subjective Clinical Evaluation

Three experienced clinicians (¿10 years) performed a single-blind, randomized evaluation of all 49 case pairs. They graded the results on a 4-point scale (4: Excellent, 3: Good, 2: Fair, 1: Poor) based on occlusal contact, model integrity (penetration), and clinical acceptability.

Subjective clinical evaluation results are shown in Table 2. The original method had 23 cases (47%) rated "Poor", whereas MAGIC-OR had only 3 (6%). Our method achieved "Good" or "Excellent" ratings in 39 cases (80%), with 33 cases (67%) rated "Excellent." The mean clinical acceptability score increased significantly from 2.16 to 3.58 (p¡ 0.05), confirming the clinical utility of the proposed method.

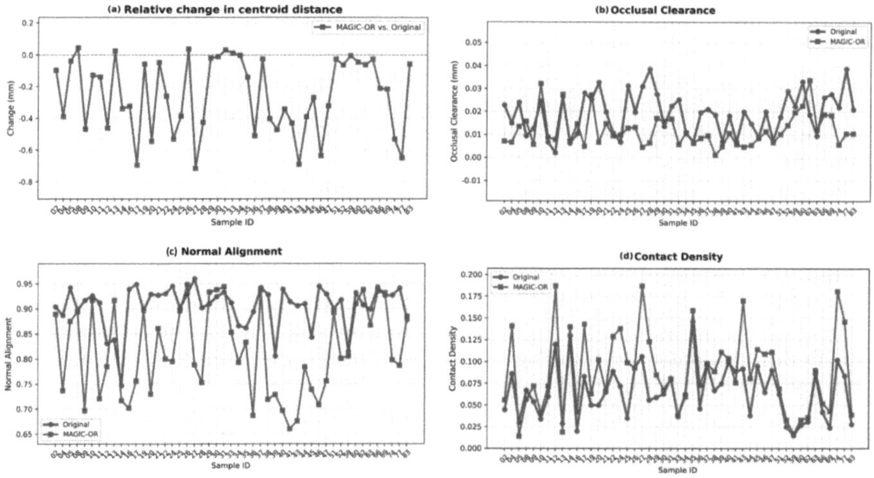

Fig. 3. Performance metrics comparison of the proposed MAGIC-OR framework against the original registration for different samples.

Table 2. Subjective clinical evaluation results.

Evaluation	Excellent	Good	Fair	Poor	Average score
Original	12	7	7	23	2.16 ± 0.74
MAGIC-OR	**33**	6	7	**3**	**3.58 ± 0.61**

4 Conclusions

This study presented MAGIC-OR, an innovative framework for maxillomandibular registration that addresses the critical challenge of limited inter-arch overlap. By integrating a dual-buccal optimization strategy with geometry-constrained refinement, our approach demonstrates significant improvements over conventional methods. Validation across 49 clinical cases confirmed the framework's robustness, showing significant improvements in both objective metrics (e.g., occlusal gap, contact density) and subjective clinical evaluations, with "excellent" ratings increasing from 24% to 67%.

Our future work will focus on a systematic parameter analysis to identify key factors that influence the accuracy of the registration, allowing adaptive parameter tuning in diverse clinical scenarios. Additionally, specialized modules will be developed to handle complex cases–such as severe tooth penetration in deep bite malocclusions and partially edentulous arches–using weighted optimization schemes.

Acknowledgments. This research was funded by the Shenzhen Science and Technology Program (grant No.JCYJ20220531103014033).This work was supported by the University-level Research Project of Shenzhen Polytechnic (No.6026310043K)

References

1. Sahab, L., Newton, J.T., Sabbah, W.: Oral health and healthy ageing: a systematic review of longitudinal studies. Dent. J. (Basel) **13**(7), 303 (2025)
2. Duong, H.Y., Roccuzzo, A., Stähli, A., et al.: Oral health-related quality of life of patients rehabilitated with fixed and removable implant-supported dental prostheses. Periodontol 2000 **88**(1), 201–237 (2022). https://doi.org/10.1111/prd.12419
3. Assoratgoon, I., Putra, R.H., Hihara, H., et al.: Occlusal contact changes in implant-supported fixed prostheses: a systematic review. J. Oral Rehabil. **52**(11), 2185–2194 (2025)
4. Siqueira, R., Galli, M., Chen, Z., Mendonça, G., Meirelles, L., Wang, H.-L., Chan, H.-L.: Intraoral scanning reduces procedure time and improves patient comfort in fixed prosthodontics and implant dentistry: a systematic review. Clin. Oral Invest. **25**(12), 6517–6531 (2021). https://doi.org/10.1007/s00784-021-04157-3
5. Besl, P.J., Mckay, N.D.: A method for registration of 3-d shapes. IEEE Trans. Pattern Anal. Mach. Intell. **14**, 239–256 (1992). https://doi.org/10.1109/34.121791
6. Chen, A., Zhuang, J., Han, X.: An improved ICP algorithm for 3D point cloud registration. In: Proceedings of the 3rd International Conference on Pattern Recognition and Machine Learning (PRML), pp. 205–210. Chengdu, China (2022). https://doi.org/10.1109/PRML56267.2022.9882220
7. Li, P., Wang, R., Wang, Y., Tao, W.: Evaluation of the ICP algorithm in 3D point cloud registration. IEEE Access **8**, 68030–68048 (2020). https://doi.org/10.1109/ACCESS.2020.2986470
8. Aoki, Y., Goforth, H., Srivatsan, R., Lucey, S.: PointNetLK: Robust & efficient point cloud registration using PointNet. In: 2019 IEEE/CVF Conference on Computer Vision and Pattern Recognition (CVPR), pp. 7156–7165. Long Beach, CA, USA (2019). https://doi.org/10.1109/CVPR.2019.00733
9. Tian, S., Dai, N., Zhang, B., Yuan, F., Yu, Q., Cheng, X.: Automatic classification and segmentation of teeth on 3D dental model using hierarchical deep learning networks. IEEE Access **7**, 84817–84828 (2019). https://doi.org/10.1109/ACCESS.2019.2924262
10. Wang, H., Huang, L., Yu, K., Song, T., et al.: Deep-learning-based multiview RGBD sensor system for 3-D face point cloud registration. IEEE Sensors Lett. **7**(5), 1–4 (2023). https://doi.org/10.1109/LSENS.2023.3267948, art no. 7001804
11. Weber, M., Wild, D., Kleesiek, J., et al.: Deep learning-based point cloud registration for augmented reality-guided surgery. In: Proceedings of the 2024 IEEE International Symposium on Biomedical Imaging (ISBI), pp. 1–5. Athens, Greece (2024). https://doi.org/10.1109/ISBI56570.2024.10635333
12. Zhang, Z., Dai, Y., Sun, J.: Deep learning based point cloud registration: an overview. VRIH **2**(3), 222–246 (2020)
13. Zhuang, S., Wei, G., Cui, Z., Zhou, Y.: Robust hybrid learning for automatic teeth segmentation and labeling on 3D dental models. IEEE Trans. Multimedia **27**, 792–803 (2025). https://doi.org/10.1109/TMM.2023.3289760

Mental Health and Disease Prediction

Breast-Rehab: A Postoperative Breast Cancer Rehabilitation Training Assessment System Based on Human Action Recognition

Zikang Chen[1], Tan Xie[2], Qinchuan Wang[2], Heming Zheng[2], and Xudong Lu[1](✉)

[1] Zhejiang University, Hangzhou 310058, China
lvxd@zju.edu.cn

[2] Zhejiang University School of Medicine Sir Run Run Shaw Hospital, Hangzhou 310058, China

Abstract. Postoperative upper limb dysfunction is prevalent among breast cancer survivors, yet their adherence to at-home rehabilitation exercises is low amidst limited nursing resources. The hardware overhead of commonly adopted VR-based mHealth solutions further hinders their widespread clinical application. Therefore, we developed Breast-Rehab, a novel, low-cost mHealth system to provide patients with out-of-hospital upper limb rehabilitation management. Breast-Rehab integrates a bespoke human action recognition algorithm with a retrieval-augmented generation (RAG) framework. By fusing visual and 3D skeletal data, our model accurately segments exercise videos recorded in uncontrolled home environments, outperforming standard models. These segmented clips, combined with a domain-specific knowledge base, guide a multi-modal large language model to generate clinically relevant assessment reports. This approach significantly reduces computational overhead and mitigates model hallucinations. We implemented the system as a WeChat Mini Program and a nurse-facing dashboard. A preliminary clinical study validated the system's feasibility and user acceptance, with patients achieving an average exercise frequency of 0.59 sessions/day over a two-week period. This work thus presents a complete, validated pipeline for AI-driven, at-home rehabilitation monitoring.

Keywords: Breast cancer · Postoperative rehabilitation · Human action recognition · Multi-modal large language model · mHealth

1 Introduction

Up to 82% of breast cancer survivors may suffer from treatment-related morbidities, especially upper limb dysfunction. Approximately 10% to 60% of women report symptoms related to upper limb dysfunction from 2 months to 3 years after surgery [10], and these symptoms often persist. Clinical experiments have

Y. Zhang et al. (Eds.): CHIP 2025, CCIS 2884, pp. 141–159, 2026.
https://doi.org/10.1007/978-981-95-7299-1_9

shown that nursing interventions, such as evidence-based care [15] and continuous personalized care [7], can effectively improve survivors' quality of life and shoulder mobility. However, the sheer volume of breast cancer survivors means that health institutions lack sufficient human resources to provide such services to all patients. In response, Brennan et al. [2] argued for the urgent need for mHealth systems to help patients adhere to correct postoperative exercises.

In the field of breast cancer limb rehabilitation, some studies have explored using Virtual Reality (VR) to enhance interactivity and guide patients through correct rehabilitation movements. A 2024 meta-analysis by Chen et al. [5] of seven studies in this area concluded that VR-based interventions could improve upper limb function and reduce postoperative pain, but did not show statistically significant differences in lymphedema. The paper noted that the small sample sizes in the field might introduce bias in the conclusions. Furthermore, the high cost of VR equipment currently limits its widespread clinical adoption.

With the development of multi-modal large language models (mm-LLMs), research related to exercise and rehabilitation has begun to incorporate multimodal information such as vision. The UbiPhysio system, developed by Wang et al. [12] at Tsinghua University, first collected joint skeletal data for 18 actions such as "sweeping the floor" and "getting out of bed" using multiple sensors. Then it used this skeletal information to classify actions and fed the skeletal data, action classification, and retrieved knowledge base information into a unimodal LLM to provide feedback to the user. Wang et al. [13] from Zhejiang Lab designed RehabGPT, a system intended to provide action analysis and guidance based on training plans and videos, using image feature extraction, human mesh reconstruction, and text-video matching. However, their paper lacked detailed methodological descriptions and was not tested in a real clinical setting. Sun et al. [11] from Tsinghua University, Shenzhen, designed a Rehabilitation Exercise Guidance System (REGS) to assess the correctness of movements based on temporal skeletal data against standards provided by physical therapists and to offer intervention information. This study included five actions, such as the "glute bridge," and used GPT-generated simulated consultation requests to test the system, comparing its feedback with expert responses.

While these studies have explored the potential of mm-LLMs in the health and fitness domain, no intelligent system specifically for postoperative breast cancer rehabilitation has been developed and applied. For the scenario addressed in this study, postoperative rehabilitation for breast cancer involves numerous exercises, some requiring additional equipment such as resistance bands. Videos uploaded by patients at home often have complex backgrounds and contain a lot of irrelevant information [8]. Directly inputting these videos into an mm-LLM would make it difficult for the model to align action information with the actual video frames, leading to inaccurate assessments and even severe hallucinations [1], such as evaluating actions that were not performed. This observation is also substantiated in the Fig. 5 of this study. Moreover, the long video lengths impose a significant computational burden, making the system's time and economic costs prohibitive. To address this, both Wang et al. [12] and Sun et al. [11] employed action recognition algorithms. However, Wang et al.'s research relied on sensor data collection, which is resource-intensive. Sun et al.'s study was conducted in a more controlled environment with a fixed background and less complex actions compared to the at-home management scenario, making direct application of their methods unfeasible.

Furthermore, existing mm-LLMs have not been specifically trained for the breast cancer domain, resulting in generic and superficial evaluations of postoperative rehabilitation exercises that lack sufficient domain knowledge. Therefore, a knowledge-enhancement process is needed to enable the mm-LLM to generate clinically valuable assessment reports. The primary challenge in building this system is to accurately recognize and evaluate the diverse set of upper limb rehabilitation exercises from videos recorded by patients in complex home environments.

To address these challenges, this study developed the Breast-Rehab system, which is based on an action recognition algorithm and an mm-LLM. The system processes postoperative exercise videos uploaded by patients from a WeChat Mini Program, accurately identifying and segmenting key exercise frames. By integrating a breast cancer knowledge base and a retrieval-augmented generation (RAG) algorithm, it employs prompt engineering to drive an mm-LLM to generate a detailed assessment report for each exercise session. This report is displayed on both the patient's interface and a dashboard for healthcare professionals, aiding patients in improving their exercises and facilitating remote monitoring and management.

The main contributions of this study are threefold:

1. We designed an action recognition algorithm that fuses image information and 3D skeleton data. On a small-sample dataset of patient postoperative exercise videos, this algorithm outperformed mainstream mm-LLMs in zero-shot and few-shot settings, as well as other existing action classification models.
2. We conducted a subjective human evaluation of assessment reports generated for 11 real exercise videos and compared the performance with other models. The results showed that the Breast-Rehab system reduces computational overhead, minimizes model hallucinations, and improves report quality.
3. Building upon the algorithmic achievements, we implemented a patient-facing WeChat Mini Program and a clinician-facing dashboard. A subsequent two-week preliminary clinical study with 15 enrolled patients demonstrated that the system helped users maintain an average exercise frequency of 0.5 sessions per day.

2 Method

2.1 System Workflow

The workflow of the Breast-Rehab system is illustrated in Fig. 1a. Patients register and link their postoperative exercise plan through a WeChat Mini Program. They then use their phone's front camera to record and upload their exercise videos to the server. The server invokes an action recognition algorithm to identify and extract action sub-videos, filtering out background noise irrelevant to the exercise. These sub-videos, along with a knowledge base of 1 million chunks developed in our prior Breast-CRAG [6] study, are fed into an mm-LLM to generate an assessment report. The report is then presented to both the patient and the healthcare provider via the WeChat Mini Program and a web dashboard, respectively.

This study received ethical approval from the Sir Run Run Shaw Hospital, affiliated with Zhejiang University School of Medicine (Approval No. 2025-0529, Acceptance No. 2025-2535-01). All participating patients provided signed informed consent.

Next, we will detail the action recognition and RAG report generation algorithms, followed by the system implementation of Breast-Rehab. Codes are available at https://github.com/Maxin-C/Breast-Rehab.

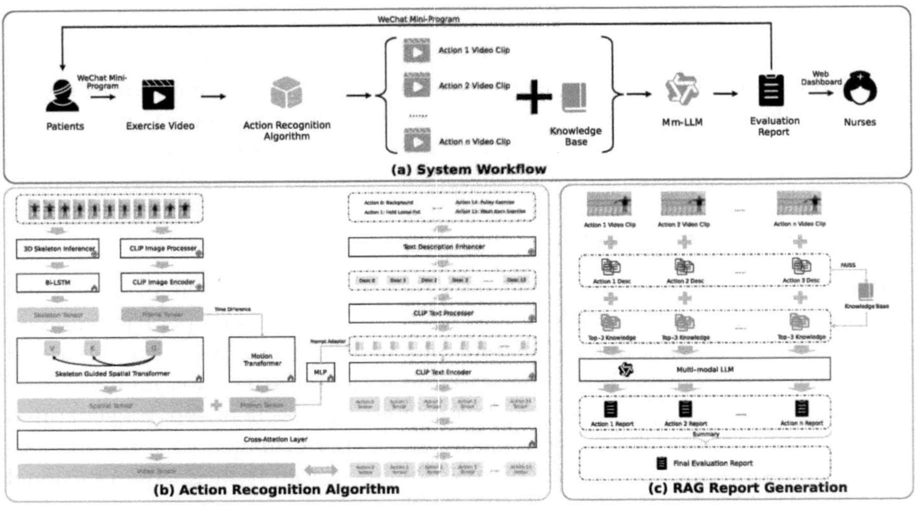

Fig. 1. Breast-Rehab method overview

2.2 Action Recognition Algorithm

Our algorithm design was inspired by the work of Wang et al. [14], incorporating the motion transformer and MCB as core components, and was enhanced with skeleton information to focus the algorithm's attention on the upper body movements, thereby improving action classification accuracy. Our proposed model recognizes human actions by deeply integrating visual, skeletal, and textual modalities through a novel skeleton-guided and motion-prompted architecture. The model takes two primary inputs: a video clip, represented as a sequence of N_f

frames $I \in \mathbb{R}^{B \times N_f \times 3 \times H \times W}$, and a corresponding sequence of processed skeleton features $S \in \mathbb{R}^{B \times N_f \times 17}$, where B is the batch size. The skeleton features were meticulously engineered from 3D human pose data extracted using OpenPose [3]. For each frame, we selected 13 keypoints corresponding to the upper body. From these keypoints, we computed four biomechanically significant joint angles: the left elbow, right elbow, left shoulder, and right shoulder angles. The angle θ_b at a joint b formed by adjacent joints a and c was calculated using the dot product between the vectors connecting the joints, based on their 3D coordinates $(\boldsymbol{p}_a, \boldsymbol{p}_b, \boldsymbol{p}_c)$:

$$\theta_b = \arccos\left(\frac{(\boldsymbol{p}_a - \boldsymbol{p}_b) \cdot (\boldsymbol{p}_c - \boldsymbol{p}_b)}{\|\boldsymbol{p}_a - \boldsymbol{p}_b\| \|\boldsymbol{p}_c - \boldsymbol{p}_b\| + \epsilon}\right) \tag{1}$$

ϵ is a very small value used to ensure that the denominator is not zero. The final 17-dimensional feature vector for each frame is a concatenation of features derived from the 13 selected keypoints and these four calculated angles.

The model architecture is a dual-stream process generating distinct spatial and motion representations. The spatial stream begins by processing the frame sequence I through a pre-trained CLIP vision encoder, Φ_I, to obtain frame-level visual features, $V_{seq} \in \mathbb{R}^{B \times N_f \times D}$, where D is the embedding dimension. In parallel, the engineered skeleton sequence S is fed into a Skeleton Temporal Encoder, comprising a bidirectional LSTM, to capture its temporal dynamics, yielding skeleton features $K_s \in \mathbb{R}^{B \times N_f \times D}$. These modalities are fused using a Guided Spatial Transformer, which functions as a Transformer decoder, using V_{seq} as the query and K_s as the key and value. This produces a spatially-aware feature sequence T_s. Concurrently, the motion stream models temporal changes by applying a Motion Transformer to the pairwise differences of V_{seq}, learning a high-level motion representation $T_m \in \mathbb{R}^{B \times N_m \times D}$. The final video representation $V \in \mathbb{R}^{B \times 1 \times D}$ is obtained by summing the mean-pooled features from both streams: $V = \text{AvgPool}(T_s) + \text{AvgPool}(T_m)$.

To achieve a fine-grained, domain-specific alignment between video and text, we utilized class descriptions generated in a novel manner. Instead of generic labels, our text prompts are detailed motion descriptions produced by an mm-LLM. This model was prompted with the official illustrated manual for post-operative upper limb rehabilitation exercises for breast cancer patients, which was originally compiled by nursing staff. This ensures our text modality is rich with clinical context and precise terminology. To make these descriptions video-specific, we inject a dynamic motion prompt $P_m = \text{MotionAdapter}(T_m)$ generated from the video's motion features T_m. For each video, this prompt P_m is prepended to the token embeddings of every class description, $[P_m; E_{text}]$. The concatenated sequence is processed by our custom CLIP text transformer, Φ_T^{cus}, yielding a set of motion-aware text features $T \in \mathbb{R}^{B \times N_c \times D}$ for all N_c classes.

Finally, to further enhance alignment, both the video feature V and text features T are fed into a cross-attention layer. This layer employs two parallel cross-attention layers to refine each modality using information from the other:

$$T' = \text{LayerNorm}(T + \text{CrossAttention}(Q = T, K = V, V = V)), \quad (2)$$
$$V' = \text{LayerNorm}(V + \text{CrossAttention}(Q = V, K = T, V = T)). \quad (3)$$

The final classification is performed by computing the cosine similarity between the enhanced video feature V' and text features T'. The resulting logits are scaled by a learnable temperature parameter τ and optimized using a cross-entropy loss.

$$\text{logits} = \exp(\tau) \cdot \frac{V' \cdot T'}{\|V'\| \|T'\|} \quad (4)$$

2.3 RAG Report Generation

The process of RAG report generation is shown in Fig. 1c. The knowledge base for RAG was derived from the breast cancer knowledge base designed in our previous Breast-CRAG study. This knowledge base contains 1 million chunks, each 100 tokens long, from English and Chinese books and guidelines on breast cancer (including nursing-related literature). These chunks were encoded using a retriever fine-tuned in the Breast-CRAG [6] study, and a FAISS database was constructed using the chunk embeddings as indices for retrieval.

For each segmented sub-video, the corresponding action description for its action class was identified. The embedding of this text description was then used as a query to search the database, retrieving the top 3 most relevant content chunks as a source for knowledge enhancement. Since the retrieval process in this RAG task is static, we consolidated the retrieved knowledge chunks during the experiment to reduce computational overhead during inference.

Considering the limited video input window of the mm-LLM, we first processed each action's sub-video by feeding it into the mm-LLM along with its corresponding action description and related knowledge to obtain an assessment for that single action. These individual assessments were then integrated into a comprehensive report. The prompt design is detailed in Appendix A.

2.4 System Implement

The front end of the Breast-Rehab system was developed using HTML, JS, and CSS. The server uses MySQL as the database and Flask as the backend. The system comprises a patient-side WeChat Mini Program and a nurse-side dashboard (as shown in Fig. 2).

After registration, users can record their exercise sessions on the exercise page by activating the front camera. During recording, the position of the user's upper body is monitored at a rate 1 Hz. If the skeleton nodes of the left and right shoulders move out of the camera's field of view, the recording is paused, and the patient is prompted to reposition themselves within the frame (Fig. 2a). When logging into the system, users can choose whether to subscribe to an exercise reminder at 8 a.m. the next day, helping patients manage their personal exercise progress. The mini-program includes exercise tutorial videos filmed by the nursing team of Sir Run Run Shaw Hospital, allowing patients to learn exercise movements at any time. Figure 2b shows the interaction page for a specific patient on the nurse's dashboard, accessible from the patient list. This page displays the user's basic information, exercise records, segmented exercise videos, and the intelligent report. Nurses can evaluate and provide feedback on the generated reports to help with future system optimization.

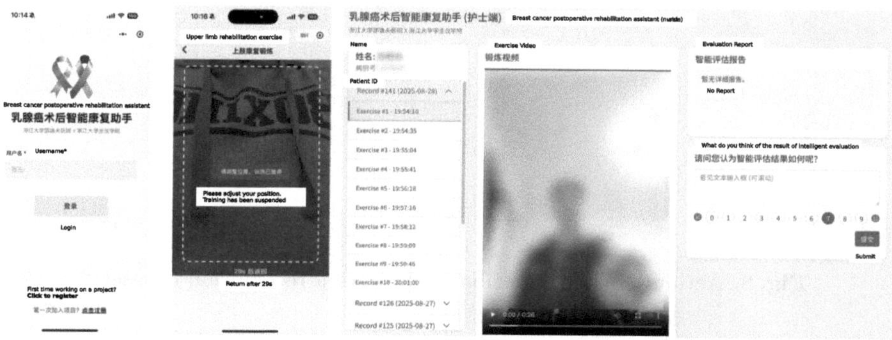

(a) Patient Side Wechat Miniprogram (b) Nurse Side Dashboard

Fig. 2. Breast-Rehab user interface

3 Experiment

3.1 Action Recognition Algorithm

Based on the definitions and requirements for postoperative upper limb functional exercises for breast cancer patients from the Sir Run Run Shaw Hospital's manual, we included 15 different rehabilitation exercises. Before clinical deployment, we collected 14 portrait-mode videos (30 fps) shot with smartphones in real-world scenarios, where the exerciser's upper body was visible throughout. Using these videos, we manually annotated the action classes on the timeline with the open-source software labelU, including 15 action labels and one "no action" label.

Based on the annotations, we constructed a dataset by extracting video frames using a sliding window approach. The rule was to sample one frame every 6 frames, with a window size of 60 frames and a stride of 21 frames. This resulted in a dataset of 10-frame sequences, where each sequence had a label for each frame and an overall label. If the labels within a 10-frame sequence were inconsistent, the most frequent label was chosen as the overall label. In case of a tie, the action label was prioritized over the "no action" label. The first 10 videos were used as the training set, and the remaining 4 videos were shuffled and split equally into validation and test sets. There was no data overlap between the training and test sets. Ultimately, this process yielded 5,445 training samples and 902 samples each for the validation and test sets. The label distribution of the dataset is shown in Fig. 3.

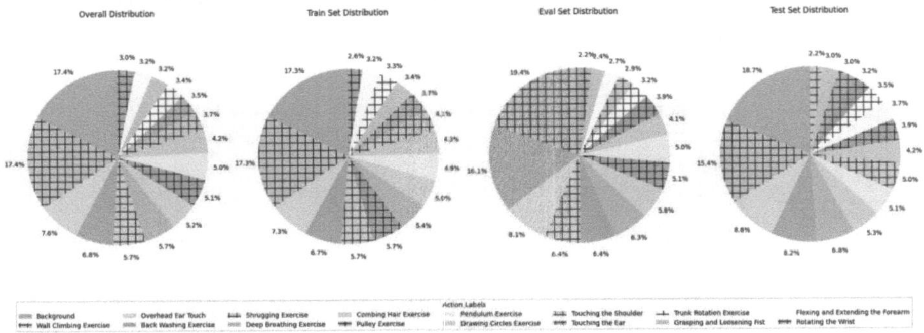

Fig. 3. Action label distribution in the action recognition dataset.

On the test set, we compared our model against several baselines, including action recognition models from pre-trained mm-LLMs and an established action recognition model. The mm-LLMs included were Qwen-VL-Max (Qwen-VL) [16] and GPT-4o-2024-08-06 (GPT-4o) [9], evaluated in both zero-shot and few-shot settings (prompt designs in Appendix B). The established action recognition model was the one proposed by Wang et al. [14] (abbreviated as CLIP-AR), which we reference. For a fair comparison, this model was trained on our training set. Evaluation metrics included F1-score (weighted), top-1 accuracy, and top-3 accuracy. (Top-3 accuracy was not considered for mm-LLMs as they output direct results).

To validate the value of our algorithm design without repeating the evaluation of the referenced design, we conducted an ablation study. We sequentially removed the skeleton-related components: skeleton information, the Skeleton Temporal Encoder, and the Guided Spatial Transformer. Without skeleton information, our model is identical to CLIP-AR, so we could reuse its results. When the Skeleton Temporal Encoder was removed, an MLP (with a hidden layer dimension matching the encoder) was used to map the 17-dimensional skeleton data to K_s. When the Guided Spatial Transformer was removed, an MLP (with a hidden layer dimension matching the transformer) was used to map the concatenated vector of V_{seq} and K_s to a vector with the same dimension as T_s.

3.2 RAG Report Generation

The dataset for report evaluation consisted of 11 real exercise videos collected from users during clinical application. The objective was to compare the quality of reports generated by an open-source action understanding model, standard mm-LLMs, and mm-LLMs enhanced by the Breast-Rehab system using real-world videos. The open-source action understanding model included was motion-LLM [4], a model released in 2024 capable of understanding actions from video input. The standard mm-LLMs were Qwen-VL and GPT-4o, as in the previous experiment. The Breast-Rehab enhanced models were the same mm-LLMs.

Given that exercise videos are often around 10 min long, feeding the entire video into a model at once would overload the input. Therefore, we divided the videos into 45-second chunks, sampling one frame per second, and fed them into the models batch by batch. The results were then aggregated by a large language model (for motionLLM, we used Qwen-VL for aggregation). Similarly, although Breast-Rehab segments the videos into action-specific sub-videos, these can still be too long. Thus, longer sub-videos also followed the batch processing approach before their reports were aggregated. The prompts used for processing sub-videos and integrating their reports are shown in Appendix A.

Due to the lack of a benchmark, the reports were evaluated manually. We asked nurses from the breast surgery department at Sir Run Run Shaw Hospital to first watch the videos and then evaluate the content generated by the five models. The evaluation was single-blinded; the evaluators were unaware of which model produced which content. A 10-point Likert scale was used for quantitative assessment (see Table 1). A higher score indicates greater agreement with the statement, signifying better model performance on that dimension. Data was collected via Tencent Questionnaire, and all user faces in the videos were blurred.

Table 1. Likert scale design for human evaluation of reports.

Dimension	Content
Accuracy	The model accurately identified and described the errors that occurred in the exercise videos
Completeness	Compared to the critical issues you observe in the video, the model does not appear to miss significant points
Practicability	The corrective suggestions given by the model are specific and practical
Safety	There is no potential risk of harm in the assessment recommendations given by the model
Language quality	The assessment report is fluent and easy to understand

Based on the evaluation results, we first performed descriptive statistics on the mean and variance of the scores for each model across the five dimensions. Then, after conducting a Shapiro-Wilk test for normality, we used either an independent samples t-test or a Mann-Whitney U test to compare whether there was a statistically significant difference in the scores of the same mm-LLM with and without Breast-Rehab enhancement.

3.3 System Implement

We promoted the system and recruited postoperative breast cancer patients for a two-week study from August 23, 2025, to September 6, 2025, by distributing flyers. To verify patients' compliance with upper limb rehabilitation exercises for breast cancer under the Breast-Rehab system, this study objectively measures this indicator based on the average number of exercise sessions and the average exercise frequency. The average number of exercise sessions is calculated by dividing the total number of exercise sessions recorded by all enrolled patients using the system during the experimental period by the total number of enrolled patients. The exercise frequency is calculated by dividing the number of exercise sessions of a single patient by the number of days they were enrolled. The average exercise frequency is obtained by dividing the total exercise frequency by the total number of enrolled patients. For subjective evaluation, this study collected feedback from nurses and patients who used the Breast-Rehab system and summarized the current strengths and weaknesses of the system.

4 Result

4.1 Action Recognition Algorithm

The evaluation results on the test set are shown in Fig. 4a. The results indicate that Qwen-VL and GPT-4o achieved an accuracy of less than 50% on this dataset. Although few-shot learning with contextual information improved accuracy by about 10%, it was still insufficient for practical application. Furthermore, the inference speed of these models was excessively slow for long contexts and multiple video inputs. Qwen-VL (few-shot) averaged 11 s per data point (10 frames), while GPT-4o (few-shot) averaged 140 s per case. Even considering that GPT-4o's performance might be affected by network issues in China, the inference time of the domestic mm-LLM was still prohibitive. After training on the training set, the CLIP-AR model achieved a better accuracy (0.60) than the mm-LLMs, with a top-3 accuracy of 0.80. By incorporating skeleton information, our model's accuracy improved by about 10%, reaching 0.72.

The confusion matrix for our model (showing precision percentages) is depicted in Fig. 4c. The model achieved a precision of over 50% for all classes. The three actions with the lowest precision were "touching the ear" (0.548), "combing hair exercise" (0.576), and "shrugging exercise" (0.523). "Touching the ear" was most frequently misclassified as "touching the shoulder". This is partly because these two exercises can be performed interchangeably according to the manual, leading to frequent switching between them in the dataset, which biased the model towards predicting "touching the shoulder". Additionally, the only difference between these two actions is whether the affected limb touches the ipsilateral ear or the contralateral shoulder, with other body parts remaining consistent. This distinction is even less clear when the patient alternates between the two, making it difficult for the model to differentiate. "Combing hair exercise" was misclassified as "touching the ear" and "overhead ear touch".

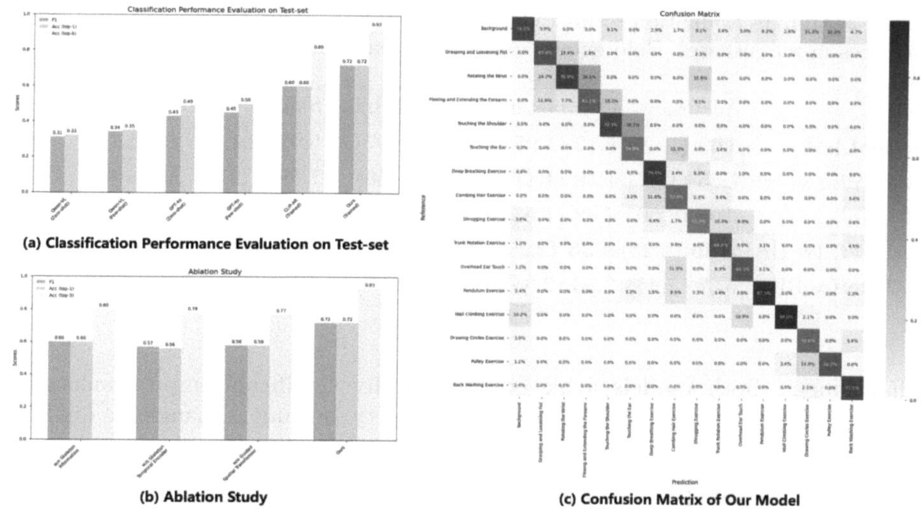

Fig. 4. Action recognition algorithm evaluation result

The arm movement in "combing hair exercise" is similar to the other two, with the hand just positioned slightly higher (touching the top of the head instead of the ear). The model needs to precisely distinguish the hand's position relative to the head to separate these actions, hence the lower precision. The challenge with "shrugging exercise" lies in its subtle range of motion. During shrugging, only the shoulder joint moves slightly. When recorded from the front, both skeleton and image data show only minor vertical movement of the shoulder, providing very weak features and causing the model to misclassify it as other actions.

4.2 Report Evaluation

For the human evaluation, five nurses assessed the outputs of five models on forms created from 11 sets of videos. The evaluation results for the reports from the five models are shown in Table 2. The results indicate that motionLLM performed the worst in this experiment. From a mean score perspective, Breast-Rehab improved the performance of both Qwen-VL and GPT-4o across all five dimensions. Furthermore, Qwen-VL performed better than GPT-4o in both with and without Breast-Rehab scenarios and achieved the highest scores on four of the five metrics.

A Shapiro-Wilk test was used to assess the normality of the evaluation results for the four models excluding motionLLM. The results showed that all p-values were greater than 0.05, indicating that the data did not follow a normal distribution. Therefore, the Mann-Whitney U test was used to compare the performance difference of the models with and without Breast-Rehab enhancement. The results are shown in Table 3. The results indicate that with Breast-Rehab

Table 2. Human evaluation result (The values in the table are the mean scores, with variances in parentheses. Bold entries are the optimal scores).

	Accuracy	Completeness	Practicability	Safety	Language quality
MotionLLM	5.69 (1.98)	5.12 (1.95)	5.73 (1.97)	5.92 (2.11)	7.10 (2.01)
Qwen-VL	7.55 (1.47)	7.49 (1.17)	7.42 (1.50)	7.59 (1.37)	7.66 (1.45)
GPT-4o	7.05 (2.30)	7.48 (1.67)	7.30 (2.14)	7.40 (1.03)	7.63 (1.09)
Qwen-VL (w BR)	**7.89** (2.25)	**8.33** (2.25)	**8.00** (1.78)	7.89 (3.36)	**8.00** (0.75)
GPT-4o (w BR)	7.87 (2.45)	7.93 (2.55)	7.64 (1.27)	**7.93** (1.58)	7.53 (1.98)

enhancement, both models achieved statistically significant improvements in Accuracy, Completeness, Practicability and Safety, but not in Language quality.

Table 3. P-values of Mann-Whitney U test (Bold values indicate statistical differences, α=0.05)

	Accuracy	Completeness	Practicability	Safety	Language quality
Qwen-VL	**0.0415**	**0.0028**	0.5086	**0.0496**	0.5037
GPT-4o	**0.0008**	0.2577	**0.0241**	0.1212	0.7306

A detailed analysis of the output content revealed several issues with models that did not have Breast-Rehab enhancement, as shown in Fig. 5: (1) Recognition Failure: The model struggled to correctly understand and extract information from the video content. This was most evident in motionLLM's analysis. The initial failure in recognition led to a lack of informative content in the final report, resulting in poor quality. (2) Hallucination: For standard mm-LLMs, due to their limited action recognition capabilities, they often misclassified action types during segmented analysis. This led to the hallucination of non-existent actions and their evaluation in the summary report. (3) Evaluation Error: Without the enhancement of additional action descriptions and related knowledge, the mm-LLM might judge an incorrect action as correct, leading to erroneous evaluations in the final report.

4.3 System Implement

During the experiment, flyers were distributed to a total of 25 patients, 15 of whom joined the Breast-Rehab program, representing a participation rate of 60% (15/25). According to the definition of objective indicators in the Experiment section, the total number of exercise sessions recorded by patients during the study was 57, with an average of 3.8 sessions per patient (57/15). Four patients exercised more than 5 times, with the highest number of sessions being 12. The average exercise frequency was 0.59. The highest and lowest exercise frequencies

Recognition failure	✖ MotionLLM: The motion doesn't provide specific details about the motion, but it's likely that the person is performing a series of movements to simulate the actions of a person walking.
Hallucination	Video 8: Contains Action [6,7,8,9,10,11,12,13,14,15] ✖ **GPT-4o: (Hallucinated action 5, missing actions 6, 7, and 9)** Movement Evaluation and Feedback - Action 8: Shoulder Shrugs: Standardization Analysis: ... - Action 5: Touching the Ear: ... - Action 10: Overhead Ear Touch: ... - Action 11: Pendulum Exercise: ... - Action 12: Wall Climbing Exercise: ... - Action 13: Arm Circles: ... - Action 14: Pulley Exercise: ... - Action 15: Towel Stretch (Washing the Back) : ... ☑ **GPT-4o (w Breast-Rehab):** - Exercise 6: Deep Breathing Exercise: ... - Exercise 7: Hair Combing Exercise: ... - Exercise 8: Shoulder Shrugs: ... - Exercise 9: Torso Twists: ... - Exercise 10: Overhead Ear Touch: ... - Exercise 11: Pendulum Exercise: ... - Exercise 12: Wall Climbing Exercise: ... - Exercise 13: Arm Circles: ... - Exercise 14: Pulley Exercise: ... - Exercise 15: Towel Stretch (Washing the Back) : ...
Evaluation error	Video 10: The nurse determined that the patient's arm was not open during the Pendulum Exercise ✖ **GPT-4o:** **Movement Name**: Pendulum Exercise - **Itemized Evaluation**: - **Standardization**: The movement meets the description, performed with a bent-over standing posture and arms abducting and adducting in a crossed motion. - **Quality of Execution**: The movement is completed smoothly with a moderate range of motion. - **Potential Risks**: The range of motion is moderate, posing a low risk. - **Feedback**: - **Strengths**: The movement rhythm is even, and good balance is maintained. - **Suggestions for Improvement**: Consider increasing the range and frequency of the movement to further enhance shoulder flexibility. ☑ **GPT-4o (w Breast-Rehab):** ## Exercise 11: Pendulum Exercise ### Itemized Evaluation - **Standardization**: The forward bending of the body is not pronounced enough, and the range of motion of the arms is limited. - **Quality of Execution**: The movement lacks fluidity and is performed at a moderate speed. ### Feedback - **Strengths**: The basic movement is completed. - **Suggestions for Improvement**: Increase the degree of forward bending and the range of motion of the arms, focusing on improving fluidity.

Fig. 5. Typical error examples of mm-LLMs without Breast-Rehab enhancement.

were 1 session/day (3/3) and 0.25 sessions/day (1/4), respectively. This indicates that, on average, patients used the system for upper limb rehabilitation exercises once every two days. The best-case scenario involved daily exercise, while the worst-case scenario involved exercising only once over four days.

Qualitative feedback on the Breast-Rehab application was gathered through discussions with two enrolled patients and three nurses. From the patients' perspective, the greatest benefits of the system were its ability to provide exercise reminders and guidance, as well as the convenience of starting exercises at any time once they had developed a habit of using it. However, for patients who had just undergone surgery, the limited range of postoperative exercises and the lack of adequate space for exercising during hospitalization made it difficult for them to persist with using Breast-Rehab. The nurses noted that remotely monitoring patients through analytical reports allowed for a more quantitative understanding of their rehabilitation progress. This data not only facilitated better patient management but also held potential for further clinical research. Additionally, the nurses believed that providing real-time exercise guidance and feedback tailored to patients' treatment progress would further enhance user engagement.

5 Discussion

5.1 Action Recognition Algorithm

The algorithm evaluation results show that directly inputting video and prompts into current large language models suffers from two main issues: insufficient accuracy and high time and economic costs. The low accuracy may be due to the difficulty of fully describing an action with prompts, making it hard for the model to correspond. The few-shot approach improved accuracy to some extent because video-based examples better described the action categories. Furthermore, there is a gap between the embedding spaces of text prompts and video or image sequences. For the specific research scenario in this study, large models have been trained on very little relevant data, making image classification based solely on model performance difficult. By training on a small number of labeled samples, even with completely different video recording environments between the training and test sets, the model can achieve good classification performance in a specific scenario, which is intuitive.

The ablation study results indicate that adding skeleton information to the reference algorithm allows the model to focus more on the specific actions, reducing interference from environmental information and thus significantly improving accuracy. Additionally, the ablation study showed that simply mapping skeleton information with an MLP is ineffective and even detrimental to the model. Directly transforming the vector dimensions instead of using a Skeleton Temporal Encoder prevents the expression of temporal information in the skeleton data. Similarly, simply concatenating vectors instead of using a Guided Spatial Transformer fuses skeleton information as noise into the image information, not only failing to increase focus on the person but also interfering with the input vector information.

The confusion matrix results show that the model's performance significantly drops for classification tasks with small motion amplitudes or similar actions. Such tasks require the model to filter out key subtle perturbations from environmental noise for accurate recognition. Therefore, adding extra feature enhancement information, such as optical flow to focus on changes in person's movements, or increasing features of the relative positions of skeleton nodes, could potentially improve model performance, but would also increase the model's overhead. Moreover, the training set included in this experiment was relatively small for the number of action categories. Increasing model complexity on a small sample size will lead to overfitting. Therefore, future research could consider continuously collecting and annotating data during experiments to form a larger benchmark to improve model performance.

5.2 RAG Report Generation

The human evaluation of the reports shows that action understanding models like motionLLM have limited ability to understand complex videos and instructions in application scenarios beyond their benchmarks. Among the five dimensions, only language quality was close to that of other models. However, this report was generated by Qwen-VL integrating motionLLM's analysis of video clips, so the higher score in this aspect is more dependent on the summarizing model's polishing of the report. Among the typical errors, motionLLM's inability to recognize video content was particularly prominent, making it unsuitable for direct use as a local report processor.

By comparing the performance of Qwen-VL and GPT-4o with and without Breast-Rehab, it is evident that the system proposed in this study can effectively improve the accuracy of the reports generated by the model, but it has little impact on the language quality of the report itself, as language quality is more related to the language generation capabilities of the large model itself. With clear action classification, mm-LLMs are much less likely to miss or hallucinate action content, although this is limited by the accuracy of the action recognition model. Furthermore, by filtering out irrelevant background information, the model's inference overhead is also greatly reduced.

5.3 System Implement

The preliminary clinical study demonstrates that it helps patients adhere to exercise at an average frequency of approximately once every two days, with the maximum number of exercise sessions reaching 12. This indicates that the system operates stably and effectively guides patients in consistently performing rehabilitation exercises. However, based on patient feedback, those who have just undergone surgery often struggle with compliance due to inadequate hospital environments, highlighting the need for enhanced in-hospital education and improved system interaction. These improvements would help patients better understand the value of Breast-Rehab and derive positive feedback from using the system. The nurses' suggestions regarding real-time interaction can further enhance the system's interactive performance, though generating personalized interactive content and achieving high-speed inference capabilities–key to enabling real-time interaction–pose significant challenges for the next phase of Breast-Rehab's development.

However, it must be acknowledged that this experiment lacks rigorous control groups to compare changes in various indicators before and after using Breast-Rehab. Currently, we are conducting a randomized controlled trial (RCT) involving more than 50 participants, monitoring indicators such as joint range of motion over a six-week period. The study will ultimately validate the system's usability. The experimental results will be made publicly available, and related papers will be published in due course.

6 Conclusion

This study, in the field of upper limb rehabilitation exercises after breast cancer surgery, designed a motion recognition algorithm incorporating skeletal information to improve accuracy, and established a RAG-based report generation framework that integrates a knowledge base with motion recognition data. This approach reduces hallucinations in rehabilitation exercise assessment reports generated by mm-LLMs while also decreasing time and economic costs. Based on the aforementioned algorithms, a clinically applicable system was developed and deployed in a hospital for a two-week preliminary clinical study. The system helped patients maintain an average upper limb rehabilitation exercise frequency of once every two days, demonstrating its usability. This work paves the way for further clinical application and improvement of postoperative rehabilitation outcomes for patients.

A Breast-Rehab RAG Report Generation Prompt Design

```
Single action prompt:
# Role
You are a professional post-operative breast cancer rehabilitation trainer.
# Task
Please evaluate a video of a [specific individual action]. Your evaluation
needs to be highly focused and specific.
# Evaluation Subject
* Action Name: Action {action_id}
* Standard Action Description: {action_desc}
# Evaluation Instructions
Based on the standard description above and the series of video frames
provided next, conduct a detailed evaluation of the patient's action
from the following three dimensions:
1. Action Standardization: Does the posture, range of motion, and
   trajectory comply with the standard?
2. Completion Quality: Is the action complete and smooth? Is the speed
   appropriate? Is there any compensation?
3. Feedback and Suggestions: Clearly point out what was done well (strengths)
   and areas needing improvement (suggestions for improvement).
Please present your analysis in clear bullet points.

Chunk evaluation prompt:
# Role
You are a professional rehabilitation trainer analyzing a
[segment of a long video].
# Task
Please analyze only the patient's performance in the current video segment.
Your analysis will be used for subsequent summarization.
# Evaluation Subject
* Action Name: Action {action_id}
* Standard Action Description: {action_desc}
# Segment Analysis Instructions
Briefly describe the observed standardization of the patient's movement,
completion quality, strengths, and areas for improvement in this segment.

Action synthesis prompt:
# Role
You are a rehabilitation trainer tasked with synthesizing multiple video
segment analyses of a [single action].
# Task
The following are analyses of consecutive segments from a [long video].
Please integrate them into a coherent and complete evaluation report
for this [one action].
# Evaluation Subject
* Action Name: Action {action_id}
* Standard Action Description: {action_desc}
# Synthesis Instructions
Synthesize the observations from all segments to summarize the overall
performance of this action, including standardization, quality, strengths,
```

```
and suggestions for improvement.
# Below are the independent analyses of all segments:
{chunk_evaluations}

Final synthesis prompt:
# Role
You are a senior post-operative breast cancer rehabilitation trainer,
tasked with writing a summary report for a patient's rehabilitation training.
# Task
You have received independent evaluation reports for multiple rehabilitation
actions completed by the patient. Please synthesize these reports into a
comprehensive and coherent final summary.
# Summary Instructions
1. Review all independent evaluations to understand the patient's overall
   performance.
2. In the ``Overall Overview'' section, summarize the patient's common
   strengths and the most critical recurring issues.
3. In the ``Detailed Breakdown of Individual Actions'' section, organize the
   independent evaluation results for each action.
4. Ensure the report is professional, positive, and encouraging in tone.
# Below are all the independent evaluation reports:
{all_evaluations}
# Please generate the final summary report based on the above information.
```

B Action Recognition Zero-Shot and Few-Shot Prompt Design

```
Zero-shot prompt:
You are a helpful expert in action recognition. Your task is to identify
the action being performed by the person in the video. Please select the
most appropriate description from the numbered list provided below.

Action options:
{class_list_str}

Now, please identify the action in this new video.

Your response must only contain the action number. For example: 3

Few-shot prompt:
You are a helpful expert in action recognition. Your task is to identify
the action being performed by the person in the video. Please select the
most appropriate description from the numbered list provided below.

Action options:
{class_list_str}

Here are some examples:
{action_1 video} Action: 1
{action_2 video} Action: 2
```

```
...
{action_n video} Action: n

Now, please identify the action in this new video.

Your response must only contain the action number. For example: 3
```

References

1. Bae, K., Kim, J., Lee, S., Lee, S., Lee, G., Choi, J.: MASH-VLM: mitigating action-scene hallucination in video-LLMs through disentangled spatial-temporal representations. In: Proceedings of the IEEE/CVF Conference on Computer Vision and Pattern Recognition, pp. 13744–13753 (2025)
2. Brennan, L., Kessie, T., Caulfield, B.: Patient experiences of rehabilitation and the potential for an mHealth system with biofeedback after breast cancer surgery: qualitative study. JMIR Mhealth Uhealth **8**(7), e19721 (2020). https://doi.org/10.2196/19721
3. Cao, Z., Hidalgo, G., Simon, T., Wei, S.E., Sheikh, Y.: OpenPose: realtime multi-person 2D pose estimation using part affinity fields. IEEE Trans. Pattern Anal. Mach. Intell. **43**(1), 172–186 (2021). https://doi.org/10.1109/TPAMI.2019.2929257
4. Chen, L.H., Lu, S., Zeng, A., Zhang, H., Wang, B., Zhang, R., Zhang, L.: Motion-LLM: Understanding Human Behaviors from Human Motions and Videos (2024). https://doi.org/10.48550/arXiv.2405.20340
5. Chen, Y., Zhou, Z., Wu, N., Du, S., Luan, Z., Peng, X.: Effectiveness of virtual reality-based interventions for upper limb rehabilitation in breast cancer patients: systematic review and meta-analysis. Games Health J. **13**(3), 149–163 (2024). https://doi.org/10.1089/g4h.2023.0040
6. Chen, Z., Wang, Q., Liu, J., Sun, Y., Zheng, H., Li, H., Duan, H., Lu, X.: Breast-CRAG: A Breast Cancer Large Language Model Leveraging Retrieval-Augmented Generation. In: Bellazzi, R., Juarez Herrero, J.M., Sacchi, L., Zupan, B. (eds.) Artificial Intelligence in Medicine. pp. 99–104. Springer Nature Switzerland, Cham (2025). https://doi.org/10.1007/978-3-031-95841-0_19
7. Kong, L.X., Zhao, Y.H., Feng, Z.L., Liu, T.T.: Personalized and continuous care intervention affects rehabilitation, living quality, and negative emotions of patients with breast cancer. World J. Psych. **14**(6), 876–883 (2024). https://doi.org/10.5498/wjp.v14.i6.876
8. Li, D., Jiang, T., Jiang, M.: Quality assessment of in-the-wild videos. In: Proceedings of the 27th ACM International Conference on Multimedia, pp. 2351–2359. ACM, Nice France (2019). https://doi.org/10.1145/3343031.3351028
9. OpenAI, Achiam, J., Adler, S., et al.: GPT-4 Technical Report (2024). https://doi.org/10.48550/arXiv.2303.08774
10. Shamley, D., Lascurain-Aguirrebeña, I., Oskrochi, R., Srinaganathan, R.: Shoulder morbidity after treatment for breast cancer is bilateral and greater after mastectomy. Acta Oncol. **51**(8), 1045–1053 (2012). https://doi.org/10.3109/0284186X.2012.695087
11. Sun, J., Zheng, M., Xian, J., Xie, R., Ni, X., Zhang, S., Yuan, K., Pan, Y.: Research on rehabilitation exercise guidance system based on action quality assessment. In:

2024 17th International Convention on Rehabilitation Engineering and Assistive Technology (i-CREATe), pp. 1–5 (2024). https://doi.org/10.1109/i-CREATe62067.2024.10776381
12. Wang, C., Feng, Y., Zhong, L., Zhu, S., Zhang, C., Zheng, S., Liang, C., Wang, Y., He, C., Yu, C., Shi, Y.: UbiPhysio: support daily functioning, fitness, and rehabilitation with action understanding and feedback in natural language. Proc. ACM Inter. Mobile Wear. Ubiquitous Technol. **8**(1), 1–27 (2024). https://doi.org/10.1145/3643552
13. Wang, H., Zhong, Z., Dai, L., Wu, F., Ma, X., Xue, J., Pavel, S., Lam, P., Zhang, Q., Lin, F.: RehabGPT: A MaaS-based solution to large model building for digital rehabilitation. In: International Workshop on Advanced Imaging Technology (IWAIT) 2024, vol. 13164, pp. 579–584. SPIE (2024). https://doi.org/10.1117/12.3019532
14. Wang, Q., Du, J., Yan, K., Ding, S.: Seeing in flowing: adapting CLIP for action recognition with motion prompts learning. In: Proceedings of the 31st ACM International Conference on Multimedia, pp. 5339–5347. ACM, Ottawa ON Canada (2023). https://doi.org/10.1145/3581783.3612490
15. Wang, S., He, P., Liu, Q., Mao, J., Shen, S.: Impact of evidence-based nursing on postoperative psychological state, quality of life, and function of affected limbs in breast cancer patients: An observational study. Medicine **103**(1), e36788 (2024). https://doi.org/10.1097/MD.0000000000036788
16. Yang, A., Li, A., Yang, B., et al.: Qwen3 Technical Report (2025). https://doi.org/10.48550/arXiv.2505.09388

CDMFuse: A Multi-modal Fusion Framework for Skin Lesion Classification

Xianghao Dong[1], Long Yu[2], Shengwei Tian[1], Qimeng Yang[1(✉)], Dezhi Zhang[3,4,5], and Shirong Yu[3,4,5]

[1] School of Software, Xinjiang University, Urumqi, China
yangqm@xju.edu.cn

[2] School of Information Science and Engineering, Xinjiang University, Urumqi, China

[3] Department of Dermatology and Venereology, People's Hospital of Xinjiang Uygur Autonomous Region, Urumqi, China

[4] Xinjiang Clinical Research Center for Dermatologic Diseases, Urumqi, China

[5] Xinjiang Key Laboratory of Dermatology Research (XJYS1707), Urumqi, China

Abstract. Skin lesion classification is a core task in automated dermatological analysis. Compared to single modalities, multi-modal data can provide complementary information, accelerating the progress of dermatological classification research. However, multi-modal integration faces challenges of insufficient feature interaction and modality heterogeneity. In this study, we propose a multi-modal fusion framework, CDMFuse, for multi-modal skin lesion classification. CDMFuse driven by two novel modules: the Sum-Difference Feature Interaction Module (SDF) and the Patch-Metadata Cross-Attention Fusion Module (PMCA). The SDF module addresses the insufficient integration of dermoscopic and clinical images in existing methods, which typically fuse features only at late stages, leading to information loss. By introducing sum and difference branches, SDF hierarchically models complementary spatial-channel interactions: the sum branch enhances shared structural features (e.g., lesion boundaries), while the difference branch captures modality-specific details (e.g., microvascular patterns in dermoscopy). The PMCA module tackles the heterogeneity gap between image modalities and metadata, where direct concatenation amplifies redundancy and noise. PMCA employs a cross-attention mechanism to dynamically align image patches with metadata embeddings, resolving structural mismatches. It further integrates content-aware multi-scale convolutions to adaptively adjust receptive fields. The effectiveness of our approach is validated on the publicly available Derm7pt multi-modal skin lesion dataset, achieving an average accuracy of 77.69%, surpassing current state-of-the-art methods and improving the test set accuracy by 1.35%. The method also demonstrates strong performance on XJU-MMSD, further verifying its robustness and superiority in multi-modal skin lesion classification.

Keywords: Multi-modal learning · Fusion framework · Skin lesion classification · Feature processing

Y. Zhang et al. (Eds.): CHIP 2025, CCIS 2884, pp. 160–177, 2026.
https://doi.org/10.1007/978-981-95-7299-1_10

1 Introduction

Skin cancer is a globally prevalent malignant tumor, with its incidence rate increasing significantly since the late 20th century. In 2020, more than 1.5 million cases of skin cancer were diagnosed, and this number is expected to rise to over 2.3 million by 2040 [1]. Early detection and timely intervention can significantly reduce the fatality rate of skin cancer [2]. For instance, in the case of melanoma, timely treatment can dramatically increase the survival rate from 14% to 99% [3]. Machine learning techniques, especially when combined with pre-trained deep learning models [4], have demonstrated great potential in improving the accuracy of skin cancer detection [5]. The significant achievement of Alex Krizhevsky et al. using deep convolutional neural networks(CNNs) in the ImageNet competition marked the advent of deep learning in the field of image recognition.

As research has progressed, some studies have started to apply deep learning techniques to dermatological detection [6], such as using CNN for skin cancer image recognition [3,7]. Subsequently, researchers have begun constructing larger-scale dermatological image datasets, such as the International Skin Imaging Collaboration (ISIC) dataset [8,9], which provides a solid foundation for training and validating deep learning models. Previously, due to challenges in data acquisition and other factors, many studies focused primarily on the use of unimodal data [10,11]. However, in practical diagnostic scenarios, multimodal data are often required for information complementation to ensure the reliability of diagnostic outcomes [12]. To address this issue, Kawahara and colleagues were the first to propose and use the multimodal Derm7pt dataset, developing the first model capable of predicting the complete "7-point checklist" in a single optimization process [13]. Compared to other dermatological datasets, the Derm7pt dataset offers more comprehensive and diverse data types. The combination of dermoscopic images, clinical images, and metadata for pathological classification provides higher reliability and accuracy than unimodal data [14].

In the early applications of the Derm7pt dataset, the primary approach involved using CNN to extract image features, with metadata encoded using One-hot encoding and then concatenated with the image features [15]. With the introduction of Swin-Transformer, diagnostic outcomes saw significant improvements. Zhang et al. employed Swin-Transformer as the backbone for feature extraction from image modalities (clinical and dermoscopic images) and used multilayer perceptrons (MLP) to process metadata features [16]. This method was capable of extracting richer shallow image features, enabling more effective integration with metadata features. Despite the significant progress achieved by current multimodal recognition methods in skin disease classification, several issues remain [17]. First, the integration between dermoscopic and clinical images is insufficient. Existing multimodal models typically extract features from dermoscopic and clinical images separately through feature extraction backbones and then fuse the final features [15,18,19]. However, this approach can result in information loss before the final fusion, preventing complete integration of the relevant information from dermoscopic and clinical images. Second, the influence of metadata on the final result is limited. Metadata, after being One-hot encoded and fed into the MLP for simple fusion, can yield satisfactory results but reduces the utilization of metadata information, leading to resource inefficiency, increased model complexity, and reduced robustness to noise, which ultimately weakens the model's generalization capability [20].

To address the two core issues of insufficient feature interaction and limited metadata utilization in existing multi-modal skin lesion classification methods, this paper proposes a novel multi-modal fusion framework (CDMFuse) featuring multi-stage feature extraction, hierarchical information interaction, and adaptive heterogeneous fusion–this framework innovatively redefines the way multi-modal data is processed in dermatological analysis. In feature extraction, we do not simply adopt the Long Short Distance Attention (LSDA) mechanism [21], instead, we optimize it for skin lesion data characteristics: by integrating LSDA into the multi-modal feature extraction process, we enable the network to capture both fine-grained lesion details (e.g., microvascular patterns) and global structural information (e.g., lesion boundaries) simultaneously–a capability that traditional single-scale feature extraction backbones (such as ResNet or Swin-Transformer) lack. More importantly, we design two exclusive modules for multi-modal fusion: the SDF module and PMCA module. The SDF module innovatively embeds feature interaction into each stage of image feature extraction (rather than only at the final fusion step), minimizing information loss during the fusion process; the PMCA module, for the first time, uses dermoscopic features as guidance to integrate metadata with image features, which solves the problem of feature redundancy caused by direct fusion of heterogeneous data and restores masked fine-grained features that are critical for lesion classification.

The contributions of this paper can be summarized as follows:

- We propose a new multi-modal fusion method that utilizes a multi-scale attention mechanism to balance the extraction of local and global features, improving the fusion strategy.
- We introduce the SDF block and PMCA block to address the issues of insufficient feature fusion and significant differences between heterogeneous data, effectively leveraging the complementary nature of features across different modalities.
- The proposed method achieves superior performance compared to existing methods on both the custom dataset and the Derm7pt dataset. Ablation experiments further validate the effectiveness of the proposed modules.

2 Related Works

2.1 Skin Lesion Classification Based on Multi-modal Methods

With the emergence and development of multi-modal techniques, research in the field of dermatology has extended beyond dermoscopic and clinical images to include the combination of images and metadata for improved outcomes [22,23]. Kawahara et al. introduced the large MSLD dataset Derm7pt, which includes dermoscopic images, clinical images, and metadata, facilitating multi-modal skin lesion diagnosis research and improving the accuracy and reliability of computer-aided diagnosis (CAD) results. This is currently the only publicly available dermatological dataset containing three types of modality data [13]. Classification methods based on tri-modal data can be broadly divided into post-fusion and end-to-end approaches.

In recent years, most research on the Derm7pt dataset has adopted end-to-end approaches, among which the TFormer method is particularly notable [16]. It aims to address the issue of insufficient information fusion in multi-modal skin lesion diagnosis, employing Transformer-based feature extraction and hierarchical multi-modal Transformer for image modality fusion, along with post-fusion of image and non-image modalities. This method comprehensively integrates multi-modal information from shallow to deep layers [24], effectively utilizing the complementary nature of different modalities and addressing the data type differences between image and non-image modalities. It also provides inspiration for subsequent methods regarding the stacking of modules for deeper feature extraction.

Existing multi-modal methods (e.g., FusionM4Net [15] and TFormer [16]) have made progress in skin lesion classification, but their fusion mechanisms still remain at the 'passive combination' level. In contrast, our CDMFuse proposes an 'active interaction' fusion paradigm, the specific implementation process is introduced in Sect. 3. To our knowledge, this is the first end-to-end framework that simultaneously solves the two core problems of image-image feature interaction and image-metadata heterogeneous fusion in multi-modal skin lesion classification.

2.2 CrossFormer: Advancing Multi-scale Attention for Visual Feature Interaction

CrossFormer is an innovative visual Transformer architecture that enhances feature representation through the introduction of cross-scale attention mechanisms [21]. Existing visual Transformers face limitations in handling interactions between different scales of features, primarily due to input embeddings having the same scale, which fails to effectively capture dependencies between fine-grained and large-scale features [25,26]. CrossFormer addresses this issue through the design of the Cross-scale Embedding Layer (CEL) [27] and the Long Short Distance Attention (LSDA) module.

CrossFormer introduced novel insights for visual feature interaction through its cross-scale attention mechanism (LSDA). Building upon this foundation, our work further optimizes these concepts by integrating CrossFormer's multi-scale attention mechanism into the skin lesion diagnosis task. The SDF module enhances the balance between local and global features, while the PMCA module addresses structural discrepancies between images and metadata. In contrast to traditional vision Transformers relying on single-scale interactions, our method achieves more flexible cross-modal adaptive fusion through Dynamic Position Bias (DPB) and content-aware multi-scale convolutions, tailored for the unique challenges of dermatological data.

3 Methods

3.1 Overall Architecture of CDMFuse

The overall architecture of CDMFuse is shown in Fig. 1. The architecture is divided into two main parts: the first part extracts and fuses features from dermoscopic and clinical images, while the second part extracts metadata features and performs the final fusion with image features.

First, dermoscopic data (derm) and clinical image data (clin) are input into the model, using the Long Short Distance Attention module for feature extraction from the image modalities, allowing the extraction of multi-scale features. To effectively fuse the features between the two image modalities, we designed a convolution-based dual-branch hierarchical multi-modal transformer, SDF block, which facilitates the fusion of image modality features. Due to the significant difference between metadata and image modalities, direct fusion may introduce redundancy and reduce final classification accuracy. Therefore, we choose to process the metadata separately before fusion. To fully fuse the features between image and metadata, we designed a cross-attention mechanism-based feature fusion block, PMCA. Before entering the PMCA module, the metadata undergoes one-hot encoding and MLP operations, followed by an upsampling operation with dermoscopic features (derm) to align with clinical image features (Fclin), dermoscopic features (Fderm), and fused features (Ffuse). Finally, after fusion in the PMCA module, the resulting feature vector is flattened and passed through a classification layer to generate the final classification result.

3.2 Sum-Difference Feature Interaction Module

The SDF block is the core innovation for solving insufficient fusion between dermoscopic and clinical images–it is the first module designed to fuse features generated at each stage of feature extraction (rather than only the final features) for multi-modal skin lesion classification, as shown in the Fig. 2. We stack the SDF block throughout the network to fully utilize the hierarchical features extracted from the backbone network at different scales. The specific process is as follows: After f_{clin} and f_{derm} enter the SDF block, a concat operation is performed on the inputs, followed by downsampling to obtain $\aleph$. Then, $\aleph$ is subjected to a Reduction operation together with the output from the previous SDF block, $\aleph_{pre}$ (for the first SDF block, only f_{clin} and f_{derm} are input). The Reduction operation reduces the channel number of the input data by applying a 1×1 convolution layer, which can be expressed as:

$$\widetilde{\aleph} = ReLU(BN(Conv_{1\times1}(\aleph))) \tag{1}$$

$$\widetilde{\aleph}_{pre} = ReLU(BN(Conv_{1\times1}(\aleph_{pre}))) \tag{2}$$

where $Conv_{1\times1}$ refers to the 1×1 convolution operation, BN is batch normalization, and $ReLU$ is the activation function. The final outputs, $\widetilde{\aleph}$ and $\widetilde{\aleph}_{pre}$ are each subjected to three convolution operations, with each convolution followed

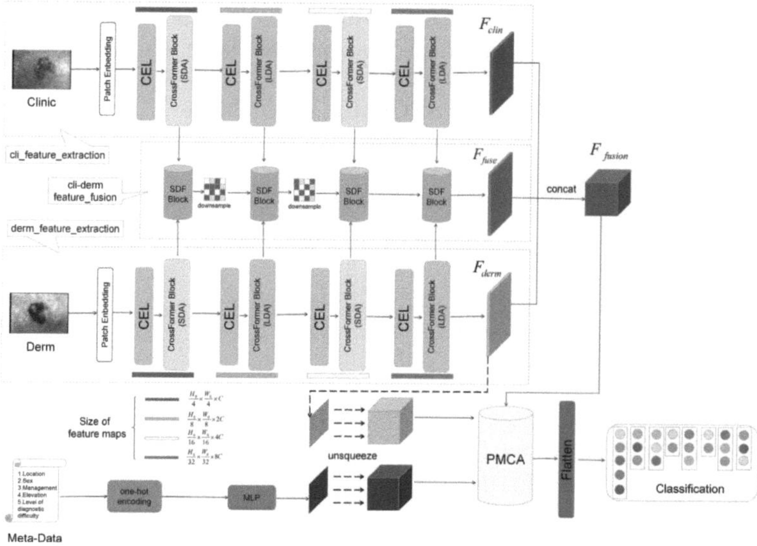

Fig. 1. The overall architecture of CDMFuse, the input data are clinical images, dermoscopic images and metadata

by a *ReLU* activation function. The output of each convolution operation is represented as ϑ:

$$\vartheta^{(1)} = ReLU(Conv_{3\times3}(\widetilde{\aleph}))$$

$$\vartheta^{(2)} = ReLU(Conv_{3\times3}(\vartheta^{(1)}))$$

$$\vartheta^{(3)} = ReLU(Conv_{3\times3}(\vartheta^{(1)} + \vartheta^{(2)})) \tag{3}$$

$$\vartheta^{(1)}_{pre} = ReLU(Conv_{3\times3}(\widetilde{\aleph}_{pre}))$$

$$\vartheta^{(2)}_{pre} = ReLU(Conv_{3\times3}(\vartheta^{(1)}_{pre}))$$

$$\vartheta^{(3)}_{pre} = ReLU(Conv_{3\times3}(\vartheta^{(1)}_{pre} + \vartheta^{(2)}_{pre})) \tag{4}$$

Then, the clinical image features and dermoscopic features are added together, followed by a 1×1 convolution to generate the fused output feature map:

$$\daleth_{add} = ReLU(BN(Conv_{1\times1}(\Xi^{(1)(2)(3)}_{\vartheta} + \Xi^{(1)(2)(3)}_{\vartheta_{pre}}))) \tag{5}$$

where $\daleth_{add}$ means the result of additive feature fusion, Ξ means adding all the convolutional outputs on a path. At this point, additive feature fusion is complete. Next, we introduce differential feature fusion, which follows a similar process to additive feature fusion, except that the input feature maps are fused using their differences. The specific operations are as follows:

$$\daleth_{diff} = ReLU(BN(Conv_{1\times1}(|\Xi^{(1)(2)(3)}_{\vartheta} - \Xi^{(1)(2)(3)}_{\vartheta_{pre}}|))) \tag{6}$$

The results of the additive feature fusion and the differential feature fusion are summed and then passed through a convolutional layer to generate the final output:

$$\aleph_{final} = ReLU(BN(Conv_{3\times3}(\neg_{diff}))) + \neg_{add} \tag{7}$$

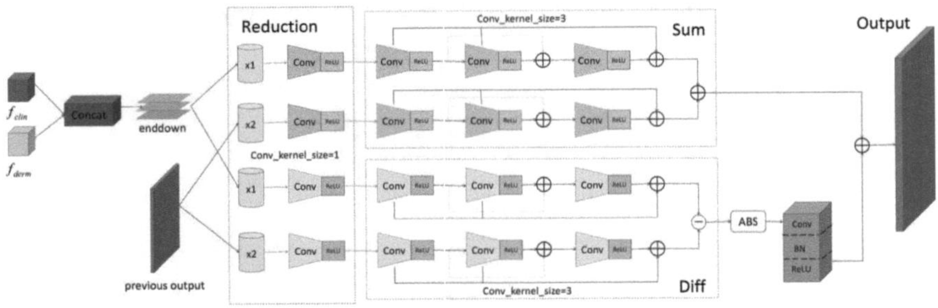

Fig. 2. The architecture of Sum-Difference Feature Interaction Module

3.3 Patch-Metadata Cross-Attention Fusion Module

The PMCA module, as shown in Fig. 3, is an innovative solution to the heterogeneity gap between image modalities and metadata–a problem that has plagued multi-modal skin lesion classification for a long time. The PMCA module proposes a three-step adaptive fusion mechanism. First, it applies a dual-path feature interaction based on multi-head attention to fused image features and metadata, this is the first work to calculate attention weights between image patches and metadata embeddings, realizing dynamic alignment of heterogeneous features rather than rigid concatenation. Next, we introduce the dermal features (derm) and perform content-based convolution operations. By integrating multi-scale information within the same layer, we can adaptively adjust the receptive field size of the neurons. The specific process is as follows: we calculate the contextual matrices ct_{fusion} and ct_{meta}.

$$ct_{fusion} = softmax(K_{fusion}^{T} \cdot V_{fusion}) \cdot V_{fusion} \tag{8}$$

$$ct_{meta} = softmax(K_{meta}^{T} \cdot V_{meta}) \cdot V_{meta} \tag{9}$$

The softmax function is used to normalize the attention weights, ensuring that information at each position interacts accurately with features from other positions. Subsequently, the cross-attention mechanism combines ct_{fusion}, ct_{meta}, and the query vector q to perform the following update operations:

$$\beth_{fusion} = q \cdot ct_{meta} \tag{10}$$

$$\beth_{meta} = q \cdot ct_{meta} \tag{11}$$

where $\beth$ represents the features after cross-attention processing, the query matrix q is obtained by concatenating the input features and applying a linear transformation.

Through this operation, F_{fusion} and F_{meta}interact and update their information. Next, the process enters the second part. The outputs from the first part, $\beth_{fusion}$, $\beth_{meta}$ and F_{derm}, are first concatenated to produce C. Subsequently, C undergoes multi-scale convolution operations, where convolution kernels of different sizes (k_i) are used to extract features at various scales. The resulting k feature maps are then stacked by performing element-wise addition, producing the fused feature U. Finally, global average pooling is applied to U along the height and width dimensions to compute the channel descriptor S. This process can be expressed as:

$$U = \sum_{i=1}^{K} Conv(C, k_i) \tag{12}$$

$$S = \frac{1}{H \times W} \sum_{h=1}^{H} \sum_{w=1}^{W} U \tag{13}$$

Using a fully connected layer (FC), the channel descriptor S is reduced in dimension to generate the weights for each scale. For each scale k_i, the corresponding fully connected layer (FC_i)produces the scale-specific weight W_i. These weights are then normalized using softmax to generate the final scale weights. Finally, each scale's feature map is multiplied by its corresponding weight, and all are summed to produce the final output V:

$$V = \sum_{i=1}^{K} \frac{exp(W_i)}{\sum_{j=1}^{K} exp(W_j)} \cdot Conv(C, k_i) \tag{14}$$

3.4 Multi-label Classification Layer

Through the above modules, we obtain a feature vector that integrates information from three modalities: clinical images, dermoscopic images, and metadata. This feature vector is fed into a multi-label classification layer consisting of 8 fully connected layers, with the outputs corresponding to the diagnostic results for BWV, PIG, DAG, VS, STR, RS, PN, and DIAG. To optimize the multi-label classification task, we adopt the cross-entropy loss function, defined as follows:

$$Loss = \frac{1}{N} \sum_{i=1}^{N} CE(p_i, y_i) \tag{15}$$

where p_i and y_i are the predicted value and true value of the i-th label respectively, N represents the number of multi-labels(8 in this study), and CE represents the cross-entropy loss.

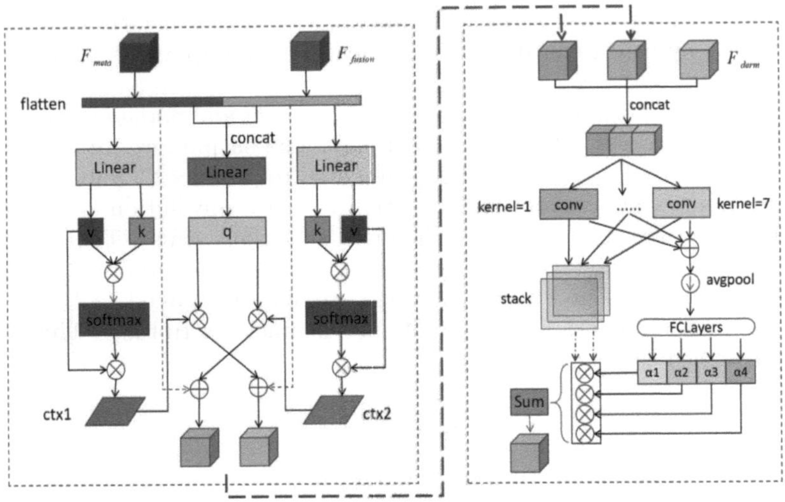

Fig. 3. The architecture of Patch-Metadata Cross-Attention Fusion Module

4 Experiments

In this section, we first introduce the dataset and evaluation metrics. Then, we present the experimental results, including a comparison between single-modal and multi-modal performance, multiple ablation experiments on the key modules of the CDMFuse model, and a comparison of our method with several state-of-the-art methods.

4.1 Datasets

Our method was evaluated on the Derm7pt dataset [13]. The Derm7pt dataset contains 413 training samples, 203 validation samples, and 395 testing samples. Each sample includes dermoscopic images, clinical images, diagnostic labels (DIAG), and Seven-Point Checklist (SPC) labels. The diagnostic labels are divided into five categories: (1) Melanoma (MEL), (2) Nevus (NEV), (3) Seborrheic Keratosis (SK), (4) Basal Cell Carcinoma (BCC), and (5) Miscellaneous Cancer (MISC). The SPC labels cover the following seven features: (1) Pigment Network (PN), (2)Striae (STR), (3) Pigmentation (PIG), (4) Regression Structures (RS), (5) Dots and Glomeruli(DaG), (6) Vascular Structures (VS), and (7) Blue-White Veil (BWV). These diagnostic types and SPC classification standards were defined by Kawahara et al.

To supplement the experiments and validate the generalization ability of the model, we conducted experiments on our private dataset, XJU-MMSD. Since the XJU-MMSD dataset contains only diagnostic categories without SPC labels, only the Diag metric was evaluated.

4.2 Evaluation Metrics

We selected five commonly used evaluation metrics: Accuracy (ACC), Precision, Sensitivity (SEN), Specificity (SPE), and F1-Score (F1), to evaluate and compare the performance of multi-modal methods. Among these, Accuracy is the primary comparison metric as it provides a comprehensive assessment of the model's overall classification performance. The definitions and calculation formulas for these metrics are as follows:

$$Accuracy = \frac{TP + TN}{TP + TN + FP + FN} \tag{16}$$

$$Precision = \frac{TP}{TP + FP} \tag{17}$$

$$Sensitivity = \frac{TP}{TP + FN} \tag{18}$$

$$Specificity = \frac{TN}{TN + FP} \tag{19}$$

$$F1 - score = 2 \times \frac{Precision \times Sensitivity}{Precision + Sensitivity} \tag{20}$$

where *TP*, *TN*, *FP*, and *FN* correspond to the number of True Positives, True Negatives, False Positives, and False Negatives, respectively, in the classification task.

4.3 Implementation Details

Our method was implemented using PyTorch and trained on an Nvidia GeForce RTX 3090 GPU with 24GB RAM. The input image size to the network was 224×224×3, and patient metadata, after one-hot encoding, had a length of 20. The batch size during training was 32, with an initial learning rate of 1e-5. The learning rate was updated using the Step Decay method, decaying to 90% of its original value every 30 epochs. Additionally, an early stopping strategy was applied to prevent overfitting. The model was trained for a total of 100 epochs. In the model, the first SDF block received dermoscopic and clinical images as input, thus omitting the concat operation to reduce unnecessary computation. Considering the small size of the dataset, we employed Crossformer-S as the feature extraction network and applied data augmentation, including edge cropping and recombination, random cropping and padding, translation, and flipping. The experimental results were obtained by averaging the results of 10 independent runs, and standard deviation was reported to assess the stability of the experiments.

4.4 Comparison Between Single-Modal and Multi-modal Learning

We first conducted experiments under single-modal settings to compare with multi-modal learning. In the single-modal experiments, each modality was fed into the model independently to obtain the final classification results. In the multi-modal experiments, we employed two data fusion methods: a simple concat operation and our proposed CDMFuse model for multi-modal data integration. The specific experimental results are shown in Table 1.

In the multi-modal experiments, when using the CDMFuse model, the Average Accuracy of any combination of two modalities exceeded that of single-modal experiments. The results further demonstrate that our proposed CDMFuse model is highly effective in feature extraction, integration, and noise suppression, achieving the highest Average Accuracy of 77.69%.

Table 1. Comparison of single-modal and multi-modal (accuracy%).

	Cli	Derm	Meta	BWV	PIG	DAG	VS	STR	RS	PN	DIAG	AVG
Single-Modality	✓			81.33±2.60	66.79±1.62	60.02±1.37	74.65±2.38	67.55±1.93	70.55±2.62	68.32±2.11	70.21±3.62	69.93±1.82
		✓		86.23±1.20	68.75±0.50	62.63±0.75	81.45±0.33	75.60±1.56	79.63±0.94	71.28±0.91	74.05±1.03	74.85±0.76
			✓	83.06±1.13	60.21±0.64	61.78±1.35	78.68±0.43	69.66±0.25	72.01±0.21	58.51±1.60	70.05±0.40	69.24±0.55
Multi-Modality	✓	✓		86.74±0.26	68.23±1.02	61.52±0.54	82.01±0.92	75.24±0.70	78.87±1.52	70.08±1.63	71.86±0.68	74.28±0.77
(Concat)	✓		✓	84.50±1.33	64.12±0.52	54.96±2.35	79.68±0.38	67.43±0.52	74.06±1.73	60.56±0.50	67.49±0.97	69.10±1.12
		✓	✓	86.52±0.78	67.63±0.48	62.74±0.65	81.05±0.90	75.84±1.32	80.56±0.40	70.87±0.66	72.03±0.71	74.55±0.88
	✓	✓	✓	87.06±1.52	66.43±0.79	62.83±0.74	82.12±0.68	74.10±0.65	80.03±0.32	71.13±0.82	71.98±0.71	74.46±0.42
Multi-Modality	✓	✓		86.58±0.94	68.30±0.64	64.68±0.45	82.08±0.72	76.58±0.87	**81.08±0.53**	72.36±0.82	75.26±0.77	75.76±0.85
(CDMFuse)	✓		✓	86.03±0.76	64.87±0.63	59.33±0.42	80.72±0.80	68.06±1.34	77.68±0.94	67.88±0.83	72.30±0.81	72.08±0.71
		✓	✓	87.44±0.60	66.82±0.54	65.74±0.83	81.78±0.64	75.70±1.87	80.12±0.65	72.55±0.53	76.52±0.66	75.89±0.51
	✓	✓	✓	**89.01±0.92**	**71.42±1.27**	**66.87±0.75**	**82.19±1.06**	**77.04±0.65**	80.03±1.23	**75.14±0.60**	**79.91±0.54**	**77.69±0.46**

4.5 Ablation Experiment

In this section, we conducted experiments and analyses to verify the effectiveness of the SDF and PMCA modules. We also explored the impact of using different modalities as guidance on the final classification performance.

Effectiveness of SDF and PMCA Modules We incrementally added SDF blocks starting from the first CrossFormer block, and the experimental results are shown in Table 2. It can be observed that as the number of SDF blocks increased, the model performance gradually improved. For the PMCA module, the experimental results demonstrate that its inclusion leads to a significant performance improvement compared to not using it. This indicates that cross-attention facilitates the effective fusion of different modal features, while multi-scale feature selection helps maintain the orderliness of the fused features, avoiding the interference of irrelevant or redundant information. The PMCA module is particularly effective for integrating features with significant structural differences, such as metadata and image features.

Table 2. The results of ablation study for SDF and PMCA (accuracy%).

	Stages of joining the SDF 1	2	3	4	BWV	PIG	DAG	VS	STR	RS	PN	DIAG	AVG
Replace PMCA					87.06±1.52	66.43±0.79	62.83±0.74	82.12±0.68	74.10±0.65	80.03±0.32	71.13±0.82	71.98±0.71	74.46±0.42
with Concat	✓				87.12±0.98	66.62±0.74	63.11±0.64	82.10±0.57	74.56±0.42	80.51±0.60	71.65±0.78	72.70±0.84	74.81±0.77
	✓	✓			87.45±0.82	66.43±0.85	63.78±0.70	81.93±0.58	74.63±0.92	81.42±0.67	72.89±0.36	73.82±1.04	75.29±0.85
	✓	✓	✓		87.32±0.65	66.18±1.36	64.30±0.62	81.76±0.47	74.75±0.82	80.94±1.08	73.62±0.75	74.38±1.09	75.40±0.57
	✓	✓	✓	✓	87.99±0.40	67.37±0.77	65.01±0.82	81.51±0.75	74.83±0.72	81.77±0.97	73.86±0.22	75.06±0.82	75.96±0.63
PMCA					87.66±0.67	64.21±0.65	64.03±0.84	81.63±0.36	75.04±1.25	79.68±0.86	72.89±0.46	74.38±0.44	74.96±0.79
	✓				88.23±1.03	69.11±2.10	63.54±0.47	81.77±0.66	75.19±0.32	81.01±1.65	73.16±0.87	78.73±0.31	76.34±0.82
	✓	✓			88.22±0.54	69.01±1.58	64.40±0.50	82.06±0.68	76.68±0.45	**82.71±0.75**	74.93±0.63	79.21±0.50	77.12±0.67
	✓	✓	✓		88.16±0.82	68.61±0.99	66.85±0.86	81.31±0.83	75.93±0.60	81.50±0.74	73.15±0.79	77.22±0.62	76.62±0.45
	✓	✓	✓	✓	**89.01±0.92**	**71.42±1.27**	**66.87±0.75**	**82.19±1.06**	**77.04±0.65**	80.03±1.23	**75.14±0.60**	**79.91±0.54**	**77.69±0.46**

Impact of Guiding Data Selection on Classification Performance(accuracy%) The single-modal Average Accuracy of dermoscopic images is higher than that of clinical images and metadata, indicating its superior feature representation. Dermoscopic images reveal microstructures of skin lesions, such as blood vessels, hair, and pigmentation, which are often imperceptible in clinical images or metadata. Additionally, dermoscopic images focus on specific lesion areas, reducing interference from surrounding skin and environmental factors. These characteristics make dermoscopic features less noisy and more detailed compared to clinical images and metadata.

However, during the exchange of complementary information between image features and metadata via cross-attention, the importance of certain subtle features may be diminished. This phenomenon can cause confusion in classifying lesion types where such subtle features are crucial. To address this issue, we incorporated dermoscopic features into the PMCA module as auxiliary data to restore these masked subtle features and enable the model to better capture non-linear relationships and complex structures in the data. The experimental results are shown in Table 3.

Table 3. The results of using different Guiding Data(accuracy%).

Guidance	BWV	PIG	DAG	VS	STR	RS	PN	DIAG	AVG
	87.72±0.21	69.54±0.84	65.91±0.72	81.36±0.49	76.36±0.78	82.27±1.47	73.63±0.33	79.54±0.54	77.05±0.55
Cli	88.85±1.04	67.39±1.32	56.52±0.80	**84.06±0.64**	71.01±0.62	**84.78±0.83**	73.91±0.77	78.98±0.91	75.82±0.43
Cli+derm	87.35±0.66	69.88±1.06	62.04±0.57	81.92±1.37	74.49±0.78	83.13±0.92	73.49±0.45	79.72±0.66	76.51±0.62
derm	**89.01±0.92**	**71.42±1.27**	**66.87±0.75**	82.19±1.06	**77.04±0.65**	80.03±1.23	**75.14±0.60**	**79.91±0.54**	**77.69±0.46**

4.6 Comparison with State-of-the-Art Methods

We compared CDMFuse with the current state-of-the-art methods used on the Derm7pt dataset, including initial-based methods (initial imbalance, initial balance, and initial combination) [13], MmA [28], TripleNet [18], Embedding-Net [29], HcCNN [30], FusionM4Net [15], AMFAM [31], T-Former [16], and MSMA

[32]. The experimental results are shown in the Table 4. The results for CDM-Fuse were obtained from our experiments, while those for TFormer and MSMA were reproduced using the authors' code. The results for the other methods were sourced from their respective papers. The table reports the Average Accuracy for all eight classification tasks as well as the overall average.

These methods can be categorized into two types: post-fusion methods and end-to-end methods. Among existing end-to-end methods, TFormer and MSMA are the best-performing ones. However, they still face issues related to insufficient local feature extraction and noise handling. TFormer, based on the Swin-Transformer architecture, struggles to fully capture fine details and local features. MSMA addresses some of TFormer's shortcomings by combining CNNs and Transformers and incorporating noise reduction mechanisms. However, during the lengthy feature extraction process, some important features may still be suppressed. Our method addresses these issues through several improvements. Sum-Diff branches and cross-attention mechanisms ensure effective fusion of multi-modal data. CrossFormer's Long Short Distance Attention (LSDA) mechanism balances local and global feature extraction. Before feeding fused features into the PMCA module, dermoscopic (derm) features are incorporated to guide the fusion process. As shown in the Table 4, our method outperforms all existing methods in almost every classification task, achieving an overall average accuracy improvement of 1.35%.

Table 4. Comparison of CDMFuse and state-of-the-art methods(accuracy%).

Method	BWV	PIG	DAG	VS	STR	RS	PN	DIAG	AVG
Inception-unbalanced	87.6	65.6	56.7	81.3	75.9	78.2	68.1	68.4	72.7
Inception-balanced	87.3	64.8	60.3	81.5	75.7	78.2	68.9	70.8	73.4
Inception-combine	87.1	66.1	60.0	79.7	74.2	77.2	70.9	74.2	73.7
MmA	83.0	61.3	59.2	75.7	69.4	73.9	65.6	70.6	69.8
EmbeddingNet	84.3	64.3	57.5	82.5	73.4	78.0	65.1	68.6	71.7
TripleNet	87.9	67.3	61.3	83.0	74.4	76.0	63.3	68.6	72.7
HcCNN	87.1	68.6	65.6	**84.8**	71.6	80.8	70.6	69.9	74.9
FusionM4Net-SS	88.50±0.40	71.30±1.30	64.40±1.30	81.60±0.50	76.10±1.10	81.40±0.80	69.20±1.50	77.60±1.50	76.30 ±0.70
TFormer	86.07±0.61	69.11±1.56	64.05±0.98	82.53±0.76	75.70±0.82	80.51±1.04	70.63±1.20	78.22±0.64	75.85±0.66
MSMA	87.08±1.29	66.07±2.03	66.58±0.76	82.78±0.69	75.18±1.50	**81.61±0.79**	72.65±0.96	79.24±0.85	76.34±0.72
CDMFuse	**89.01±0.92**	**71.42±1.27**	**66.87±0.75**	82.19±1.06	**77.04±0.65**	80.03±1.23	**75.14±0.60**	**79.91±0.54**	**77.69±0.46**

In addition, to provide a more comprehensive comparison, we calculated the sensitivity (SEN), specificity (SPE), precision (PRE), and F1-score for each method. The results are shown in the Table 5. The data for TFormer, MSMA, and our method (CDMFuse) were obtained from our experiments, while the results for FusionM4Net-SS were derived from the data reported in the literature [15]. Our method outperforms other methods in most evaluation metrics. Additionally, we plotted radar charts based on the data in the Table 5, which visualizes the overall performance of each method across multiple metrics. As shown in Fig. 4, our method demonstrates greater stability in most classification tasks, further validating its effectiveness.

Table 5. Comparisons of CDMFuse and state-of-the-art methods via different metrics.

Method	Metric	BWV	PIG	DAG	VS	STR	RS	PN	DIAG	AVG
FusionM4Net-SS	SEN	79.20	54.43	**64.20**	42.40	64.80	69.75	68.43	54.62	62.23
	SPE	79.20	79.50	82.37	75.07	84.53	69.75	85.17	92.26	80.98
	PRE	**82.25**	**69.97**	65.20	62.57	71.33	79.15	69.53	70.64	71.39
	F1-score	80.58	56.64	63.34	42.88	67.35	72.26	68.67	57.70	63.68
TFormer	SEN	75.58	**59.09**	60.41	53.51	**67.52**	71.14	69.39	66.55	65.40
	SPE	75.58	80.32	81.37	80.66	**85.31**	71.14	85.03	92.49	81.49
	PRE	77.62	65.12	61.74	61.76	67.65	75.94	69.60	71.64	68.88
	F1-score	76.92	**61.95**	61.57	58.01	67.43	72.01	69.98	69.01	67.11
MSMA	SEN	82.65	55.90	63.50	54.68	63.94	**73.20**	71.06	63.41	66.04
	SPE	82.65	79.02	82.66	**83.36**	83.07	**73.20**	86.14	92.85	**82.87**
	PRE	78.13	60.63	65.35	61.13	67.61	79.17	71.23	**77.16**	70.05
	F1-score	80.33	57.97	**64.38**	58.56	65.92	**72.83**	72.04	69.32	67.67
CDMFuse	SEN	**84.05**	56.82	63.14	**60.81**	67.47	63.36	**76.80**	**67.36**	**67.48**
	SPE	**84.05**	**80.54**	**82.80**	81.83	84.61	63.36	**88.70**	**93.59**	82.44
	PRE	81.84	62.77	**65.45**	**68.84**	**71.75**	**79.24**	**76.14**	73.73	**72.47**
	F1-score	**82.87**	58.63	63.61	**64.57**	**69.31**	65.11	**76.33**	**70.36**	**68.85**

4.7 Supplemental Experiments

To further validate the effectiveness and generalization ability of our model, we conducted supplemental experiments on the XJU-MMSD dataset. Since this dataset does not include Seven-Point Checklist (SPC) metrics, we evaluated the model solely on diagnostic labels (DIAG). The detailed results are shown in the Table 6, which reports the classification performance on the DIAG metric.

The experimental results indicate that our method outperforms the comparison methods on the XJU-MMSD dataset, further demonstrating the robustness and adaptability of CDMFuse across different datasets.

Table 6. The results on the XJU-MMSD dataset.

Method	DIAG	SEN	SPE	PRE	F1-score
TFormer	79.41	73.19	93.69	74.87	73.12
MSMA	79.70	75.57	93.89	75.67	74.87
CDMFuse	**81.31**	**75.77**	**93.99**	**76.03**	**75.17**

5 Conclusions

In this paper, we propose CDMFuse, a multi-modal skin disease classification method based on dermoscopic images, clinical images, and metadata. To enhance the feature fusion process, we integrate the Sum-Diff branch into SDF blocks. For the fusion of metadata and image features, we utilize dermoscopic features as guidance. Coupled with the cross-attention mechanism, this approach ensures that data entering the PMCA block achieves effective multi-scale fusion while suppressing noise. Experimental results on the publicly available Derm7pt dataset and the XJU-MMSD dataset demonstrate that our method outperforms existing approaches in most classification tasks. These results highlight the robustness and effectiveness of CDMFuse in handling multi-modal skin disease classification challenges.

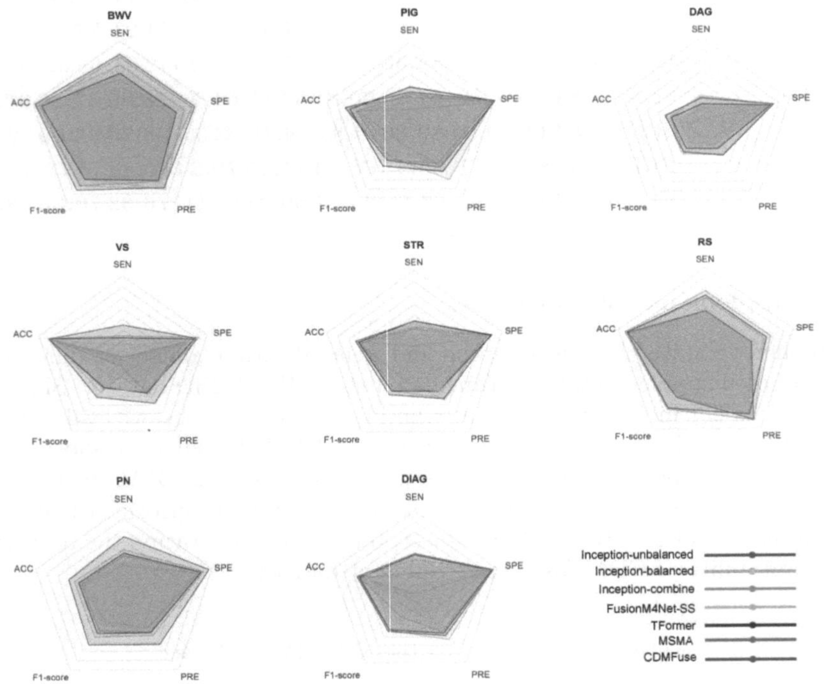

Fig. 4. The radar charts of all metrics

Declarations

Competing Interest

The authors declare that they have no known competing financial interests or personal relationships that could have appeared to influence the work reported in this paper.

Data Availability

The datasets used in this study consist of both publicly available and confidential data.

Funding

This work was supported by the National Natural Science Foundation of China 62362061, Tianshan Talent Training Program 2023TSYCLJ0023 and the Xinjiang Uygur Autonomous Region Key R & D program under Grant 2021B03001-4.

References

1. Chatzilakou, E., Hu, Y., Jiang N., et al.: Biosensors for melanoma skin cancer diagnostics[J]. Biosens. Bioelectr. 116045 (2024)
2. Aladhadh, S., Alsanea, M., Aloraini, M., et al.: An effective skin cancer classification mechanism via medical vision transformer[J]. Sensors **22**(11), 4008 (2022)
3. Esteva, A., Kuprel, B., Novoa, R.A., et al.: Dermatologist-level classification of skin cancer with deep neural networks[J]. Nature **542**(7639), 115–118 (2017)
4. Maron, R.C., Weichenthal, M., Utikal, J.S., et al.: Systematic outperformance of 112 dermatologists in multiclass skin cancer image classification by convolutional neural networks[J]. Eur. J. Cancer **119**, 57–65 (2019)
5. Naqvi, M., Gilani, S.Q., Syed, T., et al.: Skin cancer detection using deep learning—a review[J]. Diagnostics **13**(11), 1911 (2023)
6. Goyal, M., Knackstedt, T., Yan, S., et al.: Artificial intelligence-based image classification methods for diagnosis of skin cancer: Challenges and opportunities[J]. Comput. Biol. Med. **127**, 104065 (2020)
7. Attallah, O.: Skin-CAD: Explainable deep learning classification of skin cancer from dermoscopic images by feature selection of dual high-level CNNs features and transfer learning[J]. Comput. Biol. Med. **178**, 108798 (2024)
8. Codella, N.C.F., Gutman, D., Celebi, M.E.: Skin lesion analysis toward melanoma detection: a challenge at the, et al.: international symposium on biomedical imaging (isbi), hosted by the international skin imaging collaboration (isic)[C]. In: 2018 IEEE 15th International Symposium on Biomedical Imaging (ISBI 2018). IEEE 2018, pp. 168–172 (2017)
9. Alenezi, F., Armghan, A., Polat, K.: Wavelet transform based deep residual neural network and ReLU based Extreme Learning Machine for skin lesion classification[J]. Expert Syst. Appl. **213**, 119064 (2023)
10. Yue, Y., Li, Z.: Medmamba: vision mamba for medical image classification[J] (2024). preprint arXiv:2403.03849
11. Li, A., Zhang, D., Yu, L., et al.: Residual cosine similar attention and bidirectional convolution in dual-branch network for skin lesion image classification[J]. Eng. Appl. Artif. Intell. **133**, 108386 (2024)
12. Brancaccio, G., Balato, A., Malvehy, J., et al.: Artificial intelligence in skin cancer diagnosis: a reality check[J]. J. Investig. Dermatol. **144**(3), 492–499 (2024)
13. Kawahara, J., Daneshvar, S., Argenziano, G., et al.: Seven-point checklist and skin lesion classification using multitask multimodal neural nets[J]. IEEE J. Biomed. Health Inform. **23**(2), 538–546 (2018)

14. Farea, E., Saleh, R.A.A., AbuAlkebash, H., et al.: A hybrid deep learning skin cancer prediction framework[J]. Eng. Sci. Technol. Int. J. **57**, 101818 (2024)
15. Tang, P., Yan, X., Nan, Y., et al.: FusionM4Net: a multi-stage multi-modal learning algorithm for multi-label skin lesion classification[J]. Med. Image Anal. **76**, 102307 (2022)
16. Zhang, Y., Xie, F., Chen, J.: TFormer: a throughout fusion transformer for multi-modal skin lesion diagnosis[J]. Comput. Biol. Med. **157**, 106712 (2023)
17. Ain, Q.U., Al-Sahaf, H., Xue, B., et al.: Genetic programming for automatic skin cancer image classification[J]. Expert Syst. Appl. **197**, 116680 (2022)
18. Ge, Z., Demyanov, S., Chakravorty, R.: Skin disease recognition using deep saliency features and multimodal learning of dermoscopy and clinical images[C]. Medical Image Computing and Computer Assisted Intervention- MICCAI, et al. In: 20th International Conference, Quebec City, QC, Canada, September 11–13 (2017), Proceedings, Part III 20. Springer International Publishing, pp. 250–258 (2017)
19. Nunnari, F., Bhuvaneshwara, C., Ezema, A.O., et al.: A study on the fusion of pixels and patient metadata in CNN-based classification of skin lesion images[C]. In: International Cross-Domain Conference for Machine Learning and Knowledge Extraction, pp. 191–208. Springer International Publishing, Cham (2020)
20. Yi, X., Xu, H., Zhang, H., et al.: Text-IF: Leveraging semantic text guidance for degradation-aware and interactive image fusion[C]. In: Proceedings of the IEEE/CVF Conference on Computer Vision and Pattern Recognition, pp. 27026–27035 (2024)
21. Wang W, Chen W, Qiu Q, et al. Crossformer++: A versatile vision transformer hinging on cross-scale attention[J]. IEEE Trans. Pattern Anal. Mach. Intell. (2023)
22. Yap, J., Yolland, W., Tschandl, P.: Multimodal skin lesion classification using deep learning[J]. Exp. Dermatol. **27**(11), 1261–1267 (2018)
23. Walter, F.M., Prevost, A.T., Vasconcelos, J., et al.: Using the 7-point checklist as a diagnostic aid for pigmented skin lesions in general practice: a diagnostic validation study[J]. Br. J. Gen. Pract. **63**(610), e345–e353 (2013)
24. Shamshad, F., Khan, S., Zamir, S.W., et al.: Transformers in medical imaging: a survey[J]. Med. Image Anal. **88**, 102802 (2023)
25. Dosovitskiy, A.: An image is worth 16x16 words: transformers for image recognition at scale[J] (2020). arXiv:2010.11929
26. Touvron, H., Cord, M., Douze, M., et al.: Training data-efficient image transformers & distillation through attention[C]. In: International Conference on Machine Learning, pp. 10347–10357. PMLR (2021)
27. Wang, W., Xie, E., Li, X., et al.: Pyramid vision transformer: a versatile backbone for dense prediction without convolutions[C]. In: Proceedings of the IEEE/CVF International Conference on Computer Vision, pp. 568–578 (2021)
28. Ngiam, J., Khosla, A., Kim, M., et al.: Multimodal deep learning[C]. In: Proceedings of the 28th International Conference on Machine Learning (ICML-11), pp. 689–696 (2011)
29. Bi, L., Feng, D.D., Fulham, M., et al.: Multi-label classification of multi-modality skin lesion via hyper-connected convolutional neural network[J]. Pattern Recogn. **107**, 107502 (2020)
30. Yap, J., Yolland, W., Tschandl, P.: Multimodal skin lesion classification using deep learning[J]. Exp. Dermatol. **27**(11), 1261–1267 (2018)
31. Wang, Y., Feng, Y., Zhang, L., et al.: Adversarial multimodal fusion with attention mechanism for skin lesion classification using clinical and dermoscopic images[J]. Med. Image Anal. **81**, 102535 (2022)

32. Shu, C., Yu, L., Tian, S., et al.: MSMA: A multi-stage and multi-attention algorithm for the classification of multimodal skin lesions[J]. Biomed. Signal Process. Control **93**, 106180 (2024)

Composite Inflammatory Indices from Peripheral Blood Tests for Early Prediction of EBV-Associated Hemophagocytic Lymphohistiocytosis in Children

Li Xiao[1(✉)], Lin Chen[2], Ruijue Wang[3], Wanxing Liu[1], and Jie Yu[4]

[1] Ministry of Education Key Laboratory of Child Development and Disorders, Big Data Center for Children's Medical Care, Children's Hospital of Chongqing Medical University, National Clinical Research Center for Child Health and Disorders, Intelligent Application of Big Data in Pediatrics Engineering Research Center of Chongqing Education Commission of China, Chongqing, China
feeceebee@hospital.cqmu.edu.cn

[2] Department of Respiratory Children's Hospital of Chongqing Medical University, Ministry of Education Key Laboratory of Child Development and Disorders, Chongqing Key Laboratory of Child Rare Diseases in Infection and Immunity, National Clinical Research Center for Child Health and Disorders, Children's Hospital of Chongqing Medical University, Chongqing, China

[3] Department of Hepatobiliary Surgery, Ministry of Education Key Laboratory of Child Development and Disorders, Chongqing Key Laboratory of Pediatrics, Children's Hospital of Chongqing Medical University, National Clinical Research Center for Child Health and Disorders, Chongqing, China

[4] Department of Hematology and Oncology, Ministry of Education Key Laboratory of Child Development and Disorders, Children's Hospital of Chongqing Medical University, National Clinical Research Center for Child Health and Disorders, Intelligent Application of Big Data in Pediatrics Engineering Research Center of Chongqing Education Commission of China, Chongqing, China

Abstract. Objective: To evaluate the predictive value of 12 composite inflammatory indices for early identification of Epstein-Barr virus-associated hemophagocytic lymphohistiocytosis (EBV-HLH) in children. Methods: This retrospective study analyzed 3,431 children with EBV infection (2,917 with EBV-IM and 514 with EBV-HLH). Logistic regression and receiver operating characteristic (ROC) curve analyses were employed to assess the diagnostic performance of 12 inflammatory indices derived from routine blood parameters. Results: Patients with EBV-HLH exhibited significantly lower hemoglobin, lymphocyte, neutrophil, monocyte, and platelet counts, as well as reduced albumin levels, compared to those with EBV-IM (all $p < 0.001$). The platelet-to-albumin ratio (PAR; AUC = 0.901), pan-immune-inflammation value (PIV; AUC = 0.904), and combination of albumin, lymphocyte and lymphocyte counts (CALLY; AUC = 0.887) demonstrated the highest discriminatory power. The C-reactive protein-to-lymphocyte ratio (CLR) also showed excellent performance (AUC = 0.867). Patients in the highest quartiles of CAR and CLR had 7-fold (OR = 7.09) and 32-fold (OR = 31.83) increased risks of EBV-HLH, respectively. Conclusion: Composite inflammatory indices, particularly PAR, PIV, and CALLY, serve as effective and practical tools for early

Y. Zhang et al. (Eds.): CHIP 2025, CCIS 2884, pp. 178–191, 2026.
https://doi.org/10.1007/978-981-95-7299-1_11

prediction of EBV-HLH in children. These readily accessible biomarkers can significantly improve risk stratification and support timely clinical decision-making, especially in resource-limited settings.

Keywords: EBV-HLH · EBV-IM · Composite inflammatory indices · Early prediction

1 Introduction

Epstein-Barr virus (EBV) is a double-stranded DNA herpesvirus belonging to the Gammaherpesvirinae subfamily. Globally, approximately 90% of adults have been infected with EBV, making it one of the major herpesviruses causing human diseases [1, 2]. Primary infection often occurs during childhood. While EBV infection can be asymptomatic, about 50% of infected adolescents may develop infectious mononucleosis (EBV-IM) [3]. EBV-IM is a benign, self-limiting disease characterized by persistent fever, membranous tonsillitis, cervical lymphadenopathy, hepatosplenomegaly, and atypical lymphocytosis in peripheral blood [3]. Although most children with EBV-IM have a favorable prognosis, a small subset may progress to severe complications, such as EBV-associated hemophagocytic lymphohistiocytosis (EBV-HLH) [4]. EBV-HLH refers to HLH occurring in the context of EBV infection without primary genetic abnormalities related to HLH. It is a hyperinflammatory syndrome driven by excessively activated cytotoxic T cells (CTLs) and macrophages, with high mortality rates [5–9]. The mortality of EBV-HLH is significantly higher than that of EBV-IM; however, these two conditions sometimes exhibit similar symptoms in the early stages. Therefore, early identification and treatment are critical for saving lives [10].

The current diagnosis of EBV-HLH primarily relies on the Histiocyte Society's HLH-94/HLH-2004 criteria, which depend on several laboratory parameters (e.g., hyperferritinemia, elevated sCD25) [6, 11]. However, these specific indicators (such as sCD25 and NK cell activity assays) require advanced laboratory platforms, which are often unavailable in primary healthcare settings, potentially leading to diagnostic delays [6, 11]. Although studies suggest that cytokine profiles (e.g., Th1/Th2 ratio) can serve as early assessment tools, their complex detection methods and high costs limit widespread clinical application [12, 13]. Thus, there is an urgent need to identify predictive indicators based on easily accessible and low-cost parameters to address the challenge of early EBV-HLH detection.

In recent years, composite inflammatory indices derived from routine blood parameters have demonstrated significant predictive value in inflammatory diseases. Inflammatory indicators can be categorized into single indicators and composite indices, which are calculated based on multiple single indicators. Numerous relevant inflammatory indices exist, among which the Systemic Immune-Inflammation Index (SII), Neutrophil-to-Lymphocyte Ratio (NLR), Platelet-to-Lymphocyte Ratio (PLR), Lymphocyte-to-Monocyte Ratio (LMR), Neutrophil-to-Platelet Ratio (NPR), Systemic Inflammation Response Index (SIRI), Platelet-to-Albumin Ratio (PAR), C-reactive protein-to-Albumin Ratio (CAR), C-reactive protein-to-Lymphocyte Ratio (CLR), Combination of Albumin, Lymphocyte and Lymphocyte Counts (CALLY), Pan-Immune-Inflammation

Value (PIV), and Hemoglobin, Albumin, Lymphocyte, and Platelet Score (HALP) have an evidence-based foundation for predicting systemic inflammation [14–16]. These indices, derived from routine blood tests, offer a non-invasive and cost-effective approach to assessing systemic inflammation and immune status [17–19]. Their low cost and high accessibility make them particularly suitable for clinical settings with limited resources. However, although inflammatory storm is recognized as a core pathological mechanism of EBV-HLH, existing studies have mostly focused on isolated analysis of single indicators. There is a lack of systematic comparison of multiple composite inflammatory indices, and their efficacy in distinguishing EBV-IM from EBV-HLH in children remains unclear.

This study aims to systematically evaluate the early predictive value of 12 composite inflammatory indices (including SII, NLR, PLR, LMR, SIRI, PIV, CAR, CLR, CALLY, PAR, NPR, and HALP) for EBV-HLH in children, based on low-cost and highly accessible peripheral blood parameters. We seek to explore whether these routine blood-based indices can serve as early warning tools for EBV-HLH in primary healthcare settings and provide data-driven support for optimizing hierarchical diagnosis and treatment strategies.

2 Materials and Methods

2.1 Study Design and Population

This retrospective cross-sectional study was conducted using data from the Clinical Science Research Big Data Platform (CSRBDP) of the Children's Hospital of Chongqing Medical University (as of June 2025). The study protocol was reviewed and approved by the Ethics Committee of the Children's Hospital of Chongqing Medical University (approval number: 2022(135)) with a waiver of informed consent and was performed in accordance with the Declaration of Helsinki.

Strict inclusion and exclusion criteria were applied. Eligible participants met the following criteria: (1) confirmed diagnosis of Epstein–Barr virus–related infectious mononucleosis (EBV-IM) according to the 2021 Expert Consensus on the Diagnosis and Treatment of Epstein–Barr Virus Infection-Related Diseases in Children [20]; (2) confirmed diagnosis of EBV-associated hemophagocytic lymphohistiocytosis (EBV-HLH) fulfilling the HLH-2004 criteria[6] with evidence of active EBV infection; and (3) age <18 years at the time of admission. Exclusion criteria were: (1) severe co-infection with other pathogens (e.g., bacterial sepsis, COVID-19); (2) HLH not triggered by EBV (e.g., primary HLH, malignancy-associated HLH); and (3) missing data necessary to calculate inflammatory indices or confirm the diagnosis. Finally, 3,431 children were included in this study.

2.2 Definition and Calculation of Composite Inflammatory Indices

Peripheral blood laboratory parameters were extracted, including neutrophil count ($\times 10^9$/L), lymphocyte count ($\times 10^9$/L), monocyte count ($\times 10^9$/L), platelet count ($\times 10^9$/L), hemoglobin concentration (g/L), serum albumin concentration (g/L), and C-reactive protein (CRP, mg/L). Composite inflammatory indices were calculated as follows:

$$\mathbf{SII} = \text{platelet count} \times \text{neutrophil count/lymphocyte count} \tag{1}$$

$$\mathbf{NLR} = \text{neutrophil count/lymphocyte count} \tag{2}$$

$$\mathbf{PLR} = \text{platelet count/lymphocyte count} \tag{3}$$

$$\mathbf{LMR} = \text{lymphocyte count/monocyte count} \tag{4}$$

$$\mathbf{NPR} = \text{neutrophil count/platelet count} \tag{5}$$

$$\mathbf{SIRI} = \text{neutrophil count} \times \text{monocyte count/lymphocyte count} \tag{6}$$

$$\mathbf{PAR} = \text{platelet count/albumin concentration} \tag{7}$$

$$\mathbf{CAR} = \text{CRP/albumin concentration} \tag{8}$$

$$\mathbf{CLR} = \text{CRP/lymphocyte count} \tag{9}$$

$$\mathbf{CALLY} = \text{albumin concentration} \times \text{lymphocyte count/(CRP} \times 10) \tag{10}$$

$$\mathbf{PIV} = \text{neutrophil count} \times \text{monocyte count} \times \text{platelet count/lymphocyte count} \tag{11}$$

$$\mathbf{HALP} = \text{hemoglobin concentration} \times \text{albumin concentration} \times \text{lymphocyte count/platelet count} \tag{12}$$

2.3 Statistical Analysis

Categorical variables were summarized as counts and percentages and compared between groups using the χ^2 test. Continuous variables were assessed for normality; non-normally distributed variables were expressed as medians with interquartile ranges (IQRs) and compared using the Mann–Whitney U test. Each inflammatory index was categorized into quartiles (Q1: $\leq$ 25th percentile; Q2: 25–50th percentile; Q3: 50–75th percentile; Q4: $>$ 75th percentile). Logistic regression models adjusted for age and sex were used to evaluate associations between each index and EBV-related disease, reporting odds ratios (ORs) with 95% confidence intervals (CIs). Tests for linear trend across quartiles were performed by modeling the median value of each quartile as a continuous variable.

To further assess the discriminatory ability of each index for differentiating EBV-HLH from EBV-IM, receiver operating characteristic (ROC) curves were constructed, and the area under the curve (AUC) with 95% CIs was calculated. Optimal diagnostic cut-off points were determined using the Youden index, and corresponding sensitivity and specificity were reported. ROC curves for all indices were plotted together to allow direct visual comparison of diagnostic performance.

All statistical analyses were performed using R software (version 4.5.0; http://www.R-project.org). A two-sided p value <0.05 was considered statistically significant.

3 Result

3.1 Patients' Characteristic

Among 3,431 patients, 2,917 had EBV-IM and 514 had EBV-HLH. EBV-HLH patients were younger (62.4 vs. 67.9 months) and more often male (49.4% vs. 43.0%). Compared with EBV-IM, EBV-HLH patients had markedly lower hemoglobin, lymphocyte, neutrophil, monocyte, and platelet counts, and reduced albumin levels (all $p < 0.001$). Composite inflammatory indices (SII, SIRI, PAR, PIV, CALLY) were lower in HLH, whereas ratio-based indices (LMR, CAR, CLR) were higher (all $p < 0.001$). CRP was modestly elevated (14.0 vs. 9.0 mg/L; $p < 0.001$) (Table 1).

3.2 Associations of Composite Inflammation Indices with Risk of EBV-HLH

We assessed the association between quartiles of various composite inflammatory indices and the EBV-HLH. For each index, the lowest quartile (Q1) served as the reference. Indices such as SII, SIRI, PAR, CALLY, and PIV showed strong inverse associations, with ORs for Q2–Q4 ranging from 0.01 to 0.20 ($p < 1 \times 10^{-32}$), indicating that higher quartiles were markedly protective. Trend analyses confirmed highly significant dose–response relationships. NLR, PLR, LMR, and NPR exhibited non-linear associations. Middle quartiles (Q2–Q3) were generally protective (ORs 0.21–0.83), while the highest quartile (Q4) sometimes showed increased risk, suggesting threshold or U-shaped effects. Conversely, CAR and CLR demonstrated strong positive associations with the outcome. Patients in the highest quartile of CAR had an OR of 7.09 (95% CI 4.99–10.07), and CLR Q4 had an OR of 31.83 (95% CI 20.69–48.96), indicating these indices are potent predictors of high risk. HALP showed mostly protective effects in Q2–Q3 (ORs 0.16–0.20), with attenuation at Q4 (OR 0.50), suggesting a moderate protective effect that diminishes at extreme values (Table 2 and Fig. 1).

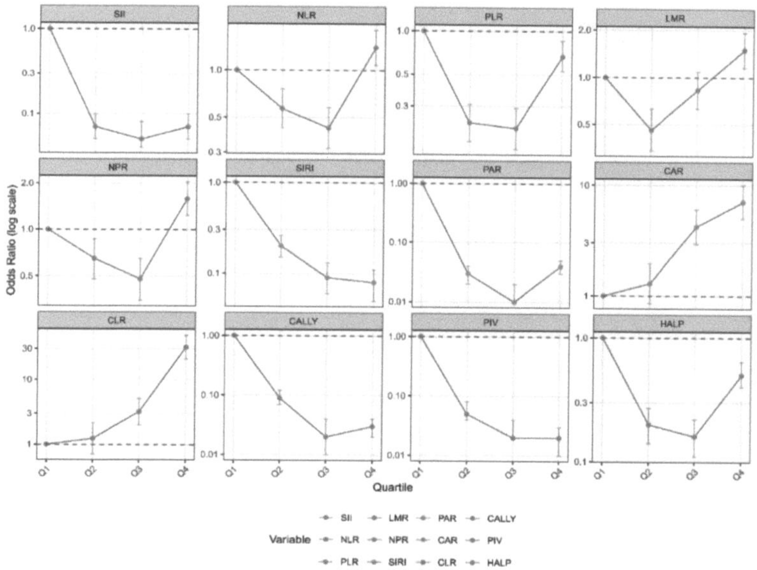

Fig. 1. Forest plots display the risk association between composite inflammatory indices and risk of EBV-HLH. The levels of composite inflammatory indices were divided into quartiles. The ORs and 95% confidence intervals for different subgroups are listed, with the lowest level group as a reference. Vertical dashed line indicates the null reference value of "1".

3.3 Predictive Performance of Composite Inflammatory Indices

We evaluated the diagnostic performance of 12 composite inflammatory indices using receiver operating characteristic (ROC) curve analysis after adjustment for age and gender (Table 3 and Fig. 2). Among all indices, PAR, PIV, and CALLY demonstrated the highest discriminative ability, with AUCs of 0.901 (95% CI 0.879–0.922), 0.904 (95% CI 0.887–0.921), and 0.887 (95% CI 0.869–0.905), respectively, and corresponding specificities exceeding 0.84. CLR also showed excellent performance (AUC 0.867, 95% CI 0.846–0.888) with high specificity (0.868). Moderate predictive values were observed for SII (AUC 0.777, 95% CI 0.750–0.803), SIRI (AUC 0.761, 95% CI 0.735–0.786), and CAR (AUC 0.709, 95% CI 0.683–0.735). Conversely, NLR, PLR, LMR, and HALP yielded AUCs below 0.65, indicating limited discriminatory power.

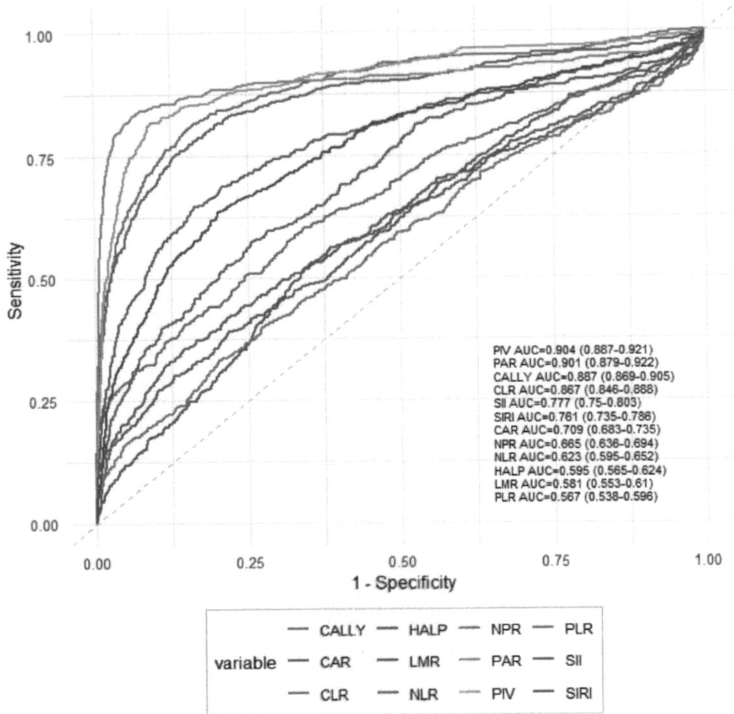

Fig. 2. ROC curve analysis of the potential value of inflammatory indicators in predicting for EBV-HLH.in children.

Table 1. Baseline characteristics of patients with EBV-IM and EBV-HLH

Variable	EBV-IM(n = 2917)	EBV-HLH (n = 514)	p
Gender (%)			0.008
Male	1255 (43.0)	254 (49.4)	
Female	1662 (57.0)	260 (50.6)	
Age(months) (mean (SD))	67.93 (35.16)	62.37 (45.51)	0.002
HBG (g/L) (median [IQR])	118.00 [111.00, 125.00]	85.00 [73.00, 97.00]	<0.001
LYMPH (×10^9/L) (median [IQR])	6.82 [4.98, 9.20]	1.44 [0.69, 2.70]	<0.001
NEUT(×10^9/L) (median [IQR])	3.36 [2.23, 4.83]	0.79 [0.37, 1.58]	<0.001
PLATELET(×10^9/L) (median [IQR])	220.00 [178.00, 272.00]	35.00 [16.00, 74.75]	<0.001

(continued)

Table 1. *(continued)*

Variable	EBV-IM(n = 2917)	EBV-HLH (n = 514)	p
MONO (×10^9/L) (median [IQR])	0.54 [0.35, 0.84]	0.10 [0.04, 0.24]	<0.001
CRP (mg/L) (median [IQR])	9.00 [8.00, 16.92]	13.96 [8.00, 29.00]	<0.001
ALB (g/L) (median [IQR])	40.10 [37.80, 42.30]	30.40 [25.70, 34.60]	<0.001
SII (median [IQR])	102.60 [64.21, 171.86]	16.81 [4.04, 59.11]	<0.001
NLR (median [IQR])	0.47 [0.31, 0.72]	0.52 [0.26, 1.17]	0.028
PLR (median [IQR])	32.03 [21.81, 48.02]	24.34 [8.76, 62.02]	<0.001
LMR (median [IQR])	12.00 [8.24, 17.95]	15.34 [7.81, 27.29]	<0.001
NPR (median [IQR])	0.02 [0.01, 0.02]	0.02 [0.01, 0.05]	<0.001
SIRI (median [IQR])	0.27 [0.13, 0.50]	0.05 [0.02, 0.17]	<0.001
PAR (median [IQR])	5.51 [4.45, 6.82]	1.21 [0.57, 2.41]	<0.001
CAR (median [IQR])	0.23 [0.19, 0.42]	0.44 [0.27, 1.04]	<0.001
CLR (median [IQR])	1.51 [0.89, 2.90]	10.55 [4.17, 27.79]	<0.001
CALLY (median [IQR])	2.67 [1.37, 4.51]	0.29 [0.10, 0.75]	<0.001
PIV (median [IQR])	56.57 [28.53, 112.14]	1.37 [0.26, 8.62]	<0.001
HALP (median [IQR])	144.94 [96.89, 220.70]	95.93 [40.65, 266.77]	<0.001

Note EBV-IM, Epstein–Barr virus–associated infectious mononucleosis; EBV-HLH, Epstein–Barr virus–associated hemophagocytic lymphohistiocytosis; HBG, hemoglobin; LYMPH, lymphocyte count; NEUT, neutrophil count; PLATELET, platelet count; MONO, monocyte count; CRP, C-reactive protein; ALB, albumin; SII, systemic immune-inflammation index; NLR, neutrophil-to-lymphocyte ratio; PLR, platelet-to-lymphocyte ratio; LMR, lymphocyte-to-monocyte ratio; NPR, neutrophil-to-platelet ratio; SIRI, systemic inflammation response index; PAR, platelet-to-albumin ratio; CAR, C-reactive protein-to-albumin ratio; CLR, C-reactive protein-to-lymphocyte ratio; CALLY, combination of albumin, lymphocyte and lymphocyte counts; PIV, pan-immune-inflammation value; HALP, hemoglobin, albumin, lymphocyte, platelet score

Table 2. Association of composite inflammatory indices quartiles with risk of EBV-HLH

Group	OR (95% CI)	P	P for trend
SII Q1	1.00 (ref)		<0.001
SII Q2	0.07 (0.05–0.1)	<0.001	
SII Q3	0.05 (0.04–0.08)	<0.001	
SII Q4	0.07 (0.05–0.1)	<0.001	
NLR Q1	1.00 (ref)		0.02
NLR Q2	0.57 (0.43–0.76)	<0.001	

(continued)

Table 2. (*continued*)

Group	OR (95% CI)	P	P for trend
NLR Q3	0.43 (0.32–0.58)	<0.001	
NLR Q4	1.39 (1.08–1.79)	0.01	
PLR Q1	1.00 (ref)		<0.001
PLR Q2	0.23 (0.17–0.31)	<0.001	
PLR Q3	0.21 (0.15–0.29)	<0.001	
PLR Q4	0.67 (0.53–0.86)	0.001	
LMR Q1	1.00 (ref)		<0.001
LMR Q2	0.46 (0.34–0.63)	<0.001	
LMR Q3	0.83 (0.63–1.09)	0.18	
LMR Q4	1.5 (1.16–1.93)	0.002	
NPR Q1	1.00 (ref)		<0.001
NPR Q2	0.65 (0.48–0.87)	0.004	
NPR Q3	0.48 (0.35–0.65)	<0.001	
NPR Q4	1.59 (1.24–2.05)	<0.001	
SIRI Q1	1.00 (ref)		<0.001
SIRI Q2	0.2 (0.15–0.26)	<0.001	
SIRI Q3	0.09 (0.06–0.13)	<0.001	
SIRI Q4	0.08 (0.05–0.11)	<0.001	
PAR Q1	1.00 (ref)		<0.001
PAR Q2	0.03 (0.02–0.04)	<0.001	
PAR Q3	0.01 (0.01–0.02)	<0.001	
PAR Q4	0.04 (0.03–0.05)	<0.001	
CAR Q1	1.00 (ref)		<0.001
CAR Q2	1.29 (0.86–1.95)	0.22	
CAR Q3	4.2 (2.93–6.03)	<0.001	
CAR Q4	7.09 (4.99–10.07)	<0.001	
CLR Q1	1.00 (ref)		<0.001
CLR Q2	1.24 (0.71–2.15)	0.45	
CLR Q3	3.2 (1.99–5.13)	<0.001	
CLR Q4	31.83 (20.69–48.96)	<0.001	
CALLY Q1	1.00 (ref)		<0.001
CALLY Q2	0.09 (0.07–0.12)	<0.001	
CALLY Q3	0.02 (0.01–0.04)	<0.001	
CALLY Q4	0.03 (0.02–0.04)	<0.001	

(*continued*)

Table 2. (*continued*)

Group	OR (95% CI)	P	P for trend
PIV Q1	1.00 (ref)		<0.001
PIV Q2	0.05 (0.04–0.08)	<0.001	
PIV Q3	0.02 (0.02–0.04)	<0.001	
PIV Q4	0.02 (0.01–0.03)	<0.001	
HALP Q1	1.00 (ref)		<0.001
HALP Q2	0.2 (0.14–0.27)	<0.001	
HALP Q3	0.16 (0.11–0.22)	<0.001	
HALP Q4	0.5 (0.4–0.64)	<0.001	

Table 3. ROC analysis of composite inflammatory indices for predicting EBV-HLH.in children.

Variable	AUC (95% CI)	Threshold	Sensitivity	Specificity
SII	0.777 (0.750–0.803)	38.317	0.646	0.837
NLR	0.623 (0.595–0.652)	1.015	0.354	0.855
PLR	0.567 (0.538–0.596)	15.118	0.331	0.799
LMR	0.581 (0.553–0.610)	18.121	0.531	0.647
NPR	0.665 (0.636–0.694)	0.0365	0.601	0.66
SIRI	0.761 (0.735–0.786)	0.095	0.636	0.798
PAR	0.901 (0.879–0.922)	3.140	0.839	0.930
CAR	0.709 (0.683–0.735)	0.251	0.578	0.740
CLR	0.867 (0.846–0.888)	4.029	0.753	0.868
CALLY	0.887 (0.869–0.905)	0.758	0.807	0.846
PIV	0.904 (0.887–0.921)	11.503	0.819	0.907
HALP	0.595 (0.565–0.624)	65.454	0.300	0.872

4 Discussion

Most primary EBV infections manifest as infectious mononucleosis (IM) in children, while a subset of patients may progress to EBV-associated hemophagocytic lymphohistiocytosis (EBV-HLH) [21]. Patients with acute EBV infection exhibit many clinical and biochemical features of HLH, such as fever, splenomegaly, and liver dysfunction, making it challenging to distinguish EBV-HLH from EBV-IM in certain cases [7]. To our knowledge, this represents the first comprehensive evaluation of multiple composite inflammatory indices derived from routine peripheral blood parameters for early prediction of EBV-HLH in children. Our findings demonstrate that PAR, PIV, and CALLY exhibit superior discriminatory ability in differentiating EBV-IM from EBV-HLH, providing a practical solution for early risk stratification in clinical settings.

This study reveals significant differences in hematological parameters between EBV-IM and EBV-HLH patients. EBV-HLH patients demonstrated comprehensive cytopenia and hypoalbuminemia, reflecting the core features of HLH: hemophagocytosis and bone marrow suppression mediated by hyperinflammatory states [6]. The marked decrease in platelet counts was particularly consistent with the cytopenia criteria in HLH-2004 diagnostic guidelines [6]. Regarding composite inflammatory indices, SII, SIRI, PAR, PIV, and CALLY were significantly lower in the EBV-HLH group, directly correlating with HLH pathophysiology. The reduction in SII and SIRI primarily reflected neutrophil and platelet consumption, consistent with hemophagocytosis due to macrophage activation and cytokine-mediated bone marrow suppression [6]. Previous studies have shown that EBV-HLH patients exhibit significantly lower CD8 + T-cell proportions but higher IFN-γ levels compared to EBV-IM patients, indicating the complex pathophysiology of HLH [22].

The excellent performance of composite indices in our study corresponds with emerging evidence on inflammatory biomarkers in HLH pathogenesis. We found that CAR (CRP/albumin concentration) and CLR (CRP/lymphocyte count) showed strong positive associations with EBV-HLH risk (ORs 7.09 and 31.83 for the highest quartiles, respectively), corroborating the findings of Huang et al., who identified IL-6 and IL-10 as independent predictors in their nomogram model (ORs 71.505 and 213.139, respectively) [23]. While ferritin ≥500 μg/L remains an HLH-2004 criterion, higher cut-off values (≥10,000 μg/L) improve specificity [24]. D-dimer levels may serve as a valuable prognostic indicator for EBV-HLH caused by EBV [25].This consistency across studies underscores the critical role of cytokine storms and CRP in EBV-HLH pathophysiology. The inverse associations observed for SII, SIRI, and PIV with EBV-HLH risk reflect the characteristic consumptive cytopenia of HLH. This pattern parallels the findings of Li et al., whose EBV-HLH screening score incorporated hemoglobin, platelet, and neutrophil parameters with similar predictive value [26]. Our multivariate analysis revealed that the highest quartiles of these indices had significant protective effects, indicating their ability to effectively capture hematological abnormalities preceding full-blown HLH.

The exceptional performance of PAR (platelet count/albumin concentration) in our study (AUC 0.901) can be attributed to the extensive platelet consumption in HLH due to macrophage activation and disseminated intravascular coagulation, while hypoalbuminemia reflects both hepatic dysfunction and systemic inflammatory response. This combination effectively captures the dual impact of consumptive coagulopathy and organ damage, making PAR a more comprehensive marker than any single parameter alone. The strong predictive value of CALLY (albumin × lymphocyte count/CRP) and PIV (neutrophil count × monocyte count × platelet count/lymphocyte count) further supports the multifactorial nature of HLH pathogenesis. These indices simultaneously assess nutritional status (albumin), immune competence (lymphocytes), and inflammatory activation (platelets/neutrophils/CRP), providing a comprehensive evaluation of the patient's physiological state. This approach aligns with the complex interplay of immune dysregulation, cytokine storms, and organ dysfunction during HLH development.

The temporal advantages of these indices deserve emphasis. Many advanced HLH diagnostic methods (ferritin, sCD25, NK cell activity, genetic testing) require specialized platforms and substantial turnaround time. In contrast, the parameters needed for these indices are routinely available in most clinical settings within hours, enabling real-time risk assessment. This addresses the critical need for early identification highlighted by Li et al., who found that diagnostic delays significantly impact prognosis [26]. The quartile-based risk stratification demonstrated in our study provides clinically actionable thresholds. For instance, patients with CAR values in the highest quartile had a 7-fold increased HLH risk, while those with CLR in the highest quartile had a remarkable 32-fold risk increase. These pronounced gradients enable meaningful risk categorization that can guide monitoring intensity and diagnostic urgency.

Our results complement recent advances in EBV-HLH prediction. Developing a points-based scoring system like that proposed by Li et al. [26] could further enhance clinical utility. Their EBV-HLH screening score (incorporating hemoglobin, platelet, neutrophil, albumin, and LDH) achieved a sensitivity of 89.2% and specificity of 89.5% in validation cohorts. Our findings suggest that incorporating additional ratio-based indices might further improve performance. Shi et al. identified D-dimer as a valuable predictor (sensitivity 88.9%, specificity 90.2% at cut-off 1721.500 μg/L) [25], while Huang et al. developed a nomogram incorporating ferritin, CD3CD16 + CD56 + %, anti-EBV-NA-IgG, IL-6, and IL-10 with exceptional discriminatory ability (AUC 0.997) [23]. Each approach has distinct advantages: D-dimer reflects coagulopathy, cytokine profiles capture immune activation, and our composite indices reflect hematological and inflammatory integration. The choice of predictive tools should consider clinical context. In primary care settings with limited resources, our composite indices derived from routine blood tests offer practical advantages. In tertiary centers, multimodal approaches combining multiple biomarker classes may provide optimal performance.

Several limitations warrant acknowledgment in this study. The retrospective design introduces potential selection bias, and the single-center nature limits generalizability. The timing of testing relative to disease progression requires standardization, as biomarker dynamics during HLH evolution remain incompletely characterized. Future studies should include: (1) prospective validation of these indices in multicenter cohorts; (2) development of standardized scoring systems incorporating the most predictive indicators; (3) exploration of dynamic monitoring during disease progression; and (4) evaluation of the cost-effectiveness of implementing these indices in different healthcare settings.

5 Conclusion

This study demonstrates that composite inflammatory indices derived from routine blood parameters provide valuable tools for early identification of EBV-HLH in children. Their strong performance, practicality, and cost-effectiveness address critical needs in HLH diagnosis, particularly in resource-limited settings.

Disclosure of Interests. The authors have no competing interests to declare that are relevant to the content of this article.

References

1. Cohen, J.I.: Epstein-Barr virus infection. N. Engl. J. Med. **343**(7), 481–492 (2000)
2. Thompson, M.P., Kurzrock, R.: Epstein-Barr virus and cancer. Clin. Cancer Res. **10**(3), 803–821 (2004)
3. Dunmire, S.K., Verghese, P.S., Balfour, H.H., Jr.: Primary Epstein-Barr virus infection. J. Clin. Virol. **102**, 84–92 (2018)
4. Young, L.S., Rickinson, A.B.: Epstein-Barr virus: 40 years on. Nat. Rev. Cancer **4**(10), 757–768 (2004)
5. Si, S.J., et al.: Diagnostic challenges in pediatric hemophagocytic lymphohistiocytosis. J. Clin. Immunol. **41**(6), 1213–1218 (2021)
6. Henter, J.I., et al.: HLH-2004: diagnostic and therapeutic guidelines for hemophagocytic lymphohistiocytosis. Pediatr. Blood Cancer **48**(2), 124–131 (2007)
7. Marsh, R.A.: Epstein-barr virus and hemophagocytic lymphohistiocytosis. Front. Immunol. **8**, 1902 (2017)
8. Canna, S.W., Marsh, R.A.: Pediatric hemophagocytic lymphohistiocytosis. Blood **135**(16), 1332–1343 (2020)
9. Risma, K.A., Marsh, R.A.: Hemophagocytic Lymphohistiocytosis: clinical presentations and diagnosis. J. Allergy Clin. Immunol. Pract. **7**(3), 824–832 (2019)
10. Huang, S.C., Chen, J.S., Cheng, C.N., Yang, Y.J.: Hypoalbuminaemia is an independent predictor for hemophagocytic lymphohistiocytosis in childhood Epstein-Barr virus-associated infectious mononucleosis. Eur. J. Haematol. **89**(5), 417–422 (2012)
11. Henter, J.I., Aricò, M., Egeler, R.M., Elinder, G., Favara, B.E., Filipovich, A.H., Gadner, H., Imashuku, S., Janka-Schaub, G., Komp, D., Ladisch, S., Webb, D.: HLH-94: a treatment protocol for hemophagocytic lymphohistiocytosis. HLH study group of the histiocyte society. Med Pediatr Oncol **28**(5), 342–347 (1997)
12. Chen, Y., Wang, Z., Luo, Z., Zhao, N., Yang, S., Tang, Y.: Comparison of Th1/Th2 cytokine profiles between primary and secondary haemophagocytic lymphohistiocytosis. Ital. J. Pediatr. **42**(1), 50 (2016)
13. Xu, X.J., et al.: Simple evaluation of clinical situation and subtypes of pediatric hemophagocytic lymphohistiocytosis by cytokine patterns. Front. Immunol. **13**, 850443 (2022)
14. Liu, Y.C., Chuang, S.H., Chen, Y.P., Shih, Y.H.: Associations of novel complete blood count-derived inflammatory markers with psoriasis: a systematic review and meta-analysis. Arch. Dermatol. Res. **316**(6), 228 (2024)
15. Guo, B., et al.: Associations of CBC-Derived inflammatory indicators with sarcopenia and mortality in adults: evidence from Nhanes 1999–2006. BMC Geriatr. **24**(1), 432 (2024)
16. Erre, G.L., et al.: Meta-analysis of neutrophil-to-lymphocyte and platelet-to-lymphocyte ratio in rheumatoid arthritis. Eur. J. Clin. Invest. **49**(1), e13037 (2019)
17. Yeniceri, A., Cayonu, M.: Outcomes of inflammatory markers in the diagnosis of complicated rhinosinusitis in children. Eur. Arch. Otorhinolaryngol. **282**(5), 2381–2387 (2025)
18. Li, Y., Shao, X.: Mediating role of inflammatory markers (NLR, PLR, SII, SIRI) in the association between 25(OH)D deficiency and obesity in children and adolescents. J. Health Popul. Nutr. **44**(1), 215 (2025)
19. Han, B., Li, X., Zhang, L., Zhang, H., Wang, B.: Clinical value of C-reactive protein to albumin ratio, aspartate aminotransferase, and platelet-to-lymphocyte ratio in predicting the severity of community-acquired pneumonia in children. Front. Pediatr. **13**, 1611792 (2025)
20. Kunling, S.: Subspecialty Group of Infectious Diseases Society of Pediatrics, Chinese Medical Association, Group National Children's EBV Infection Cooperative: Expert consensus on the diagnosis and treatment principles of Epstein-Barr virus-associated diseases in children. Zhonghua Er Ke Za Zhi **59**, 905–911 (2021). [in Chinese]

21. Taylor, G.S., Long, H.M., Brooks, J.M., Rickinson, A.B., Hislop, A.D.: The immunology of Epstein-Barr virus-induced disease. Annu. Rev. Immunol. **33**, 787–821 (2015)
22. Cai, L., et al.: Comparative study of biomarkers for the early identification of Epstein-Barr virus-associated hemophagocytic lymphohistiocytosis in infectious mononucleosis. BMC Infect. Dis. **23**(1), 728 (2023)
23. Huang, R., et al.: A predictive model for Epstein-Barr virus-associated hemophagocytic lymphohistiocytosis. Front. Immunol. **15**, 1503118 (2024)
24. Allen, C.E., Yu, X., Kozinetz, C.A., McClain, K.L.: Highly elevated ferritin levels and the diagnosis of hemophagocytic lymphohistiocytosis. Pediatr. Blood Cancer **50**(6), 1227–1235 (2008)
25. Shi, J., et al.: Clinical warning of hemophagocytic syndrome caused by Epstein-Barr virus. Ital. J. Pediatr. **47**(1), 3 (2021)
26. Li, X., et al.: Development of a screening score for Hemophagocytic Lymphohistiocytosis among pediatric patients with acute infection of Epstein-Barr virus. Front. Immunol. **13**, 981251 (2022)

A Verification-Enhanced Large Model Framework for Diabetes Knowledge Graph Construction

Kejun Wu, Yu Song, Kaixuan Yuan, Xinyang Li, Bohan Yu, Aoze Zheng, and Kunli Zhang(✉)

School of Computer Science and Artificial Intelligence, Zhengzhou University, Henan 450001, China
ieklzhang@zzu.edu.cn

Abstract. Diabetes is a common major chronic disease characterized by high incidence rates and complex complications. This paper constructs a Diabetes Knowledge Graph (DKG). At the schema layer, DKG defines 17 entity types and 85 relation types centered around diseases. At the data layer, we develop a verification-enhanced large language model framework for the medical field (MED-VerifyKG). This framework integrates LLM-based candidate triple extraction, rule-based filtering, and expert validation, with iterative prompt and rule refinement. Triple fusion is ultimately prioritized based on expert validation confidence. The constructed DKG contains 18,720 entities and 24,249 triples, providing robust data support for diabetes-related intelligent question answering and clinical decision support.

Keywords: Knowledge graph · Diabetes · Verification-Enhanced · LLM

1 Introduction

Diabetes is a major global public health challenge that significantly increases the risk of morbidity, disability, and mortality, with its incidence and prevalence rising rapidly over the past decades [1]. According to the International Diabetes Federation (IDF) *Diabetes Atlas 2025* [2], there were 589 million adults aged 20–79 living with diabetes worldwide in 2024, and the total number of patients is projected to climb to 853 million by 2050 [3]. In recent years, with the rapid growth of China's economy, the prevalence of diabetes in China has also increased sharply. Along with advances in medical research and the rapid development of big data technologies, diabetes has received widespread global attention as a critical public health issue [4]. In recent years, multiple guidelines for diabetes prevention and treatment have been issued domestically and internationally, such as the *Chinese Guidelines for the Prevention and Treatment of Diabetes* and the American Diabetes Association (ADA) standards, which have

Y. Zhang et al. (Eds.): CHIP 2025, CCIS 2884, pp. 192–205, 2026.
https://doi.org/10.1007/978-981-95-7299-1_12

promoted the standardization of diabetes care [5]. Despite progress in diabetes knowledge graph research, relatively few such graphs exist due to the disease's complex pathological mechanisms, wide range of complications, and individualized treatment needs [6]. This scarcity hinders the dissemination and sharing of medical resources and impedes research progress in diabetes.

Effective prevention and management of diabetes rely heavily on the deep integration and intelligent utilization of vast, multi-source medical knowledge [7]. Knowledge graphs (KGs) [8], with their strong semantic representation and relational reasoning capabilities, provide an ideal technological pathway for structuring medical knowledge, supporting next-generation clinical decision support systems, and enabling intelligent question-answering systems [9]. Although several medical knowledge graphs and diabetes-related datasets have been developed and released in recent years [10], serving as valuable resources for research, their construction methods still largely depend on traditional manual annotation or supervised learning paradigms [11]. While these methods have achieved significant progress, their further application and dissemination face practical challenges. First, manual construction strategies that rely on domain experts ensure accuracy but are highly time- and labor-intensive in practice [12]. Second, supervised learning methods usually depend on large-scale, high-quality annotated datasets for model training, and their performance is strongly tied to the size and quality of training data. Moreover, when confronted with new domains or relationship types, the transferability and adaptability of models remain limited [13]. Therefore, exploring a construction method for domain-specific knowledge graphs that balances automation with accuracy is of great importance for advancing medical artificial intelligence.

With the remarkable performance of large language models (LLMs) [14] in natural language processing tasks, new opportunities have emerged for automated knowledge graph construction. However, directly applying LLMs to specialized medical knowledge extraction faces three challenges: (1) high annotation costs and scarcity of expert resources [15]; (2) hallucination and inconsistency issues [16]; and (3) difficulties in ensuring quality under complex semantics [17].

This paper addresses the construction of a diabetes knowledge graph by proposing and implementing a verification-enhanced collaborative framework, termed **MED-VerifyKG**. The main contributions are as follows:

- **MED-VerifyKG framework:** We propose a verification-enhanced framework integrating large language models with multi-round verification. Its closed-loop process–"initial extraction–multi-round verification–intelligent optimization"–combines automated extraction, rule-based filtering, and expert validation, addressing reliability and efficiency challenges in knowledge graph construction.
- **High-quality diabetes knowledge graph:** Using *Practical Diabetology (4th Edition)* as the primary data source, we construct a large-scale knowledge graph covering key entities such as diseases, symptoms, medications, and examinations, along with their relationships.

- **Empirical validation:** Comparative studies show that MED-VerifyKG achieves high accuracy while reducing reliance on expert annotation, providing an efficient and reliable approach for domain-specific knowledge graph construction.

2 Related Work

With the continuous development of artificial intelligence, the construction of domain-specific knowledge graphs has gradually extended from general domains to specific diseases [18], resulting in a variety of specialized knowledge bases. In the case of diabetes [2], a major global chronic disease, building a high-quality knowledge graph is of great significance for integrating fragmented knowledge and supporting clinical decision-making.

Currently, scholars worldwide have built large-scale medical knowledge bases. For example, Aodema et al. [19] constructed the Chinese Medical Knowledge Graph (CMeKG), which contains 6,310 diseases and more than one million medical concept–relation instances. Cheng et al. [20] proposed a method that utilizes similarity metrics to link existing knowledge graphs and constructed a stroke medical knowledge graph. Chang et al. [21] released a dataset for constructing a Chinese medical knowledge graph specifically for diabetes (DiaKG), which includes 22,050 entities and 6,890 relations, by building a high-quality annotated corpus. Liu et al. [22] constructed a medical knowledge graph for diabetes prevention and control by integrating multi-source heterogeneous medical data with natural language processing techniques. Costanzo et al. [23] developed the Type 2 Diabetes Knowledge Portal (T2DKP), an open platform that integrates multi-omics data with interactive analysis tools, specifically for type 2 diabetes research. Wang et al. [24] created an evidence-based knowledge graph for diabetes complications by combining evidence-based medicine with a logistic regression risk prediction model.

Although existing diabetes knowledge graphs provide valuable resources for research, their construction methods still face two major challenges: (1) most current knowledge graphs focus on basic entity recognition and simple relation extraction [25], making it difficult to capture the complex pathological mechanisms and individualized treatment knowledge of diabetes; and (2) traditional construction approaches rely heavily on manual annotation, leading to high costs, poor adaptability, and delayed updates [26].

To address these issues, this paper constructs the MED-VerifyKG framework, a verification-enhanced approach that integrates large language model–based automated extraction, rule-based medical validation [27], and expert feedback optimization. The framework enables the construction of a high-quality, dynamically updatable diabetes knowledge graph, providing a reliable knowledge foundation for clinical intelligent applications.

3 Construction Process of the Diabetes Knowledge Graph

3.1 Overview of the Process

Knowledge graph construction generally follows top-down or bottom-up approaches [28]. In this study, the Diabetes Knowledge Graph (DKG) is built top-down, comprising a **schema layer** and a **data layer**. The schema layer defines entity and relation classifications, providing constraints for the data layer, which encodes knowledge as entity–relation triples.

As shown in **Fig.** 1, the schema layer is designed based on authoritative medical sources, including official documents issued by the National Health Commission and the National Standardization Administration, and reviewed by experts. Annotation guidelines for symptoms, treatments, and other diabetes aspects are established to complete the schema.

At the data layer, diabetes-related information is collected as **structured** (electronic medical records) and **unstructured** (textbook chapters from *Practical Diabetology*) data. Structured data are processed with large language models (LLMs) to create the *Corpus for Entity and Relation Annotation in Diabetes Domain* (CERD), manually proofread and used to build the medical rule base. Unstructured data are extracted using LLMs, as detailed in Sect. 4.

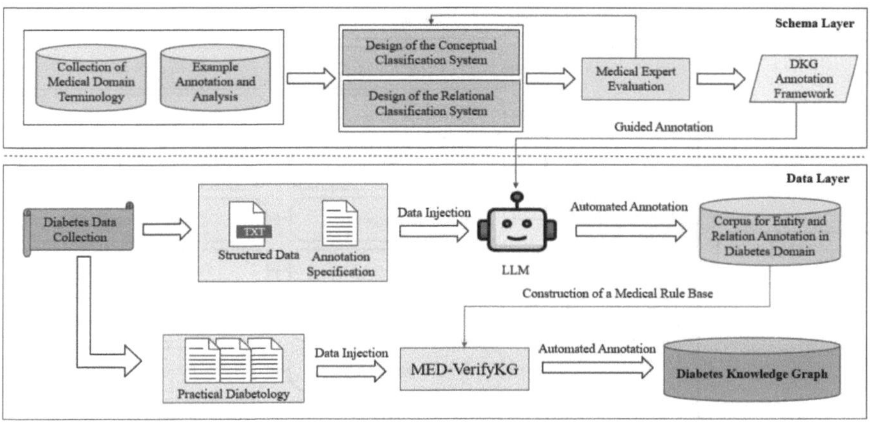

Fig. 1. DKG constructs the overall framework

3.2 Schema Layer Construction

In the schema layer, this study established a rigorous ontology for the DKG by systematically analyzing diabetes. The framework defines 17 entity types (e.g., diseases, symptoms, examinations, drugs, prognosis, treatments) and 85 relation types, forming a richly connected semantic network with fine-grained entity distinctions and precise relation semantics. Under physician guidance and by referencing clinical guidelines, treatment cases, and literature, a disease-centered conceptual classification system was developed, covering symptoms, diseases, drugs, examinations, treatments, prognosis, epidemiology, body parts, physiological parameters, chemical substances, procedures, test reagents, and others. This abstraction and categorization provide a structured description of diabetes pathogenesis, clinical manifestations, diagnostic methods, and treatment pathways, supporting accurate clinical reasoning and decision-making.

Conceptual relations capture semantic links between entities and are mapped to 85 well-defined types in the diabetes domain. Typical relations include AKO between diseases, differential diagnosis, complication, synonym, entity grouping, and causal relations. Examinations such as blood glucose, HbA1c, and fundus photography are classified as laboratory, imaging, pathological, or other types, while disease–drug relations include drug treatment and drug-induced disease. This multi-level relational system spans pathophysiology to clinical interventions, providing a structured knowledge foundation for accurate diagnosis and treatment. **Figure** 2 illustrates the disease-centered knowledge representation framework using "type 2 diabetes" as an example.

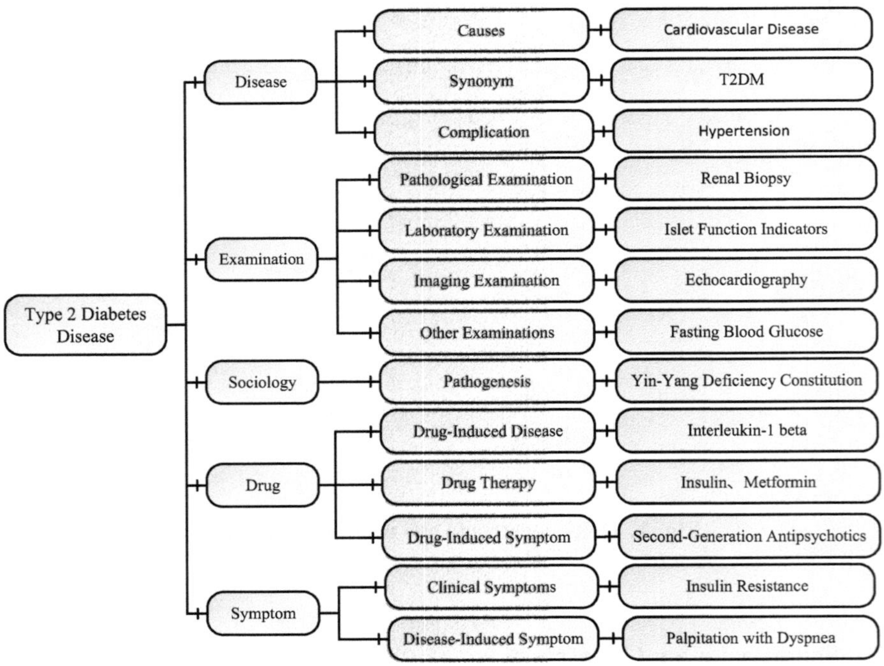

Fig. 2. Example of DKG relationship description

3.3 Data Layer Construction

The construction of the DKG data layer is the key step in operationalizing the knowledge graph. It mainly involves collecting, preprocessing, annotating, and proofreading multi-source data in the diabetes domain.

Data Collection and Preprocessing Diabetes knowledge data were collected from two sources: structured EMRs and unstructured textbook data. EMRs from partner hospitals included 800 records with symptoms, examinations, diagnoses, and treatments, processed with large language models to build the CERD corpus. Textbook data came from *Practical Diabetology (4th Edition)*, covering pathophysiology, clinical features, diagnostics, treatments, and complications.

Textbook data required preprocessing to handle headers, footers, tables/figures, special characters, formatting issues, and inconsistent terminology (e.g., "T2DM" vs. "type 2 diabetes"). Steps included removing non-text content, correcting formatting, unifying terms via a medical dictionary, and coreference resolution to ensure completeness.

Processing Structured Data Structured EMR data are often tabular. LLM-based extraction methods were employed to transform tabular information into corpus data for further use. Prompt templates were carefully designed to align LLM output with annotation specifications and required formats. As shown in Table 1, our prompts are set with Role Description, Input, and Task Definition.

Table 1. Prompting LLM for knowledge extraction

Role	Content
Role description	You are a diabetes expert. Your task is to extract entity-relation triples from the given information. Entity types: <disease, symptom, examination, prognosis>; Relation types: <disease – clinical symptom – symptom>, <disease – prognosis status – prognosis>.
Input	Please perform named entity recognition on the currently given information. Table: {...}.
Task definition	Extract triples from the given text. Please only output the triples in the format: <head entity, head entity type — relation — tail entity type, tail entity>. Separate multiple triples with semicolons. Example: <Type 2 diabetes, disease — drug treatment — drug, metformin>; ...

This resolves the limitations of LLMs in accuracy for domain-specific extraction while leveraging their ability to incorporate external knowledge. After annotation, the CERD corpus was formed.

Processing Unstructured Data Unstructured data primarily include medical textbooks, clinical guidelines, and research literature. These texts, while systematic, contain complex terminology, cross-chapter knowledge, and implicit references, requiring preprocessing before effective extraction.

Because medical knowledge demands extremely high accuracy and lacks large-scale annotated datasets, building a diabetes knowledge graph usually requires extensive expert annotation. Furthermore, the complexity of diabetes knowledge poses challenges to comprehensive collection and integration. The data sources are rich in terminology, professional concepts, and complex pathological relationships. Direct extraction using LLMs often results in errors in entity recognition, relation extraction, and semantic interpretation. To overcome these challenges, this study proposes the MED-VerifyKG framework, which combines CERD corpus knowledge with the reasoning power of LLMs. By employing multi-round verification and intelligent optimization, a domain-specific workflow for knowledge extraction in diabetes is established.

4 MED-VerifyKG Verification-Enhanced Framework

This paper proposes the MED-VerifyKG framework, a verification-enhanced processing system specifically designed for knowledge extraction tasks in the diabetes domain. The core idea is to integrate the automated extraction capability of large language models (LLMs) with professional medical knowledge through a multi-level, iterative verification mechanism, thereby achieving reliable extraction results. The innovation of this framework lies in its organic combination of automated processing and manual verification: it fully exploits the efficiency of LLMs while ensuring accuracy through medical rule bases and expert feedback. Such a design is highly suitable for medical domains like diabetes, where accuracy requirements are stringent, as it improves knowledge extraction efficiency while maintaining quality.The structure of MED-VerifyKG is shown in the **Fig.** 3.

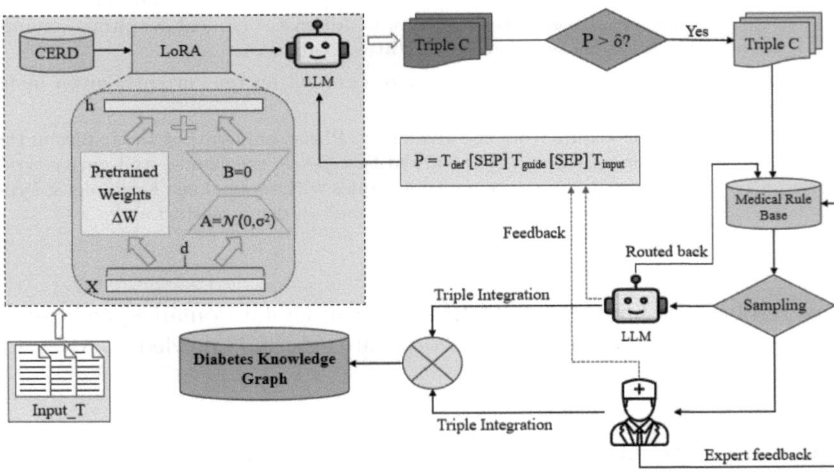

Fig. 3. MED-VerifyKG architecture diagram

The mathematical formulation of MED-VerifyKG can be defined as follows: let the input medical text be T and the final output be the triple set G, then the entire process can be formalized as shown in Eq. 1.

$$G = F_{\text{verify}}\big(F_{\text{extract}}(T;\theta); R, H\big) \tag{1}$$

where F_{extract} denotes the initial extraction function, θ represents the model parameters, F_{verify} is the verification function, R denotes the medical rule base, and H represents the involvement of expert knowledge.

4.1 Initial Extraction and Candidate Generation

Because general-purpose LLMs often exhibit insufficient understanding of diabetes terminology and weak logical reasoning, this study adapted the base model to the domain. Instead of computationally expensive full-parameter fine-tuning, we employed a parameter-efficient method, Low-Rank Adaptation (LoRA). LoRA freezes pretrained weights while training low-rank decomposition matrices, which are then combined with the original weights to achieve efficient fine-tuning.

Let the pretrained weight matrix be W. Its update process can be expressed as shown in Eq. 2.

$$W' = W + \Delta W \equiv W + BA, \tag{2}$$

where $B \in \mathbb{R}^{d\times r}$, $A \in \mathbb{R}^{r\times k}$, and the rank $r \ll \min(d,k)$.Here, A is initialized as a Gaussian random matrix and B as a zero matrix, ensuring that the adapter output is initially zero and does not affect the model's original capability.

The fine-tuned model possesses domain knowledge but requires precise instructions to execute tasks. For this, we designed a structured prompt template as shown in Eq. 3.

$$\text{P} = T_{\text{def}}\ [\text{SEP}]\ T_{\text{guide}}\ [\text{SEP}]\ T_{\text{input}} \tag{3}$$

where T_{def} defines the extraction task, T_{guide} provides output guidance, and T_{input} represents the input corpus for extraction. [SEP] is used to separate different parts of the prompt.

Using this structured prompt, the fine-tuned model performs semantic parsing and reasoning on the input text T, generating an initial candidate triple set C. To balance recall and precision, we set a probability threshold $\delta = 0.7$ and retain only those triples with confidence greater than δ, as shown in Eq. 4.

$$C = \big\{(h,r,t) \mid P_{\text{LLM}}(h,r,t \mid T) > \delta\big\} \tag{4}$$

where h denotes the head entity, r the relation, and t the tail entity; $P_{\text{LLM}}(h,r,t \mid T)$ is the confidence score assigned by the large language model indicating that the triple (h,r,t) is correct given the input text T.

4.2 Multi-round Verification Enhancement Loop

The multi-round verification loop is the core quality control of MED-VerifyKG, refining the candidate triple set C via a closed-loop process of automated validation, human–machine collaborative checking, and system self-evolution. This loop is formalized as shown in Eq. 5.

$$C_{\text{verified}} = F_{\text{verify}}(C; R, H) \tag{5}$$

where R is the medical rule base and H is expert knowledge.

Initially, candidate triples are batch-processed using structured medical knowledge to filter out those violating commonsense or logical consistency, reducing expert workload. Triples are checked against the medical rule set R from the CERD corpus, which includes declarative rules (ensuring terminology consistency, e.g., ``T2DM'' → ``Type 2 Diabetes'') and reasoning-based rules (embedding domain knowledge via IF-THEN statements for automatic verification and correction, e.g., deleting invalid drug–non-symptom relations or relabeling erroneous causal relations like "IF (entity A == Insulin) AND (entity B == Diabetes) AND (relation == causes) THEN RELABEL(relation, treats)"). Each triple $(h, r, t) \in C$ is verified against all rules, as shown in Eq. 6.

$$C_{\text{filtered}} = \{(h, r, t) \in C \mid \forall r_i \in R,\ r_i(h, r, t) = \text{True}\} \tag{6}$$

where r_i denotes a specific verification rule. Triples in C_{filtered} move to expert verification, while invalid triples are removed, efficiently eliminating most low-level errors.

Expert verification ensures knowledge accuracy by combining human judgment with LLM assistance and generating structured feedback H for system optimization. Hierarchical sampling prioritizes uncertain, high-risk, and rare triples. Sampled triples are classified: simple errors are corrected directly, and complex cases are refined via LLM with natural language guidance. Corrected triples are added to the final dataset, while LLM-assisted corrections are re-verified by rules, forming an iterative loop that maintains clinical reliability and logical consistency.

Finally, expert feedback H enables prompt and rule optimization. For prompts, the system finds optimal P^* and model parameters θ^* to maximize expected extraction performance, as shown in Eq. 7.

$$(P^*, \theta^*) = \arg\max_{P,\theta} \mathbb{E}_{(x,y)\sim H}\left[\text{Sim}(\text{F}_{\text{extract}}(x; P, \theta), y)\right] \tag{7}$$

where (x, y) are expert-corrected samples, and Sim measures similarity between model output and expert targets.

For rules, new expert knowledge is distilled as shown in Eq. 8.

$$R_{\text{new}} = R_{\text{old}} \cup \{\Delta R \mid \Delta R = F_{\text{generate}}(H)\} \tag{8}$$

where F_{generate} derives new rules ΔR from feedback H and incorporates them into R_{old}. This closed-loop "verification–feedback–optimization" progressively enhances extraction precision, rule coverage, and clinical-grade knowledge graph quality.

4.3 Triple Integration and Graph Formation

In the final integration phase of MED-VerifyKG, high-quality triples from multi-round verification are consolidated into a structured diabetes knowledge graph through triple fusion and graph construction. Triple fusion removes redundant records and resolves conflicting relations using expert-validated confidence scores, ensuring consistency and reliability. The resulting graph contains 17 disease-centered entity types and 85 relation types, with detailed entity information provided in the Table 2.

Table 2. DKG entity quantity statistics

Entity type	Number	Entity type	Number
Symptom	2,753	Epidemiology	563
Disease	2,719	Drug treatment	558
Others	2,068	Body part	398
Drug	1,827	Physiological parameter	287
Interpretation	1,696	Chemical substance	253
Sociology	1,481	Procedure	127
Examination	1,266	Surgical treatment	63
Other treatment	803	Test reagent	63
Prognosis	35		

The refined triples are batch-imported into a lightweight graph database, where predefined templates convert them into nodes and edges, forming a coherent network. An Echarts-based [29] interactive interface visualizes key entities–diseases, drugs, and symptoms–enabling node-level exploration and enhancing interpretability.The visualization results are shown in **Fig.** 4.

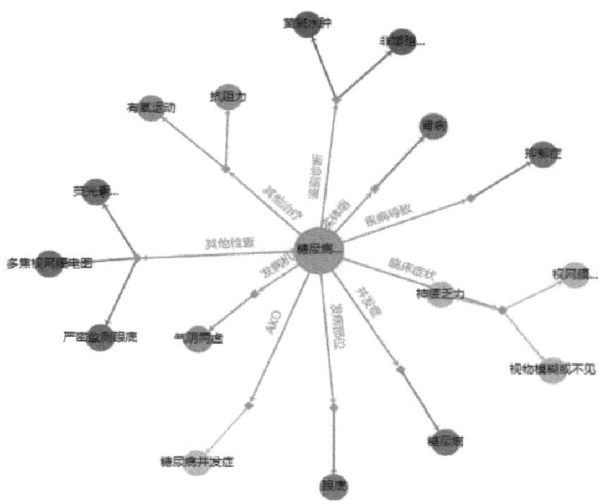

Fig. 4. DKG visualization example

5 Experiments

5.1 Experimental Data

In this study, the electronic medical records (EMRs) of diabetes patients and the medical textbook *Practical Diabetology (4th Edition)* were used as research samples. Since the textbook *Practical Diabetology (4th Edition)* contains a large amount of content, it was divided by chapters into 81 TXT files for the purpose of experimentation, as detailed in the table.

To clearly illustrate the data composition, the statistical information of the dataset is summarized in Table 3.

Table 3. Data sources used in the experiment

Data source	Data format	Quantity	Data structure
Electronic medical records	EXL file	800	Structured data
Medical textbook	TXT file	81	Unstructured data

5.2 Experimental Setup

The experimental parameter settings are shown in Table 4.We employed widely used metrics in knowledge extraction tasks: precision (P), recall (R), and F1 score.

Table 4. Unstructured knowledge extraction experimental parameter settings

Parameters	Value
CUDA version	11.7
Python version	3.8.17
GPU	NVIDIA-RTX-4090
Batch size	8
Gradient accumulation steps	16
Learning rate	2.0e-5
LoRA rank	16
LoRA alpha	32

5.3 Comparison Experiment

To validate the effectiveness of the proposed MED-VerifyKG verification-enhanced framework, we conducted comparative experiments on two base models, DeepSeek-V3-7B [30] and DeepSeek-R1-7B [31]. The results are shown in the Table 5.

Several observations can be drawn from the experimental results:

The MED-VerifyKG framework significantly improves performance on both entity recognition (NER) and relation extraction (RE) tasks across the two base models. For example, in the case of DeepSeek-V3-7B, without the framework, its F1 scores for NER and RE were 0.667 and 0.545, respectively; after being enhanced by MED-VerifyKG, they increased to 0.780 and 0.696, corresponding to relative improvements of 16.9.

Table 5. Performance of different models on NER and RE tasks

Model	Task	P	R	F	MED-VerifyKG
DeepSeek-V3-7B	NER	0.750	0.600	0.667	No
	RE	0.600	0.500	0.545	
	NER	**0.852**	**0.720**	**0.780**	Yes
	RE	**0.748**	**0.650**	**0.696**	
DeepSeek-R1-7B	NER	0.452	0.382	0.414	No
	RE	0.321	0.281	0.299	
	NER	**0.537**	**0.461**	**0.496**	Yes
	RE	**0.428**	**0.372**	**0.398**	

All base models achieved performance improvements after the integration of MED-VerifyKG, with DeepSeek-V3-7B showing stronger baseline performance and greater gains, demonstrating the synergistic effect between the framework and more powerful base models. At the task level, relation extraction exhibited more substantial improvements, validating the effectiveness of rule-based verification and expert feedback mechanisms in complex relation reasoning. Although the gains in entity recognition were smaller, the framework still enhanced recall while maintaining precision. Overall, the experimental results confirm the effectiveness and necessity of MED-VerifyKG in diabetes knowledge extraction, providing a scalable solution for constructing high-quality domain-specific knowledge graphs.

6 Conclusion

This study constructed a diabetes-oriented knowledge graph (DKG) based on a verification-enhanced large language model framework. To address the characteristics of diabetes-related medical texts, we proposed MED-VerifyKG, an automatic extraction method that integrates a multi-round verification mechanism.

By employing a closed-loop process of initial extraction–rule-based filtering–expert validation–iterative optimization, the framework enables the acquisition of high-quality medical knowledge. Experimental results demonstrate that the proposed method significantly improves knowledge extraction performance on the diabetes dataset, achieving an F1 score of 0.696 for relation extraction (RE) and 0.780 for named entity recognition (NER), thereby ensuring both the accuracy and reliability of knowledge graph construction.

The resulting diabetes knowledge graph encompasses 17 entity types and 85 relation types, forming a large-scale and well-structured medical knowledge system. This graph provides solid knowledge support for applications such as intelligent diabetes diagnosis and treatment systems as well as clinical decision support. Looking ahead, future work will focus on enhancing the automation of the verification mechanism, improving the extraction of complex medical relations, and exploring the deeper application of knowledge graphs in clinical decision-making.

References

1. Malick, R.A.S., Munir, S., Jami, S.I., et al.: DbKB a knowledge graph dataset for diabetes: a system biology approach. Data Brief **52**, 110003 (2024)
2. International Diabetes Federation: IDF Diabetes Atlas, 10th edn. International Diabetes Federation, Brussels (2025). https://diabetesatlas.org/atlas/tenth-edition/. Accessed 30 Sept 2025
3. ZhangSun, J., Yang, Y.X., Zou, B., et al.: Tuck-KGC: based on tensor decomposition for diabetes knowledge graph completion model integrating Chinese and Western medicine. PeerJ Comput. Sci. **11**, e2522 (2025)
4. Singh, S., Siwach, M.: Evaluating diabetes dataset for knowledge graph embedding based link prediction. Data Knowl. Eng. **157**, 102414 (2025)
5. Arsenyan, V., Bughdaryan, S., Shaya, F., et al.: Large language models for biomedical knowledge graph construction: information extraction from EMR notes (2023). arXiv:2301.12473
6. Gao, S., Yu, K., Yang, Y., et al.: Large language model powered knowledge graph construction for mental health exploration. Nat. Commun. **16**(1), 7526 (2025)
7. Yang, H., Li, J., Zhang, C., et al.: Large language model-driven knowledge graph construction in sepsis care using multicenter clinical databases: development and usability study. J. Med. Internet Res. **27**, e65537 (2025)
8. Hogan, A., Blomqvist, E., Cochez, M., et al.: Knowledge graphs. ACM Comput. Surv. (CSUR) **54**(4), 1–37 (2021)
9. Zuo, K., Jiang, Y., Mo, F., et al.: KG4Diagnosis: a hierarchical multi-agent LLM framework with knowledge graph enhancement for medical diagnosis. AAAI Bridge Program on AI for Medicine and Healthcare, pp. 195–204. PMLR (2025)
10. Zhang, D., Wang, Z., Li, Z.Z., et al.: MedKGent: a large language model agent framework for constructing temporally evolving medical knowledge graph (2025). arXiv:2508.12393
11. Liu, K., Zhang, Y., Martin, C., et al.: Translational bioinformatics for human reproductive biology research: examples, opportunities and challenges for a future reproductive medicine. Int. J. Mol. Sci. **24**(1), 4 (2022)

12. Mavridis, A., Tegos, S., Anastasiou, C., et al.: Large language models for intelligent RDF knowledge graph construction: results from medical ontology mapping. Front. Artif. Intell. **8**, 1546179 (2025)
13. Rezaei, M.R., Fard, R.S., Parker, J.L., et al.: Agentic medical knowledge graphs enhance medical question answering: bridging the gap between LLMs and evolving medical knowledge (2025). arXiv:2502.13010
14. Zhao, W.X., Zhou, K., Li, J., et al.: A survey of large language models **1**(2) (2023). arXiv:2303.18223
15. Wang, Q., Zhou, K., Qiao, Q., et al.: Improving unsupervised relation extraction by augmenting diverse sentence pairs (2023). arXiv:2312.00552
16. Farquhar, S., Kossen, J., Kuhn, L., et al.: Detecting hallucinations in large language models using semantic entropy. Nature **630**(8017), 625–630 (2024)
17. Asgari, E., Montaña-Brown, N., Dubois, M., et al.: A framework to assess clinical safety and hallucination rates of LLMs for medical text summarisation. NPJ Digit. Med. **8**(1), 274 (2025)
18. Abu-Salih, B.: Domain-specific knowledge graphs: a survey. J. Netw. Comput. Appl. **185**, 103076 (2021)
19. Byambasuren, O., Yang, Y., Sui, Z., et al.: Preliminary study on the construction of Chinese medical knowledge graph. J. Chin. Inf. Process. **33**(10), 1–9 (2019)
20. Cheng, B., Zhang, J., Liu, H., et al.: Research on medical knowledge graph for stroke. J. Healthc. Eng. **2021**(1), 5531327 (2021)
21. Chang, D., Chen, M., Liu, C., et al.: DiaKG: an annotated diabetes dataset for medical knowledge graph construction. In: China Conference on Knowledge Graph and Semantic Computing, pp. 308–314. Springer Singapore, Singapore (2021)
22. Liu, F., Liu, M., Li, M., et al.: Automatic knowledge extraction from Chinese electronic medical records and rheumatoid arthritis knowledge graph construction. Quant. Imaging Med. Surg. **13**(6), 3873 (2023)
23. Costanzo, M.C., von Grotthuss, M., Massung, J., et al.: The type 2 diabetes knowledge portal: an open access genetic resource dedicated to type 2 diabetes and related traits. Cell Metabolism **35**(4), 695–710. e6 (2023)
24. Wang, L., Xie, H., Han, W., et al.: Construction of a knowledge graph for diabetes complications from expert-reviewed clinical evidences. Comput. Assist. Surg. **25**(1), 29–35 (2020)
25. Yang, Z., Huang, Y., Feng, J.: Learning to leverage high-order medical knowledge graph for joint entity and relation extraction. In: Findings of the Association for Computational Linguistics: ACL 2023, pp. 9023–9035 (2023)
26. Liu, F., Liu, M., Li, M., et al.: Automatic knowledge extraction from Chinese electronic medical records and rheumatoid arthritis knowledge graph construction. Quant. Imaging Med. Surg. **13**(6), 3873 (2023)
27. Knauf, R., Gonzalez, A.J., Abel, T.: A framework for validation of rule-based systems. IEEE Trans. Syst., Man, Cybern., Part B (Cybern.) **32**(3), 281–295 (2002)
28. Wallach, W., Allen, C., Smit, I.: Machine morality: bottom-up and top-down approaches for modelling human moral faculties. In: Machine Ethics and Robot Ethics, pp. 249–266. Routledge (2020)
29. Li, D., Mei, H., Shen, Y., et al.: ECharts: a declarative framework for rapid construction of web-based visualization. Vis. Inform. **2**(2), 136–146 (2018)
30. Liu, A., Feng, B., Xue, B., et al.: Deepseek-v3 technical report (2024). arXiv:2412.19437
31. Guo, D., Yang, D., Zhang, H., et al.: Deepseek-R1: incentivizing reasoning capability in LLMS via reinforcement learning (2025). arXiv:2501.12948

Meta-Learning Enhance the Influenza Surveillance Across Spatio-Temporal Heterogeneous Scenario by Recommending Suitable Statistical Models

Yifei Li[1,2], Xin Lai[1,2(✉)], Tianci Wang[1,2], Shenjie Wang[1,2,3], and Jiayin Wang[1,2,3(✉)]

[1] School of Computer Science and Technology, Xi'an Jiaotong University, 28 Xianning West Road, Beilin, Xi'an 710049, China
laixin@xjtu.edu.cn, wangjiayin@mail.xjtu.edu.cn

[2] Shaanxi Engineering Research Center of Medical and Health Big Data, Xi'an Jiaotong University, 28 Xianning West Road, Beilin, Xi'an 710049, China

[3] Department of Respiratory Medicine, The Second Affiliated Hospital of Xi'an Jiaotong University, No. 157, Xiwu Road, Xincheng District, Xi'an 710003, China

Abstract. Public health events monitoring, e.g. influenza surveillance, is a fundamental public service. Statistical Process Control (SPC) charts are widely adopted methods for analyzing medical time-series data in this domain. Public health monitoring is inherently complex due to spatio-temporal heterogeneous, particularly evident in influenza surveillance. Thus, numerous statistical models have been developed; some prioritize detection sensitivity, while others are tailored to specific scenarios, such as varying data distributions. Selecting and configuring the appropriate statistical model presents a significant challenge, particularly for non-experts. Given that the strong spatio-temporal heterogeneity of influenza data implies no universally optimal chart exists, selection remains a critical and urgently needed computational problem.To address this challenge, we introduce the Pandemic Monitoring Control chart Automated Recommendation Model (PMcharm). This model resolves two primary computational issues: (1) the difficulty in defining an suitable chart selection due to the absence of explicit features or labels; and (2) the implementation of a meta-learning-based recommendation framework while addressing severe class imbalance problem. PMcharm extracts features by integrating classical statistical descriptors with an LSTM encoder and generate meta-targets. Additionally, the SMOTE technique is employed to address the class imbalance issue.Evaluated using U.S. state-level influenza surveillance data, PMcharm significantly outperforms fixed selection strategies, achieving an average recommendation accuracy (RA) of 0.97. Furthermore, real-time application during the 2024–2025 U.S. influenza season confirmed PMcharm's ability to recommend the suitable control chart. For instance, in Alabama, the recommended Shewhart control chart achieved a run length of 9, compared to 12 and 13 for alternative methods. In conclusion, the proposed method significantly enhances monitoring performance under such complex scenarios.

Keywords: Control chart recommendation · Influenza surveillance · Meta-learning

Y. Zhang et al. (Eds.): CHIP 2025, CCIS 2884, pp. 206–222, 2026.
https://doi.org/10.1007/978-981-95-7299-1_13

1 Introduction

Monitoring public health events is a major challenge in health statistics, relying on the analysis of time-series health-event data [1]. Statistical Process Control (SPC) charts are widely used in public health surveillance [2]. Despite the steady development of SPC, many applications rely on a fixed selection of one or two standard control charts, depending entirely on the inherent performance [3, 4]. Alternatively, some approaches utilize multiple charts simultaneously, employing voting mechanisms for decision-making [5]. For experts, they may conduct extensive simulations to identify the optimal chart for a specific context or develop entirely novel control chart models. However, these approaches have significant limitations. Relying on a fixed set of charts is sub-optimal, as the diversity of SPC methodologies indicates that no single chart is universally optimal [4, 6]. Voting strategies fail to resolve the fundamental selection challenge, merely transfer the computational burden to the decision-making process [7]. Furthermore, reliance on expert-driven simulations is often time-consuming, and the development of new models rarely generalize beyond the specific setting they target [8]. Crucially, choosing the right control chart is a critical decision, as a poor choice can trigger false alarms, miss true outbreaks, or delay response [9]. Given that the amount of existing control charts is enough to cover most common scenarios, the key challenge is how to select the chart that best fits the specific data or event-without requiring specialized expertise.

Take seasonal influenza as an example; it continues to cause substantial morbidity and mortality worldwide [10]. Consequently, monitoring, early detection, and warning of influenza outbreaks are essential public health functions worldwide [11]. Over the past decades, research has established four primary categories of statistical control charts for influenza surveillance: the Shewhart chart [12], the cumulative sum (CUSUM) chart [13, 14], the exponentially weighted moving average (EWMA) chart [15], and the generalized likelihood ratio (GLR) chart [16, 17]. Each category employs unique control limits tailored to its statistical approach [18]. Epidemic dynamics vary significantly across regions and years, so a single chart rarely fits all monitoring units [19]. For instance, one study demonstrated that under identical EWMA parameters, the outbreak detection rate in Iran differed drastically between years (approximately 50% in 2010 versus 100% in 2011) [19]. This variability is associated with spatial factors—such as population size, density, distribution, mobility, demographics, and herd immunity environments—as well as temporal factors, including seasonality and holidays. These factors interact in a complex, coupled way, resulting in significant variations in observed data patterns, such as peak intensity, volatility, and baseline rates [20]. Identifying the relationship between these underlying data patterns and the performance of different control charts and their respective control limits can significantly improve surveillance efficacy [21]. Therefore, effectively addressing this surveillance challenge requires a complex analysis of the relationship between data heterogeneity and chart performance [21].

A second key challenge involves generating corresponding labels. While the "best" chart is defined by its overall performance, specifically, which chart signals an outbreak earliest, the large number of available control charts makes selection into a complex multi-label problem. However, the principal distinctions among the four major categories of charts reside in their respective control limits [22], and research suggests that modifying these limits can sometimes render different types of control charts functionally equivalent. Therefore, we re-frame this extensive multi-label challenge into a two-stage, four-category classification task: the first stage identifies the optimal chart category, and the second determines the corresponding control limits.

To address these challenges, this study proposes the Pandemic Monitoring Control chart Automated Recommendation Model (PMcharm), which formulates the chart selection problem as a meta-learning task. The fundamental advantage of this approach is its ability to empirically learn the complex relationship between underlying data characteristics and chart performance, providing an automated, data-driven mechanism to navigate heterogeneity without requiring extensive manual simulations for every new scenario. Specifically, first, meta-features are extracted using a hybrid strategy that combines classical statistical metrics and deep representations from an LSTM encoder [23]. Second, for the candidate control charts, they are calibrated to a standardized false alarm level, and their average detection delay is then assessed across a diverse set of simulated outbreak perturbations [24]. The chart with the best overall performance is subsequently designated as the optimal label. To mitigate bias from the resulting class imbalance, the Synthetic Minority Over-sampling Technique (SMOTE) is applied to the training data. On this balanced dataset, a Random Forest meta-model is trained to learn the mapping from data characteristics to the optimal chart. When presented with new surveillance data, the final trained model leverages this learned relationship to provide an automated, data-driven recommendation for the most suitable control chart configuration.

We conducted experiments on real influenza data provided by the U.S. Centers for Disease Control and Prevention (CDC). Based on Average Run Length (*ARL*) simulations used to generate the meta-targets, confirmed significant performance heterogeneity across different regions and outbreak patterns. Also, when evaluating PMcharm using a rigorous temporal validation strategy, results show that compared with random and fixed strategies, the proposed method consistently recommends more effective control charts, achieving an average recommendation accuracy exceeding 90%. Furthermore, we applied the model to real-time monitoring during the 2024–2025 influenza season. Case studies across diverse states confirmed that PMcharm successfully adapts to local epidemic dynamics and consistently recommends the control chart offering the earliest outbreak detection.

2 Methods

The selection of an appropriate control chart configuration (c, θ) can be framed as a meta-learning problem. To address the heterogeneity of surveillance data x, an integrated framework composed of three key functions is adopted. A feature extractor g maps data x to descriptive meta-features m. A dynamic calibration procedure q ensures that control limits adapt to local data characteristics while meeting required statistical constraints. A meta-model f is trained to map these meta-features to the optimal chart type. Crucially, the optimization of f accounts for the impact of both g and the subsequent calibration q on the final surveillance performance. The learning objective is thus formalized as finding the optimal f^* by minimizing a loss function L dependent on the entire configuration.

$$f^* = \underset{f:M \to C}{argmin} L(f; g, q) \tag{1}$$

In this framework, the function f is defined to map the meta-features $m = g(x)$ of a given time-series surveillance data x to an optimal control chart c. The objective is to maximize the performance metric y, which depends on the control limit θ. To accommodate heterogeneity, θ is set dynamically by the calibration function $q(x, c)$. Therefore, the meta-learning task is formalized as selecting the chart that maximizes performance under this calibration constraint:

$$f(g(x)) \rightarrow C : maxy(c, \theta, x) \in Y, where\theta = q(x, c)(x \in P, g(x) \in M) \quad (2)$$

Here, P, M, C, Θ and Y denote the problem space, meta-feature space, control chart space, control-limit space, and performance space, respectively. By decomposing the problem using the above equation, the framework separates the learning task from the statistical calibration task. The key challenge addressed by the meta-model is determining which chart type performs best for a given instance x when optimally calibrated.

Based on the above analysis, the meta-model for control chart recommendation can be built using classification algorithms. The mapping is learned exclusively from off-season data and is then applied to flu-season surveillance. Off-season data reflect normal baseline conditions, enabling the robust labeling of the performance of candidate charts at a fixed false-alarm level [15, 25]. The learned correspondence between data characteristics and performance can then be applied to real-time flu-season monitoring [25]. Therefore, the overall framework consists of several stages: extracting meta-features and identifying the optimal control chart from historical off-season instances; training a meta-model that captures the relationship between data features and the optimal chart; then applying this framework to recommend the chart type and dynamically calibrate its control limits for the upcoming influenza season. Figure 1 illustrates this approach.

2.1 Meta-Data Collection

The first step in the influenza surveillance control chart recommendation methodology is meta-data collection, which is divided into two phases: meta-feature extraction and meta-target identification.

Meta-feature Extraction. In this study, meta-features are defined as time-series features that can effectively discriminate the performance of different Statistical Process Control (SPC) charts. In general, time-series feature-extraction methods have been widely studied but often struggle to fully capture the complex dynamics in influenza surveillance data, such as seasonality, autocorrelation, and nonlinear fluctuations [26]. These characteristics are known to significantly impact the sensitivity and specificity of different control charts. Based on literature review, we identified a set of meta-features highly correlated with control chart performance. This study employs a strategy that combines classical statistical analysis with deep learning, aiming to capture both explicit statistical features and implicit non-linear dynamics. The final feature set spans five key dimensions, summarized in Table 1.

First, standard statistical methods were used to extract features from the time series data. These features describe four aspects: the completeness of observations, autocorrelation, seasonal patterns, and the noise level and overall predictability.

Studies indicate that LSTMs learn low-dimensional latent representations from high-dimensional time series, revealing underlying dynamic features [23]. To capture complex

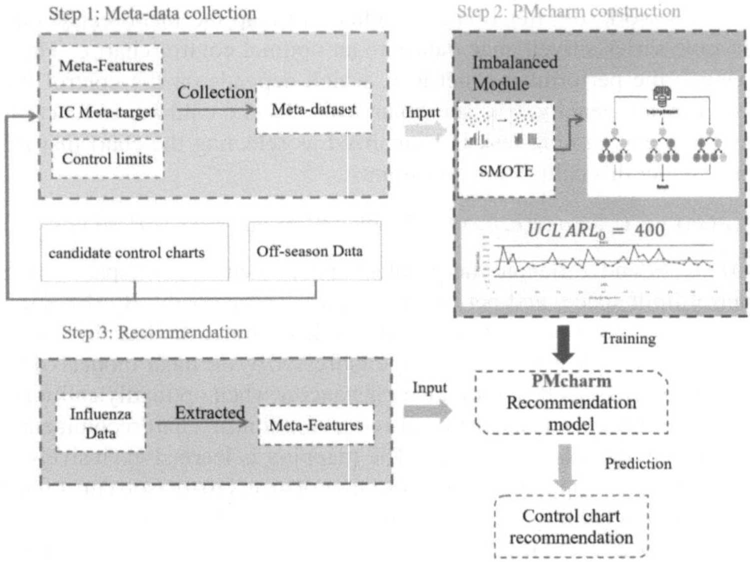

Fig. 1. Framework for automated recommendation of optimal control charts based on time-series data characteristics.

non-linear patterns and high-dimensional dynamic features, a single-layer LSTM is trained to minimize the overall Mean Squared Prediction Error (MSE):

$$\mathcal{L}_{pred} = E[(z_{t+1} - \hat{z}_{t+1})^2] \tag{3}$$

where z_{t+1} and $\hat{z}_{t+1}$ represent the standardized true value and the predicted value, respectively.

Three categories of features are extracted. The first includes prediction-performance features from the prediction residuals, such as Root Mean Square Error (RMSE) and residual summary statistics, which indicate the series' predictability. The second covers hidden-state dynamics. The temporal evolution of the LSTM hidden state norm, $r_t = \|h_t\|_2$, is analyzed. The variance of $\{r_t\}$ is calculated to measure dynamic stability. Volatility is measured by the maximum absolute first difference, defined as $\underset{t}{max}|r_t - r_{t-1}|$. Furthermore, an AR(1) model is fitted to $\{r_t\}$:

$$r_t = \alpha + \phi\, r_{t-1} + \varepsilon_t \tag{4}$$

Based on this, the persistence timescale is defined as:

$$\tau_p = \frac{1}{1-\phi} \tag{5}$$

This metric quantifies the memory length of the latent dynamics.

The third category includes low-dimensional embedding features. For each sequence, compute the mean hidden-state vector $\overline{h}$. Then, Principal Component Analysis (PCA) is

Table 1. Summary of meta-features extracted for influenza surveillance time series

Feature dimension	Category	Definition
Data coverage	Temporal coverage	Number of valid observations
Sequential dependency	Short-term Correlation	Lag-1 autocorrelation
Seasonal pattern	Seasonal strength and stability	Harmonic-regression amplitude; stability of the estimate; share of spectral power at the dominant frequency
Noise and predictability	Statistical noise and predictability	Normalized residual variance after AR(1) prewhitening; Coefficient of variation of the surveillance denominator
	Model prediction error	One-step LSTM RMSE; residual diagnostics
Latent dynamic representation	Dynamic stability and volatility	Variance of hidden state norms; maximum absolute first difference
	Persistence timescale	Characteristic timescale from the AR(1) coefficient of the hidden-state norms
	Low-dimensional embedding	PCA scores of the mean hidden-state vector

applied to the set of across instances and retain the first three principal components as meta-features, capturing the dominant directions of variation in the dynamics.

Meta-target Identification. The meta-target identification aims to generate supervisory labels for meta-learning through performance evaluation. The candidate control chart set is denoted as

$$C = \{E, S, G, W\}$$

corresponding to four common classical control chart types: EWMA, Shewhart, GLR, and CUSUM, respectively. Average Run Length (ARL) is used as the performance evaluation criterion [18], where ARL_0 measures the interval between false alarms, and ARL_1 measures the detection delay. To ensure comparability across control charts at the same false alarm rate, we perform in-control calibration, this procedure is the practical implementation of the dynamic calibration function $q(x, c)$: using off-season data as baseline, tune the control limit parameters θ_c for each chart $c \in C$ are tuned so that ARL_0 is standardized to a predefined constant τ:

$$ARL_0(c; \theta_c|x) = \tau, \tau = 400 \tag{6}$$

Given the in-control calibration ARL_0, a smaller ARL_1 indicates superior performance. ARL is estimated using Monte Carlo simulation, and the control limit θ_c is determined via the bisection search algorithm. The resulting control limit θ_c is thus inherently dependent on the specific data instance x, enabling adaptation to local heterogeneity.

The candidate control charts can be categorized into two classes. EWMA and Shewhart charts are constructed from standardized residuals of the baseline model. Considering the prevalent overdispersion in influenza surveillance count data, the GLR and CUSUM charts are derived directly from the negative binomial likelihood.

EWMA: For the standardized residual z_t, denote,

$$E_t = (1 - \lambda)E_{t-1} + \lambda z_t \tag{7}$$

Shewhart: Using asymptotic regression to provide the baseline value μ_t and the prediction error σ_t,

$$z_t = \frac{x_t - \mu_t}{\sigma_t} \tag{8}$$

GLR: using the generalized likelihood ratio test to detect an unknown mean shift within a time window. Its statistic G_t is defined as the maximized log-likelihood ratio over the window range and shift size,

$$G_t = \max_{t-w+1 \le s \le t} \left\{ \max_{r \ge 1} \sum_{i=s}^{t} w_i(r) \right\} \tag{9}$$

where w is the maximum window length, and $w_i(r)$ is the log-likelihood ratio increment.

CUSUM: Given a design shift $r > 1$, its log-likelihood ratio increment $w_t(r)$ is defined as,

$$w_t(r) = x_t \ln(r) + (x_t + k)\ln(k + \mu_t) - (x_t + k)\ln(k + r\mu_t) \tag{10}$$

the statistic is:

$$S_t = \max(0, S_{t-1} + w_t(r)) \tag{11}$$

Let the region-year pair be (u, y). The weekly off-season observation sequence is denoted as $x_{u,y}^{\mathrm{off}} = \{x_{u,y,t}\}, t \in \Omega_{\mathrm{off}}$, where Ω_{off} is the index set of off-season weeks. The evaluation of ARL_1 is conducted by superimposing simulated "out-of-control perturbations" onto the baseline model. To enhance robustness, a perturbation set $\Delta = \{\Delta_k\}_{k=1}^{K}$ is defined. We then use a chart-specific scheme: apply additive shifts to residual-based charts and multiplicative (mean-scaling) perturbations to likelihood-based charts.

$$z_t^{'} = z_t + \delta, \delta \in \Delta_z \tag{12}$$

$$\mu_t^{'} = r\mu_t, r = exp(\eta), \eta \in \Delta_\mu \tag{13}$$

For the region-year (u, y), the overall performance $A_c^{(u,y)}$ of control chart c is obtained by equally weighted averaging of ARL_1 over the perturbation set Δ:

$$A_c^{(u,y)} = \frac{1}{K} \sum_{k=1}^{K} ARL_1\left(c; \Delta_k \middle| x_{u,y}^{off}\right) \tag{14}$$

Finally, the optimal control chart (meta-target) $\ell_{u,y}$ for this instance is defined as the method with the minimum average ARL_1:

$$\ell_{u,y} = \underset{c \in \mathcal{C}}{argmin} A_c^{(u,y)} \tag{15}$$

This constitutes the meta-learning dataset $\mathcal{D} = \{(m_{u,y}, \ell_{u,y})\}_{(u,y)}$ where $m_{u,y}$ is the meta-feature vector.

Meta-dataset Balancing. To address the class imbalance observed in the constructed meta-dataset, applying the Synthetic Minority Over-sampling Technique (SMOTE) during training data preprocessing. In our meta-learning scenario, the share of instances labeled with each optimal control chart often varies widely, which can bias the meta-model toward the majority class. Specifically, for each minority class c, let $S_c = \{\boldsymbol{m}_i | \ell_i = c\}$ be the set of samples belonging to that class. The SMOTE algorithm augments the minority class by generating new samples along the line segment between a sample and one of its nearest neighbors of the same class:

$$m^{new} = m_i + \lambda\left(m_j - m_i\right), \lambda \sim Uniform(0,1), m_i, m_j \in \mathcal{S}_c \tag{16}$$

This process is repeated until all minority classes reach the majority-class size. Let the balanced dataset be denoted as $D_{bal} = \{(m_i^{bal}, l_i^{bal})\}_i$, then we have:

$$|\{i | l_i^{bal} = c\}| = n_{max} forallc \in C$$

where n_{max} represents the number of samples in the original majority class. This approach balances class labels during meta-learner training and reduces bias toward the majority class. Importantly, balancing is applied only to the training set; the test set retains its original distribution to ensure a valid performance evaluation.

2.2 Meta-Model Construction and Recommendation

Based on the meta-dataset $\mathcal{D} = \{(m_i, \ell_i)\}_{i=1}^N$ constructed above, the control chart recommendation problem is framed as a supervised multi-class classification task. The model learns a mapping $f : \mathbb{R}^d \to C$, where $m_i \in \mathbb{R}^d$ is the meta-feature vector of the data instance, $\ell_i \in C$ is its meta-target, and C is the set of candidate control charts. To handle the heterogeneity of meta-features and the potential non-linear relationships between features and targets, we use a random forest as the meta-model. The trained model outputs class-posterior probabilities $p(c|m)$ for each control chart $c \in C$.

When applying the framework to a new surveillance instance x with meta-features m, the process integrates both stages. First, the trained meta-model f is used. The recommendation follows the MAP rule, selecting the chart with the largest posterior probability $\widehat{\ell}$:

$$\widehat{\ell} = \underset{c \in \mathcal{C}}{argmax} p(c|m) \tag{17}$$

Second, the dynamic calibration function q is applied to the instance's baseline data x to determine the control limit $\theta^* = q(x, \widehat{\ell})$. The final output deployed for monitoring is the integrated configuration $(\widehat{\ell}, \theta^*)$, dynamically tailored to the local data heterogeneity.

However, maximizing classification accuracy does not always guarantee the maximum performance gain, as it ignores the performance gaps between different sub-optimal choices. Therefore, Recommendation Accuracy (RA) is introduced as a utility measure to evaluate the recommendation performance more finely. RA is defined based on performance metrics, measuring the performance of the selected control chart c relative to the best and worst control charts for that instance:

$$RA(c; m) = \frac{A_{worst}(m) - A(c; m)}{A_{worst}(m) - A_{best}(m)} \tag{18}$$

where A_{best} and A_{worst} represent the performance of the best and worst control charts for that instance, respectively. The value of RA ranges from [0, 1]; a larger value indicates performance closer to the optimum.

3 Results

This section presents a series of empirical studies designed to systematically evaluate the proposed two-stage PMcharm framework. The experiments are organized to validate the necessity, effectiveness, and practical value of this approach across three questions.

First, the experiments test whether different control charts show meaningful performance differences across monitoring scenarios, thereby establishing the necessity of both adaptive selection and instance-specific dynamic calibration. Second, examining whether the proposed recommender consistently outperforms baseline methods-measured by Recommendation Accuracy (RA) and top-k hit rate-in a temporal extrapolation setting. Finally, the practical performance of the integrated PMcharm system is evaluated by examining the Run Length (RL) of the recommended charts, which are dynamically calibrated via stage 2, when applied to actual influenza season monitoring.

3.1 Experimental Setup

Data Source and Definition. The subject of this study is the state-level weekly Influenza-like Illness (ILI) surveillance series provided by the U.S. Centers for Disease Control and Prevention (CDC). The fundamental unit of analysis for the experiments is the "region-year" pair, denoted as (u, y). Following epidemiological conventions, the Flu Season is defined as the period from week 40 of a given year to week 20 of the following year, while the Off-Season spans from week 21 to week 39 of the same year. A key design principle is information isolation: for each pair (u, y), only off-season data are used for meta-feature extraction and parameter calibration. This is because off-season data better reflect the stable baseline of the series, and using it prevents anomalous signals from the flu season from introducing bias into the model.

Validation Strategy and Data Partitioning. To ensure valid evaluation and generalization to future data, this study employs a temporal validation scheme with annual splits. Let the set of region-year indices be $\mathcal{I} = \{(u, y)\}$. This set is chronologically decomposed into disjoint training and testing subsets I_{tr} and I_{te}, respectively:

$$I = I_{tr} \cup I_{te}, I_{tr} = \{(u, y)|y \in Y_{tr}\}, I_{te} = \{(u, y)|y \in Y_{te}\} \tag{19}$$

It is ensured that $max(Y_{tr}) < min(Y_{te})$ to strictly follow the principle of using the past to predict the future. In this study, the training years are set to $Y_{tr} = \{2011, \ldots, 2023\}$, and the testing year is $Y_{te} = \{2024\}$.

Based on this partitioning, the meta-learning datasets are constructed. For any given pair (u, y), its off-season data is used to extract meta-features and the meta-target. The final datasets are defined as follows:

$$D_{tr} = \{(m_{u,y}, l_{u,y})|(u, y) \in I_{tr}\}, D_{te} = \{(m_{u,y}, l_{u,y})|(u, y) \in I_{te}\} \quad (20)$$

The training set D_{tr} after being balanced using SMOTE, is used to train the Random Forest meta-model f.

3.2 Control Chart Performance Comparison and Meta-Target Generation

This section evaluates the need for tailored chart selection across surveillance settings by systematically comparing the four candidate control charts and illustrating meta-target generation. Following the protocol described above, all control charts were aligned at the $ARL_0 = 400$ level. Crucially, this alignment was achieved by executing the dynamic calibration procedure independently for each region-year instance, ensuring the control limits were adapted to local data heterogeneity. Performance evaluation is based on a series of simulated out-of-control shifts, with intensities designed to match the statistical scale and cover a range from weak to strong signals. For the standardized residual-based EWMA and Shewhart charts, additive shifts of $\mu = \{0.5,1.0,3.0,5.0\}$ were used. For the negative binomial-based GLR and CUSUM charts, log-multiplicative shifts of $\eta = \{0.01, 0.05, 0.1, 0.3\}$ were used. These settings follow common practice in influenza-surveillance studies and reflect typical signal strengths from the early onset to the peak of an outbreak. Tables 2 and 3 report the ARL_1 results for selected representative regions.

The results show the expected monotonicity: ARL_1 decreases as the shift magnitude increases. Also, the results reveal significant performance differentiation in the sensitivity across control charts. The Shewhart chart is highly sensitive to large shifts. For example, when μ=5.0, ARL_1 universally approaches the theoretical minimum of 1.0. In contrast, the EWMA chart generally performs better for mild to moderate persistent shifts. For instance, in Louisiana, when μ=1.0 the ARL_1 for EWMA is 14.40, compared to 102.47 for Shewhart. Similarly, GLR and CUSUM demonstrate high sensitivity to sustained multiplicative increases. This phenomenon of "division of labor by shift type and magnitude" indicates that the charts have complementary strengths, which justifies the need for an adaptive selection mechanism.

Further analysis shows that the performance of control charts is strongly modulated by regional specificity, exhibiting significant regional heterogeneity. Under the same shift magnitude, ARL_1 varies widely across different states. For example, when $\mu = 0.5$, the ARL_1 for EWMA is 37.44 in Louisiana but reaches 137.48 in Texas. This heterogeneity in detection sensitivity persists even after instance-specific calibration has ensured a uniform false alarm rate. It reflects the fundamental influence of baseline statistical properties on chart performance. Crucially, the relative ranking of the charts often reverses across regions. For instance, at $\mu = 0.5$, Shewhart attains 30.83 in Florida, beating

EWMA's 43.60, whereas in Ohio, EWMA attains 73.57 and outperforms Shewhart's 120.30.

The experimental results strongly confirm that different control charts exhibit high performance complementarity in influenza surveillance, and their effectiveness heavily depends on the specific "region-year" context and the underlying outbreak pattern. This shows that no single chart is universally optimal, and fixed-selection strategies will be suboptimal in some settings. Therefore, developing a framework capable of adaptively recommending control charts based on data characteristics is necessary. In addition, defining the meta-target by minimizing the average performance across diverse perturbations provides a robust and informative training signal for subsequent meta-learning.

Table 2. Performance of EWMA and shewhart control charts under additive shifts

Region	EWMA (μ)				Shewhart (μ)			
	0.5	1.0	3.0	5.0	0.5	1.0	3.0	5.0
Florida	43.60	17.51	2.86	1.91	30.83	26.39	2.68	1.00
Arizona	66.06	26.07	3.13	1.97	50.62	25.86	2.81	1.00
NY	89.08	16.53	2.20	1.82	77.86	27.20	1.74	1.00
Louisiana	37.44	14.40	2.16	1.83	123.34	102.47	13.35	1.11
Illinois	84.46	34.73	3.72	2.04	108.42	90.27	8.44	1.08
Ohio	73.57	22.94	3.02	1.94	120.30	121.32	30.12	1.37
Tennessee	41.60	10.14	2.02	1.14	136.04	109.71	15.41	1.29
Kansas	93.94	30.28	3.81	2.11	139.25	82.33	10.52	1.00
Texas	137.48	82.68	8.15	3.71	99.40	66.95	7.08	1.00
New Jersey	52.17	13.92	2.30	1.81	217.25	108.41	6.64	1.00

3.3 Recommendation Effectiveness Evaluation

This section assesses the effectiveness of the proposed meta-learning recommender under the temporal extrapolation validation scenario. Models are trained on data from 2011 to 2023 and evaluated on an independent 2024 test set with 52 regional instances. The primary evaluation metric is Recommendation Accuracy (RA), which measures the proximity of the recommended performance to the true optimal control chart.

Necessity of Data Balancing. The meta-dataset shows inherent class imbalance in how often each control chart is labeled as optimal. To examine the impact of this imbalance on meta-model performance and the necessity of the data balancing strategy, we conduct an ablation study. Table 4 compares test-set classification results for models trained on the original, imbalanced data without SMOTE and for models trained on data balanced with SMOTE.

Table 3. Performance of GLR and CUSUM control charts under multiplicative shifts

Region	GLR (η)				CUSUM (η)			
	0.01	0.05	0.1	0.3	0.01	0.05	0.1	0.3
Florida	257.72	142.36	73.70	42.84	196.40	104.97	60.07	40.52
Arizona	245.17	136.88	77.40	42.81	196.31	99.75	57.48	38.67
NY	235.85	119.93	67.45	35.08	202.48	96.41	59.91	38.21
Louisiana	245.70	126.71	69.68	40.37	197.93	106.69	57.86	39.96
Illinois	224.48	117.04	78.32	39.64	195.49	104.34	58.25	38.39
Ohio	211.23	122.92	68.65	37.81	201.59	105.76	57.99	40.24
Tennessee	241.61	128.77	74.50	39.12	210.69	102.82	59.52	37.69
Kansas	246.56	119.08	63.56	40.35	209.94	98.84	57.19	37.41
Texas	210.05	125.11	67.17	38.52	199.93	101.30	55.45	38.12
New Jersey	289.63	153.47	83.85	40.51	218.03	109.87	59.10	40.30

Table 4. Classification performance comparison on the 2024 test set: impact of smote during training

Class	Precision	Recall	F1-score	Support
(a) *No smote*				
1	0.52	1	0.6842	26
2	1	0.125	0.2222	16
4	0	0	0	10
Accuracy	0.5385			52
Macro avg	0.5067	0.375	0.3021	52
Weighted avg	0.5677	0.5385	0.4105	52
(b) *Smote*				
1	0.8929	0.9615	0.9259	26
2	0.9286	0.8125	0.8667	16
4	1	1	1	10
Accuracy	0.9231			52
Macro avg	0.9405	0.9247	0.9309	52
Weighted avg	0.9245	0.9231	0.9219	52

The results clearly demonstrate that class imbalance severely impairs the model's ability to distinguish classes. As reported in Table 4a, the model trained without SMOTE is strongly biased toward the majority class, which is EWMA, and it attains very low recall on the minority classes. Consequently, the overall classification accuracy is only

0.5385, and the macro-average F1-score is as low as 0.3021. Under these conditions, the model fails to provide reliable recommendations for scenarios where minority classes are optimal.

As shown in Table 4b, balancing the training set with SMOTE yields a substantial improvement. The overall classification accuracy increases to 0.9231, and the macro-average F1-score reaches 0.9309. The model achieves high and balanced precision and recall across all classes, demonstrating that SMOTE effectively corrects learning bias and ensures the meta-model possesses equitable recognition capabilities for all candidate control charts. Therefore, employing data balancing strategies is crucial for building a robust recommendation system. Subsequent performance evaluations are based on the optimized model trained using SMOTE.

Overall Recommendation Performance and Comparison. We compare the optimized meta-learning recommender, referred to as Ours, with four fixed-selection baselines to assess its relative advantages. Table 5 summarizes the comparison of RA-based metrics on the 2024 test set.

The experimental results demonstrate that the proposed meta-learning recommender outperforms all fixed-selection baselines. The recommender achieved a high mean RA of 0.9799, indicating that the surveillance performance obtained through adaptive recommendation reaches, on average, 98% of the theoretical optimum. In contrast, the best-performing fixed strategy, Always-EWMA, attains a mean RA of only 0.7283, while other strategies performed significantly worse. For example, Always-GLR yields 0.1758. These findings are consistent with above section: due to the spatio-temporal heterogeneity of surveillance data, a single control chart cannot remain optimal across all scenarios.

Table 5. Recommendation Accuracy (RA) comparison between the proposed meta-learning recommender and fixed-selection baselines on the 2024 test set

(a) Our RA recommender—overall metrics

Metric	RA.mean	Median(RA)	Regret.mean	DiscMean	Top-1	Top-2
Ours	0.9799	1	0.0201	99.52	0.904	1

(b) *Always-one baselines*

Baseline	RA.mean	Regret	DiscMean	Top-1
Always EWMA.mean	0.7283	0.2717	95.96	0.5
Always Shewhart.mean	0.5018	0.4982	93.08	0.308
Always GLR.mean	0.1758	0.8242	87.31	0
Always WCUSUM.mean	0.4719	0.5281	93.65	0.192

3.4 Real-Time Monitoring During the Influenza Season

This section aims to evaluate the real-world usefulness of the meta-learning recommendation framework in influenza surveillance. The complete two-stage process was applied to the 2024–2025 influenza season: the trained meta-model selected the chart type, followed by dynamic calibration using the 2024 off-season data to determine the control limits. Figure 2 shows results for four regions with representative dynamics comparing the alert performance and displaying the dynamically calibrated control limits.

The effect and necessity of dynamic calibration are evident from the substantial variation in control limits across regions for the same chart type. For example, the EWMA limit ranges from 1.34 in Colorado to 19.5 in Wyoming, and the Shewhart limits range from 2.52 in the District of Columbia to 11.9 in Wyoming. These differences reflect variation in baseline statistical properties such as noise levels, and the framework adapts to this heterogeneity to ensure the ARL_0 constraint is met locally.

In Alabama and the District of Columbia (DC) (Fig. 2a and c), the ILI curves exhibit rapid, steep increases. The recommender selected the Shewhart chart for both regions with a run length of 9 and 13. In Alabama, Shewhart triggered an alarm at week 9 (RL = 9), precisely coinciding with the starting point of the rapid rise in the epidemic curve. In contrast, memory-based methods such as EWMA (RL = 12), CUSUM (RL = 11), and GLR (RL = 13) all exhibited delays. A similar phenomenon was observed in DC, where Shewhart (RL = 13) sensitively captured a significant week-to-week jump, alarming 4 weeks earlier than EWMA (RL = 17). This confirms that when facing large, abrupt shifts, the Shewhart chart, sensitive to single-point anomalies, offers optimal detection timeliness, and the recommender successfully identified this scenario.

Conversely, the outbreak in Colorado (Fig. 2b) exhibited a smoother, more sustained growth pattern. In this context, the recommender selected EWMA. By effectively accumulating the persistent above-baseline signals, EWMA provided timely detection (RL = 9). In contrast, the Shewhart chart, which relies on large instantaneous shifts, did not trigger an alarm until week 18 (RL = 18), near the peak, resulting in a significant delay. The responses of GLR and CUSUM (RL = 14) were also later than EWMA. This indicates that for moderate-intensity sustained shifts, EWMA provides more timely and robust early warning, whereas fixedly choosing Shewhart would miss the opportunity for early intervention.

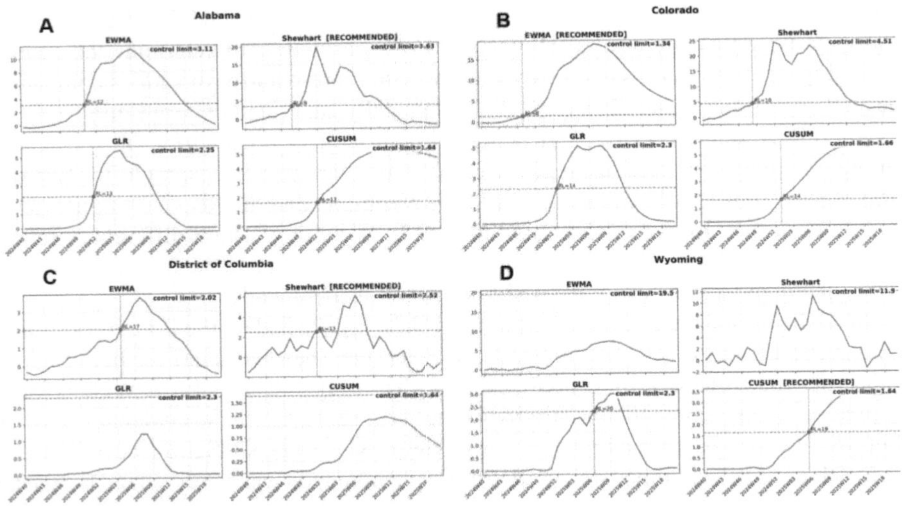

Fig. 2. Case studies of real-time influenza surveillance monitoring (2024–2025 Season) in four representative regions

The case of Wyoming (Fig. 2d) represents a pattern of slow growth starting from a low baseline. The recommender selected CUSUM. In this case, methods based on standardized residuals charts like EWMA and Shewhart failed to detect the anomaly, with their statistics remaining below the threshold. However, the likelihood-based CUSUM (RL = 11) and GLR (RL = 10) successfully issued warnings. This highlights the effectiveness of likelihood ratio-based methods in detecting weak multiplicative growth and the importance of selecting the appropriate statistical model.

Synthesizing these cases, it is evident that under a unified false alarm level, the most effective control chart type depends on the local baseline characteristics and the actual morphology of the emerging epidemic signal. The integrated PMcharm framework is capable of adapting across regional heterogeneity by combining intelligent selection with dynamic calibration to deploy the most appropriate and timely chart.

4 Conclusion

To enhance the timely monitoring capability of influenza surveillance, selecting the most suitable SPC chart configuration for heterogeneous data across regions and time periods is important. To address this, we introduce PMcharm, a two-stage meta-learning framework that integrates intelligent chart selection and dynamic control limit calibration. The framework couples classical statistical metrics with LSTM-based representations, derives robust meta-targets via in-control alignment and multi-perturbation aggregation, and applies SMOTE to mitigate class imbalance. Using U.S. CDC state-level ILI data (2011–2023 training and 2024 testing), it is confirmed that no single chart is universally optimal. PMcharm outperforms all fixed strategies, achieving a high mean RA of 0.9799. Furthermore, real-time case studies from the 2024–2025 influenza season validated the framework's practical utility, demonstrating its ability to adapt to diverse regional epidemic dynamics and consistently deploy the configuration offering the earliest outbreak detection. This approach facilitates enhanced surveillance efficiency and supports faster public health responses.

Acknowledgments. This work was supported by the National Natural Science Foundation of China [72274152,62572389].

Disclosure of Interests All authors declare that the research was conducted in the absence of any commercial or financial relationships that could be construed as a potential conflict of interest.

References

1. Hong, R., et al.: The power of public health surveillance. Delaware J. Public Health **6**(2), 60–63 (2020)
2. Suman, G., Prajapati, D.: Control chart applications in healthcare: a literature review. Int. J. Metrol. Quality Eng. **9**(9), 5 (2018)
3. Spiring, F.: Introduction to statistical quality control. Technometrics **49**(1), 108–109 (2007)
4. Woodall, W.H., Montgomery, D.C.: Some current directions in the theory and application of statistical process monitoring. J. Qual. Technol. **46**(1), 78–94 (2014)
5. Lee, I.-S., et al.: Random-forest-based real-time contrasts control chart using adaptive breakpoints with symbolic aggregate approximation. Expert Syst. Appl. **158**, 113407 (2020)
6. Kuiper, A., Goedhart, R.: Optimized control charts using indifference regions. Qual. Eng. **36**(2), 371–389 (2023)
7. Probert, W.J.M. et al.: Vote-processing rules for combining control recommendations from multiple models. Philos. Trans. R. Soc. A: Math. Phys. Eng. Sci. **380**, 2233 (2022). https://doi.org/10.1098/rsta.2021.0314
8. Wittenberg, P.: Modeling the patient mix for risk-adjusted CUSUM charts. Stat. Methods Med. Res. **31**(5), 779–800 (2022)
9. Tan, Y., et al.: Risk-adjusted zero-inflated poisson CUSUM charts for monitoring influenza surveillance data. BMC Med. Informa. Decis. Making 21, Suppl 2 (2021)
10. CDC Flu Burden. Preliminary Estimated Flu Disease Burden 2023–2024 Flu Season. https://www.cdc.gov/flu-burden/php/data-vis/2023-2024.html
11. CDC. Expanding the Global Influenza Surveillance and Response System to include other respiratory viruses with epidemic or pandemic potential (2025)
12. Muscatello, D.J., et al.: Prospective surveillance of excess mortality due to influenza in New South Wales: feasibility and statistical approach. Commun. Dis. Intell. Q. Rep. **32**(4), 435–442 (2008)
13. Lai, X., et al.: Classifier chain-based monitoring method for multivariate surgical outcomes. Comput. Ind. Eng. **194**, 110378 (2024)
14. Yu, M., et al.: A robust CUSUM scheme with a weighted likelihood ratio to monitor an overdispersed counting process. Comput. Ind. Eng. **126**, 165–174 (2018)
15. Steiner, S.H., et al.: Detecting the start of an influenza outbreak using exponentially weighted moving average charts. BMC Med. Inform. Decis. Mak. **10**, 17 (2010)
16. Lai, X., et al.: Generalized likelihood ratio based risk-adjusted control chart for zero-inflated poisson process. Qual. Reliab. Eng. Int. **39**(1), 363–381 (2022)
17. Höhle, M., Paul, M.: Count data regression charts for the monitoring of surveillance time series. Comput. Stat. Data Anal. **52**(9), 4357–4368 (2008)

18. Sonesson, C., Bock, D.: A review and discussion of prospective statistical surveillance in public health. J. R. Stat. Soc. Ser. A Stat. Soc. **166**(1), 5–21 (2003)
19. Solgi, M., et al.: Timely detection of influenza outbreaks in Iran: evaluating the performance of the exponentially weighted moving average. J. Infect. Public Health **11**(3), 389–392 (2017)
20. Gao, Y., et al.: Application of the moving epidemic method for influenza surveillance in Kunming. Front Public Health **13** (2025)
21. Saeed, N., et al.: Sensitivity and reliability comparisons of EWMA mean control chart based on robust scale estimators under non-normal process: COVID data application. Qual. Reliabil. Eng. Int.
22. Hawkins, D.M., Wu, Q.: The CUSUM and the EWMA head-to-head. Qual. Eng. **26**(2), 215–222 (2014)
23. Tadese, Z.B., Arage, F.G., Tsegaw, T.K., et al.: Forecasting tuberculosis in Ethiopia using deep learning: progress toward sustainable development goal evidence from global burden of disease 1990–2021. BMC Infect. Dis. **25**, 870 (2025)
24. Hric, P., Sabahno, H.: Developing machine learning-based control charts for monitoring different GLM-type profiles with different link functions. Appl. Artif. Intell. **38**, 1 (2024)
25. Puerto, A.M., et al.: Establishing epidemic and intensity thresholds after a major change in respiratory virus surveillance in Spain in 2020. Influenza Other Respir. Viruses **19**, 9 (2025)
26. Wiemken, T.L., et al.: Thresholds versus anomaly detection for surveillance of pneumonia and influenza mortality. Emerg. Infect. Dis. **26**(11), 2733–2735 (2020)

Construction of the Text Sentiment Analysis Model for College Students' Mental Health: Based on Machine Learning and Sentiment Dictionary

Zhaojia Chai(✉)

Institute of Language Sciences, Shanghai International Studies University, Shanghai, China
chaizhaojia0905@163.com

Abstract. The mental health problems of college students are becoming increasingly prominent. It is of great significance to detect the tendency of psychological problems as early as possible and reduce the occurrence of psychological crisis problems in order to promote the healthy development of students. Psychological health, as an important factor in the growth process of college students, is closely related to emotional changes. Social media is an important channel for college students to express their emotional attitudes, and the emotional information contained in their texts also provides data support for assessing college students' mental health. In order to analyze the mental health status of college students more intelligently and accurately from their social texts, this study constructed a text sentiment analysis model for college students' mental health, using machine learning and sentiment lexicon methods to visually display the trend of users' emotional states from two aspects: emotional polarity and emotional intensity. This study will provide a reference for identifying the mental health status and warning of psychological crises among college students.

Keywords: Mental health · College students · Text sentiment analysis · Machine learning · Sentiment dictionary

1 Introduction

With the acceleration of modern life pace and the sudden increase in learning pressure, the mental health problems of college students have become increasingly prominent, bringing huge burdens to their learning and life. The emotional characteristics of college students change rapidly, with intense intensity and significant fluctuations. However, the passivity, limited sample size, and retrospective data acquisition of traditional mental health assessment methods are not conducive to monitoring the mental health of college students to a certain extent. According to a survey report, the positive detection rate of depression in the 18–26 age group is 21.48%, and negative events such as suicide and crime caused by psychological problems are increasing year by year [1]. Therefore, it has become particularly important to assess students' mental health status and promptly identify psychological crisis issues.

Y. Zhang et al. (Eds.): CHIP 2025, CCIS 2884, pp. 223–231, 2026.
https://doi.org/10.1007/978-981-95-7299-1_14

The development of Web 2.0 has promoted the emergence of online social media that focuses on user interaction. More and more students are sharing their opinions, expressing their thoughts, and emotions through social media. The text content usually contains a lot of emotional, viewpoint, and attitude information, which provides important data support for establishing a psychological health text emotional corpus [2]. Psychological studies have shown that emotions are an important representation of mental health issues [3]. Therefore, social text data rich in emotional expression provides a new perspective for mental health assessment: based on the rich viewpoints and emotional expressions contained in social texts, combined with text sentiment analysis techniques, it can provide multidimensional references for college students' mental health assessment.

Text sentiment analysis is a hot research topic in the fields of computational linguistics and natural language processing, which can help researchers deeply explore the emotions, attitudes, and viewpoints contained in texts, and apply them to various aspects such as public opinion monitoring, psychological diagnosis, emotional dialogue, and product review analysis. In recent years, research on sentiment analysis of Chinese social texts has gradually received widespread attention. Researchers have used data mining and sentiment analysis techniques to bring new breakthroughs to mental health research driven by data [4]. The sentiment analysis technology for social texts processes the behavior, emotions, language, and other data generated by college students. Researchers can collect data in real situations without invading the subjects, providing diversified evidence for predicting psychological crisis states, identifying psychologically abnormal users, and intervening in mental health problems. This promotes the physical and mental health development of students and helps to build intelligent mental health platforms in universities. In this context, this study will focus on college students and construct a text sentiment analysis model for mental health based on social text data, in order to provide reference for the recognition and dynamic monitoring of college students' mental health status.

2 The Related Word

2.1 Current Situation of Mental Health Screening

Economic development has improved people's living standards, and people have gradually begun to pay more attention to their mental life. Mental health is an indispensable part of health. External environment and self-stress are the main causes of great fluctuations in mental state and trigger mental illness. Without prevention and timely diversion, mental health problems can arise. Screening and measurement of mental health problems are mostly in the form of scales. Existing mental health screenings can be divided into four types. Such as assessment modality (self-assessment or other assessment), target population (adolescents, adults, or the elderly), applicable scenarios (online questionnaire or active consultation), and applicable pathologies (suicidal ideation, depression, anxiety disorders, etc.) [5]. For the detection of suicidal depressive conditions, the scale for suicidal ideation (SSI-C) developed by Beck et al., and the suicide status questionnaire (SSF) are both commonly used suicide detection scales [6].

The current mental health survey is mainly conducted by sending & collecting questionnaires, active reporting to doctors, and observation by specialists. The time lag, limited population coverage, high cost, and reliance on human cooperation are not helpful for the detection of mental health crises. Many tests are done for specific diseases without constant dynamic monitoring. In addition, most patients do not have the awareness and behavior to actively seek psychological help, which makes the identification and analysis of mental health problems more difficult [7].

2.2 Sentiment Analysis Based on Social Media Big Data

Social media is a comprehensive virtual community and platform used by people to share opinions and viewpoints. The characteristics of social media data are: massive data volume, high data noise, high potential value, and fast interaction changes. The main social media platforms abroad are Facebook, Twitter, and Instagram; The main social media platforms in China are Weibo, Tieba, etc. Due to the limitation of information length, the main form of publication is short text, not exceeding 140 words. Therefore, people tend to shorten the word count as much as possible when posting messages, express them briefly, and make the emotional content of the text richer and more concentrated. Some researchers confirm the shift in people's attitudes when expressing themselves on social media, showing that the text on social media conveys the real sentiment and attitude of the poster [8]. Combining social media data for sentiment analysis is becoming increasingly popular in the field of natural language processing, involving multiple disciplines such as computer science, linguistics, psychology, and sociology, and its application value is also highlighted in different fields.

The abundance of opinion-based texts on social media is an important source for constructing sentiment analysis corpora. Many researchers have conducted extensive methodological and applied research on social text data. Ahmad et al. modeled and analyzed emotional words in consumer reviews to generate popularity rankings of product features, in order to determine consumer preferences and assist relevant companies in making decisions for product improvement [9]. Zhao Yonghua and Dou Shuqi conducted sentiment analysis on comments on Twitter, closely integrating social media big data with the social environment to gain insights into the public's speech trends and emotional characteristics in online public opinion [10].

2.3 Research on Text Sentiment Analysis for Mental Health

Text Sentiment Analysis refers to the use of computer technology to mine the subjective and objective attributes, viewpoints, emotions, etc. expressed in text, in order to determine the emotional tendency of the text [4]. Sentiment classification is one of the core tasks in text emotion analysis. The commonly used emotion classification in psychology is based on "valence-arousal", which is mapped to sentiment polarity and sentiment intensity in natural language processing. Zhang Jinwei designed a multi-level psychological warning model, using the traditional sentiment lexicon method to analyze the emotions of students' Weibo texts and screen students who may have psychological problems [11]. Li Tongtong et al. combined the stress response theory of psychology and the Big Five personality traits to calculate the emotional intensity and emotional threshold of five personality types, and constructed a psychological crisis warning model for students [12].

Based on the above literature, this article mainly uses text sentiment analysis technology to mine emotions in students' social texts, constructs a text sentiment analysis model for mental health, and visually analyzes their mental health status from the two dimensions of 'valence-arousal'.

3 Construction of Psychological Mental Health Analysis Model Based on Text Sentiment Analysis

Our study is based on the social text sentiment analysis framework [13] and constructs a text sentiment analysis model for college students' mental health, as shown in Fig. 1.

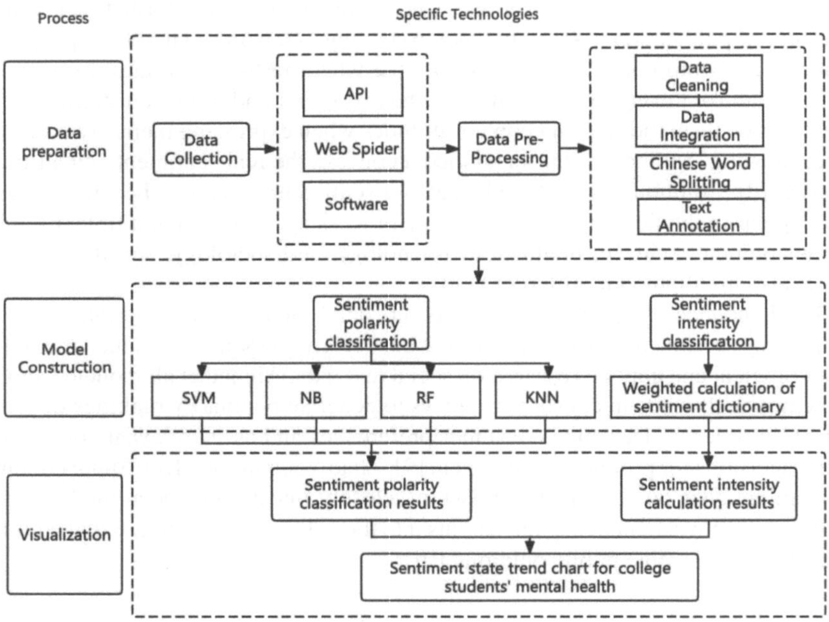

Fig. 1. Text sentiment analysis model for college students' mental health.

The first stage involves data preparation, mainly the collection and preprocessing of data. The collected data is the text of college students' Weibo social platforms, which can be accessed through three methods: calling API interfaces, using mature web crawling software, and developing web crawling frameworks based on Python. The original corpus contains redundancy, missing information, ambiguity, and other issues that cannot be directly used for sentiment analysis; therefore, text preprocessing is required. The text preprocessing process includes data cleaning, text segmentation, removal of stop words, and feature extraction. Data cleaning is the process of removing duplicate or missing data, while text segmentation is the process of breaking a sentence into multiple words. Accurate segmentation can improve a computer's ability to recognize and understand text. Removing stop words is the process of removing frequently used words that are not helpful for text analysis, such as "I," "Yes," and words that have no practical meaning, such as "Oh," "Hmm," or "En," in order to reduce the dimensionality of the text and improve the accuracy of text analysis. After preprocessing, the text remains in text format and needs to be converted into a series of vectors expressing text features through word vector encoding for feature extraction.

During the model construction phase, machine learning methods are used to classify text into three categories of sentiment polarity: positive, neutral, and negative. Four classic machine learning models, SVM, Naive Bayes, Random Forest, and KNN, were selected for model construction. The model with the best results was chosen as the output of the sentiment polarity classifier to optimize the classification performance of sentiment polarity. Meanwhile, for the calculation of sentiment intensity, a sentiment dictionary is used as the calculation standard to weight the text. The specific process is shown in Fig. 2. The sentiment dictionary is based on the Chinese sentiment vocabulary ontology library developed by Dalian University of Technology. This is a professional vocabulary library specifically designed for the field of Chinese sentiment analysis, providing basic data support for natural language processing and sentiment computing research. This dictionary covers Chinese vocabulary of various sentiment types such as positive, negative, neutral, etc. It is classified according to sentiment types and vocabulary attributes, forming a clear hierarchical ontology structure, containing thousands of words and their related attributes. Due to the polarity and intensity annotation of sentiment words in this sentiment dictionary, we use the partial polarity sentiment intensity values of their sentiment intensity to calculate and integrate degree adverbs, modal particles, emoticons, and punctuation marks to construct the sentiment intensity dictionary. The calculation process is as follows: the basic sentiment intensity score for each text is 1. At the lexical hierarchy, the judgment is first made based on keywords, and it is necessary to combine the sentiment intensity dictionary to weight the degree adverbs and sentiment words. At the sentence hierarchy, it is necessary to judge based on symbols, calculate the emoji and punctuation contained in the text separately, and finally weight the specific sentiment intensity value of the entire sentence and output the result.

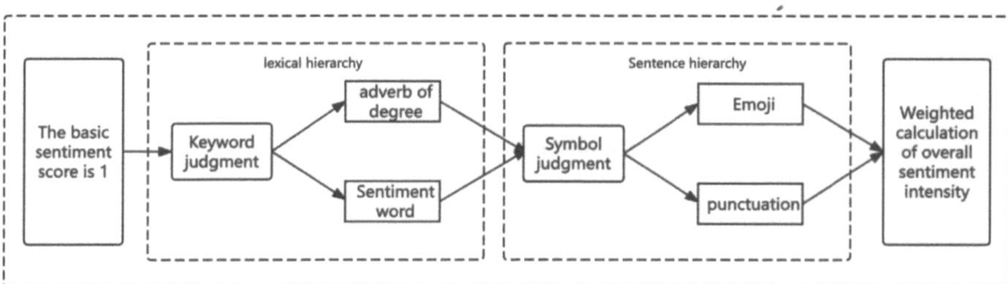

Fig. 2. Sentiment intensity calculation based on sentiment dictionary.

In the visualization stage, a two-dimensional emotional state trend chart for mental health is constructed, with the vertical axis representing the emotional intensity value of each text and the horizontal axis representing each Weibo text arranged in chronological order of posting, in order to visualize the results of emotional analysis and determine the trend of emotional changes.

4 Application of Psychological Health Analysis Model

4.1 Experimental Data Collection and Preprocessing

Our study collected Weibo social text data of 100 students from a university in East China from July 2024 to December 2024 using GooSeeker software. We collected a total of 13472 Weibo text data, including user nicknames, user IDs, Weibo texts, and posting times. After data cleaning, redundant and missing data items were removed, and 12758 Weibo text data were retained after removing meaningless data.

4.2 Sentiment Polarity Classification Results

Using machine learning algorithms for text sentiment analysis typically involves selecting the optimal algorithm based on four criteria: accuracy, F-score, precision, and recall. This study mainly evaluates the effectiveness of the model based on accuracy, with reference to Precision, Recall, and F-value. Generally, the higher the indicator value, the more effective the model. The specific calculation method is shown in Formulas (1)–(4).

$$Precision = \frac{TP}{TP + FP} \tag{1}$$

$$Recall = \frac{TP}{TP + FN} \tag{2}$$

$$F1 = \frac{2Precision * Recall}{Precision + Recall} \tag{3}$$

$$Precision = \frac{TP + TN}{TP + TN + FN + FP} \tag{4}$$

After thoroughly considering the characteristics of text data, as well as positive, neutral, and negative emotional text, the evaluation results shown in Table 1 were obtained. Analyzing the data in Table 1, it is evident that the SVM algorithm yields optimal results in terms of Accuracy, F-value, Precision, and Recall in the sentiment analysis. Therefore, we choose the SVM algorithm for sentiment polarity classification.

Table 1. Results of sentiment polarity classification model.

Model	KNN			Random forest			Naive Bayes			SVM		
Index												
	0	1	2	0	1	2	0	1	2	0	1	2
Precision	0.530	0.864	0.708	0.524	0.851	0.739	0.437	0.876	0.952	0.714	0.835	0.912
Recall	0.798	0.821	0.497	0.781	0.821	0.473	0.487	0.958	0.293	0.699	0.964	0.483
F1	0.702	0.816	0.530	0.638	0.814	0.596	0.374	0.806	0.415	0.656	0.877	0.476
Accuracy (%)	72.9376			74.7937			70.3821			79.6935		

Note 0 is neutral, 1 is positive, 2 is negative

4.3 Sentiment Intensity Calculation Results

We calculated the emotional intensity of the text based on a self-built sentiment intensity dictionary from both lexical and sentence hierarchy, and finally normalized the results. The specific pseudocode example is shown in Table 2.

Table 2. Pseudocode example for emotion intensity calculation.

```
// Sentiment Intensity Calculation Pseudocode
Define BASE_SCORE = 1.0
// Initialize dictionaries
sentiment_dict = {
   "happy": 1.5, "sad": -1.5,  // Emotion word weights
   "very": 1.8, "slightly": 0.5 // Degree adverb weights}
symbol_scores = {
   "!": 0.3, "!!": 0.5,        // Punctuation weights
   "😊": 1.0, "😢": -1.0       // Emoji weights}
Function calculate_sentiment(text):
   total_score = BASE_SCORE
   // Lexical level calculation
   words = split_text(text)
   For each word in words:
      If word in sentiment_dict:
         modifier = 1.0
         prev_word = get_previous_word(word)
         If prev_word in sentiment_dict.modifiers:
            modifier = sentiment_dict.modifiers[prev_word]
         total_score += sentiment_dict[word] * modifier
   // Symbol level calculation
   For each symbol in symbol_scores:
      If symbol in text:
         total_score += symbol_scores[symbol] * count_occurrences(symbol, text)
   Return round_to_two_decimal(total_score)
```

For the convenience of presenting the results, the obtained sentiment intensity values were linearly normalized (i.e. minimum maximum normalization) and mapped to a fixed interval of [−3, 3], thus obtaining the overall sentiment intensity value of the final sentence. Some of the results are shown in Fig. 3.

```
春天到了，我们去田野里春游吧！
情感强度分值：2.125
夏季鼻血综合症提前来临 今天洗澡洗到洗到就来了股鼻血 打响了今年夏天我战鼻血的第一枪[鄙视]
情感强度分值：2.80
又梦见khun oppa了，哇咔咔 去听讲座喽[嘻嘻]
情感强度分值：2.65
我居然还能表现出来无所谓的样子。
情感强度分值：1.545
就这样吧，也没什么大不了
情感强度分值：0.85
聊完之后就没影儿了，想问问如何解决也不知道找谁
情感强度分值：0.33
东西还行，就是听着一般般吧。
情感强度分值：0.25
```

Fig. 3. Sentiment intensity calculation results (partial)

4.4 Visual Analysis of Mental Health Status

Based on the theoretical model of "valence-arousal", we integrate the results of sentiment polarity classification and intensity calculation, and use a two-dimensional line chart to display the sentiment state trend of observed student users over a period of time. The change in sentiment state can to some extent reflect the psychological health status of students. If the sentiment polarity is positive, multiply by $+1$, and if the sentiment polarity is negative, multiply by -1, which are represented by the upper and lower parts of the red boundary line in the figure. In psychology, neutral sentiment polarity lacks clear sentiment intensity characteristics and sentiment states are uncertain. Therefore, in our study, if the sentiment polarity is neutral, it is multiplied by 0. The weighted calculation of sentiment intensity values and sentiment polarity values yields a trend chart of sentiment states towards mental health.

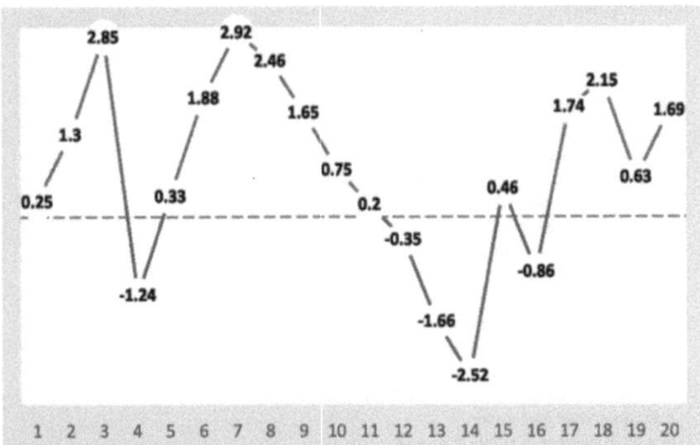

Fig. 4. Sentiment state trend chart for mental health

A normal sentiment state should be diverse, with small fluctuations and relatively stable sentiment levels, primarily characterized by a balanced expression of positive and negative emotions, as well as sentiment regulation that is adapted to life events. Taking Fig. 4 as an example, it can be seen that the sentiment state of the student user exhibits some fluctuations; however, there is no significant fluctuation in sentiment intensity or sustained negative sentiment, and the overall development trend is positive. This moderate sentiment changes and diversity are a normal part of human emotional experience. Constructing a sentiment state trend chart for mental health can provide psychologists with intuitive visual feedback on changes in students' sentiment states. If students are in a long-term negative state, timely intervention measures can be provided to reduce the occurrence of mental health crises and promote their physical and mental health development.

5 Conclusion

Our study constructed a text sentiment analysis model for college students' mental health, utilizing two methods: machine learning and sentiment dictionary. This model visualizes the sentiment state trends of college students from two aspects: sentiment polarity and intensity. The results of our study will provide a reference for the automatic assessment and intelligent monitoring of mental health. However, there are still certain limitations in this research, mainly including the following two points. Firstly, more advanced deep learning methods can be used to improve classification accuracy for sentiment polarity classification, and algorithms can also be improved for sentiment intensity to enhance the accuracy of intensity calculation; Secondly, our study will continue to improve and optimize the analysis model based on the results of sentiment analysis, combined with time dimension and psychological health theory, in order to provide support for intelligent identification of college students' psychological health status.

Acknowledgments. This work was supported by the Second Batch of Scientific Research Projects of the Advance Research Center of Education and Technology in 2025 (KX002), the Project of the Digital Culture and Media Research Base, Key Research Base of Social Sciences, Sichuan Province (No.SC25DCM04), and the Supervisor Academic Guidance Program of Shanghai International Studies University under Grant (No.2024DSYL040).

Disclosure of Interests The author declares that he has no competing interests.

References

1. Fu, X., Zhang, K.: Blue Book on mental health: report on the Development of National Mental Health in China (2021–2022). Beijing, China (2023)
2. Peng, L., Guo, L., Li, Q.: Research on psychological health education for college students from the perspective of generative artificial intelligence. J. Foshan Univ. Sci. Technol. (Soc. Sci. Ed.) 42(04), 96–100 (2024). https://doi.org/10.13797/j.cnki.jfosu.1008-018x.2024.0048
3. Dheeraj, K., Ramakrishnudu, T.: Negative emotions detection on online mental-health related patients texts using the deep learning with MHA-BCNN model. Expert Syst. Appl. **182**, 115265 (2021)
4. Liu, B.: Emotion Analysis Excavates Viewpoints, Emotions, and Emotions. Beijing, China (2018)
5. Gao, L.: Big Data driven psychological health assessment model for college students. Inf. Technol. (1), 32–36, 43 (2022)
6. Yang, L., Zhai, D.K., Zhou, Y.: Reliability and validity of the suicide status form in Chinese college students. Chinese J. Clin. Psychol. (03), 541–544+594 (2022)
7. Yu, W.: Analysis of psychological health status of college students and educational countermeasures. Educ. Career **2015**(11), 68–70 (2015)
8. Cheng, Q., Li, T.M., Kwok, C.-L., Zhu, T., Yip, P.S.: Assessing suicide risk and emotional distress in Chinese social media: A text mining and machine learning study. J. Med. Internet Res. **19**(7), e243 (2017)
9. Ahmad, S.R., Bakar, A.A., Yaakub, M.R., Yusop, N.M.M., Wook, M., Ahmad, A.: Product feature ranking and popularity model based on sentiment comments. Int. J. Adv. Comput. Sci. Appl. **9**(9) (2018)
10. Zhao, Y., Dou, S.: Research on public emotions in the international discourse space of overseas social media from the perspective of social constructivism: a computational communication analysis based on the Sino US trade dispute issue. News Enthusiast (05), 14–19. https://doi.org/10.16017/j.cnki.xwahz.2022.05.011
11. Zhang, J., Liu, X.: Research on Weibo emotion recognition based on psychological warning model. J. Hefei Univ. Technol. (Nat. Sci. Ed.) **36**(11), 1318–1322 (2013)
12. Li, T., Li, T., Guo, X.: Psychological crisis warning for college students based on social media big data. Modern Distance Educ. Res. **33**(04), 92–103 (2021)
13. Li, J., Liu, D., Wan, C., Liu, X., Qiu, X., Bao, L., Zhu, T.: A review of research on automatic assessment of psychological health of social network users Chinese J. Inf. Sci. **35**(02), 19–32 (2021)

A Review of Multimodal Large Language Model Driven Intelligent Tongue, Pulse, and Facial Diagnosis in Traditional Chinese Medicine

Bo An[1,2](✉)

[1] University of Chinese Academy of Social Sciences, Beijing, China
[2] Institute of Ethnology and Anthropology, Chinese Academy of Social Sciences, Beijing, China
anbo@cass.org.cn

Abstract. In recent years, artificial intelligence–especially large-scale foundation models–has advanced rapidly in healthcare. Traditional Chinese Medicine (TCM) diagnosis relies on the four examinations (inspection, listening/smelling, inquiry, and palpation) and is highly dependent on clinician experience, leading to subjectivity and variability. The emergence of multimodal large language model (MLLM) offers new opportunities for making TCM diagnosis more objective and standardized. This review surveys the latest progress on applying MLLM and large language models to TCM-aided diagnosis. Focusing on three representative diagnostic dimensions–tongue, pulse, and facial diagnosis–we summarize how image analysis, sensing technologies, and natural-language processing enable data acquisition, preprocessing, and analytics for these modalities. We then synthesize current applications and performance of LLMs in TCM diagnostic settings, with particular attention to systems that integrate tongue/facial images, voice-based consultations, and textual medical records for multimodal, AI-assisted decision making. We further highlight advances and open challenges in applying LLMs to multi-visit, longitudinal follow-up scenarios, and discuss how such models may enhance the scientific rigor, standardization, and verifiability of TCM clinical practice. Finally, we outline future research directions–including cross-modal alignment, knowledge enhancement, personalized prediction, and large-scale multimodal pretraining–to inform subsequent research and applications.

Keywords: Traditional Chinese Medicine diagnosis · Multimodality · Large language models (LLMs) · Tongue diagnosis · Pulse diagnosis · Facial diagnosis · Intelligent follow-up · Cross-modal fusion

Y. Zhang et al. (Eds.): CHIP 2025, CCIS 2884, pp. 232–250, 2026.
https://doi.org/10.1007/978-981-95-7299-1_15

1 Introduction

Diagnosis in Traditional Chinese Medicine (TCM) centers on the Four Examinations–inspection, listening/smelling, inquiry, and palpation–with tongue diagnosis, pulse diagnosis, and assessment of facial complexion constituting key components of inspection and palpation [1,2]. In routine practice, physicians synthesize observations of tongue features and facial complexion, auditory and olfactory cues, medical history obtained through inquiry, and tactile information from pulse palpation to infer the patient's pattern (zheng) [3]. However, this workflow is highly dependent on individual expertise and thus prone to subjectivity and inter-practitioner variability. Digitizing and objectifying the diagnostic process is therefore a critical challenge for the modernization of TCM and for improving diagnostic consistency [4,5]. Over the past decade, rapid advances in artificial intelligence (AI) have opened new avenues to address this challenge.

MLLM refers to technologies capable of processing and fusing heterogeneous data types such as images, text, speech, and sensor signals [6]. In healthcare, MLLM can integrate images, physiologic signals, and clinical narratives to provide more comprehensive decision support than any single modality alone [7]. In the TCM diagnostic setting, MLLM aligns naturally with the Four Examinations: computer vision can analyze tongue images and facial appearance; sensors can capture pulse waveforms [8]; and LLMs can process inquiry text–together enabling an integrated, intelligent analysis of "inspection, listening/smelling, inquiry, and palpation."

Concurrently, large-scale pretrained models–including Transformer-based deep learning models and LLMs–have demonstrated strong capabilities in medicine [7,9]. Generative pretrained models represented by ChatGPT exhibit outstanding performance in natural-language understanding and generation, motivating exploration of their use in medical consultation and diagnostic support [10,11]. Direct deployment of general-purpose models to TCM, however, faces domain-mismatch issues such as insufficient domain knowledge and stylistic incongruence [12]. In response, TCM-specific LLMs have emerged, for example Qihuang Wendao and the Digital TCM model based on the GLM-130B architecture. These models integrate extensive TCM knowledge and clinical data to enhance intelligent question-answering and decision support in TCM [13,14].

Existing studies suggest that LLMs possess distinct advantages for TCM [15]. On the one hand, the rich experiential knowledge embedded in TCM texts and case records can be acquired via self-supervised learning, allowing LLMs to internalize linguistic patterns from classical literature and medical cases [16]. On the other hand, TCM's paradigm of pattern identification and treatment (bianzheng lunzhi) requires synthesizing multidimensional evidence and performing nontrivial reasoning–capabilities at which LLMs and multimodal fusion excel [17,18]. For instance, recent work indicates that LLMs can adapt to the knowledge system of TCM compound prescriptions and pattern differentiation, thereby providing effective support for clinical decision-making [12,19].

In this review, we synthesize progress on applying MLLM and LLMs to TCM-aided diagnosis. Sections 2–4 survey the digitization and intelligent analysis of three representative diagnostic dimensions–tongue, pulse, and facial diagnosis–detailing how image processing, sensor acquisition, and machine-learning methods enable objective quantification of diagnostic cues [4,20,21]. Section 5 summarizes integrated applications and performance of multimodal large-model systems in TCM, including platforms that fuse tongue/facial images, voice-based inquiry, and textual medical records, as well as the construction of TCM-oriented pretrained models. Section 6 highlights advances and challenges in deploying LLMs for multi-visit and longitudinal follow-up, examining how they can track disease trajectories and optimize efficacy evaluation to enhance the scientific rigor and verifiability of TCM practice. Finally, Section 7 discusses current challenges and outlines future directions, including cross-modal alignment, knowledge-enhancement strategies grounded in TCM theory, individualized prediction, and large-scale multimodal pretraining tailored to TCM [22,23].

2 Multimodal Acquisition and Analysis for Tongue Diagnosis

Tongue diagnosis is a central component of visual inspection in Traditional Chinese Medicine (TCM) [24]. TCM posits that tongue features–including the morphology and color of the tongue body and the characteristics of the tongue coating–reflect internal pathophysiological changes. Objectifying tongue diagnosis requires acquiring and analyzing objective information about the tongue via digital imaging technologies [25]. In recent years, substantial progress has been made toward computer-aided tongue diagnosis across the full pipeline from image acquisition and preprocessing to feature extraction and intelligent classification.

2.1 Tongue-Image Acquisition and Preprocessing

High-quality image acquisition is foundational for intelligent tongue diagnosis. To ensure that images faithfully capture diagnostic information, standardized protocols typically employ uniform illumination and imaging devices, fixed shooting distance and angle, and a natural tongue protrusion posture. Empirical evidence suggests that tongue images should be clear and high-resolution, exhibit accurate color reproduction, and contain complete information about both the tongue body and coating. Because ambient lighting and device variations can affect perceived color and texture, color calibration and white balancing are commonly applied prior to analysis to mitigate environmental confounders. Early studies introduced color-difference–based standardization methods to improve cross-session consistency of chromatic features [26].

Automatic segmentation of the tongue region is a critical preprocessing step that removes background structures (face, lips) and improves the accuracy of downstream analysis. Classical approaches include thresholding, edge detection, and active contour models. More recently, deep learning has markedly improved segmentation accuracy and robustness; for example, U-Net–based convolutional neural networks have been shown to delineate tongue boundaries with high precision [27,28].

2.2 Feature Extraction and Intelligent Diagnosis

Core diagnostic cues in tongue images comprise two aspects: the *tongue body* and the *tongue coating*. Tongue-body features include chromatic categories (e.g., pale, red, crimson), morphology (e.g., enlarged, thin, prickled, fissured, teeth-marked), and moisture/luster, whereas coating features concern coating color (e.g., white, yellow), texture (e.g., thin/thick, moist/dry, greasy), and spatial distribution. Traditionally, practitioners infer cold–heat and deficiency–excess patterns from these observations.

To automate recognition of such cues, researchers combine image processing with pattern recognition. On preprocessed images, color-space transformations (e.g., RGB to CIELAB) enable computation of color histograms for the tongue body and coating, as well as quantitative indices such as the area ratio between body and coating. More advanced descriptors capture subtle differences in texture and shape–for example, gray-level co-occurrence matrices (GLCM) for texture analysis and Fourier descriptors for contour morphology. Early machine-learning pipelines typically extracted handcrafted features and employed classifiers such as support vector machines (SVMs) or random forests to predict patterns or disease categories [29].

With the advent of deep learning, convolutional neural networks (CNNs) have demonstrated superior capability to learn high-level representations of tongue images, substantially improving classification accuracy. Reviews of deep CNNs in tongue-image analysis report state-of-the-art performance in recognizing tongue-body and coating colors as well as hallmark pathological signs, and transfer learning has been successfully applied to constitution classification and disease prediction. A notable trend is multimodal (or hybrid) fusion of handcrafted and deep features: traditional color/texture descriptors can be combined with CNN-derived embeddings and then fed into a downstream classifier to leverage both expert priors and data-driven representations. For example, after precise segmentation with an improved U-Net++ model on a standardized dataset of 1,374 subjects, researchers have fused CIELAB color and texture features with a 2,048-dimensional ResNet-50 embedding and trained a multilayer perceptron to recognize five common TCM constitution types, achieving high accuracy with good generalization. Such systems promise to overcome reliance on subjective experience and questionnaires, providing objective, quantitative tools for constitution and pattern identification

2.3 Current Applications of Intelligent Tongue Diagnosis

Building on these techniques, several prototype systems and commercial products for objective tongue diagnosis have emerged. Dedicated TCM tongue-diagnosis devices integrate high-resolution cameras with standardized lighting to capture images and ship with analysis software that automatically generates reports. Typical outputs include quantitative assessments of tongue color, coating thickness, and tongue morphology, along with preliminary suggestions of likely TCM patterns or health states for clinician reference. In research settings, objective tongue analysis has been used to explore the relationship between tongue features and TCM syndromes in specific diseases–for instance, associating characteristic tongue-body and coating features in diabetes with particular pattern types to inform treatment strategies. As larger tongue-image databases are established and deep-learning algorithms continue to improve, the accuracy of intelligent tongue diagnosis is expected to increase further, with promising applications in preventive care and population-level constitution monitoring [30,31].

3 Objectification and Intelligent Recognition for Pulse Diagnosis

Pulse diagnosis (palpation) is another core component of TCM diagnosis, wherein physicians sense pulsations of the radial artery with their fingertips to identify pulse characteristics (e.g., floating vs. deep, slow vs. rapid, deficiency vs. excess). Traditional practice, however, relies heavily on tactile experience, suffers from poor inter-practitioner consistency, and uses descriptors that can be ambiguous. Since the late twentieth century, various TCM pulse-diagnosis devices have been developed to digitize pulse signals via sensors and to analyze pulse features algorithmically. With the advent of machine learning and deep learning, research on objective pulse diagnosis has entered a new stage, with steadily improving accuracy for automatic pulse-type recognition and diagnostic support.

3.1 Acquisition and Quantitative Characterization of Pulse Signals

Modern pulse-diagnosis devices typically employ pressure-sensor arrays or strain gauges to standardize fingertip location and applied force, acquiring pulse waveforms at the three canonical sites—*cun*, *guan*, and *chi*. The resulting signals are time-varying pressure traces that encode frequency, amplitude, and morphological information. A typical pulse waveform exhibits periodic peaks and troughs corresponding to the systolic peak and the diastolic phase within each cardiac cycle.

To extract informative features, a range of signal-processing techniques are used. In the time domain, one can compute the mean cycle length, rhythm stability, peak amplitude, and pulse rate. In the frequency domain, Fourier or wavelet transforms yield harmonic components and energy distributions that reflect vascular tone and elasticity. Model-based approaches further decompose the waveform into a forward (primary) wave and multiple reflected waves to derive parameters such as rise time and reflection ratios. These quantitative indices map traditional qualitative descriptors to measurable data: for example, a *floating* pulse (*fu mai*) manifests as prominent waveforms under shallow applied pressure (captured in pressure–amplitude curves), whereas a *deep* pulse (*chen mai*) requires greater pressure to elicit clear deflections. Likewise, a *slippery* pulse (*hua mai*) may correspond to smoothly rising upstrokes and faster cycles, while a *choppy* pulse (*se mai*) shows steeper, discontinuous upstrokes. Such empirical associations are being progressively validated and refined by data.

3.2 Pulse-Pattern Recognition and Classification

Given digitized waveforms, the key task is to automatically identify pulse types and their pathophysiological implications. Early studies followed a "features + classifier" paradigm: handcrafted parameters were extracted from each beat (including first- and second-derivative features), and pattern classifiers such as support vector machines (SVMs) were trained to distinguish common pulse types (e.g., deep, floating, wiry, thready), with reported accuracies of approximately 70–85%. With larger datasets and improved feature engineering, performance has continued to rise. Unsupervised clustering has also been used to relate objective pulse parameters to disease groupings, offering clues to correlations between TCM patterns and modern clinical indices.

More recently, deep learning has been applied to pulse recognition. One approach treats the waveform as a time series and uses recurrent neural networks (RNNs) or long short-term memory (LSTM) networks to model temporal dynamics and learn pulse patterns automatically. Another converts segments of the waveform into two-dimensional time–frequency representations (e.g., continuous wavelet spectra) and applies convolutional neural networks (CNNs), recasting the problem as image classification. Studies indicate that deep models capture subtle morphological variations, surpassing rule-based baselines in recognizing hallmark pulse types (e.g., *hua mai*, rapid/irregular *cu mai*). With large, expertly labeled datasets comprising tens of thousands of pulses, CNN-based classifiers have achieved average accuracies exceeding 90% across more than a dozen common pulse categories. In addition, deep models can be extended to multimodal inputs (e.g., combining pulse signals with symptom descriptors) for end-to-end prediction of likely TCM patterns. Specifically, models were trained on datasets containing over 10,000 pulse recordings collected from three hospitals, evaluated using Accuracy, F1-score, and AUC metrics.

3.3 Effectiveness and Applications of Objective Pulse Diagnosis

Preliminary clinical studies suggest that digital pulse diagnosis improves objectivity and inter-rater reliability. In one comparison between a digital device and experienced TCM physicians, diagnostic accuracy reached 90% with the device versus 78% with traditional palpation, indicating that sensors and algorithms can reduce human error and enhance consistency. Beyond hospital-based decision support, digital pulse systems are used in education to train students on standardized exemplars of pulse types. Consumer-grade, portable devices have also entered personal health management: users can collect pulse data at home via wrist-worn sensors and receive constitution and health-status assessments through mobile applications powered by AI.

These systems are often integrated with other TCM data streams—tongue and facial imaging and structured inquiry—to enable multi-parameter constitution profiling. For example, an AI-based "Four Examinations" station can acquire facial complexion, tongue features, and pulse signals within minutes and, leveraging cloud-scale data, deliver personalized constitution assessments and regimen recommendations. Reports typically cover TCM constitution types, functional states of the *zang–fu* organs, subhealth risks, and tailored advice on diet, lifestyle, acupuncture, and massage.

Challenges remain. Anatomical variability of the radial artery and hemodynamic states (e.g., blood pressure) can influence signals, motivating algorithms with subject-specific adaptation. Moreover, boundaries between pulse categories are inherently fuzzy, and label noise in current datasets can hinder supervised learning. As larger longitudinal datasets with multi-visit recordings accumulate, LLMs may better capture the evolution of pulse characteristics over time, thereby enhancing the verifiability and scientific rigor of TCM diagnosis.

4 Image-Based Recognition and Analysis for Facial Diagnosis

Observation of facial complexion and appearance is also a key component of visual inspection in TCM. According to classical doctrine—"what is internal is manifested externally"—changes in the Five Colors of the face (green/blue, red, yellow, white, black) and in facial luster are thought to correspond to the functional status of the *zang–fu* organs. Abnormal coloration at specific facial regions is further believed to map to particular organ systems (the "facial correspondence zones"). Because visual assessment is susceptible to lighting conditions and subjective bias, applying computer vision to analyze facial images can quantify complexion features and standardize facial diagnosis. Recent studies have begun to explore recognition of TCM-relevant facial and related features (e.g., tongue–face association, eyelid appearance), yielding promising preliminary results [32,33].

4.1 Facial-Image Acquisition and Preprocessing

Analogous to tongue diagnosis, digitizing facial diagnosis first requires standardized image capture. Typical protocols instruct subjects to remove makeup, adopt a natural stance, and be photographed under uniform illumination from a frontal view; some systems employ multi-light setups to reduce shadows. Captured images undergo face alignment and region-of-interest (ROI) segmentation: facial landmark detection localizes key features, and affine transformations normalize pose. ROIs are then delineated according to TCM facial theory—for example, the forehead, cheeks, and chin corresponding to the upper, middle, and lower *jiao*, respectively. Color analysis is commonly performed within each ROI to relate findings to organ-specific information. In addition, skin-tone calibration maps image colors to a reference chart to mitigate device- and lighting-induced color shifts.

4.2 Feature Extraction and Complexion Classification

TCM typically categorizes facial complexion into five principal hues (red, yellow, white, black, and green/blue), with ruddy redness often associated with yang heat or excess patterns, and dull–dark shades suggesting kidney deficiency or blood stasis. A fundamental task is therefore to classify the dominant facial hue. Methods that fuse deep learning with traditional descriptors have achieved automatic complexion classification. In one representative pipeline, a deep convolutional network detects facial landmarks and segments major facial regions; subsequently, color-space features (e.g., means and variances in HSV and CIELAB spaces), skin-texture descriptors (e.g., local binary patterns, LBP), and lip-color features are extracted and fed to a machine-learning classifier to determine complexion category. On an expert-annotated dataset of 575 standardized facial images, the fused-feature approach achieved 91.03% accuracy for four-class recognition (red, yellow, white, black), with skin color components emerging as dominant predictors. These findings indicate that computer vision can reliably distinguish complexion categories as defined in TCM.

Beyond global complexion, additional facial cues are amenable to quantitative analysis. Specular highlights can index facial glossiness, potentially reflecting the sufficiency of *qi* and blood; periocular chromaticity can be used to detect dark circles or eyelid dullness; and wrinkles or facial expressions may be considered in certain wellness contexts. Although the links between these features and TCM theory are not yet fully resolved, data-driven approaches can probe their associations. Notably, visual inspection in TCM often combines facial and tongue information; accordingly, several intelligent systems jointly analyze facial and tongue images to strengthen assessments of overall health status.

4.3 Applications and Outlook for Intelligent Facial Diagnosis

Current complexion-analysis techniques have been preliminarily applied to constitution identification and subhealth screening. For instance, models that integrate facial complexion with tongue coating and pulse features can classify biased types among the nine TCM constitutions with higher agreement than questionnaire-only methods. Some integrated health kiosks acquire facial photos alongside tongue images and pulse signals and generate multi-metric reports that include complexion analysis. Cross-validating evidence across modalities can substantially improve pattern identification: a thick, greasy tongue coating coupled with a yellowish complexion, for example, may increase confidence in a damp–heat pattern, whereas a pale, swollen tongue with a pallid complexion may suggest *qi* or yang deficiency.

Challenges remain. Skin-tone variability across ethnicities and camera models necessitates improved color standardization and cross-population adaptation. Transient facial expressions and emotional states can confound appearance and should be suppressed or corrected during analysis. While most current studies emphasize qualitative complexion categorization, future work may map specific facial subregions to particular diseases or TCM patterns to aid early screening.

Reports have begun to explore detection of conditions such as thyroid disorders or anemia from facial images. Coupled with large-scale datasets and the representational power of LLMs, such efforts may yield breakthroughs in the objectification of TCM visual diagnosis. Table 1 summarizes representative AI approaches and their reported accuracies for tongue, pulse, and facial diagnosis.

Table 1. Comparison of AI methods for tongue, pulse, and facial diagnosis

Modality	Typical models/Methods	Acc. (%)
Tongue	U-Net/U-Net++ seg.; ResNet-50+MLP; handcrafted+deep fusion	≈88–92
Pulse	Pressure-sensor arrays; CNN/LSTM waveform clf.; digital vs. manual	90/78
Facial	CNN + HSV/CIELAB + LBP (four-class complexion)	91.03

In summary, tongue, pulse, and facial diagnosis—three pillars of TCM inspection and palpation—are progressively moving toward objectivity and intelligence through multimodal data acquisition and AI-driven analysis.

5 Applications of Multimodal LLMs in TCM Diagnosis

With the maturation of single-modality analytics for tongue, pulse, and facial diagnosis, researchers have begun to fuse multiple modalities to emulate the clinical decision-making process of the Four Examinations in TCM. Applications of multimodal LLMs in this setting fall broadly into two categories: (i) multimodal TCM decision-support systems that ingest tongue/facial images, pulse signals, and inquiry text on a unified platform and produce diagnostic suggestions via algorithmic fusion; and (ii) TCM-oriented LLMs pretrained on extensive domain data and capable of accepting heterogeneous inputs (text and images) to generate professional diagnostic recommendations [19,42] (Fig. 1).

5.1 Multimodal Fusion Systems for the Four Examinations

Industry and academia have developed prototype systems and products that integrate diverse TCM diagnostic information, often termed "intelligent Four Examinations stations" or "digital TCM decision-support systems." Typical configurations include hardware such as tongue-image and facial-image capture devices and pulse-detection modules, coupled with cloud-based big-data and AI algorithms.

As a representative example, an AI-enabled Four Examinations station uses high-resolution cameras and controlled lighting to acquire tongue and facial images, from which computer-vision algorithms extract tongue-body/coating features, facial complexion, and sublingual venation. An integrated pulse module with high-precision pressure sensors emulates the technique of experienced physicians to record waveforms at *cun*, *guan*, and *chi*, deriving indices such as

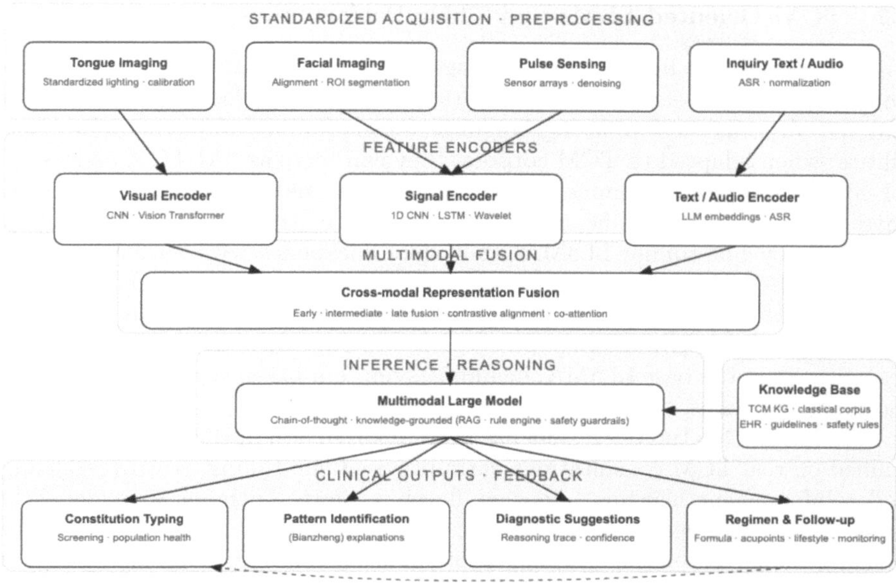

Fig. 1. Overall framework of multimodal large-model–driven intelligent TCM diagnosis.

rate, amplitude, and rhythm. A digital inquiry module collects subjective information on symptoms, sleep, and diet via questionnaires or voice interaction. These multimodal data streams are transmitted to a cloud analytics backend, where pretrained fusion models perform cross-validation and joint inference.

When tongue, facial, and pulse cues concordantly indicate, for instance, "spleen deficiency with predominant dampness," the model outputs the corresponding pattern with high confidence; when modalities conflict, the system balances evidence using inquiry-derived symptoms and knowledge-based rules. The final report typically includes constitution typing, primary pattern identification, probable TCM disease categories, and regimen recommendations. Reports suggest that cross-confirmation among modalities significantly improves pattern recognition compared with single-modality approaches. Standardized data acquisition further reduces subjective bias and enhances comparability across patients. Such digital TCM systems have been piloted in hospitals and community clinics for physician decision support and trainee education. In a municipal primary-care demonstration, the platform supported the entire workflow: rapid pre-visit data capture to improve throughput, in-visit suggestions grounded in an expert-knowledge library with auto-generated structured records, and post-visit longitudinal follow-up with efficacy assessment–collectively enabling an intelligent upgrade of the TCM care pathway. These deployments underscore the potential of multimodal fusion to enhance objectivity, efficiency, and patient experience.

5.2 TCM-Oriented LLMs and Their Performance

Another prominent line of work leverages LLMs for TCM dialogue and decision support. Foundation models such as GPT-3 and ChatGPT, trained on massive corpora, possess strong language understanding and generation capabilities; when adapted to TCM corpora, they can serve as "AI TCM assistants" for consultation and recommendation. Since 2023, multiple China-based teams have released TCM-specific models. For example, the *ShenNong-TCM-LLM* [34], built by fine-tuning LLaMA-family [35] backbones with an entity-centric self-instruction dataset exceeding 110,000 TCM prompts, integrates entities from a TCM knowledge graph with medical QA dialogues, markedly improving domain specificity. Evaluations indicate more TCM-consistent, human-centered responses than the base LLaMA, including symptom-based suggestions of classic formulae and herbs.

Similarly, "HuaTuo GPT" [36] has been reported as a medical-dialogue model trained on real TCM consultations via supervised fine-tuning, reward modeling, and reinforcement learning. Another flagship effort, *Qihuang Wendao: TCM Large Model* [37]–described as a vertical, domain-specific TCM model–reports a rich training corpus comprising approximately 11 million knowledge-graph entries, 1,500 classical texts, 100,000 expert case records, around 100,000 objective tongue/pulse samples, and millions of clinical records. A four-stage training pipeline (pretraining, supervised fine-tuning, reward modeling, and reinforcement learning) aims to couple mastery of TCM theory with multi-pronged therapeutic planning. Demonstrations show that, given symptoms such as "fear of cold," the model can generate integrated regimens spanning herbal prescriptions, meridian/acupoint modulation, and diet/tea therapy. Even with symptom-only inputs lacking explicit diagnoses, the system can propose plausible pattern identifications and treatment suggestions, reflecting elements of *bianzheng lunzhi*. A dialogue interface lowers the barrier to use, allowing patients to interact in a conversational manner.

On the evaluation front, some TCM models have reported strong performance on professional benchmarks, such as MedBench [38]. A mixture-of-experts (MoE) architecture is used to handle the breadth of TCM knowledge; chain-of-thought (CoT) prompting emulates diagnostic reasoning; and retrieval-augmented generation (RAG) [39] keeps the knowledge base current [33]. Crucially, the model supports multimodal understanding and reasoning, jointly leveraging text, images (e.g., tongue/facial), and pulse signals for comprehensive pattern identification. It can further provide stepwise rationales to improve transparency and clinician trust. By deeply integrating classical TCM theory with modern medical knowledge, the system has reportedly gained recognition from frontline TCM practitioners as a bellwether of "smart TCM."

Notwithstanding this promise, several challenges remain. *Safety and accuracy* are paramount: models may produce suggestions that conflict with TCM theory or entail clinical risk (e.g., dosing errors), necessitating rigorous expert review and iterative feedback. *Explainability* is crucial for clinical adoption; practitioners expect models to justify diagnoses and recommendations, motivating interpretable AI (e.g., citation of knowledge sources or analogous cases). *Data and compute barriers* persist, as curating high-quality, multimodal TCM datasets is difficult and training LLMs is resource-intensive–even vertical domain models require sustained investment. Finally, *regulatory compliance* regarding privacy and safety is essential for clinical deployment.

Overall, multimodal LLMs show substantial potential to advance TCM decision support. Whether as integrated hardware–software stations or AI-enabled consultations, such systems can improve efficiency and standardization in TCM practice. In the next section, we discuss the role of LLMs in multi-visit longitudinal follow-up and how these technologies can strengthen the evidentiary basis of TCM clinical research.

6 Applications and Challenges of LLMs in Multi-visit Follow-Up

Clinical practice in TCM emphasizes *bianzheng lunzhi* (pattern identification and treatment) and dynamic evaluation of therapeutic efficacy, which often requires multiple return visits and longitudinal follow-up to adjust regimens. This repeated process of inquiry and observation is central to TCM. In traditional workflows, however, information from different visits is documented by different clinicians and rarely integrated systematically, hindering quantitative analysis of disease trajectories. Large-model techniques provide a new pathway: by cumulatively learning from and globally analyzing data across visits, models can help physicians track pattern evolution and evaluate efficacy, thereby enhancing the scientific basis of clinical decision-making.

6.1 Longitudinal Record Memory and Integrated Analysis

A notable strength of LLMs is their ability to process long contexts and extract useful knowledge. In multi-visit scenarios, each encounter produces new Four Examinations data and an updated treatment plan. Feeding these data to a large model sequentially endows the AI with a longitudinal "memory" of the patient record [41]. The model can link information across encounters—for example, whether symptoms have improved or worsened, how tongue and pulse features have changed, and what feedback followed the previous prescription. Based on such evidence, the system may, for instance, suggest: "The cough markedly improved after the last treatment, but the yellow, greasy coating persists; this visit should continue to strengthen the spleen and resolve dampness." Multimodal TCM models have highlighted capabilities for automatic, continuous comparison of tongue–pulse data to reveal trends. Meanwhile, the model can retain the entirety of physician–patient interactions during follow-up, including each chief complaint and the clinician's reasoning. Curated longitudinal corpora of this kind can further serve training, expanding clinical TCM data by orders of magnitude and, in turn, improving model performance. Thus, in multi-visit settings, LLMs function not only as decision-support tools but also as continually learning systems.

6.2 Efficacy Evaluation and Decision Support

Efficacy assessment is pivotal during follow-up. Traditionally, TCM outcome evaluation has relied on clinician judgment and patient self-report, with limited quantification. LLMs enable more standardized appraisal: by integrating objective changes (e.g., temperature, symptom scores) with subjective reports, a model can categorize responses as “markedly effective,” “effective,” or “ineffective” for clinician review. Intelligent follow-up systems also define endpoints (e.g., laboratory or imaging changes) that can be logged in digital TCM platforms. Aggregating these data, LLMs can assist in judging regimen effectiveness; if multiple visits show no improvement, the system may prompt reconsideration of the pattern identification or prescription. Conversely, recommendations can be dynamically updated as new information arrives. For example, if a patient initially assessed as kidney yang deficiency received warming therapy but returns with altered symptoms, the model may suggest adding *qi*-regulating herbs or screening for complications. In this way, the AI extends clinical reasoning, improving the accuracy and timeliness of decisions during follow-up.

6.3 Enhancing Scientific Rigor and Verifiability in TCM

Applying LLMs to longitudinal follow-up benefits not only individual cases but also enables clinical big-data research in TCM. Historically, experience regarding therapeutic efficacy and pattern transitions has been textual and difficult to quantify. With standardized, multimodal data capture, models can extract common regularities—for example, typical trajectories of pattern evolution for a given disease—to test the prognostic statements of classical texts; they can also compare prescription-adjustment strategies across schools to provide quantitative evidence for TCM lineage and inheritance. This makes experiential knowledge more “verifiable.” In practice, digital follow-up data have been used to study objective changes in tongue and pulse after TCM treatment (e.g., in coronary heart disease) and their correlations with biomedical indices, often supporting the plausibility of TCM pattern differentiation and offering scientific interpretations. LLMs act as a bridge between massive clinical datasets and traditional theory: through deep learning on longitudinal data, they can uncover latent patterns and test hypotheses, accelerating research in TCM.

6.4 Challenges and Countermeasures

Despite these advantages, several challenges require attention when deploying LLMs for multi-visit follow-up. *Data quality and privacy* are foundational: longitudinal data are dispersed across institutions and clinicians, so interoperability and patient-privacy safeguards are prerequisites for data linkage. *Temporal modeling* must be strengthened: unlike pure text, follow-up records include time intervals, external interventions, and other complex factors that demand suitable representations beyond standard language modeling. *Trust and adoption* also matter: clinicians need interpretable outputs, especially when model suggestions diverge from experience. A pragmatic approach is human–AI collaboration: the model provides longitudinal summaries, candidate regimen adjustments, and supporting rationales; clinicians make final decisions and feed outcomes back for learning. Such a closed loop can progressively align model behavior with clinical realities.

In summary, deploying LLMs in multi-visit follow-up promises end-to-end patient management and cumulative knowledge building from first visit to recovery, with substantial implications for improving clinical efficacy and advancing TCM research. With continued pilots and technical refinements, this direction is expected to mature.

7 Future Research Directions and Outlook

Although multimodal large-model–driven TCM decision support has achieved impressive progress, the field remains nascent, with many avenues warranting deeper investigation. Building on the foregoing review and open challenges, we outline priority directions below.

7.1 Cross-Modal Alignment and Fusion

While current multimodal models can fuse tongue, pulse, facial, and textual information, precise alignment across modalities remains a bottleneck. For example, how can features of a pulse waveform at a specific moment be linked to synchronous changes in tongue appearance? How can a model reliably map "an image of a red tongue" to the textual description "red tongue with scant coating"? Future work should develop advanced alignment strategies by collecting paired multimodal data (e.g., synchronized tongue photos and pulse recordings at the same visit, clinician narratives aligned with images) to learn mappings between visual features and TCM terminology. Methods inspired by visual question answering can be adapted to the TCM context. Another direction is adversarial or contrastive learning to determine whether heterogeneous inputs originate from the same patient and visit, thereby learning consistent cross-modal representations. Solving alignment will make fusion more accurate and efficient, enabling truly integrated, intelligent diagnosis across the Four Examinations.

7.2 Knowledge Enhancement and Explainability

TCM diagnosis is grounded in rich theoretical knowledge (meridian theory, *zang–fu* correlations, formula–pattern correspondences), which data-only models may not fully internalize. Incorporating TCM knowledge graphs and classical literature into LLMs is thus essential. Retrieval-augmented generation (RAG) can automatically surface relevant passages from classical texts and modern references to substantiate answers, improving both accuracy and explainability. In parallel, knowledge injection—encoding rules such as the Eight-Principle logic or incompatibility constraints in prescriptions as decoding constraints or post-processing—can prevent outputs that violate domain common sense. Building large TCM knowledge bases (e.g., repositories of classical formulae and pattern features) will further support traceable reasoning: when a model proposes a diagnosis, it can cite pertinent classics or expert case records, making recommendations more acceptable to clinicians. Knowledge-enhanced models will also benefit TCM education by supplying theoretically grounded explanations in tutoring scenarios.

7.3 Individualized Prediction and Precision TCM

TCM emphasizes personalization ("treating the same disease differently and different diseases similarly"). Future LLMs should strengthen individualized prediction, delivering differentiated plans for different patients. This requires accounting for patient-specific attributes (age, sex, constitution, living environment) when reasoning about diagnosis and therapy, potentially by integrating structured electronic health records (EHRs) or by prompting with background context. Reinforcement learning or meta-learning can enable continual adaptation to a single patient: the model updates its internal representation of constitution and disease trajectory based on prior responses, yielding progressively more tailored suggestions during follow-up. This mirrors the "mental model" a physician forms over longitudinal care and aspires to **"one person, one prescription"** at scale.

7.4 Large-Scale Multimodal Pretraining

Most current TCM AI systems process modalities separately and fuse only at the decision layer; genuinely unified multimodal pretraining remains rare. Future research should develop foundational TCM models pretrained on large-scale triplets of tongue images, pulse signals, and text, endowing a single backbone with both visual and linguistic representations. Once trained, such a model—analogous to GPT-4 [40] in capability to accept mixed text–image prompts—could directly output diagnostic recommendations, simplifying fusion pipelines and uncovering deeper cross-modal relationships. Achieving this goal requires large, expertly annotated datasets (e.g., pattern-labeled tongue/facial photos and pulse recordings at scale). Existing industrial corpora with tens of thousands of objective tongue–pulse samples suggest feasibility. Unified multimodal pretraining is expected to surpass naive ensembles by learning modality correspondences via self-supervision, improving data efficiency and transfer to downstream tasks such as disease-specific diagnosis and efficacy prediction.

7.5 Data Sharing and Evaluation Frameworks

Beyond algorithms, realizing this vision calls for sector-wide collaboration to establish open TCM multimodal data platforms and objective evaluation protocols. Today, datasets are siloed with heterogeneous standards, impeding progress.

National-level initiatives for de-identified data sharing and standards for formats and annotations (tongue, pulse, and case records) would greatly expand training resources and reduce duplication. On evaluation, benchmarks inspired by medical LLM suites (e.g., MedBench) should be tailored to TCM, covering competencies such as pattern-classification accuracy, prescription rationality, and longitudinal follow-up analytics, thereby motivating healthy competition and continuous improvement.

In sum, multimodal LLMs are propelling TCM toward a **"data-driven + knowledge-driven"** convergent paradigm. Future research—from cross-modal learning and knowledge-graph integration to personalization and unified pretraining—will further erode subjective barriers and render TCM diagnosis more scientific, standardized, and verifiable. We anticipate that, in the near future, a TCM AI system will perform the Four Examinations with seasoned proficiency and robust analogical reasoning, assisting clinicians and enabling the public to access more precise, intelligent TCM services. The ancient treasury of Chinese medicine is poised to radiate renewed vitality through the infusion of multimodal LLMs.

8 Conclusion

Multimodal large-model technologies offer unprecedented opportunities to render TCM-assisted diagnosis objective and intelligent. By applying computer vision, sensor-signal processing, and large-scale data analytics, key features of traditional tongue, pulse, and facial diagnosis can be digitized and quantitatively analyzed, substantially improving diagnostic consistency and accuracy. Furthermore, introducing deep learning and LLMs that fuse multi-source information enables integrated interpretation of the Four Examinations, demonstrating strong capabilities in assisting pattern identification and in the automated generation of therapeutic plans. In multi-visit follow-up and efficacy assessment, LLMs can retain long-term clinical context and analyze disease evolution, steering TCM practice toward greater scientific rigor.

Challenges remain, including incomplete cross-modal alignment, insufficient integration of medical knowledge, and the need to enhance the explainability and safety of model decisions. Looking ahead, the advent of larger-scale multimodal pretraining, deeper incorporation of TCM knowledge, and the establishment of data-sharing mechanisms and robust evaluation frameworks will further amplify the role of multimodal LLMs in TCM, advancing precision, standardization, and modernization of clinical practice. We anticipate that the fusion of TCM and AI will open new avenues for the inheritance and innovation of traditional medicine, revitalizing this ancient discipline and delivering more intelligent and efficient healthcare services.

References

1. Matos, L.C., Machado, J.P., Monteiro, F.J., Greten, H.J.: Can traditional Chinese medicine diagnosis be parameterized and standardized? a narrative review. In: Healthcare, vol. 9, no. 2, p. 177. MDPI (2021)
2. Sang, X., Wang, Z., Liu, S., Wang, R.: Relationship between traditional Chinese medicine (TCM) constitution and TCM syndrome in the diagnosis and treatment of chronic diseases. Chin. Med. Sci. J. **33**(2), 114–119 (1 June 2018)
3. Tian, D., Chen, W., Xu, D., Xu, L., Xu, G., Guo, Y., Yao, Y.: A review of traditional Chinese medicine diagnosis using machine learning: inspection, auscultation - olfaction, inquiry, and palpation. Comput. Biol. Med. **170**, 108074 (1 Mar 2024)
4. Zhao, C., Li, G.Z., Li, F., Wang, Z., Liu, C.: Qualitative and quantitative analysis for facial complexion in traditional Chinese medicine. Biomed. Res. Int. **2014**(1), 207589 (2014)
5. Xie, J., Jing, C., Zhang, Z., Xu, J., Duan, Y., Xu, D.: Digital tongue image analyses for health assessment. Med. Rev. **1**(2), 172–198 (20 Dec 2021)
6. Baltrušaitis, T., Ahuja, C., Morency, L.P.: Multimodal machine learning: a survey and taxonomy. IEEE Trans. Pattern Anal. Mach. Intell. **41**(2), 423–443 (25 Jan 2018)
7. AlSaad, R., Abd-Alrazaq, A., Boughorbel, S., Ahmed, A., Renault, M.A., Damseh, R., Sheikh, J.: Multimodal large language models in health care: applications, challenges, and future outlook. J. Med. Internet Res. **26**, e59505 (25 Sept 2024)
8. Tiryaki, B., Torenek-Agirman, K., Miloglu, O., Korkmaz, B., Ozbek, İ.Y., Oral, E.A.: Artificial intelligence in tongue diagnosis: classification of tongue lesions and normal tongue images using deep convolutional neural network. BMC Med. Imaging **24**(1), 59 (8 Mar 2024)
9. Thirunavukarasu, A.J., Ting, D.S., Elangovan, K., Gutierrez, L., Tan, T.F., Ting, D.S.: Large language models in medicine. Nat. Med. **29**(8), 1930–1940 (2023)
10. Kung, T.H., Cheatham, M., Medenilla, A., Sillos, C., De Leon, L., Elepaño, C., Madriaga, M., Aggabao, R., Diaz-Candido, G., Maningo, J., Tseng, V.: Performance of ChatGPT on USMLE: potential for AI-assisted medical education using large language models. PLoS Digit. Health **2**(2), e0000198 (9 Feb 2023). https://doi.org/10.1371/journal.pdig.0000198
11. Rao, A., Pang, M., Kim, J., Kamineni, M., Lie, W., Prasad, A.K., Landman, A., Dreyer, K., Succi, M.D.: Assessing the utility of ChatGPT throughout the entire clinical workflow: development and usability study. J. Med. Internet Res. **25**, e48659 (22 Aug 2023). https://doi.org/10.2196/48659
12. Ren, Y., Luo, X., Wang, Y., Li, H., Zhang, H., Li, Z., Lai, H., Li, X., Ge, L., Estill, J., Zhang, L.: Large language models in traditional Chinese medicine: a scoping review. J. Evid. Based Med. **18**(1), e12658 (2025). https://doi.org/10.1111/jebm.12658. Mar
13. Zhou, X., Dong, X., Li, C., Bai, Y., Xu, Y., Cheung, K.C., Se, S., Song, X., Zhang, R., Zho, X., Zhang, N.L.: TCM-FTP: fine-tuning large language models for herbal prescription prediction. In: 2024 IEEE International Conference on Bioinformatics and Biomedicine (BIBM), pp. 4092-4097. IEEE (3 Dec 2024)
14. Zeng, A., Liu, X., Du, Z., Wang, Z., Lai, H., Ding, M., Yang, Z., Xu, Y., Zheng, W., Xia, X., Tam, W.L.: Glm-130b: an open bilingual pre-trained model (2022). arXiv:2210.02414
15. Yip, H.F., Li, Z., Zhang, L., Lyu, A.: Large language models in integrative medicine: progress, challenges, and opportunities. J. Evid. Based Med. **18**(2), e70031 (2025). https://doi.org/10.1111/jebm.70031. Jun

16. Zhang, H., Wang, X., Meng, Z., Chen, Z., Zhuang, P., Jia, Y., Xu, D., Guo, W.: Qibo: a large language model for traditional Chinese medicine (2024). arXiv:2403.16056
17. Matos, L.C., Machado, J.P., Monteiro, F.J., Greten, H.J.: Can traditional Chinese medicine diagnosis be parameterized and standardized? a narrative review. In: Healthcare, vol. 9, no. 2, p. 177. MDPI (7 Feb 2021). https://doi.org/10.3390/healthcare9020177
18. Wei, J., Wang, X., Schuurmans, D., Bosma, M., Xia, F., Chi, E., Le, Q.V., Zhou, D.: Chain-of-thought prompting elicits reasoning in large language models. In: Advances in Neural Information Processing Systems, vol. 35, pp. 24824–24837 (6 Dec 2022)
19. Liu, Y., Yuan, Y., Yan, K., Li, Y., Sacca, V., Hodges, S., Cannistra, M., Jeong, P., Wu, J., Kong, J.: Evaluating the role of large language models in traditional Chinese medicine diagnosis and treatment recommendations. NPJ Digit. Med. **8**(1), 466 (21 July 2025). https://doi.org/10.1038/s41746-025-00920-7
20. Yang, Z., Zhao, Y., Yu, J., Mao, X., Xu, H., Huang, L.: An intelligent tongue diagnosis system via deep learning on the android platform. Diagnostics **12**(10), 2451 (2022). https://doi.org/10.3390/diagnostics12102451
21. Velik, R.: An objective review of the technological developments for radial pulse diagnosis in traditional Chinese medicine. Eur. J. Integr. Med. **7**(4), 321–331 (2015). https://doi.org/10.1016/j.eujim.2015.04.005. Aug
22. Feng, L., Huang, Z.H., Zhong, Y.M., Xiao, W., Wen, C.B., Song, H.B., Guo, J.H.: Research and application of tongue and face diagnosis based on deep learning. Digital Health **8**, 20552076221124436 (2022). https://doi.org/10.1177/20552076221124436. Sep
23. Yang, Z., Mitra, A., Liu, W., Berlowitz, D., Yu, H.: TransformEHR: transformer-based encoder-decoder generative model to enhance prediction of disease outcomes using electronic health records. Nat. Commun. **14**(1), 7857 (29 Nov 2023). https://doi.org/10.1038/s41467-023-43376-8
24. Zhang, D., Zhang, H., Zhang, B.: Tongue image analysis for appendicitis diagnosis. In: Tongue Image Analysis, pp. 281–293. Springer Singapore (2017). https://doi.org/10.1007/978-981-10-2167-1_15
25. Wei, L.I., Jinming, C.H., Bo, L.I., Wei, H.U., Xingjin, W.U., Hui, Z.H.: Tongue image segmentation and tongue color classification based on deep learning. Digit. Chin. Med. **5**(3), 253–263 (1 Sept 2022). https://doi.org/10.1016/j.dcmed.2022.08.002
26. Jiatuo, X.U., Tao, J.I., Shi, L.I.: Research status and prospect of tongue image diagnosis analysis based on machine learning. Digit. Chin. Med. **7**(1), 3–12 (1 Mar 2024). https://doi.org/10.1016/j.dcmed.2023.12.002
27. Huang, Z., Miao, J., Song, H., Yang, S., Zhong, Y., Xu, Q., Tan, Y., Wen, C., Guo, J.: A novel tongue segmentation method based on improved U-Net. Neurocomputing **500**, 73–89 (21 Aug 2022). https://doi.org/10.1016/j.neucom.2022.05.056
28. Wang, X., Cao, Y., Chen, Y., Li, H., Han, A., Tang, Y.: An improved lightweight tongue segmentation model with self-attention parallel network and progressive upsampling. Sci. Rep. **15**(1), 27622 (29 July 2025). https://doi.org/10.1038/s41598-025-79865-x
29. Liu, Y., Fan, L., Zhao, M., Wei, D., Zhao, M., Dong, Y., Zhang, X.: Study on a Traditional Chinese Medicine constitution recognition model using tongue image characteristics and deep learning: a prospective dual-center investigation. Chin. Med. **20**(1), 84 (12 June 2025). https://doi.org/10.1186/s13020-025-01062-2

30. Chen, T., Chen, Y., Zhou, Z., Zhu, Y., He, L., Zhang, J.: Deep learning-based automated tongue analysis system for assisted Chinese medicine diagnosis. Front. Physiol. **16**, 1559389 (28 Apr 2025). https://doi.org/10.3389/fphys.2025.1559389
31. Segawa, M., Iizuka, N., Ogihara, H., Tanaka, K., Nakae, H., Usuku, K., Yamaguchi, K., Wada, K., Uchizono, A., Nakamura, Y., Nishida, Y.: Objective evaluation of tongue diagnosis ability using a tongue diagnosis e-learning/e-assessment system based on a standardized tongue image database. Front. Med. Technol. **5**, 1050909 (13 Mar 2023). https://doi.org/10.3389/fmedt.2023.1050909
32. Liu, Y., Fan, L., Zhao, M., Wei, D., Zhao, M., Dong, Y., Zhang, X.: Study on a Traditional Chinese Medicine constitution recognition model using tongue image characteristics and deep learning: a prospective dual-center investigation. Chin. Med. **20**(1), 84 (12 June 2025). https://doi.org/10.1186/s13020-025-01062-2
33. Chen, Z., Wang, H., Li, C., Liu, C., Yang, F., Zhang, D., Fauci, A.J., Zhang, J.: Large language models in traditional Chinese medicine: a systematic review. Acupunct. Herb. Med. **5**(1), 57–67 (1 Mar 2025). https://doi.org/10.1016/j.ahm.2025.01.005
34. Li, J., Luo, L., Lv, T., Liu, C., Qi, J., Yang, Z., Wang, J., Lin, H.: Instruction fine-tuning of large language models for traditional Chinese medicine. In: China Conference on Knowledge Graph and Semantic Computing, pp. 419–430. Singapore: Springer Nature Singapore (20 Sept 2024). https://doi.org/10.1007/978-981-97-8648-7_32
35. Touvron, H., Lavril, T., Izacard, G., Martinet, X., Lachaux, M.A., Lacroix, T., Rozière, B., Goyal, N., Hambro, E., Azhar, F., Rodriguez, A.: Llama: Open and efficient foundation language models (27 Feb 2023). arXiv:2302.13971
36. Wang, H., Liu, C., Xi, N., Qiang, Z., Zhao, S., Qin, B., Liu, T.: Huatuo: Tuning llama model with Chinese medical knowledge (14 Apr 2023). arXiv:2304.06975
37. Linda, Y.L., Qinghua, P.E., Darrel, D.D.: Unveiling the digital renaissance of traditional Chinese medicine: a leap towards holistic healthcare and precision medicine. Digit. Chin. Med. **8**(1), 1–3 (25 Mar 2025). https://doi.org/10.1016/j.dcmed.2025.02.001
38. Liu, M., Hu, W., Ding, J., Xu, J., Li, X., Zhu, L., Bai, Z., Shi, X., Wang, B., Song, H., Liu, P.: Medbench: a comprehensive, standardized, and reliable benchmarking system for evaluating Chinese medical large language models. Big Data Min. Anal. **7**(4), 1116–1128 (4 Dec 2024). https://doi.org/10.26599/BDMA.2024.9020014
39. Lewis, P., Perez, E., Piktus, A., Petroni, F., Karpukhin, V., Goyal, N., Küttler, H., Lewis, M., Yih, W.T., Rocktäschel, T., Riedel, S.: Retrieval-augmented generation for knowledge-intensive NLP tasks. Adv. Neural. Inf. Process. Syst. **33**, 9459–9474 (2020)
40. Achiam, J., Adler, S., Agarwal, S., Ahmad, L., Akkaya, I., Aleman, F.L., Almeida, D., Altenschmidt, J., Altman, S., Anadkat, S., Avila, R.: Gpt-4 technical report (15 Mar 2023). arXiv:2303.08774
41. Chae, S., Street, W.N., Ramaraju, N., Gilbertson-White, S.: Prediction of cancer symptom trajectory using longitudinal electronic health record data and long short-term memory neural network. JCO Clin. Cancer Inform. **8**, e2300039 (2024). https://doi.org/10.1200/CCI.23.00039. Mar
42. Bai, S., Chen, K., Liu, X., Wang, J., Ge, W., Song, S., Dang, K., Wang, P., Wang, S., Tang, J., Zhong, H.: Qwen2.5-vl technical report (19 Feb 2025). arXiv:2502.13923

Drug Prediction and Knowledge Map

KD4FIRE: A Knowledge Distillation Approach for Fine-Grained Medical Relation Extraction in Low-Resource Settings

Wenjing Li, Shijie Li(✉), Jintao Tang(✉), Shasha Li, and Ting Wang

College of Computer Science and Technology, National University of Defense Technology, Changsha 410073, China
{liwenjing,tangjintao}@nudt.edu.cn, lishijienudt@163.com
{liwenjing,tangjintao}@nudt.edu.cn

Abstract. Medical relation extraction (MRE) is a critical foundation for intelligent healthcare tasks such as clinical text analysis and drug repositioning. Although large language models (LLMs) with massive parameter counts have achieved significant progress in general relation extraction, they still face challenges in the medical domain due to the specialized and fine-grained nature of medical relation types, as well as the scarcity of high-quality annotated data. In contrast, smaller models, while offering the advantage of fine-tunability, are limited by their foundational capabilities, failing to capture certain relatively complex semantic patterns in medical relation extraction. Inspired by human cognitive learning, in which individuals reinforce strengths through self-practice and overcome weaknesses with external guidance and repeated practice, this paper proposes a knowledge distillation (KD) framework named KD4FIRE, which integrates the complementary strengths of larger teacher models and smaller student models. Specifically, KD4FIRE first divides samples into easy and hard categories based on the smaller student model's performance on an initial seed set. For easy samples, chain-of-thought (CoT) self-reinforcement is applied to consolidate the student model's existing knowledge. For hard samples, we propose an error-aware chain-of-thought refinement method and an abstraction-based data augmentation approach to explicitly address the student model's knowledge gaps. Experimental results demonstrate that KD4FIRE significantly improves model performance in low-resource scenarios, providing a practical and efficient solution for fine-grained medical relation extraction.

Keywords: Medical relation extraction · Knowledge distillation · Integration of large and small models

Y. Zhang et al. (Eds.): CHIP 2025, CCIS 2884, pp. 253–269, 2026.
https://doi.org/10.1007/978-981-95-7299-1_16

1 Introduction

Medical texts contain a wealth of knowledge about diseases, treatments, and clinical practices, serving as a critical resource for scientific research and healthcare applications. Extracting information from medical texts and transforming it into structured forms holds significant practical value for various health-related applications. Among these efforts, medical relation extraction is a key step in the process of medical information extraction, aiming to identify semantic relations between entities in unstructured medical texts.

Medical relation extraction is widely recognized as a challenging task. First, medical relations are highly specialized and fine-grained, characterized by subtle differences between different relation types, ambiguous semantic boundaries, and the involvement of complex medical concepts. These characteristics make it difficult for models to accurately distinguish between them. Second, the medical domain generally faces issues such as high annotation costs and strict privacy constraints, which result in a scarcity of high-quality annotated resources, further increasing the difficulty of the task.

In recent years, large language models with massive parameters have achieved remarkable success in open-domain natural language processing tasks, owing to their powerful semantic modeling and reasoning capabilities [1–3]. However, relying solely on instructions and in-context prompts, general-purpose large language models often struggle to adequately handle specialized terminology in the medical domain. Meanwhile, their ability to distinguish fine-grained relations also has limitations [4]: The input examples in the prompts may fail to cover the diverse contexts of all relation types; therefore, when encountering highly similar relations with blurred semantic boundaries, these models frequently produce classification errors. On the other hand, the scarcity of high-quality annotated data in the medical domain, along with computational constraints, poses significant challenges to the effective fine-tuning of larger language models. In contrast, smaller language models benefit from their lightweight architectures, demonstrating strong task adaptability and the ability to quickly learn salient semantic patterns from limited annotated data through fine-tuning. However, these smaller models exhibit limited representational capacity and generalization ability, making it difficult to adapt to data involving complex semantic structures. That is, smaller language models have certain capability boundaries under limited annotated data. These observations indicate that larger and smaller language models exhibit inherent complementarity in fine-grained medical relation extraction: large models possess powerful semantic modeling and reasoning capabilities but weaker task adaptability and low-resource fine-tuning feasibility; small models, although limited in capability, are efficient learners in low-resource scenarios and offer flexible deployment.

Knowledge Distillation provides a natural pathway to combine the strengths of larger and smaller models, by transferring knowledge from a larger teacher model to a smaller student model [17], thereby enhancing the smaller student model's performance on target tasks. In recent years, most research has focused on extracting specific knowledge or capabilities from advanced large language models using heuristic and carefully designed prompts. Among these, some studies, such as LLM2LLM [22], attempt to enhance the student model by synthesizing data from the teacher model on instances where the student model makes incorrect predictions. However, these methods do not explicitly model the chain of thought. They typically involve the teacher model directly generating new data for hard samples that the student model fails to handle, leading to passive imitation by the student. This approach fails to adequately expose the student model's knowledge weaknesses, and the teacher model struggles to provide more targeted corrections. Moreover, the student model lacks opportunities to independently practice and consolidate on simpler samples, preventing it from fully leveraging its own advantages.

Based on this, this paper proposes KD4FIRE, a knowledge distillation framework designed for fine-grained medical relation extraction in low-resource settings. The framework draws inspiration from human cognitive learning mechanisms, where individuals reinforce their proficiencies through self-practice, and address weaknesses through external guidance and repeated practice. Specifically, we first partition samples into easy and hard categories based on the student model's performance on an initial seed set. For easy samples, we employ chain-of-thought self-reinforcement to help the student model further consolidate its existing knowledge and capabilities. For hard samples, a larger teacher model is introduced to correct the erroneous chains of thought generated by the student and to synthesize diverse new samples. This allows the student model to learn from the teacher's guidance and repeated practice to remediate its weaknesses. The experimental results show that the proposed distillation framework significantly improves the performance of small models in low-resource scenarios, confirming the effectiveness of the approach.

The main contributions of this paper are summarized as follows:

•We propose KD4FIRE, a knowledge distillation framework designed for low-resource fine-grained medical relation extraction. By categorizing sample difficulty based on the student model's performance, KD4FIRE implements a collaborative learning mechanism of "self-practice + teacher guidance" to enhance the capability of small models in fine-grained medical relation extraction tasks.

•We design an error-aware chain-of-thought refinement method and an abstraction-based data augmentation strategy. On hard samples, the teacher model corrects flawed reasoning chains and synthesizes diverse data, thereby explicitly exposing and addressing the student model's knowledge gaps.

•A series of experiments on a fine-grained medical relation extraction dataset demonstrate the effectiveness of KD4FIRE in low-resource fine-grained medical relation extraction scenarios.

2 Related Work

2.1 Biomedical Relation Extraction

Natural language processing techniques have been widely applied in the biomedical domain, driving significant progress in both research and practical applications [5,6]. Among these, biomedical relation extraction focuses on identifying semantic relationships between entities in biomedical texts. As a foundational technology, it plays a crucial role in supporting downstream tasks such as medical knowledge graph construction, clinical decision support, and drug repositioning.With the continuous advancement of NLP, methods for biomedical relation extraction have evolved through several stages, ranging from rule-based approaches and statistical learning methods to deep learning techniques and large-scale pretrained language models.

Early approaches relied primarily on expert-crafted rules or patterns to extract relations from sentences [7,8]. While these methods achieved high precision in specific domains, they suffered from poor generalizability and were not well suited for the diverse expressions found in open-domain texts. Subsequently, statistical machine learning methods became mainstream. These approaches depended heavily on manually designed features [9] and kernel functions [10] to perform biomedical relation classification. Although they improved automation to some extent, their performance remained highly dependent on feature engineering and corpus quality, and they struggled to model deeper semantic relationships.The emergence of deep learning brought new opportunities for medical relation extraction. Deep learning-based methods [11,12], which are typically trained in an end-to-end manner, can automatically learn features from large-scale data, thus eliminating the reliance on handcrafted features. In particular, pretrained language models such as BioBERT [12] have significantly enhanced biomedical semantic understanding through deep bidirectional encoding and large-scale pretraining on biomedical literature.

In recent years, the rapid development of large language models (LLMs) has demonstrated remarkable capabilities in tasks such as medical question answering and reasoning [6,13], offering new technological pathways for biomedical relation extraction. Existing research has primarily enhanced the performance of large language models in biomedical relation extraction tasks through approaches such as prompt engineering and fine-tuning. First, prompt-based techniques have been explored to guide models in recognizing biomedical relations. For example, Chang et al. [14] designed six progressive prompt templates to evaluate the performance of general-purpose LLMs in the task of proteinprotein interaction extraction. Labrak et al. [15] investigated the use of instruction-tuned LLMs in clinical and biomedical tasks, particularly focusing on zero-shot and few-shot learning scenarios. Second, task-specific fine-tuning has been employed to enhance model adaptability. For example, Y-Mol [16] was trained on a large-scale biomedical corpus and instruction set, effectively integrating biomedical knowledge and improving performance across various stages of drug development.

Despite progress achieved through prompt engineering and instruction tuning, these approaches still face significant challenges. Prompt-based methods often rely heavily on the model scale, and most large-scale LLMs are accessible only via external APIs, raising concerns regarding data privacy. Furthermore, annotated biomedical data are often scarce, and under such low-resource conditions, larger language models often fail to undergo effective fine-tuning;

meanwhile, trainable models with smaller parameter sizes are limited by their capabilities and thus struggle to effectively tackle complex tasks.

2.2 Knowledge Distillation from Large Language Models

Knowledge distillation aims to transfer knowledge from a large and complex teacher model to a smaller, more efficient student model. In recent years, research in this area has focused on extracting specific knowledge or capabilities from advanced LLMs using heuristic and carefully designed prompts, and transferring this knowledge to smaller models [17]. For example, Chen and Feng [18] proposed a conditional prompt distillation method that significantly improves the reasoning ability and overall performance of student models by distilling the reasoning capabilities of LLMs. This approach also has advantages in terms of data efficiency, interpretability, and cross-domain generalizability. Tian et al. [19] introduced TinyLLM, a novel knowledge distillation paradigm in which student models learn from multiple teacher models, thereby acquiring diverse reasoning skills across different LLMs. Despite the reduced model size, TinyLLM outperforms individual large teacher models on multiple tasks. Zhang et al. [20] proposed a new distillation framework that trains student models by jointly distilling teacher-generated outputs and self-supervised reward signals, highlighting the potential of scalable and efficient distillation through structured self-supervised reward learning. However, most of these approaches focus on unidirectional, static knowledge transfer from teacher to student, often overlooking the intrinsic learning capabilities of the student model itself.

To address this, some studies have explored methods that provide more targeted feedback based on the student's weaknesses. For example, Lion [21] leverages a teacher model to identify instructions that are challenging for the student model and samples additional difficult tasks specifically targeting those the student fails to solve. LLM2LLM [22] proposes a novel targeted and iterative data augmentation framework that leverages a teacher LLM to expand the training dataset in a targeted and iterative manner. Similarly, PERsD [23] uses a teacher model to provide customized improvement feedback on erroneous code snippets generated by the student model based on specific execution errors, further demonstrating the effectiveness of feedback-based distillation.

Nevertheless, most of these methods primarily focus on leveraging teacher models to provide feedback and data augmentation for hard samples that student models fail to solve. The student models do not explicitly model the chain of thought, making it difficult to fully expose their own knowledge weaknesses, and teachers struggle to offer more targeted corrections. At the same time, student models lack opportunities to independently practice and consolidate on simpler samples, preventing them from fully leveraging their own strengths.

3 Method

In this section, we first present a formal definition of the Medical Relation Extraction task. Subsequently, we elaborate on the proposed KD4FIRE framework, whose overall architecture is illustrated in Fig. 1. This framework consists of three sequentially coupled modules:(1) Chain-of-Thought Generation and Sample Difficulty Stratification;(2) Teacher-Student Collaborative Knowledge Distillation;(3) Student Model Fine-Tuning.

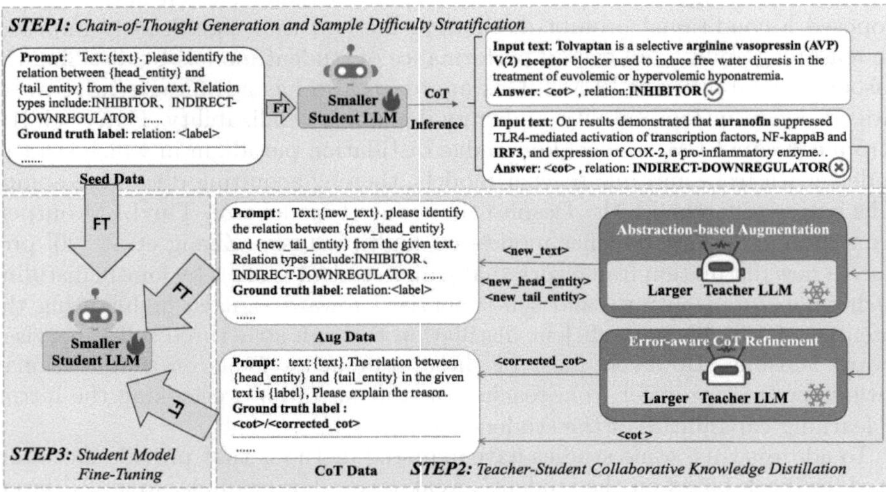

Fig. 1. The overall architecture of KD4FIRE.

3.1 Task Definition

Medical relation extraction aims to predict the predefined medical relation ($r \in R$) between a head entity (e_h) and a tail entity (e_t) based on a medical text (t) that contains these two entities. Formally, the input is represented as $x = (t, e_h, e_t)$, and the model is required to output the predicted relation r. Compared with general relation extraction, medical relations are typically highly fine-grained. They involve a large number of predefined relation categories, and the semantic differences between these relations are minimal. Additionally, the scarcity of annotated samples makes relation prediction more challenging under low-resource conditions. An example from the ChemProt dataset is illustrated in Fig. 2. Where the relation between "auranofin" and "IRF3" is labeled as "INHIBITOR".

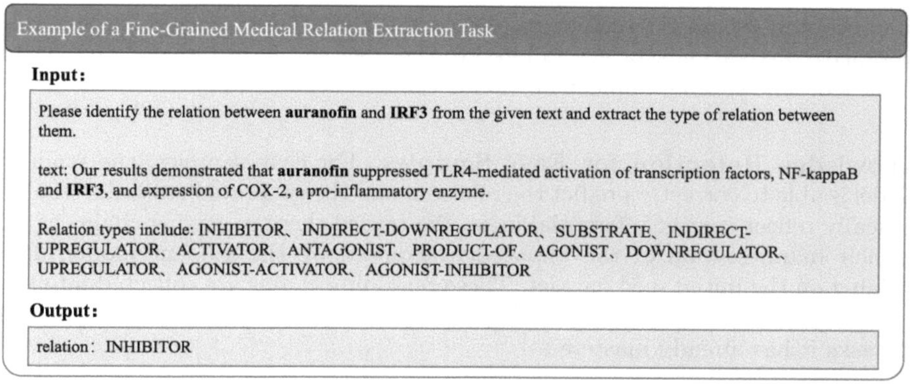

Fig. 2. Example of a Fine-Grained Medical Relation Extraction Task.

3.2 Chain-of-Thought Generation and Sample Difficulty Stratification

Student Model Fine-Tuning and Chain-of-Thought Generation Assume that a seed dataset for fine-grained relation extraction is given, denoted as $D_{seed} = \{(x_i, r_i)\}_{i=1}^{N}$, where each task instance consists of an input instruction x_i and a corresponding label r_i.

In the initial stage, we perform supervised fine-tuning of the student model on the original seed dataset D_{seed} to enable the model to acquire foundational domain-specific knowledge and task-solving capabilities for fine-grained medical relation extraction.

After the initial fine-tuning of the student model, in order to uncover the reasoning logic of the student model and distinguish the difficulty of samples, we conduct inference tests on the same batch of samples. Specifically, we employ the "think step by step" instruction to guide the student model to generate reasoning over the samples in D_{seed}. For each sample, the model outputs (cot_{pred}, r_{pred}), producing not only the final predicted relation but also the corresponding reasoning process.

Sample Difficulty Stratification After generating the reasoning chains and prediction results, we filter the samples based on the correctness of the predictions. Specifically, if the student model's predicted relation matches the ground-truth label, meaning the model predicts the relation correctly, the corresponding sample is defined as an easy sample. Conversely, if the student model's prediction does not match the ground-truth label, the sample is categorized as a hard sample, representing instances that the student model struggles with.

3.3 Teacher-Student Collaborative Knowledge Distillation

Inspired by the cognitive principle observed in human learning, where individuals reinforce strengths through self-practice and overcome weaknesses with external guidance and repeated practice, we design a differentiated teacher-student collaborative distillation strategy tailored to the easy and hard samples previously identified. The specific implementation details are as follows:

Knowledge Retention for Easy Samples. For easy samples, the student model is able to correctly predict the relation, and the generated reasoning chains typically reflect correct inferential logic. We regard these reasoning chains as an explicit manifestation of the knowledge acquired by the student model after training on the initial seed dataset. These reasoning chains are collected into the set $D_{cot\_correct}$ and are used to further reinforce the student model's performance on tasks it has already mastered.

Error-Aware Chain-of-Thought Refinement For hard samples, where the student model's predicted relation does not match the ground-truth label, we submit the reasoning chains generated by the student model on these samples to the teacher model for targeted intervention. Given that fine-tuning is essentially a form of imitation learning, our goal is to guide the student model to focus more on the substantive content of the reasoning chains rather than merely mimicking their surface language style or structural form. To achieve this, we introduce an error-aware chain-of-thought refinement mechanism. Under label supervision, the teacher model is used to correct the defective reasoning paths generated by the student model on hard samples. This correction process improves the accuracy of the reasoning content while preserving the student model's original linguistic style and expression patterns, thereby producing corrected reasoning chains that are both characteristic of the student model and more "learnable". This mechanism is intended to provide more targeted learning signals, which are expected to enhance the student model's reasoning capability and learning efficiency.

Specifically, the task instruction, the erroneous reasoning chain generated by the student model, and the corresponding label are fed into the teacher model. Guided by prompts (as shown in Fig. 3), the teacher model revises the reasoning chain under the constraint of the label while attempting to preserve the original style and structural characteristics of the student's reasoning. The inclusion of the correct label not only provides answer-level supervision but also effectively constrains the direction of the correction, ensuring that the logical derivation process aligns with the task objectives.

Leveraging this correction mechanism, we first construct a revised sample set denoted as $D_{cot\_corrected}$, which is combined with the set of originally correct reasoning samples $D_{cot\_correct}$ to form a high-quality chain-of-thought dataset D_{cot}. During training, this dataset provides explicit reasoning supervision, enhancing the student model's understanding of task-specific knowledge.

Semantic Abstraction-Based Data Augmentation. After performing knowledge retention and correction on both easy and hard samples, we fur-

Prompt for Error-aware CoT Refinement

The student was given the following question:
{question}
The answer has this as the chains of thought and relation:
{results}

The answer generated by the student is wrong. Please correct the wrong content in the student's chain of thought that leads to the wrong relation and generate a chain of thought that can lead to the correct relation.
the correct relation is: {label}
The generated new chain of thought should try to maintain the original structure and expression style of the student's chain of thought.

Fig. 3. Prompt for Error-aware CoT Refinement.

ther introduce a data abstraction-based augmentation mechanism. By increasing sample diversity, this mechanism enables the student model to repeatedly learn various expressions of the same relation, thereby enhancing its generalization capability and robustness in fine-grained relation extraction tasks. Drawing upon previous studies [24,25], we leverage the teacher model to extract high-level semantic information from the seed data and summarize latent relation patterns, thereby generating structurally diverse new samples. This augmentation process is primarily applied to hard samples, aiming to specifically address the knowledge gaps of the student model.

Considering the varying impact of samples with different difficulty levels on model learning, we introduce an augmentation ratio coefficient $\beta \in [0, 1]$ to control the extent of augmentation for easy samples. The specific strategy is as follows: for hard samples, we apply full augmentation, generating one abstract sample per original sample; for easy samples, we perform augmentation only on a stratified subset based on class distribution, selected at a ratio of β, to avoid introducing redundant information or reducing training efficiency.

To increase training data diversity while maintaining semantic consistency, we adopt a four-stage prompting strategy (as illustrated in Fig. 4) to guide the teacher model in generating diverse new samples for augmentation. The steps are as follows.

Step 1: Entity Replacement. This stage aims to generate semantically diverse samples by replacing head and tail entities, providing rich foundational data for subsequent abstraction stages. Specifically, the original text, head entity, tail entity, and corresponding relation label are input into the teacher model, which is instructed to replace the head and tail entities with alternatives while preserving the original semantic relation.

Step 2: Relation Abstraction. In this stage, the teacher model is prompted to abstract and summarize the samples generated in Step 1. This involves identifying structural commonalities and providing an explanatory representation of the relation type. The resulting abstraction captures the essential semantics of

Prompt for Abstraction-based Augmentation

Step 1-Entity Replacement:

Text: {text}, where the head entity is {head_entity}, the tail entity is {tail_entity}, and the relation between the head and tail entities is {relation}. Please replace only the head and tail entities without changing their relation, and generate three new texts along with their head and tail entities.

Step2-Relation Abstraction:

{Examples after entity replacement}
Based on the three examples provided, generate an explanation for the relation {relation}, and summarize the common characteristics among these examples.
The output structure should be: Explanation of the relation: ...; Common features: ...

Step3-Abstract Augmentation:

Please generate a new text. The generated text should be constructed according to the {Common_features}. The text should include new words of the same type as {head_entity} and new words of the same type as {tail_entity}, ensuring that these two entities consistently conform to the relation: {relation}. The explanation of the relation is: {Explanation_of_the_relation}.The new text that is generated needs to be diverse.
The output structure should be:text:...;head_entity:....;tail_entity:...

Step4-Confidence Estimation:

Text: {text}, Candidate relation: {candidate_relation}
Based on the given text, judge the confidence level (0~10) that the relation between the head entity ({head_entity}) and the tail entity ({tail_entity}) is {label}. Please express your confidence in this answer on a scale from 0 to 10.

Fig. 4. Prompt for Abstraction-based Augmentation.

the relation, serving as a structural and conceptual guide for sample generation in the final stage.

Step 3: Abstract Augmentation. Guided by the abstracted concept produced in Step 2, the teacher model is instructed to generate new samples that conform to the semantic and structural characteristics of the given relation type. Unlike simple surface-level paraphrasing, this process is grounded in the conceptual understanding of the relation. As a result, the newly generated samples preserve the core meaning while exhibiting greater surface-level diversity, enabling the student model to learn relation structures at a higher level of abstraction, thereby enhancing its generalization capability and robustness to unseen patterns.

Step 4: Quality Control of Samples. After generating diverse augmented samples, it is necessary to perform quality filtering to ensure their semantic reliability. To this end, we employ the teacher model to evaluate the confidence of each generated sample, which measures its semantic consistency with the target relation. Only samples with non-zero confidence are retained and included in the final augmented dataset D_{aug}. This filtering mechanism helps control noisy data and ensures that the student model receives high-quality supervision signals during training.

3.4 Student Model Fine-Tuning

Finally, we merge the original seed dataset, the high-quality chain-of-thought dataset, and the augmented dataset to construct the final training set. The final representation of the training set D_{train} is as follows:

$$D_{train} = D_{seed} \cup D_{cot} \cup D_{aug}. \tag{1}$$

Here, D_{cot} contains correct and teacher-corrected chain-of-thought samples, while D_{aug} denotes diversified augmented samples generated via semantic abstraction.

We perform supervised fine-tuning of the student model on D_{train}. During training, the model is required not only to accurately predict relation labels but also to generate reasoning processes that resemble the target chains of thought. This encourages a deeper mastery of task-specific knowledge and reasoning logic. By simultaneously leveraging high-quality chain-of-thought data and diversified augmented samples, this strategy consolidates existing knowledge, improves comprehension of challenging examples, and enhances overall generalization performance.

4 Experiments

4.1 Experimental Setup

Dataset and Evaluation Metrics We conduct experiments on the publicly available biomedical relation extraction dataset ChemProt [26], which contains a total of 10,065 instances divided into 4,169 instances for training, 2,427 instances for development, and 3,469 instances for testing. To evaluate model performance comprehensively, we adopt standard metrics used in prior studies, including micro-averaged precision (micro-P), micro-averaged recall (micro-R), micro-averaged F1 score (micro-F1), and macro-averaged F1 score (macro-F1) as the primary evaluation metrics. Micro-P measures the proportion of correctly predicted positive instances among all instances predicted as positive, reflecting the overall precision of the model. Micro-R quantifies the proportion of true positive instances successfully identified by the model among all actual positive instances, indicating the model's coverage capability for positive relations. Micro-F1 combines micro-P and micro-R to provide a balanced measure of the model's overall performance. In contrast, macro-F1 calculates the F1 score independently for each relation type and then averages them, placing greater emphasis on the model's performance across different categories. This is particularly suitable for datasets with imbalanced class distributions, such as those commonly found in biomedical domains with long-tail characteristics.

Training Parameter Settings In this study, we fine-tune the student model using the LoRA method. During LoRA fine-tuning, the batch size is set to 1, with a gradient accumulation step of 8. The LoRA α and LoRA rank are set to 16 and 64, respectively. For learning rate scheduling, we adopt a cosine scheduler with an initial learning rate of 1×10^{-5} and a warm-up ratio of 0.01.

Baselines We compare KD4FIRE with a range of baseline methods, including the following: (1) Inference-only: Inference is performed directly using the untrained student model (Qwen2.5 7B). (2) LoRA-fine-tuning: Inference is performed using the student model fine-tuned on the original seed dataset via LoRA. (3) Teacher: Inference is conducted using the teacher model (DeepSeek-R1).

4.2 Main Results

Table 1 compares the performance of the KD4FIRE and baseline methods on the ChemProt dataset with different proportions of training data. We observe that the untrained teacher model significantly outperforms the untrained student model, highlighting the strong reasoning and generation capabilities of the teacher. However, when relying solely on in-context learning, the teacher model's performance remains constrained to some extent. In contrast, LoRA fine-tuning notably enhances the student model's ability to adapt to the fine-grained biomedical relation extraction task. Remarkably, with only 30% of the seed data (approximately 1,000 instances), the fine-tuned student model already outperforms the large-scale DeepSeek-R1 teacher model in terms of Micro-F1, demonstrating the student's advantage in task-specific adaptation.

To harness the complementary strengths of both models, our proposed method integrates the teacher's capacity for complex semantic reasoning and the student's efficiency and adaptability. The experimental results show that KD4FIRE consistently achieves superior performance across all levels of seed data. Specifically, in the 30% seed training data setting, our method outperforms LoRA fine-tuning by approximately 4.1% in terms of Micro-F1 and 2.6% in terms of Macro-F1, indicating its effectiveness in enhancing student model performance in low-resource scenarios. Under the 60% condition, Micro-F1 and Macro-F1 are improved by approximately 2.5% and 2.2% respectively. Even with 100% of the seed training data, our method still results in consistent increases in Micro-F1 and Macro-F1 of around 1.6% and 1.7% respectively, demonstrating its continued benefit as the data volume increases.

4.3 Ablation Study

In this section, we investigate the effectiveness of our proposed method by ablating each key component individually. The results are presented in Table 2. Removing the chain-of-thought supervision dataset leads to a decrease in Micro-F1 and Macro-F1 of approximately 3.6% and 1.3% respectively, indicating the critical role of guided reasoning in improving model understanding. Similarly, removing the abstracted data augmentation dataset results in a decrease in Micro-F1 and Macro-F1 of approximately 0.6% and 1.3% respectively, highlighting the contribution of semantically diverse samples to model generalization. Furthermore, the simultaneous removal of both modules results in a more pronounced degradation in performance, indicating that each component of the proposed method plays an effective role in enhancing the model's overall performance.

Table 1. Comparison of the performance of various methods with different seed training data scales. To adapt to different data volume requirements, β (Augmentation Ratio) under 30%/60%/100%: 0.7/0.4/0.2.

Seed data proportion	Method	Micro-P	Micro-R	Micro-F1	Macro-F1
–	Teacher	0.7175	0.7132	0.7153	0.5229
	Inference-only	0.6162	0.6077	0.6119	0.3727
30%	LoRA-fine-tuning	0.7482	0.7469	0.7475	0.5159
	ours	**0.7890**	**0.7881**	**0.7886**	**0.5415**
60%	LoRA-fine-tuning	0.7865	0.7835	0.7850	0.5419
	ours	**0.8105**	**0.8086**	**0.8095**	**0.5643**
100%	LoRA-fine-tuning	0.8138	0.8115	0.8126	0.5660
	ours	**0.8310**	**0.8262**	**0.8286**	**0.5825**

Table 2. Results of the ablation study with 30% seed training data.

Method	Micro-P	Micro-R	Micro-F1	Macro-F1
Ours	**0.7890**	**0.7881**	**0.7886**	**0.5415**
- w/o D_{cot}	0.7543	0.7504	0.7523	0.5282
- w/o D_{aug}	0.7826	0.7824	0.7825	0.5282
- w/o D_{cot}+D_{aug}	0.7482	0.7469	0.7475	0.5159

4.4 Further Analysis

Effectiveness of Self-Distilled and Corrected Chain-of-Thought Data. To further evaluate the effectiveness of chain-of-thought distillation, we conducted a series of ablation experiments focusing on the self-distilled chain-of-thought generated by the student model for correctly answered instances and the teacher-corrected chain-of-thought. Table 3 presents the impact of different types of distilled data on student model performance under the 30% seed training data condition. When the self-distilled chain-of-thought data $D_{correct}$ are removed, the Micro-F1 score decreases by approximately 0.9%, suggesting that these samples play an important role in reinforcing the student's existing knowledge structure and serve as a key source of "self-reinforcement". Similarly, removing the corrected chain-of-thought data results in a larger performance drop of approximately 1.4%, indicating that reasoning chains revised by the teacher model are effective in addressing the student model's cognitive blind spots for challenging samples. These findings confirm that both types of reasoning data contribute meaningfully to improving the student model's ability to understand and extract fine-grained biomedical relations.

Comparison Between Directly Generated and Corrected Reasoning Data To further analyze the effectiveness of the teacher's corrections for the

Table 3. Verification of the effectiveness of self-distilled and corrected chain-of-thought data under 30% seed training data conditions.

Method	Micro-P	Micro-R	Micro-F1
$D_{seed}+D_{cot}$	**0.7826**	**0.7824**	**0.7825**
- w/o $D_{cot\_correct}$	0.7745	0.7723	0.7734
- w/o $D_{cot\_corrected}$	0.7691	0.7679	0.7685
- w/o $D_{cot\_correct}+D_{cot\_corrected}$	0.7482	0.7469	0.7475

student model's erroneous reasoning chains, we conducted comparative experiments by replacing the corrected data $D_{cot\_corrected}$ in D_{cot} with reasoning chain data D_{llm} generated directly by the large model. Table 4 compares the performances obtained in the 30% seed data setting for two types of distilled data: (1) a combination of the seed data, verified correct chain-of-thoughts, and teacher-corrected reasoning data and (2) a combination of the seed set, verified correct chain-of-thoughts, and chain-of-thoughts directly generated by a large language model without feedback-based correction. The results show that our approach achieves superior performance in terms of Micro-P, Micro-R, and Micro-F1, providing further evidence for the effectiveness of incorporating teacher feedback in correcting reasoning paths.

Table 4. Comparison between raw LLM-generated chain-of-thought data and corrected chain-of-thought data under 30% seed training data conditions.

Method	Micro-P	Micro-R	Micro-F1
$D_{seed}+D_{cot}$	**0.7826**	**0.7824**	**0.7825**
$D_{seed}+D_{cot\_correct}+D_{llm}$	0.7762	0.7757	0.7760

Comparison Between Full Fine-Tuning and Continued Fine-Tuning As shown in Table 5, we further investigate the performance differences between full fine-tuning and continued fine-tuning. Specifically, full fine-tuning refers to retraining the original student model from scratch using the combined dataset that includes both the original seed data and the augmented data (i.e., chain-of-thought distillation data and abstracted data). Continued fine-tuning involves further training from the checkpoint obtained after chain-of-thought distillation, which uses only the abstracted augmentation data.

We observe that full fine-tuning outperforms continued fine-tuning, with an increase in Micro-F1 of approximately 0.7%. This performance gap may be attributed to catastrophic forgetting that occurs during continued fine-tuning, where the model, when exposed only to augmented data, tends to overfit to new patterns and forget part of the knowledge acquired during earlier training on

Table 5. Comparison between full fine-tuning and continual fine-tuning under 30% seed training data conditions.

Method	Micro-P	Micro-R	Micro-F1
Full fine-tuning	**0.7890**	**0.7881**	**0.7886**
Continual fine-tuning	0.7816	0.7809	0.7813

the original task. This suggests that full fine-tuning allows for better integration and balance of both original and augmented knowledge.

Case Study. To further validate the effectiveness of KD4FIRE in low-resource fine-grained medical relation extraction tasks, we conducted a case study focusing on the relation identification between "prostate-specific antigen" and "estramustine".

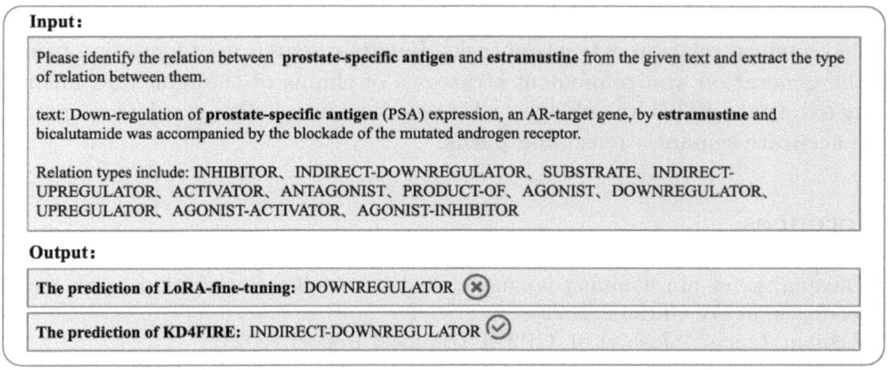

Fig. 5. Comparison of LoRA-Fine-tuning and KD4FIRE on a Fine-Grained Relation Extraction Case under 30% seed training data conditions.

As shown in Fig. 5, the model fine-tuned using only seed data via LoRA, constrained by its foundational semantic understanding capabilities, tended to rely on superficial lexical cues such as "down-regulation". It failed to adequately recognize the complex mechanism by which estramustine indirectly regulates the expression of prostate-specific antigen by blocking the mutated androgen receptor. Consequently, it incorrectly classified the relation as DOWNREGULATOR. In contrast, the KD4FIRE method correctly identified the relation as INDIRECT-DOWNREGULATOR, demonstrating its stronger capability to capture relatively complex semantic patterns. This result verifies that KD4FIRE, through its collaborative learning mechanism of "self-practice + teacher guidance", effectively combines the strengths of both large and small models, thereby enhancing the performance of the small model in fine-grained medical relation extraction tasks.

5 Conclusion

This paper addresses the task of low-resource fine-grained medical relation extraction and proposes a novel knowledge distillation framework named KD4FIRE. Inspired by the human cognitive learning process, this framework implements a collaborative learning mechanism of "self-practice + teacher guidance" through the division of sample difficulty based on the performance of the student model. For hard samples, an error-aware chain-of-thought refinement mechanism and an abstraction-based data augmentation method are further designed to explicitly identify and address the student model's knowledge gaps, thereby enabling more effective knowledge transfer. The experimental results obtained on the ChemProt dataset for fine-grained medical relation extraction demonstrate that the proposed method outperforms various baseline approaches in low-resource settings, confirming the effectiveness of the framework in fine-grained medical relation extraction tasks. Future research may focus on optimizing the generation and refinement strategies of chains of thought, and incorporating external reliable knowledge such as medical knowledge graphs to construct more accurate semantic reasoning paths.

References

1. Ouyang, L. et al.: Training language models to follow instructions with human feedback. arXiv e-prints (2022)
2. Achiam, OpenAI Josh et al. GPT-4 Technical Report (2023)
3. DeepSeek-AI et al. DeepSeek-R1: Incentivizing Reasoning Capability in LLMs via Reinforcement Learning. ArXiv abs/2501.12948 (2025): n. pag
4. Ma, Y. et al.: Large Language Model Is Not a Good Few-shot Information Extractor, but a Good Reranker for Hard Samples!. ArXiv abs/2303.08559 (2023)
5. Singhal, K., Tu, T., Gottweis, J., et al.: Toward expert-level medical question answering with large language models. Nat. Med. **31**, 943–950 (2025). https://doi.org/10.1038/s41591-024-03423-7
6. Wang, H. et al.: HuaTuo: Tuning LLaMA Model with Chinese Medical Knowledge. ArXiv: abs/2304.06975 (2023)
7. Huang, M., et al.: Discovering patterns to extract protein-protein interactions from full texts. Bioinformatics **20**(18), 3604–3612 (2004)
8. Fundel, K., Kuffner, R., Zimmer, R.: RelEx-Relation extraction using dependency parse trees, BIOINFORMATICS -OXFORD- (2007)
9. Peng, Y. et al.: An extended dependency graph for relation extraction in biomedical texts. In: Bionlp Workshop (2015)
10. Airola, A. et al.: All-paths graph kernel for protein-protein interaction extraction with evaluation of cross-corpus learning. Bmc Bioinf. **9** Suppl 11 (2008)

11. Spandana, S., Prakash, R.V.: Multiple features-based adverse drug reaction detection from social media using deep convolutional neural networks (DCNN). Multimed. Tools Appl. **83**(26) (2024)
12. Lee, J. et al.: BioBERT: a pre-trained biomedical language representation model for biomedical text mining. Bioinformatics (2019)
13. Bao, Z. et al.: DISC-MedLLM: Bridging General Large Language Models and Real-World Medical Consultation (2023)
14. Chang, Y.C., Huang, M.S., Huang, Y.H., et al.: The influence of prompt engineering on large language models for protein–protein interaction identification in biomedical literature. Sci. Rep. **15**, 15493 (2025). https://doi.org/10.1038/s41598-025-99290-4
15. Labrak, Y., Rouvier, M., Dufour, R.: A Zero-shot and Few-shot Study of Instruction-Finetuned Large Language Models Applied to Clinical and Biomedical Tasks. arXiv: abs/2307.12114 (2023)
16. Ma, T. et al.: Y-Mol: A Multiscale Biomedical Knowledge-Guided Large Language Model for Drug Development (2024)
17. Xu, X. et al.: A Survey on Knowledge Distillation of Large Language Models. ArXiv: abs/2402.13116 (2024)
18. Chen, F., Feng, Y.: Chain-of-Thought Prompt Distillation for Multimodal Named Entity Recognition and Multimodal Relation Extraction (2023)
19. Tian, Y. et al.: Beyond answers: transferring reasoning capabilities to smaller llms using multi-teacher knowledge distillation. In: Proceedings of the Eighteenth ACM International Conference on Web Search and Data Mining (2024)
20. Zhang, Y. et al.: Distill Not Only Data but Also Rewards: Can Smaller Language Models Surpass Larger Ones? ArXiv: abs/2502.19557 (2025)
21. Jiang, Y. et al.: Lion: Adversarial distillation of proprietary large language models. In: Conference on Empirical Methods in Natural Language Processing (2023)
22. Lee, N. et al.: LLM2LLM: Boosting LLMs with Novel Iterative Data Enhancement. ArXiv: abs/2403.15042 (2024)
23. Chen, H. et al.: Personalised Distillation: Empowering Open-Sourced LLMs with Adaptive Learning for Code Generation. ArXiv: abs/2310.18628 (2023)
24. Zheng, H.S. et al.: Take a Step Back: Evoking Reasoning via Abstraction in Large Language Models. ArXiv:abs/2310.06117 (2023)
25. Kang, H. et al.: Guidance-Based Prompt Data Augmentation in Specialized Domains for Named Entity Recognition. ArXiv: abs/2407.18442 (2024)
26. Cheng, D. et al.: Adapting Large Language Models to Domains via Reading Comprehension (2023)

Zero-Shot Knowledge Distillation for Chinese Clinical Diagnosis: Enhancing Small LLMs via Prompting and Loss-Based Filtering

Zhongtian Hua[1], Xia Liu[1], Mengyuan Wang[1], Meijia Yu[2], Yi Luo[1], Kunli Zhang[1], and Yingjie Han[1](✉)

[1] Zhengzhou University, No. 100 Science Avenue, Zhengzhou, China
{hzt1113,xliu,wangmengyuan}@gs.zzu.edu.cn, nancetide@stu.zzu.edu.cn, {ieklzhang,ieyjhan}@zzu.edu.cn

[2] Henan University of Science and Technology, No. 263 Kaiyuan Avenue, Luoyang, China

Abstract. Accurate clinical diagnosis is of vital importance in the medical field. Large Language Models (LLMs) usually need to be fine-tuned and improved before they can be applied in the medical vertical field, and this process means additional data annotation and huge computing power overhead. Small Language Models (SLMs) can serving as an efficient alternative to fine-tuning LLMs through model distillation. However, during the distillation process, the teacher models often fail to stimulate their own vertical domain knowledge due to the lack of guidance, thereby causing the performance bottleneck problem of the student model. Aiming at the problems of incomplete internal knowledge stimulation of the teacher model and low quality of knowledge samples in model distillation, this paper proposes a zero-shot knowledge distillation framework PeKDiL (**P**rompt-**e**nhanced **K**nowledge **Di**stillation with **L**oss-based filtering) for Chinese clinical diagnosis, aiming to enhance the performance of SLMs through prompt engineering and loss-based data filtering, meanwhile reducing training costs and avoid manual annotation. This framework first guides LLMs to generate higher-quality knowledge through prompt engineering, and then uses a detection model to screen the confidence level of the generated knowledge data, retaining high-quality samples for the final model distillation. The experimental results show that SLMs distilled by PeKDiL perform better than general LLMs and other methods, verifying the effectiveness of this framework in improving the diagnostic accuracy and generalization ability of the model.

Keywords: Knowledge distillation · Zero-shot learning · Clinical diagnosis

Y. Zhang et al. (Eds.): CHIP 2025, CCIS 2884, pp. 270–283, 2026.
https://doi.org/10.1007/978-981-95-7299-1_17

1 Introduction

Accurate diagnosis is vitally important in the field of healthcare [1]. The diagnostic process usually involves identifying diseases by analyzing symptoms, signs and examination results, and formulating diagnoses and differential diagnoses based on this [2]. Even though doctors have received extensive medical training, errors in diagnosis are still inevitable [27]. With the rapid development of electronic information technology, electronic medical record has become a widely popularized research topic in major medical institutions. The pathological feature information and health indicators of patients contained in electronic medical records not only enable doctors to make more accurate judgments, but also promote the rapid development of deep learning models in the field of clinical. diagnosis [3].

In recent years, Large Language Models (LLMs) have demonstrated powerful emergent capabilities in multiple fields. Through techniques such as prompt learning and Chain-of-Thought(CoT) [30], LLMS can demonstrate strong diagnostic performance and reasoning capabilities in the field of assisted diagnosis [4–6]. However, in real clinical deployment scenarios, LLMs still face major challenges such as high computational costs and a lack of knowledge in the medical professional field [28]. Especially when deploying models with a large number of parameters (>72B), if one wants to enhance their performance through fine-tuning, it requires a high resource cost [7].

Small Language Model (SLM) has become a more computatively efficient alternative through methods such as model distillation and prompt learning [8–10]. These methods enable SLM to inherit the reasoning capabilities driven by large language models with large parameter scale and enhance generalization performance through instruction-based adaptation. However, these methods still face two major challenges: First, in the distillation process, large-scale parameter LLMs serving as teacher models are generally general-purpose models, lacking auxiliary diagnostic thinking and reasoning methods, which leads to poor quality of distillation data. And the second question that follows is the distillation data generated by the teacher model cannot be used directly and requires further cleaning and adjustment before it can be used as knowledge for the student model to conduct distillation learning.

In response to the above problems, we propose a **P**rompt-**e**nhanced **K**nowledge **Di**stillation framework with **L**oss-based Filtering (PeKDiL). In this framework, we first integrate multiple prompt enhancement methods into the prompt template to enable the teacher model to better extract the pathological features of patients from electronic medical records in accordance with the reasoning method of doctors' diagnoses, and conduct more logical diagnostic reasoning in line with reality, generating high-quality diagnostic reasoning knowledge. Then, we fine-tune the lightweight LLMs through this high-quality knowledge to obtain a checking model with certain domain knowledge. We use this model to calculate the cross-entropy loss for each piece of data in the teacher knowledge data and use the obtained loss as the confidence index to clean the knowledge data, thereby obtaining a final high-quality knowledge database. And it was used to conduct distillation fine-tuning again on the student model with small-scale parameters, and finally applied in the clinical diagnosis. To sum up, our contributions are as follows:

I. We propose a model distillation framework, PeKDiL. This framework stimulates the reasoning ability of the teacher model in the field of clinical diagnosis through prompt engineering, enabling it to produce higher-quality diagnostic knowledge. At the same time, data cleaning is introduced to improve the quality of distillation knowledge, and the data screening work was completed under the condition of zero labeling.
II. We utilize the cross-entropy loss during the forward propagation of the model as an evaluation index for data screening. This index reflects from the inherent perspective of the model whether the input data is reliable, thereby achieving efficient, stable and accurate data cleaning.
III. We conduct comparative experiments and ablation experiments on the C-EMRs dataset. Demonstrating the necessity of the two sub-modules through ablation experiments, and at the same time, we prove the advanced nature of the lightweight LLMs distilled through the PeKDiL framework in the field of clinical diagnosis through comparative experiments.

2 Related Work

2.1 Clinical Diagnosis

Auxiliary clinical diagnosis is a comprehensive technology that integrates artificial intelligence, data analysis and clinical medical knowledge, aiming to enhance the efficiency and accuracy of disease identification. For decades, researchers and medical professionals have invested a great deal of resources and energy dedicated to breaking through the limitations of traditional diagnosis and treatment models [11]. From the early clinical decision support systems (CDSS) [12] constructed based on clear medical rules to the clinical prediction models developed in recent years using structured feature extraction and machine learning algorithms [24], the technical path has been constantly evolving. In recent The proposal and iteration of Pre-trained Language Models (PLMs) and Large Language Models (LLMs)have significantly accelerated Natural Language Processing(NLP). The research progress in the field of NLP has stimulated extensive research on the application of LLMs in the biomedical field. Specialized models for medical scenarios such as ClinicalBERT [13], NYUTron [14], GatorTron [15], and BioGPT [16] have emerged one after another, demonstrating significant potential in complex tasks such as medical predictive analysis. However, the practical application of LLM in the medical field is still in the exploratory stage [17]. Generally speaking, the expansion of the model parameter scale can simultaneously enhance the model's semantic understanding and generation capabilities. However, given the strict requirements for knowledge accuracy in the medical field, the application of LLMs with large-scale parameters in disease diagnosis often requires fine-tuning, knowledge injection [29] or other means to supplement professional medical knowledge. This process is accompanied by high computing costs and resource consumption, which has become a key bottleneck that restricts its wide implementation.

2.2 Knowledge Distillation

Benefit from the advantages of a streamlined parameter scale and lower inference latency, Small Language Models (SLMs) have been regarded as an efficient alternative to LLMs in many vertical fields [18,19]. One of the core topics of the current research is how to achieve the precise transfer of LLM knowledge to SLM at a lower cost. Recent work has generally adopted "rationale distillation" to transfer the complex reasoning ability of LLM to SLM. Furthermore, chain-of-thought prompting was further introduced to activate and enhance the multi-step reasoning performance of SLM.

However, the existing distillation frameworks generally have a "teacher model capability bottleneck": The teacher models serving as knowledge sources are mostly general LLMs that have not undergone domain fine-tuning and lack factual knowledge of professional scenarios such as medical diagnosis, resulting in limited quality of the generated knowledge data [31]. Low-quality distillation knowledge, if used for SLM fine-tuning without strict screening, will introduce significant noise and lead to performance degradation. Therefore, it is urgently necessary to establish an efficient cleaning mechanism for distillation data. Regrettably, the current mainstream cleaning strategies still rely on manual review or gold label verification, which leads to high labor costs or large-scale data annotation requirements, seriously restricting the scalability of the distillation process.

3 Methodology

An overview of our approach is illustrated in Fig. 1. To achieve higher-quality model distillation, we designed a model distillation framework called PeKDiL. The PeKDiL framework consists of two sub-modules, namely, high-quality knowledge extraction based on prompts and loss-based distillation data filtering. In high-quality knowledge extraction, we integrated multiple prompt methods in the prompt template based on the task characteristics of pathological diagnosis, enabling LLMs with large-scale parameters to better extract the pathological features of patients from electronic medical records, thereby conducting more accurate diagnostic reasoning and generating high-quality diagnostic reasoning knowledge. In the loss-based distillation data filtering, we first fine-tune the large language model with small-scale parameters using the obtained high-quality diagnostic knowledge data, thereby obtaining a filtering model for loss value filtering. Then, we used this model to calculate the loss for each piece of data in the diagnostic knowledge data. The loss was used as the confidence index to clean and screen the diagnostic knowledge data. Eventually, a high-quality knowledge database is obtained, and it is used to distill and fine-tune the lightweight small-scale model, which was finally applied in the clinical diagnosis.

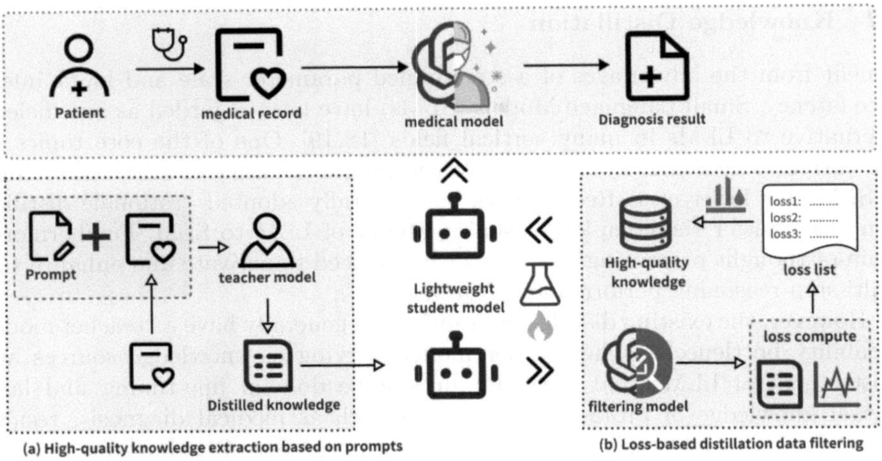

Fig. 1. The overview of our method. We design a knowledge distillation framework called PeKDiL, which has two sub-modules. Among them, the high-quality knowledge extraction module based on prompts obtains high-quality knowledge from the teacher model through carefully designed prompt templates, while the distillation data filtering module based on loss further screens the distillation data through cross-entropy loss, thereby obtaining the final knowledge data to better distill the SLM.

3.1 High-Quality Knowledge Extraction Based on Prompts

In order to obtain higher-quality knowledge from teacher models with large-scale parameters, we carefully design a prompt template that integrates multiple prompt enhancement methods [26]. Specifically, we first constructed a model inference step process prompt framework using markdown syntax. This framework consists of four major parts: core task definition, model logic inference steps, special case handling, and input/output examples. In the core task definition, we detail the task background of pathological diagnosis and instruct the LLM to play the role. In the model logic reasoning step, we integrate multiple reasoning enhancement methods such as Chain-of-Thought and Chain-of-Tree, thereby guiding the teacher model to use a thinking mode closer to real diagnosis to extract and feature about the medical record information in electronic medical records, thereby generating higher-quality distilled knowledge data. The overall structure of the prompt template is shown in the Fig. 2. The complete improvement template is provided in the appendix.

3.2 Loss-Based Distillation Data Filtering

After obtaining the knowledge data generated by the large-scale parameter model, we find that there are still errors in the knowledge data generated by the teacher model. Therefore, it is necessary to screen the knowledge data. We performed parameter-efficient fine-tuning on a lightweight LLM using existing knowledge data, thereby obtaining a filtering model capable of screening of

```
### ** Medical Diagnosis Instruction Manual **

#### **1. Core task definition **
** objective ** : XXXXXX
 ** Diagnostic basis ** :XXXXXX

#### **2. Input data specification **
** input format ** : XXXXXX

#### **3. Model reasoning logic instructions **
** phased analysis ** :
1. ** Key information extraction :XXXXXX
2. ** Generate a list of differential diagnoses ** :XXXXXX
3. ** Pathophysiological verification ** :XXXXXX
4. ** Diagnostic Decision Tree ** :XXXXXX

#### **4. Special Scenario handling rules **:XXXXXX
1. ** Fuzzy Expression Handling **:XXXXXX
2.** Logical Control for Coexistence of multiple diseases ** :XXXXXX

#### **5. Final output format requirements **
XXXXXX
```

Fig. 2. The framework of the prompt template we designed. It consists of four parts: core task definition, model logical reasoning, special scenario handling, and input/output instances. It integrates multiple prompt enhancement methods to help LLM better generate diagnostic reasoning knowledge.

knowledge data. Specifically, we first pre-process the diagnostic instructions and the output knowledge of the teacher model, converting them into a structured dataset. Then, we use this dataset to conduct LoRA efficient fine-tuning of the student model. At the same time, during the fine-tuning process, we apply label smoothing technology to prevent overfitting of the student model and enhance its generalization ability. The fine-tuned model, through distillation, retains some of its own original knowledge while acquiring certain pathological diagnosis knowledge of the teacher model, thereby being able to screen the knowledge data of teachers.

Checkpoints that performed best during training is selected as the inspection model and re-input the knowledge into the model in the training manner. The returned loss is used as the metric to screen the data. We believe that data with a lower loss value reflects that the model is more confident in the output of this piece of data, with a high level of confidence; conversely, it indicates a lower level of confidence. Specifically, we first switched the model to training mode and removed the weight update and gradient optimization functions in the optimizer to prevent the weight update from affecting the model's loss output result. Then, we distinguish the input data during model training into the instruction part and the output part through special start and end flags, and hide the instruction part by masking. During the calculation, only the loss of the output part of the model is calculated, which can save GPU's memory space and accelerate the training efficiency when calculating the loss. For the input instruction sequence X and the predicted label sequence T = $[t_1,t_2,...,t_n]$, we take the cross-entropy loss of the next token in the output label part as the confidence index, and the formula is as follows:

$$Loss = -\frac{1}{n}\sum_{i=1}^{n}\log P(t_i|t_1,t_2,...,t_{i-1}) \tag{1}$$

This formula calculates the conditional probability log-likelihood of each predicted label ti and takes the average to obtain the overall loss value. The smaller the loss value, the higher the model's prediction confidence for the corresponding label.

After obtaining the loss of each piece of knowledge data through the detection model, we sorted them in ascending order and ultimately selected the top 50% of the data as the final high-quality knowledge dataset. We then fine-tuned a lightweight base LLM with LoRA [25], thereby obtaining a lightweight doctor model that can be used for clinical diagnosis.

4 Experiments

4.1 Experimental Setup

To verify the effectiveness of the PeKDiL framework in model distillation, we select the Qwen3-235B [20], DeepSeek-V3.1 [21] and Qwen2.5-72B [22] models as the teacher models, and at the same time select Qwen3-8B and ChatGlm4-9B [23] as the student models for the experiment. Additionally, we included several knowledge-enhanced intelligent diagnosis models as comparative methods, including MacBERT [33] (a pre-trained model based on a bidirectional Transformer encoder with more powerful encoding capabilities than BERT [36]), KAIE [34] (a model that incorporates triple-form medical knowledge on top of a BERT model with an enhanced layer), GSKN [32] (a model that incorporates graph-structured medical knowledge on top of a BERT model with an enhanced layer), and DGKE [35] (a knowledge-enhanced model based on a hierarchically information-enhanced MacBERT, incorporating disease subgraph and text subgraph forms of knowledge).

We use the original teacher and student models, along with the aforementioned knowledge-enhanced models, as baselines. Using the student models as a baseline serves to demonstrate the performance improvement of the models distilled using the PeKDiL framework compared to the original models, and also acts as a benchmark for ablation experiments to verify the necessity of the two sub-modules. Using the teacher models as a baseline helps validate that the high-quality data selected by the PeKDiL framework contains less noise and hallucination compared to the original knowledge data. The inclusion of knowledge-enhanced models for comparison aims to demonstrate that the PeKDiL framework not only eliminates the reliance on extensive manually labeled data for training required by these advanced methods, but also achieves further performance gains through knowledge distillation, highlighting its versatility and advantages in the medical diagnosis domain.

To control the influence of hyperparameters on the experimental results, we have fixed all the hyperparameters involved in the experiment, which are presented in the Table 1.

Table 1. The hyperparameters involved in the training process.

Parameter name	Parameter value
Epoch	10
Batch size	1
Gradient_accumulation	4
Learning rate	2e-5
Max grad norm	1.0
Lora_r	64
Lora_alpha	512

Furthermore, we ultimately took 50% of the knowledge data generated by the four teacher models from the lowest to the highest loss value, and performed a union operation on them to obtain the final distillation dataset.

4.2 Datasets and Metrics

To measure the effectiveness of our method in the field of clinical diagnosis, we cite the clinical diagnosis dataset (C-EMRs) proposed by Yang et al. [24]. This dataset contains 18,590 real-world electronic medical records, covering the most common disease types in multiple departments, including hypertension, diabetes, chronic obstructive pulmonary disease (COPD), gout, arrhythmia, asthma, gastritis and gastric polyps, etc. Each medical record, after desensitization, retains 13 key items including the chief complaint, present illness history and physical examination, and is accompanied by the doctor's final diagnosis as a label. This dataset has a certain imbalance in category distribution, but the datasets' authors have constructed a subset suitable for model training and testing through screening and balanced sampling. It has high authenticity and representativeness and is widely used in the tasks of semantic understanding and clinical diagnosis of electronic medical records.

In the original dataset, the data is divided into the training set, validation set and test set in an 8:1:1 ratio. However, our method does not require a training set for training. Instead, the LLM conducts zero-shot reasoning to obtain knowledge data, which is then used to fine-tune the SLM through distillation. Therefore, we combine the original training set, validation set and test set into a complete dataset, and then divide this dataset into a knowledge set and a test set in a 2:8

ratio. We perform zero-shot prediction on the data in the knowledge set using LLM, and then distill it with SLM.

Clinical diagnosis is essentially a classification task. Therefore, we adopt classic classification task metrics such as accuracy, recall, precision and F1 value to quantify the capabilities of our framework.

4.3 Results and Analysis

In experiments and experimental analyses, for convenience, we refer to the high-quality knowledge extraction module based on prompts as Module E(Extract) and the distillation data filtering module based on losses as Module F(Filter). Precision (P), Accuracy (A), and Recall (R) will all use their abbreviations. The comparative experimental results are shown in the Table 2, and the ablation experiments results are shown in the Table 3.

Table 2. Comparative experiments results

Model	Fine-tuning	P	A	R	F1
Qwen2.5-72B	–	0.821	0.869	0.862	0.833
Qwen3-235B	–	0.854	0.884	0.893	0.871
DeepSeek-V3.1	–	0.896	0.872	0.912	0.905
MacBERT	Train with the training set	0.898	0.894	0.874	0.883
KAIE		0.845	0.897	<u>0.935</u>	0.875
GSKN		0.879	0.899	0.859	0.868
DGKE		0.909	0.914	0.874	0.890
Qwen3-8B	–	0.845	0.336	0.483	0.612
	PekDiL	**0.922**	**0.931**	**0.938**	**0.929**
ChatGlm4-9B	–	0.811	0.479	0.502	0.593
	PekDiL	<u>0.914</u>	<u>0.929</u>	0.917	<u>0.915</u>

Overall, the qwen3-8B model distilled using the complete PeKDiL framework performed the best on the C-EMRs dataset, with an average F1 value reaching 0.924. Compared with the unfine-tuned LLM and SLM, there was a significant improvement in performance, which proved the effectiveness of the PeKDiL framework. Next, we will conduct a detailed analysis of the experimental results from two perspectives: comparative experiments and ablation experiments.

Comparative Experiments From the experimental results, we can see that the advanced large language models at the present stage have already possessed strong auxiliary diagnostic capabilities, and the overall evaluation index has reached 0.85+. However, due to the lack of knowledge in specific fields, it does not have a significant lead compared with the methods based on pre-trained models trained with dedicated domain data. This proves our viewpoints in the previous two sections and also demonstrates the necessity of fine-tuning general domain

LLMs in the field of clinical diagnosis. Then, from the comparison of the fine-tuned Qwen3-8B and the ChatGlm4-9B model with the general domain LLM, it can be seen that the performance of the fine-tuned SLM is significantly better than that of the general LLM as the teacher model. This indicates that this phenomenon occurs because PekDiL first guided the LLM to generate higher-quality knowledge data that is more in line with the real diagnostic domain through prompt enhancement, and retained higher-quality knowledge data through data cleaning, thus making the final distilled dataset closer to the real general domain dataset. This also enables SLM to achieve "taking the essence and discarding the dross" when undergoing distillation fine-tuning, thereby learning more professional diagnostic knowledge and thus achieving better diagnostic performance than general LLMs. Finally, from the comparison between the fine-tuned SLM and the methods based on pre-trained models, the performance of the fine-tuned SLM is slightly better than that of the methods based on pre-trained models. However, methods based on pre-trained models rely on large-scale training sets for training, while SLM can distill the diagnostic knowledge in LLM under zero-shot conditions, thereby avoiding reliance on training sets. This is also a major advantage of PekDiL over traditional methods.

Table 3. Ablation experiments results.

Model	Fine-tuning		P	A	R	F1
	Module E	Module F				
Qwen3-8B	–		0.845	0.336	0.483	0.612
		✓	0.726	0.697	0.731	0.730
	✓		0.877	0.905	0.879	0.873
	✓	✓	**0.922**	**0.931**	**0.938**	**0.929**
ChatGlm4-9B	–		0.811	0.479	0.502	0.593
		✓	0.853	0.683	0.892	0.877
	✓		0.894	0.905	0.862	0.876
	✓	✓	**0.914**	**0.929**	**0.917**	**0.915**

Ablation experiments From the ablation experiment, we can see the significance of the two sub-modules in the PekDiL framework. No matter which sub-module is missing, the performance of the SLM after distillation will decline. Specifically, when PekDiL only retains the high-quality knowledge extraction module based on prompts without data cleaning, even if the knowledge extracted with high quality is already relatively close to the real diagnostic domain data, there still exists "dirty data" generated by the LLM illusion phenomenon. Therefore, the performance of the distilled SLM can only be comparable to that of the teacher model And it is impossible to achieve a comprehensive surpass. When PekDiL only retains the loss-based data filtering module, due to the relatively low quality of distillation data, data cleaning loses its function and can only perform cleaning and optimization on the existing distillation data, but cannot take it further. In conclusion, through the analysis of ablation research, both sub-modules of PeKDiL are effective and necessary.

5 Conclusion

This paper address the current issue of insufficient domain knowledge of LLMs in clinical auxiliary diagnosis, which leads to performance bottlenecks in student models, and propose a novel zero-shot knowledge distillation framework, PeKDiL. By enhancing the guidance for LLM to generate high-quality diagnostic reasoning data through prompts and further purifying the knowledge base in combination with a loss-based data filtering mechanism, the performance of SLM in Chinese electronic medical record diagnosis tasks has been significantly improved.

The experimental results show that the PeKDiL framework can not only effectively improve the diagnostic accuracy of SLM, but also avoid the reliance on labeled data in a zero-shot setting, and has strong practicability and scalability. The ablation experiment further verify the necessity and complementarity of the two sub-modules of prompt enhancement and loss filtering. Future work will explore more prompt strategies and filtering mechanisms to further enhance distillation efficiency and model robustness, and promote the application of lightweight models in clinical practical scenarios.

A Appendix

See Figs. 3 and 4.

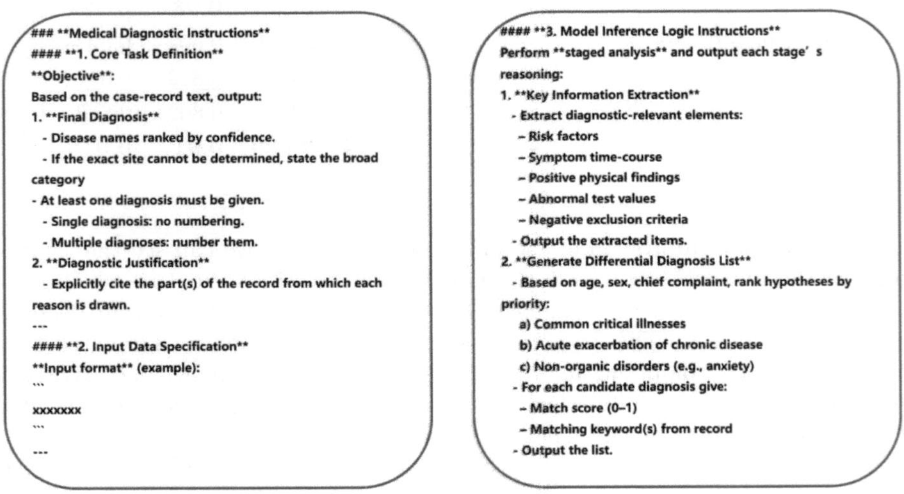

Fig. 3. This picture shows our complete prompt template (Part One).

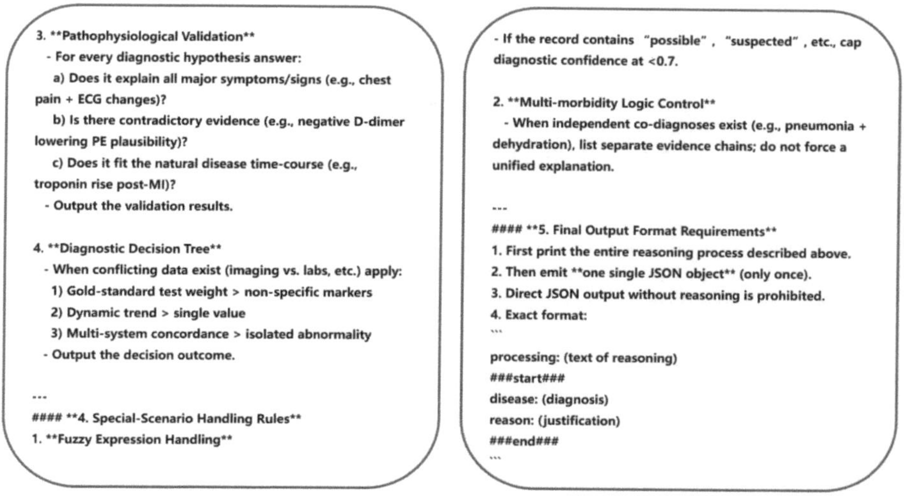

Fig. 4. This picture shows our complete prompt template (Part Two).

References

1. Scully, J.L.: What is a disease? Disease, disability and their definitions. EMBO Rep. **5**, 650–653 (2004)
2. Kaur, S., et al.: Medical diagnostic systems using artificial intelligence (AI) algorithms: principles and perspectives. IEEE Access **8**, 228049–228069 (2020). https://doi.org/10.1109/ACCESS.2020.3042273
3. Laghuvarapu, S., Lin, Z., Sun, J.: Codrug: conformal drug property prediction with density estimation under covariate shift. In: Advances in Neural Information Processing Systems, vol. 36 (2024)
4. Wei, J., et al.: Chain-of-thought prompting elicits reasoning in large language models. In: Advances in Neural Information Processing Systems, vol. 35, pp. 24824–24837 (2022)
5. Singhal, K., et al.: Large language models encode clinical knowledge. Nature **620**(7972), 172–180 (2023)
6. Chen, Z., et al.: Meditron-70b: scaling medical pretraining for large language models (2023). arXiv:2311.16079
7. Niu, S., et al.: Knowledge-augmented multimodal clinical rationale generation for disease diagnosis with small language models. In: Proceedings of the 63rd Annual Meeting of the Association for Computational Linguistics (Volume 1: Long Papers), pp. 11011–11024 (2025)
8. Hsieh, C.-Y., et al.: Distilling step-by-step! outperforming larger language models with less training data and smaller model sizes. In: Proceedings of the 61st Annual Meeting of the Association for Computational Linguistics (2023)
9. Kang, M., et al.: Knowledge-augmented reasoning distillation for small language models in knowledge-intensive tasks. In: Advances in Neural Information Processing Systems, vol. 36 (2024)

10. Kwon, T., et al.: Large language models are clinical reasoners: reasoning-aware diagnosis framework with prompt-generated rationales. In: Proceedings of the AAAI Conference on Artificial Intelligence, vol. 38, pp. 18417–18425 (2024)
11. Liu, X., et al.: A generalist medical language model for disease diagnosis assistance. Nat. Med. **31**, 932–942 (2025). https://doi.org/10.1038/s41591-024-03416-6
12. Wasylewicz, A.T., Scheepers-Hoeks, A.: Clinical decision support systems. In: Fundamentals of Clinical Data Science, pp. 153–169. Springer (2019)
13. Huang, K., Altosaar, J., Ranganath, R.: ClinicalBERT: modeling clinical notes and predicting hospital readmission (2020). arXiv:1904.05342
14. Jiang, L.Y., et al.: Health system-scale language models are all-purpose prediction engines. Nature **619**, 357–362 (2023)
15. Yang, X., et al.: A large language model for electronic health records. NPJ Digit. Med. **5**, 194 (2022)
16. Luo, R., et al.: BioGPT: generative pre-trained transformer for biomedical text generation and mining. Brief. Bioinform. **23**, bbac409 (2022)
17. Zhang, X., et al.: Alpacare: instruction-tuned large language models for medical application (2023). arXiv:2310.14558
18. Lin, H., et al.: Beneath the surface: unveiling harmful memes with multimodal reasoning distilled from large language models. In: Findings of the Association for Computational Linguistics: EMNLP 2023, pp. 9114–9128 (2023)
19. Ho, N., Schmid, L., Yun, S.-Y.: Large language models are reasoning teachers. In: Proceedings of the 61st Annual Meeting of the Association for Computational Linguistics (Volume 1: Long Papers), pp. 14852–14882 (2023)
20. Yang, A., et al.: Qwen3 technical report (2025). arXiv:2505.09388
21. DeepSeek-AI, et al.: DeepSeek-R1: incentivizing reasoning capability in LLMs via reinforcement learning (2025). arXiv:2501.12948
22. Yang, A., et al.: Qwen2 technical report (2024). arXiv:2407.10671
23. Team GLM, et al.: ChatGLM: a family of large language models from GLM-130B to GLM-4 all tools (2024). arXiv:2406.12793
24. Yang, Z., et al.: Clinical assistant diagnosis for electronic medical record based on convolutional neural network. Sci. Rep. **8**, 6329 (2018). https://doi.org/10.1038/s41598-018-24389-w
25. Hu, E.J., et al.: LoRA: low-rank adaptation of large language models (2021). arXiv:2106.09685
26. Sahoo, P., et al.: A systematic survey of prompt engineering in large language models: techniques and applications (2024). arXiv:2402.07927
27. Graber, M.L.: The incidence of diagnostic error in medicine. BMJ Qual. Saf. **22**, ii21–ii27 (2013)
28. Gaube, S., et al.: Do as AI say: susceptibility in deployment of clinical decision-aids. NPJ Digit. Med. **4**, 31 (2021)
29. Singhal, K., et al.: Large language models encode clinical knowledge. Nature **620**, 172–180 (2023)
30. Cobbe, K., et al.: Training verifiers to solve math word problems (2021). arXiv:2110.14168
31. Jiang, P., et al.: Reasoning-enhanced healthcare predictions with knowledge graph community retrieval. In: International Conference on Learning Representations (ICLR) (2025)
32. Zhang, K., et al.: Graph-based structural knowledge-aware network for diagnosis assistant. Math. Biosci. Eng. **19**(10), 10533–10549 (2022)

33. Cui, Y., et al.: Revisiting pre-trained models for Chinese natural language processing. In: Findings of the Association for Computational Linguistics: EMNLP 2020, pp. 657–668 (2020)
34. Zhang, K., et al.: Knowledge-enabled diagnosis assistant based on obstetric EMRs and knowledge graph. In: Proceedings of the 19th China National Conference on Computational Linguistics. LNCS, vol. 12522, pp. 444–457 (2020)
35. Song, Y., et al.: Research on double-graphs knowledge-enhanced intelligent diagnosis. In: China Health Information Processing Conference, pp. 317–332. Springer Nature Singapore (2023)
36. Devlin, J., et al.: BERT: Pre-training of deep bidirectional transformers for language understanding. In: Proceedings of the 2019 Conference of the North American Chapter of the Association for Computational Linguistics: Human Language Technologies (Volume 1: Long and Short Papers), pp. 4171–4186 (2019)

Enabling AI Scientists to Recognize Innovation: A Domain-Agnostic Algorithm for Assessing Novelty

Yao Wang[1,2](✉), Mingxuan Cui[3], Arthur Jiang[2], and Jun Yan[4]

[1] Department of Automation, Tsinghua University, Beijing, China
wang-yao24@mails.tsinghua.edu.cn
[2] Yidu Technology, Beijing, China
[3] Nankai University, Tianjin, China
mingxuan.cui@mail.nankai.edu.cn
[4] Department of Biostatistics, City University of Hong Kong, Hong Kong, China
yan.jun@cityu.edu.hk

Abstract. As large language models (LLMs) demonstrate increasing capability in generating research ideas, automating novelty evaluation has become a critical challenge for AI-driven scientific discovery. This paper presents Relative Neighbor Density (RND), a domain-agnostic algorithm for novelty assessment in research ideas that overcomes the limitations of existing approaches by comparing an idea's local density with its adjacent neighbors' densities. We first developed a scalable methodology to create test sets without expert labeling, addressing a fundamental challenge in novelty assessment. Using these test sets, we demonstrate that our RND algorithm achieves state-of-the-art (SOTA) performance in computer science (AUROC=0.820) and biomedical research (AUROC=0.765) domains. Most significantly, while SOTA models like Sonnet-3.7 and existing metrics show domain-specific performance degradation, RND maintains consistent accuracies across domains by its domain-invariant property, outperforming all benchmarks by a substantial margin (0.795 v.s. 0.597) on cross-domain evaluation. These results validate RND as a generalizable solution for automated novelty assessment in scientific research.

Keywords: Novelty Assessment · Large Language Models · Relative Neighbor Density · AI Scientist · Domain-Agnostic Algorithms

1 Introduction

As AI research advances toward AGI, automating scientific discovery processes becomes increasingly important. While large language models (LLMs) now demonstrate capability in generating research ideas, such as AI scientist [9], a critical challenge remains in how to pick pearls from those generated ideas,

---

Mingxuan Cui did this work during his internship at Yidu Technology.

Y. Zhang et al. (Eds.): CHIP 2025, CCIS 2884, pp. 284–328, 2026.
https://doi.org/10.1007/978-981-95-7299-1_18

i.e., how to reliably evaluate these ideas for novelty. Traditionally, novelty in research ideas has been assessed through expert evaluation, where domain specialists judge originality based on their knowledge and experience. However, such assessments are inherently subjective, time-consuming, and inconsistent across evaluators. Automated methods for novelty assessment are therefore crucial for identifying truly innovative directions, particularly as AI systems begin to participate more actively in the research process.

Existing approaches primarily fall into two categories: (1) leveraging large language models (LLMs) as judges and (2) using absolute local density-based novelty metrics. LLM-based approaches include Swiss system tournaments [6, 14] and augmented judgment using NeurIPS review guidelines and Semantic Scholar API [9,16]. Alternatively, absolute local density metrics measure novelty through Euclidean distances between embeddings, as demonstrated by Su et al.'s Overall Novelty (ON) metric [16], which combines Historical Dissimilarity, Contemporary Dissimilarity, and citation-based Contemporary Impact, showing strong correlation with human-labeled novelty.

Despite these advances, significant challenges remain. First of all, in studies of any existing approach, the validation methodologies typically rely on small, domain-specific test sets with human-labeled data that quickly become outdated as research advances, limiting scalability and long-term accuracy. Additionally, the LLM-based judgment exhibits sensitivity to input perturbations [15,19], potentially yielding inconsistent novelty ratings for semantically identical ideas. Finally, absolute local density metrics suffer from arbitrary parameter choices and lack generalizability across research domains with varying citation patterns and publication velocities.

To address these challenges, we establish comprehensive semantic embedding databases for novelty assessment, incorporating publications from two distinct domains: Pubmed, the leading biomedical literature search engine with nearly 36 million articles [8], and Arxiv, which contains more than 2.3 million scholarly articles across eight subject areas [3]. Based on these resources, we develop a methodology to create test sets with trustworthy novelty labels without requiring expert manual labeling.

Furthermore, we propose the Relative Neighbor Density (RND) algorithm, which measures novelty by analyzing the distribution patterns of semantic neighbors rather than simple absolute local density (Fig. 1). This approach proves more reliable than LLM-based judgments and more generalizable than existing absolute local density-based metrics across different research domains. Our extensive evaluations using test sets from computer science, biomedical science, and cross-domain contexts demonstrate that our proposed algorithm maintains accuracy within specific domains while scaling effectively across diverse research areas.

Our main contributions are:

- A novel neighbor density-based Relative Neighbor Density (RND) algorithm for assessing research idea novelty that is robust across domains, which holds domain-invariant property

- A scalable methodology for validating novelty metrics without expert labeling
- Comprehensive evaluations comparing SOTA reasoning models, LLMs and algorithms for assessing novelty across multiple research domains

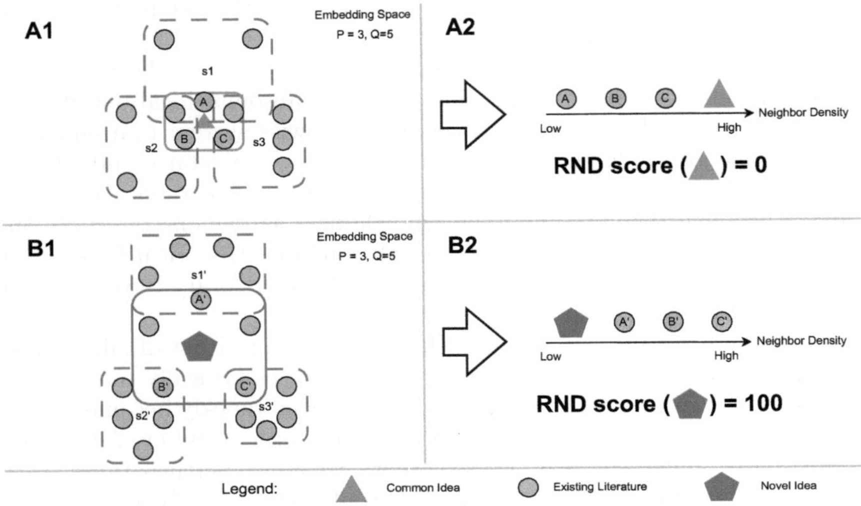

Fig. 1. Illustration of the Relative Neighbor Density (RND) algorithm. *A1/B1*: In this step, both the given idea (triangle in A1 and pentagon in B1) and all existing literature in a given research domain are represented in a semantic embedding space. The P nearest neighbors (A/B/C or A'/B'/C') of the given idea are identified. Then, for each of these neighbors, the neighbor density is computed by identifying Q nearest surrounding neighbors (neighbor sets s1–s3 in A1 and s1'–s3' in B1). *A2/B2*: The neighbor densities of the P closest pieces of literature and the given idea are sorted. The RND score of the given idea is determined based on its relative rank among these neighbor densities.

2 Related Works

2.1 LLMs for Novelty Assessment

Recent work has demonstrated promising results in using LLMs as autonomous judges for research novelty. Si et al. [14] evaluated this approach using ICLR submissions, converting them into standardized project proposals and conducting pairwise comparisons between accepted and rejected papers (Table 7). Their Swiss tournament system iteratively paired proposals based on accumulated scores, with Claude-3.5-Sonnet achieving 71.4% accuracy in predicting paper acceptance. As a control measure, they included human expert reranking, which revealed notable discrepancies between automated and human judgments.

Lu et al. [9] expanded this concept with their AI Scientist framework, integrating idea generation, evaluation, and refinement. Their system employs chain-of-thought prompting and external knowledge retrieval via Semantic Scholar API to enhance assessment quality. While showing promise in matching human-level performance, these LLM-based approaches face fundamental challenges in reliability and consistency, as highlighted by studies showing their sensitivity to input variations [15,19].

2.2 Absolute Local Density-based Metrics

An alternative approach focuses on semantic local density to evaluate novelty. Su et al. [16] used the Historical Dissimilarity (HD), which is the average Euclidean distance between the generated abstract embedding and embeddings of the 5 most similar abstracts in the historical literature base. We denote it as "Absolute Local Density" because the average distance is a metric of local density, and they use the value of density directly.

In addition to HD, they also developed Overall Novelty (ON) as below, where CI is Contemporary Impact, the average citation count of the top 5 most similar abstracts in contemporary literature base; CD is Contemporary Dissimilarity, calculated by same algorithm in contemporary literature base.

$$ON = \frac{HD \times CI}{CD} \tag{1}$$

The main challenge of local density-based metric is that the density values vary across different domains. In case of evaluating ideas from mixed research domains, the variance would cause a severe degrade in the accuracy.

2.3 Validating Novelty Metrics

A critical limitation in existing research is the lack of scalable validation methodologies. Current approaches [6,9,14,16] typically rely on small-size literature database and manually labeled test set created by domain experts. For instance, Su et al. [16] constructed an “ecosystem” for computer science (CS) using information extracted from 85,217 papers—a dataset that represents only a small fraction of the CS literature available on platforms like arXiv. While their analysis demonstrated promising correlations between novelty scores and human labels across 100 manually evaluated abstracts, the methodology's reliance on domain-specific expertise significantly constrains its generalizability, which is echoed by reviewer's comments that only validating CS is “relatively simple” [13].

3 Method

3.1 Problem Description

Given a set of ideas I,

$$I = \{idea_i\}, i \in [1, N] \tag{2}$$

Where $idea_i$ is a sequence of words or characters in nature language. $N \geq 1$ represents the number of ideas whose novelty needs to be assessed.

The objective is to design a mapping $\mathscr{F}$ from idea space to a score in real value space

$$F(idea_i) = score_i, \quad \text{where} \quad idea_i \in I,\, score_i \in \mathbb{R} \tag{3}$$

The novelty score score should be **monotonic**, meaning that for any two ideas idea_i and idea_j, if idea_i is more novel than idea_j, then their corresponding scores must satisfy:

$$\forall\, \text{idea}_i, \text{idea}_j \in I, \quad \text{idea}_i \succ \text{idea}_j \Rightarrow F(\text{idea}_i) > F(\text{idea}_j) \tag{4}$$

where $\text{idea}_i \succ \text{idea}_j$ denotes that idea_i is considered more novel than idea_j based on a given novelty criterion.

3.2 Semantic Embedding and Literature Database

Each published literature's abstract, which is also a sequence of words or characters in natural language, is denoted as a_j.

The semantic embedding model is a mapping function $\mathscr{G}$, which maps ideas and abstracts into embedding vectors:

$$\mathscr{G}(\text{idea}_i) = \mathbf{v}_i, \quad \text{where} \quad \mathbf{v}_i \in \mathbb{R}^{\text{dims}}, \tag{5}$$

$$\mathscr{G}(a_j) = \mathbf{v}_j, \quad \text{where} \quad \mathbf{v}_j \in \mathbb{R}^{\text{dims}} \tag{6}$$

Thus, the preprocessed literature semantic database is represented as a set A:

$$A = \{(a_j, \mathbf{v}_j) \mid j \in [1, M]\} \tag{7}$$

We collected 36 million academic articles from the PubMed Download API [11] and 2.6 million papers from the ArXiv dataset [4]. Among all fetched documents, only those with both a non-empty title and abstract were considered valid for the experiment, resulting in 25,360,114 papers from PubMed and 2,643,057 papers from ArXiv.

For each paper, two semantic embedding vectors were generated—one from its title and another from its abstract—using the M3-Embedding model [2]. The embedding vector dimension, denoted as *dims*, is 1024. All texts and embedding vectors were stored in Elasticsearch Version 8 for efficient retrieval.

3.3 Algorithm

For each idea idea_i and its embedding $\mathbf{v}_i$, we first find its P nearest neighbors using k-Nearest Neighbors (KNN) search:

$$\{\mathbf{v}_1, \mathbf{v}_2, \ldots, \mathbf{v}_P\} = KNN(\mathbf{v}_i, P, A) \tag{8}$$

where $\mathbf{v}_j$ is the j-th nearest neighbor of $\mathbf{v}_i$, $j \in [1, P]$.

For the idea itself $\mathbf{v}_i$ and each neighbor $\mathbf{v}_j$, the neighbor density (ND) is defined as below

$$ND = \frac{1}{Q}\sum_{k=1}^{Q} d(\mathbf{v}, \mathbf{v}_k) \tag{9}$$

where $\mathbf{v}_k$ denotes the k-th nearest article's embedding vector in the literature corpus A and $d(\cdot,\cdot)$ is the cosine distance between two vectors.

We define the set S_i that contains the neighbor density values of idea$_i$'s neighbors:

$$S_i = \{ND_j \mid j \in [1, P]\} \tag{10}$$

Finally, we compute the novelty score score$_i$ for idea$_i$ as:

$$\text{score}_i = \frac{|\{ND \in S_i \mid ND \leq ND_i\}|}{|S_i|} \times 100 \tag{11}$$

In Appendix A, the pseudocode for ND calculation is presented in Algorithm 1; and the pseudocode of complete algorithm is provided in Algorithm 2.

In this algorithm, the selection of values of P and Q is a trade-off between reliability of estimation and other cost. Refer to Appendix A for mathematical analysis and Sect. 4.3 for empirical experimental results. Based on analysis and empirical experiments, we set $P = 100$ and $Q = 50$.

3.4 Validation without Human Labeling

As a novelty evaluation algorithm, the most challenging point in past research is to find a reliable labeled test set to evaluate the algorithm. Therefore, we propose a new method to construct a convincing test set instead of relying on human experts to annotate it.

For the positive samples (a.k.a novel ideas) in the test set, we select recent articles from top journals or conferences. For the negative samples (a.k.a. non-novel ideas), highly cited articles published before the last few years were selected, also from the research domain's top journals or conferences. The fundamental principles behind such methodology were: high-quality novel ideas are more likely to be published in recent issues and top journals or conferences; while after time passes, the at-the-time novel ideas were more likely to attract attention and related works, thus become non-innovative at present.

4 Result

4.1 Experiment Setup

Test Set We have two test sets: NeurIPS, which represents the most advanced research results in the field of computer science, and Nature Medicine, which represents the most cutting-edge papers in the medical field. The sample year distribution of the test sets can be found in Table 1

NeurIPS test set: The initial corpus consists of papers that are Accept (oral) or Accept (spotlight) by Program Chairs at the 2024 NeurIPS conference, which represents the latest research results in computer science. Furthermore, we select articles from the initial corpus that explicitly mention that the papers have obvious novelty in the comments of Program Chairs to form the positive samples of the NeurIPS test set. The comments and decision information of Program Chairs can be obtained on the OpenReview.net website. At the same time, we use the Semantic Scholar API to obtain the 99 most cited papers published in the NeurIPS conference from 2015 to 2020 to form the negative samples of the test set. The titles of all samples are presented in Table 4

Nature Medicine test set: The positive samples of the Nature Medicine test set consist of articles classified as "Article" type, published in Nature Medicine from August 2024 to February 2025, according to the classification on the nature.com website. Articles related to phase 2 or phase 3 trials were excluded. And we used the same method as the negative samples of the NeurIPS test set to obtain 99 articles of Nature Medicine with the highest citation count in the past 15 years as negative samples of the test set. The titles of all samples are presented in Table 5

Mixed Test set: The mixed test set is the combination of the negative samples from NeurIPS and positive samples from Nature Medicine.

Table 1. Count of data in different time ranges for NeurIPS and nature medicine test sets. *Positive*: novel samples, *Negative*: non-novel samples.

Test set	Label	Count				
		Total	2024–2025	2019–2023	2014–2018	–2014
NeurIPS	Positive	80	80	0	0	0
	Negative	99	0	31	68	0
Nature medicine	Positive	66	66	0	0	0
	Negative	99	0	29	32	38

Baseline To evaluate our algorithm, we selected all existing novelty assessment algorithms as baselines, categorized into two groups: LLM-based and non-LLM-based. Non-LLM-based algorithms, including Relative Neighbor Density(Ours), Historical Dissimilarity(HD), and Overall Novelty(ON), rely solely on literature search and mathematical calculations. Since the output of the literature search for the same query remains consistent, we conducted a single test to assess the algorithm's performance. In contrast, for LLM-based algorithms, due to the inherent variability of LLM outputs, we ran three tests for each algorithm, calculated the average result, and included the standard deviation in the results.

For all algorithms tested, we use the abstracts of the papers as "ideas" for testing.

Table 2. AUROC Comparison of different models across research domains. Results for our proposed RND algorithm are compared against absolute local density metrics and various LLM-based configurations.

Model		NeurIPS	Nature medicine	Mixed
Relative neighbor density (Ours)		0.820	**0.765**	**0.795**
Absolute local density	HD	**0.856**	0.699	0.362
	ON	0.584	0.544	0.456
LLM + Literature search	Sonnet-3.7	0.813 ± 0.01	0.616 ± 0.006	0.597 ± 0.004
	Deepseek-R1	0.710 ± 0.027	0.673 ± 0.025	0.596 ± 0.049
	GPT-4o	0.567 ± 0.008	0.545 ± 0.02	0.522 ± 0.022
Sonnet-3.7 with guideline		0.546 ± 0.035	NaN	NaN
Sonnet-3.7 with tournament		0.496 ± 0.001	0.503 ± 0.005	0.501 ± 0.004

Historical Dissimilarity (HD) & **Overall Novelty (ON)**: Both HD and ON are described in Sect. 2.2. During calculation, the historical database contains papers from 2011 to 2021, and the contemporary database contains papers from 2021 to 2025.

LLM + literature search: Provide LLM with the titles and abstracts of the 10 most relevant papers to the given idea. The model then assesses whether the core concepts of these papers significantly overlap with the idea (Table 8). Sonnet-3.7 [1], Deepseek-r1 [5] and GPT-4o [7] were selected as the LLMs to be tested.

LLM with guideline: Utilize the NeurIPS 2024 review guidelines to assist LLM in evaluating the novelty of ideas (Table 6). Sonnet-3.7 is selected as the LLM to be tested.

LLM with tournament: First, the idea is transformed into the Standardized Project Proposal format(Table 7). Next, the novelty of all standardized ideas is assessed using the Swiss tournament method, where ideas are iteratively compared in a structured competition. Finally, each idea is assigned a score based on the number of wins it accumulates throughout the tournament. Sonnet-3.7 is selected as the LLM to be tested.

4.2 Accuracy Evaluation

As shown in Table 2, our enhanced neighbor density-based novelty measurement algorithm outperforms all baseline models on the Nature Medicine and Mixed test sets, and performs strongly on the NeurIPS test set.

By comparing the results of various LLM-related algorithms, we find that both **Sonnet-3.7 with guideline** and **Sonnet-3.7 with tournament** show limited external knowledge input, leading to inaccurate novelty judgments. In contrast, the **LLM + literature search** method, which incorporates the 10 most relevant papers based on semantic embedding, significantly improves accuracy. This method shows a higher AUROC in computer science than in biomedicine, highlighting the impact of the model's internal knowledge on judgment outcomes.

Additionally, Sonnet-3.7 and Deepseek-r1 outperform GPT-4o, suggesting that external knowledge enhances the performance of the inference model compared to autoregressive models.

We also observed that the Historical Dissimilarity (HD) metric performed similarly to our method on the Nature Medicine and NeurIPS test sets. However, on the Mixed test set, there was a significant disparity, with our method achieving an AUROC of 0.795, while HD reached only 0.362. This difference reflects the limited generalization ability of HD across domains. In contrast, the distributions of our method's scores are consistent across all test sets, indicating its robust cross-domain evaluation capability, making it applicable to various research fields.

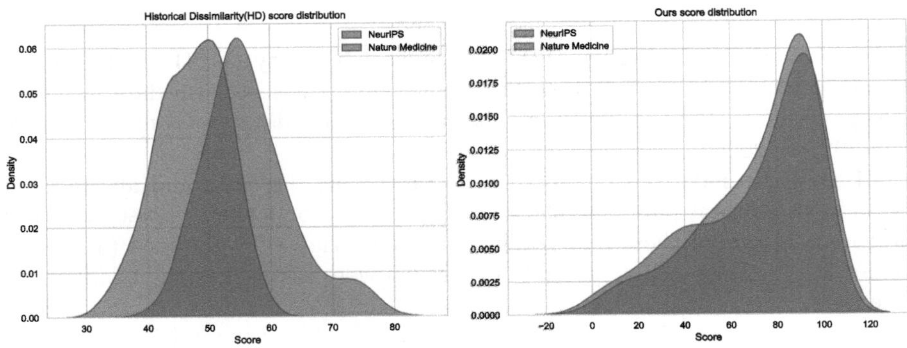

Fig. 2. Comparison of HD & Our score distributions in different domains. *1*: In the right panel, the upper and lower bounds of the score exceeded the actual score range ([0, 100]) because of linear interpolation. *2*: to make the horizontal axis comparable, we scaled the Historical Dissimilarity scores by ×100.

4.3 Sensitivity Study

Sensitivity of Hyper-Parameter As illustrated in the left panel of Fig. 3, the AUROC on each test set increases as P grows. However, when $P > 50$, the improvement in AUROC becomes marginal compared to the significant gain observed when increasing P from 10 to 50. This suggests that the marginal benefit of further increasing P diminishes while simultaneously incurring substantial computational costs, given that the algorithm's time complexity is $O(P \cdot Q)$. Additionally, the poor performance observed when $P = 10$ can be attributed to the biased estimation of novelty scores when P is too small, a phenomenon influenced by multiple factors. For a more detailed explanation, please refer to Appendix A.2.

The right panel of Fig. 3 demonstrates that when P remains constant, both excessively small and large values of Q negatively impact the algorithm's performance. This is due to the inaccuracy in local density estimation when Q is too small and the significant reduction in algorithm sensitivity when Q is too large. For further details, please refer to Appendix A.3.

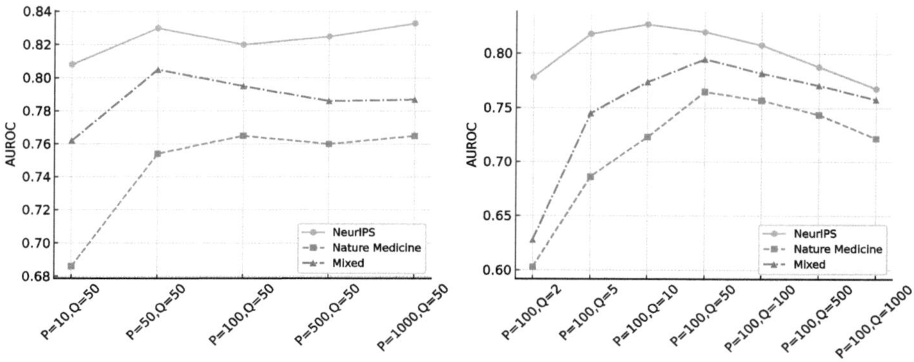

Fig. 3. Comparison of AUROC of RND algorithm with different parameters. *left*: AUROC with different P value when Q=50. *right*: AUROC with different Q value when P=100.

Sensitivity of Design In our Relative Neighbor Density algorithm, the notion "relative", i.e. comparing idea's local density with its neighbor's local densities, plays an important role. Moreover, other distance metric, such as Euclidean distance, could also be used in our algorithm. To understand the sensitivity of the current design, we conducted experiments by changing the design of the "relative" notion, and distance metric. The result presented in Table 3 validate our statement.

Table 3. AUROC comparison for different design. *Absolute local density*: Use the idea's local density as novelty score. (density calculated by mean distances between idea and idea's P first level neighbors). *Euclidean distance*: replace the cosine distance with Euclidean in RND

Test set	AUROC		
	Ours	Absolute local density	Euclidean distance
NeurIPS	0.820	**0.851**	0.815
Nature medicine	**0.765**	0.757	0.753
Mixed	**0.795**	0.395	0.78

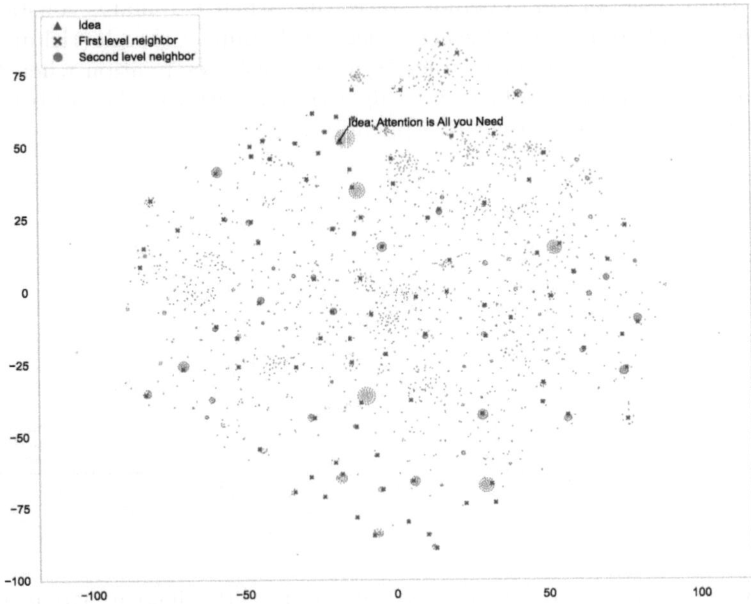

Fig. 4. Neighbor distribution of a non-novel idea in embedding space (t-SNE processed)

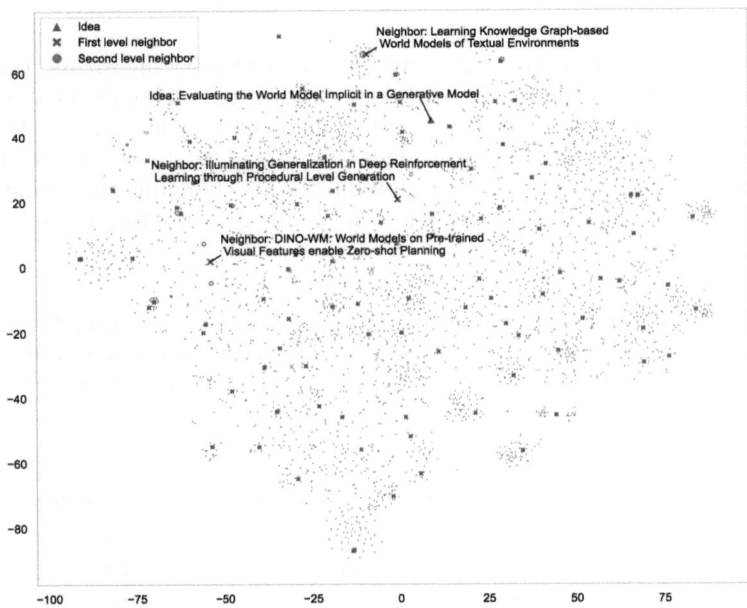

Fig. 5. Neighbor Distribution of a Novel Idea in Embedding Space (t-SNE processed).

4.4 Case Study

To visualize the geometric structure of ideas and their neighboring points in the embedding space, we selected two ideas and plotted their surrounding neighbors on a 2-D plane using t-SNE [10].

We first examine *Attention is All You Need* [18], a highly cited article, as an example of a non-novel idea from the current perspective. As shown in Figure 4, there is a dense cluster of neighbors surrounding the idea, while the neighbors around its P nearest neighbors are relatively fewer and more sparsely distributed.

Next, we analyze *Evaluating the World Model Implicit in a Generative Model* [17], an article recognized as highly novel by the NeurIPS 2024 Program Chairs based on their comments [12]. In Fig. 5, the idea's local neighborhood appears considerably sparser than that of its P nearest neighbors.

Moreover, the differences between the two figures extend beyond the local density around the central idea; the local densities of neighboring ideas also exhibit distinct patterns. In Fig. 4, multiple neighboring clusters centered around the idea's P nearest neighbors are visible, whereas such clustering patterns are absent in the novel idea's neighborhood. These observations suggest that an idea's novelty is associated not only with its own local density but also with the density distribution of its neighboring ideas.

5 Discussion

In this work, we proposed a novel neighbor density-based metric for assessing research idea novelty, addressing the limitations of LLM judgment and absolute local density-based metrics. By leveraging large-scale literature embeddings from both biomedical sciences and computer science, our approach ensures robust reliability and cross-domain generalizability. Additionally, we introduced a scalable validation framework that eliminates reliance on expert labeling, enabling objective and reproducible novelty assessment.

5.1 Why a Non-LLM Novelty Assessment Algorithm is Necessary?

While LLMs have the potential to assess novelty, the reliability of their judgment is limited, as outlined in the Introduction section (1). Our experiments (see Table 2) echoed such concern: without an integrated search tool, even the most advanced reasoning models' performance was comparable to random guessing (AUROC$\doteq$0.5). When a search tool was introduced, Sonnet-3.7 achieved similar accuracy on the NeurIPS test set (AUROC$\doteq$0.8) but experienced significant degradation (AUROC$\doteq$0.6) on both the Nature Medicine and cross-domain test sets.

In contrast, our proposed RND algorithm can produce more reliable and consistent results, as seen in Table 2. Additionally, our algorithm is better at distinguishing genuinely novel ideas from the large pool of candidates from mixing research domains (AUROC$\doteq$0.78 v.s Other's AUROC<=0.6). Such cross-domain novelty assessment capability is crucial to AI scientist, as more and more innovation happens in the intersection of research domains.

5.2 Domain-invariant Accuracy

The most significant advantage of RND algorithm is in being able to accurately compare novelty across different domains.

As demonstrated in the Table 3, though local density-based HD algorithm and LLM with literature search tools achieved 0.8+ AUROC in NeruIPS test set, their performance degraded in Nature Medicine test set (0.699 for HD, 0.673 for Deepseek-r1). Moreover, when tested in the cross-domain test set (the Mixed test set), the AUROC of HD and LLM significantly degraded below 0.6. In contrast, the AUROC of our proposed RND algorithm remained robust (0.820, 0.765, 0.795) across each single domain and mixed domain test sets.

We argue that such benefits come from RND algorithm's **domain-invariant property**, i.e. the distribution of novelty scores produced by RND is identical regardless of the tested domain, which explained why our relative density-based approach succeeds in cross-domain scenarios. According to the mathematical reasoning in Appendix A.4, we concluded the distribution of novelty score S is only subject to P (the number of neighbors considered); thus it is invariant to the validation domain. Furthermore, in Figure 2 (right panel) and Fig. 6, the actual distribution of scores echoed the theoretical analysis. Such domain-invariant property is crucial for conducting multi-disciplinary scientific research, where ideas from diverse fields must be compared and evaluated effectively.

5.3 Limitations and Future Work

First, the RND algorithm's effectiveness is inherently linked to the breadth and quality of the underlying literature database and semantic embedding model. Incomplete literature coverage or suboptimal embedding quality can impact novelty assessment accuracy. While implementing RND requires more infrastructure than LLM-as-judge approaches, this investment enables consistent, deterministic assessments that remain stable across model versions and prompting strategies.

Second, in the test set created by our validation methodology, while the need for expert labeling was avoided, the non-novel samples may be too easily distinguishable from novel ones. By using historical highly-cited papers as non-novel examples, rather than borderline cases such as recently rejected papers or incremental work from current journals, we created a simpler assessment scenario than the actual scenario in real research settings. However, the fact that none of the tested algorithms achieved saturated AUROCs even in this relatively straightforward scenario demonstrates the fundamental challenge of novelty assessment.

While acknowledging these limitations, we believe our work establishes a solid foundation for several promising research directions that could significantly advance automated scientific discovery.

1. Integration with AI Research Workflows: Incorporating our novelty evaluation algorithm into end-to-end AI scientist workflows would enable autonomous research ideation and evaluation. This integration would allow AI systems to independently generate research hypotheses, assess their novelty using our

domain-invariant RND algorithm, and prioritize the most promising directions for further investigation. Such integration could accelerate scientific discovery by efficiently navigating complex multi-disciplinary research landscapes where human intuition about novelty is often limited.

2. Enhancing Reasoning Capability for LLM: We propose utilizing our RND algorithm as a sophisticated reward mechanism within reinforcement learning frameworks for training reasoning models for AI research. By providing domain-invariant novelty signals during training, it could potentially guide models to generate more innovative scientific ideas while maintaining scientific validity.

A Appendix 1: Algorithms

A.1 Pseudocode

Algorithm 1 Find Neighbors and Calculate Neighbor Density

function NEIGHBOR(Input, P, Q)
  $\mathbf{v}_{Input} \leftarrow$ GET_EMBEDDING(Input) ▷ Using M3-Embedding model
  $C \leftarrow []$
  neighbors $\leftarrow$ GET_NEIGHBORS($\mathbf{v}_{Input}$, $\max(P, Q)$) ▷ Find $\max(P, Q)$ nearest neighbors
  neighbors_for_count $\leftarrow$ *neighbors*[: Q] ▷ Only use the Q nearest neighbors to calculate density
  neighbors_for_distribution $\leftarrow$ *neighbors*[: P] ▷ The P nearest neighbors are used to calculate distribution
  for each paper in *neighbors_for_count* **do**
    $\mathbf{v}_{paper} \leftarrow$ GET_EMBEDDING(paper)
    distance $\leftarrow$ 1 - COSINE_SIMILARITY($\mathbf{v}_{Input}, \mathbf{v}_{paper}$)
    C.Append(*distance*)
  end for
  $ND_{Input} \leftarrow$ MEAN(C)
  return ND_{Input}, *neighbors_for_distribution*
end function

Algorithm 2 Calculate Novelty Score of Given Idea

Input: Idea
Output: A score in the range of 0 to 100
$D \leftarrow []$
ND_{Idea}, *neighbors* $\leftarrow$ NEIGHBOR(Idea, P, Q)
for paper in *neighbors* **do**
  $ND_{paper}, \_ \leftarrow$ NEIGHBOR(paper, P, Q)
  D.Append(ND_{paper})
end for
$score \leftarrow \frac{|\{ND \in D | ND \leq ND_{Idea}\}|}{|D|} \times 100$
Return *score*

A.2 Effects of Parameter P

The novelty score is computed as

$$\text{score}_i = \frac{|\{ND \in S_i \mid ND \leq ND_i\}|}{P} \times 100, \tag{12}$$

where $S_i = \{ND_j \mid j = 1, 2, \ldots, P\}$ is the set of neighbor densities for the P nearest neighbors of the idea i, and ND_i is the neighbor density for idea i itself.

1. Empirical Cumulative Distribution Function (ECDF) Interpretation Define the empirical cumulative distribution function (ECDF) for the set S_i as

$$F_P(x) = \frac{1}{P} \sum_{j=1}^{P} \mathbf{1}_{\{ND_j \leq x\}},$$

where $\mathbf{1}_{\{ND_j \leq x\}}$ is the indicator function that is 1 if $ND_j \leq x$ and 0 otherwise. Then, by definition, the novelty score can be written as

$$\text{score}_i = 100 \cdot F_P(ND_i). \tag{13}$$

2. Consistency of the ECDF Let $F(x)$ be the true cumulative distribution function of the neighbor densities (assumed to be i.i.d. samples from a distribution F). By the Glivenko-Cantelli theorem, the ECDF $F_P(x)$ converges uniformly to $F(x)$ as $P \to \infty$:

$$\sup_x |F_P(x) - F(x)| \xrightarrow{P \to \infty} 0.$$

Thus, for a sufficiently large P, we have

$$F_P(ND_i) \approx F(ND_i). \tag{14}$$

This shows that the score, being proportional to $F_P(ND_i)$, converges to $100 \cdot F(ND_i)$, which is the true quantile of ND_i in the distribution of neighbor densities.

3. Variance and Sensitivity with Finite P For a finite sample size P, $F_P(ND_i)$ is a random variable whose variance depends on P. Under the assumption of i.i.d. sampling,

$$\mathrm{Var}(F_P(ND_i)) = \frac{F(ND_i)(1 - F(ND_i))}{P}.$$

Thus, the standard deviation is proportional to $\frac{1}{\sqrt{P}}$. This quantifies that:

- **Smaller P** : The variance $\mathrm{Var}(F_P(ND_i))$ is larger, leading to a noisier (less reliable) estimation of the quantile, and hence of the novelty score.
- **Larger P** : The variance decreases, yielding a more accurate estimation of the true quantile $F(ND_i)$.

The novelty score becomes less sensitive to random fluctuations when P is large, as the empirical quantile is a better estimator of the true quantile.

4. Discreteness of the Score for Small P When P is small, the possible values of $F_P(ND_i)$ are discrete, specifically:

$$F_P(ND_i) \in \left\{0, \frac{1}{P}, \frac{2}{P}, \ldots, 1\right\}.$$

For instance, if $P = 1$, then $F_1(ND_i)$ can only be 0 or 1, corresponding to a score of either 0% or 100%. This coarse granularity can result in a biased or uninformative measure of novelty. As P increases, the steps $\frac{1}{P}$ become finer, allowing the score to capture more subtle differences in the density distribution.

Conclusion The parameter P affects the final novelty score in two major ways:

1. **Accuracy:** As P increases, the empirical cumulative distribution $F_P(x)$ better approximates the true cumulative distribution $F(x)$, leading to a more accurate quantile estimate $F(ND_i)$.
2. **Variance:** The variance of the estimate $F_P(ND_i)$ is proportional to $\frac{1}{P}$. Thus, a larger P reduces the variability of the score, making it less sensitive to random noise.

In summary, a higher P leads to a more robust and sensitive measure of novelty, while a smaller P results in a discrete and noisier estimate.

A.3 Effects of Parameter Q

The neighbor density (ND) is given by:

$$ND = \frac{1}{Q} \sum_{k=1}^{Q} d_k, \tag{15}$$

where $d_k = d(\mathbf{v}, \mathbf{v}_k)$ represents the distance between the point $\mathbf{v}$ and its k-th nearest neighbor.

Assuming that d_k are independent and identically distributed (i.i.d.) random variables with mean $\mathbb{E}[d_k] = \mu_d$, we compute the expectation of ND:

$$\mathbb{E}[ND] = \mathbb{E}\left[\frac{1}{Q}\sum_{k=1}^{Q} d_k\right] = \frac{1}{Q}\sum_{k=1}^{Q}\mathbb{E}[d_k] = \frac{1}{Q}Q\mu_d = \mu_d. \tag{16}$$

The variance of ND is given by:

$$\text{Var}(ND) = \text{Var}\left(\frac{1}{Q}\sum_{k=1}^{Q} d_k\right). \tag{17}$$

Using the property that the variance of the mean of Q i.i.d. random variables is:

$$\text{Var}\left(\frac{1}{Q}\sum_{k=1}^{Q} d_k\right) = \frac{1}{Q^2}\sum_{k=1}^{Q}\text{Var}(d_k). \tag{18}$$

Since each d_k has variance σ_d^2, we obtain:

$$\text{Var}(ND) = \frac{Q\sigma_d^2}{Q^2} = \frac{\sigma_d^2}{Q}. \tag{19}$$

Interpretation of Variance Scaling The derived formula:

$$\text{Var}(ND) = \frac{\sigma_d^2}{Q} \tag{20}$$

shows that:

- As Q increases, the variance of ND decreases.
- Specifically, variance scales inversely with Q, meaning that larger Q results in a more stable estimate of ND.
- When $Q \to \infty$, $\text{Var}(ND) \to 0$, indicating that ND converges to its expected value μ_d, which would cause lost of information on local density.
- For small Q, ND exhibits higher variability, making it more sensitive to local fluctuations.

A.4 Domain-Invariant

Theoretical Analysis Consider a test set in which each idea is assigned a neighborhood density defined as

$$ND = \frac{1}{Q}\sum_{i=1}^{Q} d(\text{idea}, a_i), \tag{21}$$

where a_i denotes the ith nearest article in the literature corpus and $d(\cdot,\cdot)$ is the cosine distance.

Let $F(x)$ be the cumulative distribution function (CDF) of the neighborhood densities in the literature corpus. The percentile score for an idea is then defined by

$$S = F(ND). \tag{22}$$

By the probability integral transform, if ND is drawn from a distribution with CDF $F(x)$, then

$$S \sim \mathcal{U}(0,1). \tag{23}$$

In practice, $F(x)$ is estimated empirically using P articles from the neighborhood. The empirical CDF is given by

$$\hat{F}_P(x) = \frac{1}{P}\sum_{j=1}^{P} \mathbf{1}\{ND_j \leq x\}, \tag{24}$$

where ND_j is the neighborhood density of the jth article, and $\mathbf{1}\{\cdot\}$ is the indicator function. Since

$$\sum_{j=1}^{P} \mathbf{1}\{ND_j \leq x\} \sim \text{Binomial}(P, F(x)), \tag{25}$$

we have

$$\mathbb{E}[\hat{F}_P(x)] = F(x) \quad \text{and} \quad \text{Var}[\hat{F}_P(x)] = \frac{F(x)(1-F(x))}{P}. \tag{26}$$

Now, consider two literature corpora: a medical corpus with density distribution $F_M(x)$ and a computer science corpus with density distribution $F_C(x)$. For an idea in the test set, define its scores as

$$\hat{S}_M = \hat{F}_M(ND_M) \quad \text{and} \quad \hat{S}_C = \hat{F}_C(ND_C), \tag{27}$$

where ND_M and ND_C are the neighborhood densities computed using the respective corpora. According to equation 26, we have

$$\mathbb{E}[\hat{S}] = F(ND) \quad \text{and} \quad \text{Var}[\hat{S}] = \frac{F(ND)(1-F(ND))}{P}. \tag{28}$$

where $F(ND) \sim \mathcal{U}(0,1)$, which implies

$$\hat{S}_M \stackrel{d}{=} \hat{S}_C. \tag{29}$$

Furthermore, note that the variance of the empirical estimate $\hat{F}_P(x)$ is solely a function of P:

$$\text{Var}[\hat{F}_P(x)] = \frac{F(x)(1-F(x))}{P}. \tag{30}$$

Thus, when P changes (e.g., $P = 50$, 100, or 500), the change in variance—and hence the fluctuation in the score—is proportional to $\frac{1}{P}$ and is independent of the corpus. In other words,

$$\Delta \,\mathrm{Var} \propto \frac{1}{P}, \tag{31}$$

which holds for both the medical and the computer science datasets.

Therefore, we conclude that:

$$\boxed{\hat{S}_M \overset{d}{=} \hat{S}_C \quad \text{and} \quad \Delta\hat{S} \propto \frac{1}{P}.} \tag{32}$$

This establishes that the scoring distributions for the test set are identical across corporas, and the effect of changing P on the score variation is equivalent for all datasets.

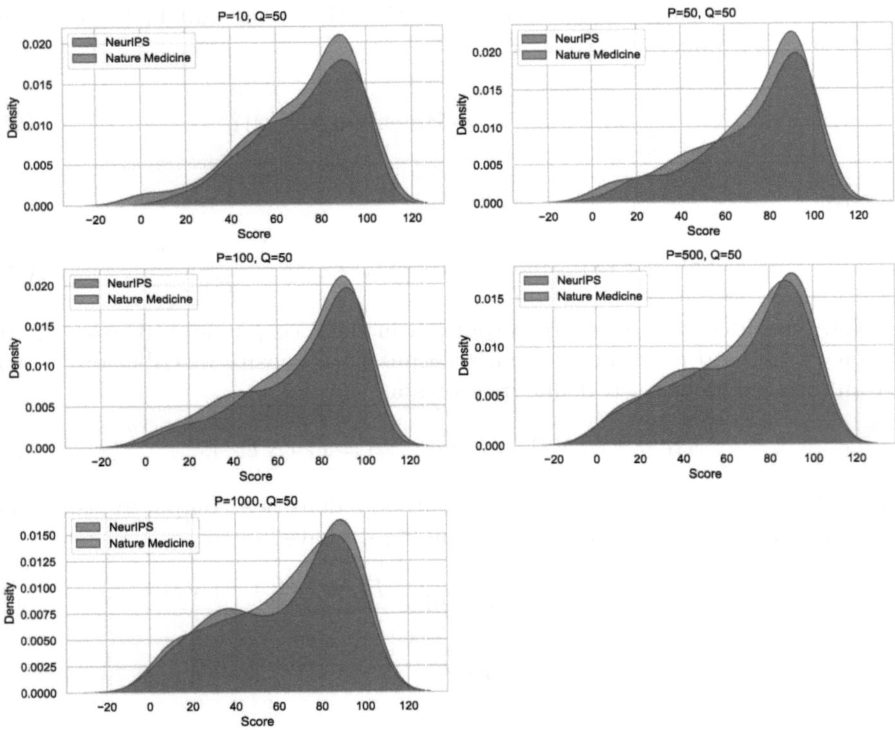

Fig. 6. Score Distribution of RND algorithm with different P value.

Experimental Evidence

B Appendix 2: Test Set

B.1 NeurIPS Test Set

Table 4. Titles of novel (Positive) and non-novel (Negative) papers in NeurIPS test set

NeurIPS Test Set	
Positive	**Negative**
1. Learning to grok: Emergence of in-context learning and skill composition in modular arithmetic tasks	1. Attention is All you Need
2. Nonlocal Attention Operator: Materializing Hidden Knowledge Towards Interpretable Physics Discovery	2. PyTorch: An Imperative Style, High-Performance Deep Learning Library
3. Emergence of Hidden Capabilities: Exploring Learning Dynamics in Concept Space	3. Language Models are Few-Shot Learners
4. Continual learning with the neural tangent ensemble	4. A Unified Approach to Interpreting Model Predictions
5. Neglected Hessian component explains mysteries in sharpness regularization	5. Inductive Representation Learning on Large Graphs
6. Generalization Analysis for Label-Specific Representation Learning	6. Denoising Diffusion Probabilistic Models
7. The Power of Resets in Online Reinforcement Learning	7. GANs Trained by a Two Time-Scale Update Rule Converge to a Local Nash Equilibrium
8. Paths to Equilibrium in Games	8. PointNet++: Deep Hierarchical Feature Learning on Point Sets in a Metric Space
9. Double-Ended Synthesis Planning with Goal-Constrained Bidirectional Search	9. LightGBM: A Highly Efficient Gradient Boosting Decision Tree
10. Time-Reversal Provides Unsupervised Feedback to LLMs	10. Improved Training of Wasserstein GANs
11. Compositional Generalization Across Distributional Shifts with Sparse Tree Operations	11. Improved Techniques for Training GANs
12. Stable Minima Cannot Overfit in Univariate ReLU Networks: Generalization by Large Step Sizes	12. XLNet: Generalized Autoregressive Pretraining for Language Understanding

(*continued*)

Table 4. (*continued*)

NeurIPS Test Set

Positive	Negative
13. Rule Extrapolation in Language Modeling: A Study of Compositional Generalization on OOD Prompts	13. Prototypical Networks for Few-shot Learning
14. A generalized neural tangent kernel for surrogate gradient learning	14. Convolutional LSTM Network: A Machine Learning Approach for Precipitation Nowcasting
15. GREATS: Online Selection of High-Quality Data for LLM Training in Every Iteration	15. Convolutional Neural Networks on Graphs with Fast Localized Spectral Filtering
16. Non-Asymptotic Uncertainty Quantification in High-Dimensional Learning	16. Spatial Transformer Networks
17. Boosting Vision-Language Models with Transduction	17. Matching Networks for One Shot Learning
18. Input-to-State Stable Coupled Oscillator Networks for Closed-form Model-based Control in Latent Space	18. Learning both Weights and Connections for Efficient Neural Network
19. Assouad, Fano, and Le Cam with Interaction: A Unifying Lower Bound Framework and Characterization for Bandit Learnability	19. Bootstrap Your Own Latent: A New Approach to Self-Supervised Learning
20. Exploring Jacobian Inexactness in Second-Order Methods for Variational Inequalities: Lower Bounds, Optimal Algorithms and Quasi-Newton Approximations	20. Character-level Convolutional Networks for Text Classification
21. Who's asking? User personas and the mechanics of latent misalignment	21. R-FCN: Object Detection via Region-based Fully Convolutional Networks
22. Self-Consuming Generative Models with Curated Data Provably Optimize Human Preferences	22. Simple and Scalable Predictive Uncertainty Estimation using Deep Ensembles
23. Selective Generation for Controllable Language Models	23. wav2vec 2.0: A Framework for Self-Supervised Learning of Speech Representations

(*continued*)

Table 4. (*continued*)

NeurIPS Test Set

Positive	Negative
24. Constrained Adaptive Attack: Effective Adversarial Attack Against Deep Neural Networks for Tabular Data	24. Neural Ordinary Differential Equations
25. Learning Generalized Linear Programming Value Functions	25. Dynamic Routing Between Capsules
26. Optimizing Automatic Differentiation with Deep Reinforcement Learning	26. What Uncertainties Do We Need in Bayesian Deep Learning for Computer Vision?
27. Overcoming Common Flaws in the Evaluation of Selective Classification Systems	27. Retrieval-Augmented Generation for Knowledge-Intensive NLP Tasks
28. Revisiting K-mer Profile for Effective and Scalable Genome Representation Learning	28. Neural Discrete Representation Learning
29. Trading Place for Space: Increasing Location Resolution Reduces Contextual Capacity in Hippocampal Codes	29. InfoGAN: Interpretable Representation Learning by Information Maximizing Generative Adversarial Nets
30. Reproducibility of predictive networks for mouse visual cortex	30. Multi-Agent Actor-Critic for Mixed Cooperative-Competitive Environments
31. Nonlinear dynamics of localization in neural receptive fields	31. Supervised Contrastive Learning
32. Learning Noisy Halfspaces with a Margin: Massart is No Harder than Random	32. Equality of Opportunity in Supervised Learning
33. Cracking the Code of Juxtaposition: Can AI Models Understand the Humorous Contradictions	33. Unsupervised Learning of Visual Features by Contrasting Cluster Assignments
34. Evaluating the World Model Implicit in a Generative Model	34. Mean teachers are better role models: Weight-averaged consistency targets improve semi-supervised deep learning results
35. TrackIME: Enhanced Video Point Tracking via Instance Motion Estimation	35. Teaching Machines to Read and Comprehend

(*continued*)

Table 4. (*continued*)

NeurIPS Test Set	
Positive	**Negative**
36. DiffLight: A Partial Rewards Conditioned Diffusion Model for Traffic Signal Control with Missing Data	36. ViLBERT: Pretraining Task-Agnostic Visiolinguistic Representations for Vision-and-Language Tasks
37. Mean-Field Langevin Dynamics for Signed Measures via a Bilevel Approach	37. Convolutional Networks on Graphs for Learning Molecular Fingerprints
38. Stabilized Proximal-Point Methods for Federated Optimization	38. Generative Modeling by Estimating Gradients of the Data Distribution
39. Reparameterization invariance in approximate Bayesian inference	39. FixMatch: Simplifying Semi-Supervised Learning with Consistency and Confidence
40. Disentangling the Roles of Distinct Cell Classes with Cell-Type Dynamical Systems	40. Learning Structured Output Representation using Deep Conditional Generative Models
41. Linear Regression using Heterogeneous Data Batches	41. Glow: Generative Flow with Invertible 1x1 Convolutions
42. A Near-optimal Algorithm for Learning Margin Halfspaces with Massart Noise	42. CatBoost: unbiased boosting with categorical features
43. Neural Krylov Iteration for Accelerating Linear System Solving	43. Man is to Computer Programmer as Woman is to Homemaker? Debiasing Word Embeddings
44. Human Expertise in Algorithmic Prediction	44. Neural Tangent Kernel: Convergence and Generalization in Neural Networks
45. Analysing Multi-Task Regression via Random Matrix Theory with Application to Time Series Forecasting	45. Generative Adversarial Imitation Learning
46. No-regret Learning in Harmonic Games: Extrapolation in the Face of Conflicting Interests	46. Pointer Networks
47. Learning diffusion at lightspeed	47. BinaryConnect: Training Deep Neural Networks with binary weights during propagations
48. Voila-A: Aligning Vision-Language Models with User's Gaze Attention	48. MixMatch: A Holistic Approach to Semi-Supervised Learning

(*continued*)

Table 4. (*continued*)

NeurIPS Test Set	
Positive	**Negative**
49. Barely Random Algorithms and Collective Metrical Task Systems	49. Unsupervised Image-to-Image Translation Networks
50. Goal Reduction with Loop-Removal Accelerates RL and Models Human Brain Activity in Goal-Directed Learning	50. Deep Reinforcement Learning from Human Preferences
51. BricksRL: A Platform for Democratizing Robotics and Reinforcement Learning Research and Education with LEGO	51. Cross-lingual Language Model Pretraining
52. Breaking Long-Tailed Learning Bottlenecks: A Controllable Paradigm with Hypernetwork-Generated Diverse Experts	52. Attention-Based Models for Speech Recognition
53. Kermut: Composite kernel regression for protein variant effects	53. End-To-End Memory Networks
54. Automatically Learning Hybrid Digital Twins of Dynamical Systems	54. Gradient Episodic Memory for Continual Learning
55. On the Identifiability of Poisson Branching Structural Causal Model Using Probability Generating Function	55. Open Graph Benchmark: Datasets for Machine Learning on Graphs
56. Weisfeiler and Leman Go Loopy: A New Hierarchy for Graph Representational Learning	56. Conditional Image Generation with PixelCNN Decoders
57. Unlocking the Capabilities of Thought: A Reasoning Boundary Framework to Quantify and Optimize Chain-of-Thought	57. Generalized Cross Entropy Loss for Training Deep Neural Networks with Noisy Labels
58. Reinforcement Learning Under Latent Dynamics: Toward Statistical and Algorithmic Modularity	58. Skip-Thought Vectors
59. Generalization Error Bounds for Two-stage Recommender Systems with Tree Structure	59. Self-Normalizing Neural Networks
60. Can Transformers Smell Like Humans?	60. PointCNN: Convolution On X-Transformed Points

(*continued*)

Table 4. (*continued*)

NeurIPS Test Set

Positive	**Negative**
61. Geodesic Optimization for Predictive Shift Adaptation on EEG data	61. Learning Structured Sparsity in Deep Neural Networks
62. Second-order forward-mode optimization of recurrent neural networks for neuroscience	62. Implicit Neural Representations with Periodic Activation Functions
63. Discrete Flow Matching	63. Deep Generative Image Models using a Laplacian Pyramid of Adversarial Networks
64. Motion Forecasting in Continuous Driving	64. Hindsight Experience Replay
65. Moving Off-the-Grid: Scene-Grounded Video Representations	65. Unsupervised Data Augmentation for Consistency Training
66. Aligner: Efficient Alignment by Learning to Correct	66. Conditional Adversarial Domain Adaptation
67. Questioning the Survey Responses of Large Language Models	67. SuperGLUE: A Stickier Benchmark for General-Purpose Language Understanding Systems
68. Saliency-driven Experience Replay for Continual Learning	68. Big Self-Supervised Models are Strong Semi-Supervised Learners
69. Adversarial Environment Design via Regret-Guided Diffusion Models	69. Fourier Features Let Networks Learn High Frequency Functions in Low Dimensional Domains
70. Localized Zeroth-Order Prompt Optimization	70. Improved Deep Metric Learning with Multi-class N-pair Loss Objective
71. Molecule Design by Latent Prompt Transformer	71. Hierarchical Graph Representation Learning with Differentiable Pooling
72. Can Learned Optimization Make Reinforcement Learning Less Difficult?	72. Scheduled Sampling for Sequence Prediction with Recurrent Neural Networks
73. Reverse Transition Kernel: A Flexible Framework to Accelerate Diffusion Inference	73. Learning to learn by gradient descent by gradient descent
74. Any2Graph: Deep End-To-End Supervised Graph Prediction With An Optimal Transport Loss	74. Co-teaching: Robust training of deep neural networks with extremely noisy labels

(*continued*)

Table 4. (*continued*)

NeurIPS Test Set

Positive	Negative
75. MInference 1.0: Accelerating Pre-filling for Long-Context LLMs via Dynamic Sparse Attention	75. Continual Learning with Deep Generative Replay
76. Ensemble Learning for Heterogeneous Large Language Models with Deep Parallel Collaboration	76. Learning a Probabilistic Latent Space of Object Shapes via 3D Generative-Adversarial Modeling
77. Humanoid Locomotion as Next Token Prediction	77. Big Bird: Transformers for Longer Sequences
78. NeoRL: Efficient Exploration for Nonepisodic RL	78. Weight Normalization: A Simple Reparameterization to Accelerate Training of Deep Neural Networks
79. Toxicity Detection for Free	79. A Simple Unified Framework for Detecting Out-of-Distribution Samples and Adversarial Attacks
80. Semi-supervised Multi-label Learning with Balanced Binary Angular Margin Loss	80. Sanity Checks for Saliency Maps
	81. When Does Label Smoothing Help?
	82. Graph Contrastive Learning with Augmentations
	83. Link Prediction Based on Graph Neural Networks
	84. Improved Variational Inference with Inverse Autoregressive Flow
	85. Training Generative Adversarial Networks with Limited Data
	86. Visualizing the Loss Landscape of Neural Nets
	87. Adversarial Examples Are Not Bugs, They Are Features
	88. HiFi-GAN: Generative Adversarial Networks for Efficient and High Fidelity Speech Synthesis
	89. Understanding the Effective Receptive Field in Deep Convolutional Neural Networks

(*continued*)

Table 4. (*continued*)

NeurIPS Test Set

Positive	Negative
	90. Learning to summarize from human feedback
	91. Federated Multi-Task Learning
	92. Training Very Deep Networks
	93. Efficient and Robust Automated Machine Learning
	94. A Theoretically Grounded Application of Dropout in Recurrent Neural Networks
	95. Generating Diverse High-Fidelity Images with VQ-VAE-2
	96. f-GAN: Training Generative Neural Samplers using Variational Divergence Minimization
	97. Coupled Generative Adversarial Networks
	98. Conservative Q-Learning for Offline Reinforcement Learning
	99. A simple neural network module for relational reasoning

B.2 Nature Medicine Test Set

Table 5. Titles of novel (Positive) and non-novel (Negative) papers in nature medicine test set

Nature Medicine Test Set	
Positive	**Negative**
1. Sleep patterns and risk of chronic disease as measured by long-term monitoring with commercial wearable devices in the All of Us Research Program.	1. Microenvironmental regulation of tumor progression and metastasis
2. Botensilimab plus balstilimab in relapsed/refractory microsatellite stable metastatic colorectal cancer: a phase 1 trial.	2. Temporal dynamics in viral shedding and transmissibility of COVID-19

(*continued*)

Table 5. (*continued*)

Nature Medicine Test Set

Positive	Negative
3. Lipidome changes due to improved dietary fat quality inform cardiometabolic risk reduction and precision nutrition.	3. The Consensus Molecular Subtypes of Colorectal Cancer
4. Fratricide-resistant CD7-CAR T cells in T-ALL.	4. High-performance medicine: the convergence of human and artificial intelligence
5. International multicenter validation of AI-driven ultrasound detection of ovarian cancer.	5. Understanding the tumor immune microenvironment (TIME) for effective therapy
6. Donor-derived GD2-specific CAR T cells in relapsed or refractory neuroblastoma.	6. Intestinal microbiota metabolism of L-carnitine, a nutrient in red meat, promotes atherosclerosis
7. Single-nucleus chromatin accessibility and transcriptomic map of breast tissues of women of diverse genetic ancestry.	7. Post-acute COVID-19 syndrome
8. Unidirectional association of clonal hematopoiesis with atherosclerosis development.	8. Melanoma exosomes educate bone marrow progenitor cells toward a pro-metastatic phenotype through MET
9. Echocardiographic screening for heart failure and optimization of the care pathway for individuals with pacemakers: a randomized controlled trial.	9. Signatures of T cell dysfunction and exclusion predict cancer immunotherapy response
10. Population-based, first-tier genomic newborn screening in the maternity ward.	10. Neutralizing antibody levels are highly predictive of immune protection from symptomatic SARS-CoV-2 infection
11. Allogeneic CD5-specific CAR-T therapy for relapsed/refractory T-ALL: a phase 1 trial.	11. Ischemia and reperfusion—from mechanism to translation
12. Transplantation of a genetically modified porcine heart into a live human.	12. Mechanisms of fibrosis: therapeutic translation for fibrotic disease

(*continued*)

Table 5. (*continued*)

Nature Medicine Test Set	
Positive	**Negative**
13. A multi-modal single-cell and spatial expression map of metastatic breast cancer biopsies across clinico-pathological features.	13. Metabolite profiles and the risk of developing diabetes
14. ctDNA-based molecular residual disease and survival in resectable colorectal cancer.	14. Mechanisms of NAFLD development and therapeutic strategies
15. Antifungal heteroresistance causes prophylaxis failure and facilitates breakthrough Candida parapsilosis infections.	15. Inflammasomes: mechanism of action, role in disease, and therapeutics
16. Subcutaneous weekly semaglutide with automated insulin delivery in type 1 diabetes: a double-blind, randomized, crossover trial.	16. Chronic inflammation in the etiology of disease across the life span
17. Combined endurance and resistance exercise training in heart failure with preserved ejection fraction: a randomized controlled trial.	17. Mutational Landscape of Metastatic Cancer Revealed from Prospective Clinical Sequencing of 10,000 Patients
18. Multi-omic profiling a defined bacterial consortium for treatment of recurrent Clostridioides difficile infection.	18. Antibody responses to SARS-CoV-2 in patients with COVID-19
19. An organotypic atlas of human vascular cells.	19. ABT-199, a potent and selective BCL-2 inhibitor, achieves antitumor activity while sparing platelets
20. Lipid profiling identifies modifiable signatures of cardiometabolic risk in children and adolescents with obesity.	20. Clinical and immunological assessment of asymptomatic SARS-CoV-2 infections
21. Ferric carboxymaltose for anemia in late pregnancy: a randomized controlled trial.	21. Extrapulmonary manifestations of COVID-19
22. Effects of conditional cash transfers on tuberculosis incidence and mortality according to race, ethnicity and socioeconomic factors in the 100 Million Brazilian Cohort.	22. A guide to deep learning in healthcare

(*continued*)

Table 5. (*continued*)

Nature Medicine Test Set

Positive	Negative
23. Phenome-wide associations of sleep characteristics in the Human Phenotype Project.	23. A global survey of potential acceptance of a COVID-19 vaccine
24. Proteomic signatures improve risk prediction for common and rare diseases.	24. The emerging role of lncRNAs in cancer
25. Remotely delivered weight management for people with long COVID and overweight: the randomized wait-list-controlled ReDIRECT trial.	25. SARS-CoV-2 Entry Genes Are Most Highly Expressed in Nasal Goblet and Ciliated Cells within Human Airways
26. Sustained effect of prasinezumab on Parkinson's disease motor progression in the open-label extension of the PASADENA trial.	26. Gut microbiota metabolism of dietary fiber influences allergic airway disease and hematopoiesis
27. Collaboration between clinicians and vision-language models in radiology report generation.	27. The immunology of stroke: from mechanisms to translation
28. Oral obeldesivir provides post-exposure protection against Marburg virus in nonhuman primates.	28. Asthma phenotypes: the evolution from clinical to molecular approaches
29. Digital consults in heart failure care: a randomized controlled trial.	29. Single-cell landscape of bronchoalveolar immune cells in patients with COVID-19
30. Increased frequency of repeat expansion mutations across different populations.	30. A small-molecule inhibitor of the NLRP3 inflammasome for the treatment of inflammatory diseases
31. Autogene cevumeran with or without atezolizumab in advanced solid tumors: a phase 1 trial.	31. Respiratory virus shedding in exhaled breath and efficacy of face masks
32. A high-performance brain-computer interface for finger decoding and quadcopter game control in an individual with paralysis.	32. Cancer stem cells revisited
33. Mapping the effectiveness and risks of GLP-1 receptor agonists.	33. Atherosclerosis: current pathogenesis and therapeutic options

(*continued*)

Table 5. (*continued*)

Nature Medicine Test Set	
Positive	**Negative**
34. Evaluating generalizability of oncology trial results to real-world patients using machine learning-based trial emulations.	34. Brown and beige fat: development, function and therapeutic potential
35. AI-based differential diagnosis of dementia etiologies on multimodal data.	35. Cardiologist-level arrhythmia detection and classification in ambulatory electrocardiograms using a deep neural network
36. Molecular classification to refine surgical and radiotherapeutic decision-making in meningioma.	36. An inflammatory cytokine signature predicts COVID-19 severity and survival
37. A framework for sharing of clinical and genetic data for precision medicine applications.	37. Classification and mutation prediction from non–small cell lung cancer histopathology images using deep learning
38. A generalist medical language model for disease diagnosis assistance.	38. CSF-1R inhibition alters macrophage polarization and blocks glioma progression
39. Subclassification of obesity for precision prediction of cardiometabolic diseases.	39. Clinically applicable deep learning for diagnosis and referral in retinal disease
40. Somatic CAG repeat expansion in blood associates with biomarkers of neurodegeneration in Huntington's disease decades before clinical motor diagnosis.	40. Development, maintenance and disruption of the blood-brain barrier
41. Genomic reanalysis of a pan-European rare-disease resource yields new diagnoses.	41. Adipocytes promote ovarian cancer metastasis and provide energy for rapid tumor growth
42. In vivo base editing extends lifespan of a humanized mouse model of prion disease.	42. An ultrasensitive method for quantitating circulating tumor DNA with broad patient coverage
43. Self-improving generative foundation model for synthetic medical image generation and clinical applications.	43. The cancer stem cell: premises, promises and challenges

(*continued*)

Table 5. (*continued*)

Nature Medicine Test Set

Positive	Negative
44. Data-driven cluster analysis identifies distinct types of metabolic dysfunction-associated steatotic liver disease.	44. Attributes and predictors of long COVID
45. The economic value of reducing avoidable mortality.	45. WNT signaling in bone homeostasis and disease: from human mutations to treatments
46. Genetic basis of early onset and progression of type 2 diabetes in South Asians.	46. The role of autophagy in neurodegenerative disease
47. Posthospitalization COVID-19 cognitive deficits at 1 year are global and associated with elevated brain injury markers and gray matter volume reduction.	47. Clinical-grade computational pathology using weakly supervised deep learning on whole slide images
48. Safety and reactogenicity of a controlled human infection model of sand fly-transmitted cutaneous leishmaniasis.	48. A human memory T-cell subset with stem cell-like properties
49. Cabozantinib and nivolumab with or without live bacterial supplementation in metastatic renal cell carcinoma: a randomized phase 1 trial.	49. Current understanding of the human microbiome
50. Seven-year performance of a clinical metagenomic next-generation sequencing test for diagnosis of central nervous system infections.	50. Molecular analysis of gastric cancer identifies subtypes associated with distinct clinical outcomes
51. Brain aging patterns in a large and diverse cohort of 49,482 individuals.	51. Cellular senescence in aging and age-related disease: from mechanisms to therapy
52. Large floods drive changes in cause-specific mortality in the United States.	52. PPARγ signaling and metabolism: the good, the bad and the future
53. Cytokine-mediated CAR T therapy resistance in AML.	53. Resting-state connectivity biomarkers define neurophysiological subtypes of depression

(*continued*)

Table 5. (*continued*)

Nature Medicine Test Set	
Positive	**Negative**
54. Prediction of brain metastasis development with DNA methylation signatures.	54. Age-dependent effects in the transmission and control of COVID-19 epidemics
55. Personalized, autologous neoantigen-specific T cell therapy in metastatic melanoma: a phase 1 trial.	55. Tumor angiogenesis: molecular pathways and therapeutic targets
56. A generalist vision-language foundation model for diverse biomedical tasks.	56. Evidence for osteocyte regulation of bone homeostasis through RANKL expression
57. DNA liquid biopsy-based prediction of cancer-associated venous thromboembolism.	57. Modelling the COVID-19 epidemic and implementation of population-wide interventions in Italy
58. Semaglutide in patients with overweight or obesity and chronic kidney disease without diabetes: a randomized double-blind placebo-controlled clinical trial.	58. Identification of the molecular basis of doxorubicin-induced cardiotoxicity
59. Intracerebroventricular B7-H3-targeting CAR T cells for diffuse intrinsic pontine glioma: a phase 1 trial.	59. New from NPG: Genome-wide association study identifies five new schizophrenia loci
60. AI-based selection of individuals for supplemental MRI in population-based breast cancer screening: the randomized ScreenTrustMRI trial.	60. Senolytics Improve Physical Function and Increase Lifespan in Old Age
61. A toolbox for surfacing health equity harms and biases in large language models.	61. Subtypes of Pancreatic Ductal Adenocarcinoma and Their Differing Responses to Therapy
62. Partitioned polygenic risk scores identify distinct types of metabolic dysfunction-associated steatotic liver disease.	62. A purified membrane protein from Akkermansia muciniphila or the pasteurized bacterium improves metabolism in obese and diabetic mice
63. Multi-omics-based mapping of decidualization resistance in patients with a history of severe preeclampsia.	63. The NALP3/NLRP3 Inflammasome Instigates Obesity-Induced Autoinflammation and Insulin Resistance

(*continued*)

Table 5. (*continued*)

Nature Medicine Test Set	
Positive	**Negative**
64. Electronic nudges for sustained influenza vaccination uptake in older adults: the nationwide randomized NUDGE-FLU-2 trial.	64. IgE and mast cells in allergic disease
65. A time-stratified, case-crossover study of heat exposure and perinatal mortality from 16 hospitals in sub-Saharan Africa.	65. Brown adipose tissue activity controls triglyceride clearance
66. SARS-CoV-2 correlates of protection from infection against variants of concern.	66. Intraoperative tumor-specific fluorescence imaging in ovarian cancer by folate receptor-α targeting: first in-human results
	67. The cellular and signaling networks linking the immune system and metabolism in disease
	68. Supplementation with Akkermansia muciniphila in overweight and obese human volunteers: a proof-of-concept exploratory study
	69. Why don't we get more cancer? A proposed role of the microenvironment in restraining cancer progression
	70. Clearance of senescent cells by ABT263 rejuvenates aged hematopoietic stem cells in mice
	71. 4-1BB Costimulation Ameliorates T Cell Exhaustion Induced by Tonic Signaling of Chimeric Antigen Receptors
	72. Characteristics of pediatric SARS-CoV-2 infection and potential evidence for persistent fecal viral shedding
	73. Molecular subtypes of diffuse large B cell lymphoma are associated with distinct pathogenic mechanisms and outcomes

(*continued*)

Table 5. (*continued*)

Nature Medicine Test Set

Positive	Negative
	74. The oral and gut microbiomes are perturbed in rheumatoid arthritis and partly normalized after treatment
	75. End-to-end lung cancer screening with three-dimensional deep learning on low-dose chest computed tomography
	76. The practical implementation of artificial intelligence technologies in medicine
	77. Estimating clinical severity of COVID-19 from the transmission dynamics in Wuhan, China
	78. Microglia emerge as central players in brain disease
	79. Organ reengineering through development of a transplantable recellularized liver graft using decellularized liver matrix
	80. RET, ROS1 and ALK fusions in lung cancer
	81. Divergent clonal evolution of castration resistant neuroendocrine prostate cancer
	82. Long-term cardiovascular outcomes of COVID-19
	83. Ketone body β-hydroxybutyrate blocks the NLRP3 inflammasome-mediated inflammatory disease
	84. Large language models in medicine
	85. In vivo photodynamic therapy using upconversion nanoparticles as remote-controlled nanotransducers
	86. Mitochondrial transfer from bone-marrow–derived stromal cells to pulmonary alveoli protects against acute lung injury

(*continued*)

Table 5. (*continued*)

Nature Medicine Test Set

Positive	Negative
	87. A single-cell atlas of the peripheral immune response in patients with severe COVID-19
	88. Determinants of response and resistance to CD19 chimeric antigen receptor (CAR) T cell therapy of chronic lymphocytic leukemia
	89. Cancer epigenetics reaches mainstream oncology
	90. Real-time tracking of self-reported symptoms to predict potential COVID-19
	91. Metformin alters the gut microbiome of individuals with treatment-naive type 2 diabetes, contributing to the therapeutic effects of the drug
	92. Synaptic plasticity and depression: new insights from stress and rapid-acting antidepressants
	93. Matrix-embedded cells control osteoclast formation
	94. Targeting EZH2 in cancer
	95. Comprehensive molecular characterization of clinical responses to PD-1 inhibition in metastatic gastric cancer
	96. Identification of miR-34a as a potent inhibitor of prostate cancer progenitor cells and metastasis by directly repressing CD44
	97. Phenotype molding of stromal cells in the lung tumor microenvironment
	98. Key roles of adjuvants in modern vaccines
	99. AI in health and medicine

C Appendix 3: Prompt

C.1 Prompt for LLM with NeurIPS 2024 Review Guideline

Table 6. Prompt for LLM with NeurIPS 2024 review guideline

Prompt
Task description: You are a researcher who is reviewing a paper that was submitted to a computer science venue. Be critical and cautious in your decision. If a paper is bad or you are unsure, give it bad scores and reject it. Below is a description of the questions you will be asked on the review form for each paper and some guidelines on what to consider when answering these questions. **Reviewer guidelines**: 1. Summary: Briefly summarize the paper and its contributions. This is not the place to critique the paper; the authors should generally agree with a well-written summary. 2. Strengths and Weaknesses: Please provide a thorough assessment of the strengths and weaknesses of the paper, touching on each of the following dimensions: - Originality: Are the tasks or methods new? Is the work a novel combination of well-known techniques? (This can be valuable!) Is it clear how this work differs from previous contributions? - Quality: Is the submission technically sound? Are claims well-supported (e.g., by theoretical analysis or experimental results)? Are the methods used appropriately? Is this a complete piece of work or a work in progress? Are the authors careful and honest about evaluating both the strengths and weaknesses of their work? - Clarity: Is the submission clearly written? Is it well organized? (If not, please make constructive suggestions for improving its clarity.) Does it adequately inform the reader? (Note that a superbly written paper provides enough information for an expert reader to reproduce its results.) - Significance: Are the results important? Are others (researchers or practitioners) likely to use the ideas or build on them? Does the submission address a difficult task in a better way than previous work? Does it advance the state of the art in a demonstrable way? Does it provide unique data, unique conclusions about existing data, or a unique theoretical or experimental approach? 3. Questions: Please list and carefully describe any questions and suggestions for the authors. Think of the things where a response from the author can change your opinion, clarify confusion, or address a limitation. This can be very important for a productive rebuttal and discussion phase with the authors. 4. Ethical concerns: If there are ethical issues with this paper, please flag the paper for an ethics review. 5 Overall· Please provide an "overall score" for this submission

(continued)

Table 6. (*continued*)

Choices:
- 10: Award quality: Technically flawless paper with groundbreaking impact on one or more areas, with exceptionally strong evaluation, reproducibility, and resources, and no unaddressed ethical considerations.
- 9: Very Strong Accept: Technically flawless paper with groundbreaking impact on at least one area and excellent impact on multiple areas, with flawless evaluation, resources, and reproducibility, and no unaddressed ethical considerations.
- 8: Strong Accept: Technically strong paper, with novel ideas, excellent impact on at least one area or high-toexcellent impact on multiple areas, with excellent evaluation, resources, and reproducibility, and no unaddressed ethical considerations.
- 7: Accept: Technically solid paper, with high impact on at least one sub-area or moderate-to-high impact on more than one area, with good-to-excellent evaluation, resources, reproducibility, and no unaddressed ethical considerations.
- 6: Weak Accept: Technically solid, moderate-to-high impact paper, with no major concerns with respect to evaluation, resources, reproducibility, and ethical considerations.
- 5: Borderline accept: Technically solid paper where reasons to accept outweigh reasons to reject, e.g., limited evaluation. Please use sparingly.
- 4: Borderline reject: Technically solid paper where reasons to reject, e.g., limited evaluation, outweigh reasons to accept, e.g., good evaluation. Please use sparingly.
- 3: Reject: For instance, a paper with technical flaws, weak evaluation, inadequate reproducibility, and incompletely addressed ethical considerations.
- 2: Strong Reject: For instance, a paper with major technical flaws, and/or poor evaluation, limited impact, poor reproducibility, and mostly unaddressed ethical considerations.
- 1: Very Strong Reject: For instance, a paper with trivial results or unaddressed ethical considerations

Provided paper:
Here is the paper you are asked to review:
{paper}
Output:
Return a JSON object:
<JSON>
template
<JSON>

C.2 Prompt for Standardized Project Proposals

Table 7. Prompt for standardized project proposals

Prompt
Role: You are a writing assistant specialized in editing academic writing. **Task**: I will give you a student's research idea and an idea template. Your task is to edit the student's idea to follow the template's format. **Student idea**: Title {title} Main Idea {paper} **Template**: 1. Title: A concise statement of the main research question to be used as the paper title. 2. Problem Statement: Clearly define the problem your research intends to address. Explain clearly why this problem is interesting and important. 3. Motivation: Explain why existing methods are not good enough to solve the problem, and explain the inspiration behind the new proposed method. You should also motivate why the proposed method would work better than existing baselines on the problem. 4. Proposed Method: Explain how the proposed method works, describe all the essential steps. 5. Step-by-Step Experiment Plan: Break down every single step of the experiments, make sure every step is executable. Cover all essential details such as the datasets, models, and metrics to be used. If the project involves prompting, give some example prompts for each step. 6. Test Case Examples: Give at least two concrete examples. The first example should show how the baseline method fails on the test case. If there are multiple baselines, give examples for all of them. The second example should show how the proposed method succeeds on the test case. For each test case, include the input (test example and the full prompt) and the expected output. You should also provide an explanation for why the outputs from the proposed prompt are better. If the proposed method has multiple steps, break them down into intermediate steps. 7. Fallback Plan: Propose some alternative plans for what should the students do if the proposed method doesn't manage to satisfy the success criteria. For example, you can suggest additional analysis to help debug why the proposed method didn't work, which could inform alternative new methods, or just turn the project into an analysis paper instead by offering some interesting ablation and insights. **Requirement**: Make sure that you only edit the wording and formatting, including things like punctuation, capitalization, linebreaks, and bullet points. Also make sure to edit any informal wording and phrasing to use vocabulary that sounds like the template's writing style. No other changes are allowed beyond these.

(continued)

Table 7. *(continued)*

You should use tab as indentation and make sure to use appropriate nested indentation for sub-bullets. All bullets should have a clear hierarchy so people can easily differentiate the sub-bullets. Only leave empty lines between sections and remove any extra line breaks. If many bullet points are clustered together in a paragraph, separate them clearly with indentation and appropriate bullet point markers. Change to a new line for each new bullet point.
For the fallback plan, do not list a bunch of bullet points. Instead, condense them into one coherent paragraph. For line breaks, avoid Raw String Literals or Double Backslashes when using "
n", and change them to spaces or tabs.
For in-line citations, if the citation mentioned the author's last name (like "(Si et al., 2023)" or "(An et al., 2024)"), you should keep them there; but if the citation is just a number (like "[1]" or "[3,4,5]"), you should just remove it and do some necessary rephrasing to make the sentence still sound coherent without the references.
Apart from minor rephrasing and changing formatting, do not change any content of the idea. You must preserve the exact meaning of the original idea, do not change, remove, or add any other details. Do not drop any sections (including test case examples). Do not rename any models, datasets, or methods. Do not drop clarification or examples in brackets and do not drop any data source mentions (e.g., Chatbot Arena or Wildchat)! Note that when indexing test case examples, each test case example could have multiple steps of inputs and outputs and you shouldn't give separate indices to them. Each test case example should be a whole set of input-output pairs for the baseline(s) and proposed method.
For the proposed method section, avoid any big changes. If the section comes in as a coherent paragraph, you don't have to break it down into bullet points. If the section is already in bullet points, you should keep it that way. If the section is a mix of both, you should keep the bullet points and the coherent paragraph as they are. Keep all the clarification and examples mentioned in all the sections and do not remove any of them (including those in brackets). For model selection, if any version of Claude is mentioned, change it to the latest version of Claude (Claude-3.5); if any version of LLaMA is mentioned, change it to the latest version LLaMA-3. Do not make any other model changes. Now directly generate the edited student idea to match the format of the template.

C.3 Prompt for LLM with Literature Search

Table 8. Prompt for LLM with literature search

Prompt
Role: You are an ambitious AI PhD student who is looking to publish a paper that will contribute significantly to the field. **Task description**: You have an idea and you want to check if it is novel or not. I.e., not overlapping significantly with existing literature or already well explored. Be a harsh critic for novelty, ensure there is a sufficient contribution in the idea for a new conference or workshop paper. You will be given the titles and abstracts of the 10 papers most relevant to your idea. Decide a paper idea is novel if after sufficient searching, you have not found a paper that significantly overlaps with your idea. Decide a paper idea is not novel, if you have found a paper that significantly overlaps with your idea. Set your decision to True if you think the idea is novel, set it to False if you think the idea is not novel. **Your Idea**: This is the idea you need to judge for novelty: {Idea} **Top 10 relevant papers**: {papers} **Output**: Return only True or False, dont return any other words.

D Appendix 4: Result in Detail

D.1 AUROC of Different LLM-Based Model in Detail

See Table 9

Table 9. AUROC of different LLM-based model in detail

		Sonnet-3.7 with guideline	Sonnet-3.7 with tournament	LLM + literature search		
				Sonnet-3.7	Deepseek-r1	Gpt-4o
Round1	NeurIPS	0.544	0.497	0.818	0.746	0.56
	Nature medicine	NaN	0.501	0.616	0.663	0.518
	Mixed	NaN	0.5	0.596	0.583	0.492
Round2	NeurIPS	0.505	0.496	0.799	0.701	0.578
	Nature medicine	NaN	0.51	0.624	0.707	0.551
	Mixed	NaN	0.497	0.603	0.661	0.535
Round3	NeurIPS	0.59	0.496	0.823	0.682	0.564
	Nature medicine	NaN	0.497	0.609	0.649	0.566
	Mixed	NaN	0.506	0.593	0.543	0.54

D.2 Comparison of AUROC of RND algorithm with different P values

Table 10. Comparison of AUROC of RND algorithm with different P values

Test set	AUROC				
	P = 10, Q = 50	P = 50, Q = 50	P = 100, Q = 50	P = 500, Q = 50	P = 1000, Q = 50
NeurIPS	0.808	0.830	0.820	0.825	0.833
Nature medicine	0.686	0.754	0.765	0.760	0.765
Mixed	0.762	0.805	0.795	0.786	0.787

D.3 Comparison of AUROC of RND algorithm with different Q values

See Table 11

Table 11. Comparison of AUROC of RND algorithm with different Q values. Results indicate that performance peaks at moderate Q values before sensitivity diminishes at higher ranges.

Test set	AUROC						
	$Q = 2$	$Q = 5$	$Q = 10$	$Q = 50$	$Q = 100$	$Q = 500$	$Q = 1000$
NeurIPS	0.778	0.818	0.827	0.820	0.808	0.788	0.768
Nature medicine	0.603	0.686	0.723	0.765	0.757	0.744	0.722
Mixed	0.628	0.745	0.774	0.795	0.782	0.771	0.758

E Appendix 5: Computing Resources

To conduct our experiment, the necessary computing resources includes

1. Literature database with embedding vector: we used a server with 16 CPU cores, 128GB RAM, 2TB SSD disk(which actually used around 1TB) to deploy an ElasticSearch version 8 as literature search engine. The embedding of each literature is obtained using public available API services.

2. Algorithm development and experiment: a server with 16 CPU cores, 128GB RAM.

References

1. Anthropic: Claude 3.7 sonnet and claude code (2025), https://www.anthropic.com/news/claude-3-7-sonnet. Last visited on 28 Feb 2025
2. Chen, J., Xiao, S., Zhang, P., Luo, K., Lian, D., Liu, Z.: Bge m3-embedding: multi-lingual, multi-functionality, multi-granularity text embeddings through self-knowledge distillation (2024). arXiv:2402.03216
3. Cornell Tech: Arxiv annual report (2023). https://info.arxiv.org/about/reports/2023_arXiv_annual_report.pdf. Last visited on 25 Feb 2025

4. Cornell University: Arxiv dataset (2025). https://www.kaggle.com/datasets/Cornell-University/arxiv. Last visited on 10 Jan 2025
5. Guo, D., Yang, D., Zhang, H., Song, J., Zhang, R., Xu, R., Zhu, Q., Ma, S., Wang, P., Bi, X., et al.: Deepseek-r1: incentivizing reasoning capability in llms via reinforcement learning (2025). arXiv:2501.12948
6. Hu, X., Fu, H., Wang, J., Wang, Y., Li, Z., Xu, R., Lu, Y., Jin, Y., Pan, L., Lan, Z.: Nova: an iterative planning and search approach to enhance novelty and diversity of LLM generated ideas (2024). arXiv:2410.14255 [cs]
7. Hurst, A., Lerer, A., Goucher, A.P., Perelman, A., Ramesh, A., Clark, A., Ostrow, A., Welihinda, A., Hayes, A., Radford, A., et al.: Gpt-4o system card (2024). arXiv:2410.21276
8. Jin, Q., Leaman, R., Lu, Z.: Pubmed and beyond: biomedical literature search in the age of artificial intelligence. EBioMedicine **100** (2024)
9. Lu, C., Lu, C., Lange, R.T., Foerster, J., Clune, J., Ha, D.: The AI scientist: towards fully automated open-ended scientific discovery (2024). arXiv:2408.06292 [cs]
10. Van der Maaten, L., Hinton, G.: Visualizing data using t-SNE. J. Mach. Learn. Res.**9**(11) (2008)
11. National Library of Medicine: Pubmed download (2025). https://pubmed.ncbi.nlm.nih.gov/download/. Last visited on 10 Jan 2025
12. openreview: Evaluating the world model implicit in a generative model (2025). https://openreview.net/forum?id=aVK4JFpegy. Last visited on 26 Feb 2025
13. Openreview Reviewer 2X9t: Official review of submission1763 (2025). https://openreview.net/forum?id=yYQLvofQ1k&noteId=SbNNx8xCH5. Last visited on 7 Mar 2025
14. Si, C., Yang, D., Hashimoto, T.: Can LLMs generate novel research ideas? a large-scale human study with 100+ NLP researchers (2024). arXiv:2409.04109 [cs]
15. Singh, A., Singh, N., Vatsal, S.: Robustness of LLMs to perturbations in text (2024). arXiv:2407.08989 [cs]
16. Su, H., Chen, R., Tang, S., Zheng, X., Li, J., Yin, Z., Ouyang, W., Dong, N.: Two heads are better than one: a multi-agent system has the potential to improve scientific idea generation (2024). arXiv:2410.09403 [cs]
17. Vafa, K., Chen, J., Rambachan, A., Kleinberg, J., Mullainathan, S.: Evaluating the world model implicit in a generative model. Adv. Neural. Inf. Process. Syst. **37**, 26941–26975 (2025)
18. Vaswani, A., Shazeer, N., Parmar, N., Uszkoreit, J., Jones, L., Gomez, A.N., Kaiser, Ł., Polosukhin, I.: Attention is all you need. In: Advances in Neural Information Processing Systems, vol. 30 (2017)
19. Zhuo, T.Y., Li, Z., Huang, Y., Shiri, F., Wang, W., Haffari, G., Li, Y.F.: On robustness of prompt-based semantic parsing with large pre-trained language model: an empirical study on codex (2023). arXiv:2301.12868 [cs]

Knowledge-Augmented Multimodal Learning for Breast Cancer Diagnosis

Luqi Li, Lun Wang, and Li Hou(✉)

Institute of Medical Information/Medical Library, Chinese Academy of Medical Sciences & Peking Union Medical College, Beijng, China
li.luqi@imicams.ac.cn

Abstract. Current methods for breast cancer diagnosis often face limitations in integrating prior knowledge, fusing multimodal data, and providing interpretability. To this end, we propose a novel knowledge-augmented multimodal learning framework. Based on a clinically guided breast cancer knowledge graph, our approach enhances patient clinical representations using Graph Attention Networks (GAT) and extracts pathological image features through weak supervision learning. A bidirectional cross-attention fusion mechanism enables interactive alignment and integration of multimodal heterogeneous information in the feature space. Extensive experiments on a real-world PathologicalEMR dataset demonstrate that our method achieves outstanding performance, with an AUC of 0.9963 in distinguishing benign from malignant cases. Further ablation studies validate the contributions of various multimodal feature combinations and knowledge enhancement strategies, underscoring the framework's effectiveness and interpretability. The proposed solution significantly advances the capability and trustworthiness of multi-source information integration for complex medical diagnostics, offering a promising tool for clinical decision support.

Keywords: Breast cancer diagnosis · Knowledge-augmented · Multimodal learning

1 Background

The latest data shows that in 2020, the number of new breast cancer cases in the world will reach 2.26 million, surpassing lung cancer (2.21 million cases) for the first time to become the world's largest cancer, which is one of the important factors threatening women's health [1]. Early detection can help reduce the mortality of breast cancer. With the popularization of medical imaging technology and electronic medical record systems, the diagnosis of breast cancer gradually relies on the fusion analysis of multimodal data (such as mammography, pathological sections, clinical reports, etc.) [2]. Many new models based on deep learning have promoted the performance of multimodal fusion, such as Transformer, graph neural network [3, 4]. Multiple fusion strategies and alignment mechanisms (collaborative training, attention mechanism, et al.) have been studied for the fusion of different modal data to fully explore complementary information between different modalities [5]. The related research results have shown great potential in scenarios such as disease diagnosis classification and cancer prognosis.

Y. Zhang et al. (Eds.): CHIP 2025, CCIS 2884, pp. 329–346, 2026.
https://doi.org/10.1007/978-981-95-7299-1_19

However, a critical gap persists in these data-driven models: the lack of integration of rich, structured clinical knowledge. Existing multi-modal models treat diagnostic tasks purely as a pattern recognition problem on pixels and signals. They fail to incorporate the foundational knowledge that guides a radiologist's reasoning. For instance, while a model might learn that certain texture features are important, it does not explicitly "know" that a "spiculated margin" is a strong indicator of malignancy, as defined by the BI-RADS standard. Many studies have pointed out that developing multimodal fusion models based on artificial intelligence aims to simulate the thinking process of clinical doctors integrating multiple information sources in the diagnosis and decision-making process. As shown in Fig. 1, the clinical diagnosis process of doctors is a complex process that combines experience and knowledge, and comprehensively considers the current multimodal characteristics of patients. This process not only requires the fusion model to have high prediction accuracy, but also demands its interpretability [6]. However, the experience of doctors is difficult to quantify, and we can only replace it with a medical knowledge graph established based on reliable sources such as clinical guidelines. Knowledge graph, due to its prior knowledge and internal hierarchical structure, has been proven by some studies to help improve the knowledge representation of diseases, thereby enhancing the accuracy and interpretability of disease prediction [7].

Therefore, this study aims to develop a novel knowledge-augmented multimodal learning framework for breast cancer diagnosis, designed to replicate the real-world clinical decision-making process by integrating imaging examinations, clinical features, and knowledge graphs, such as Fig. 1. The main contributions of our work are as follows.

(1) Medical knowledge integration: this study introduces knowledge graph technology to provide structured prior knowledge as medically informed constraints, such as symptom-disease relationships and pathological manifestations. By leveraging graph neural networks, our approach enables joint modeling of knowledge representations and clinical case features. This integration enhances the accuracy of disease diagnosis and analysis, while also improving the interpretability and credibility of diagnostic outcomes through visually explainable reasoning paths.
(2) Cross modal feature semantic feature alignment: This study proposes a dynamic feature fusion module based on bidirectional cross attention to address the deep fusion problem of heterogeneous modalities between patient pathological images and clinical features. In this module, image features and knowledge-augmented clinical features serve as mutual query-key-value pairs, enabling deep and dynamic interaction between the two types of heterogeneous information in the feature space. This design allows the model to actively retrieve relevant knowledge entities as diagnostic evidence when interpreting images, while also focusing on corresponding visual evidence in the images when reasoning with medical logic.

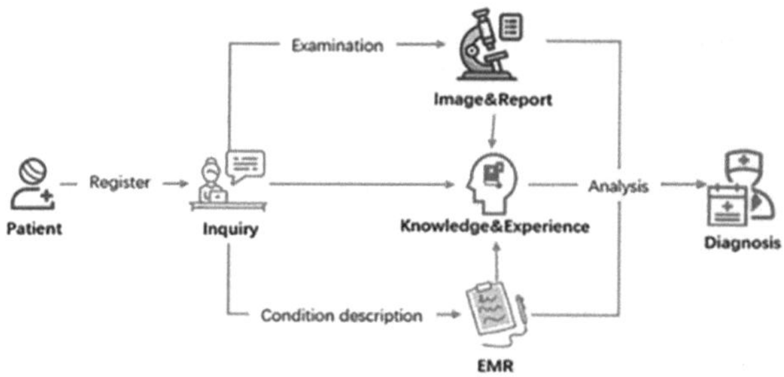

Fig. 1. A simple introduction to diagnosis workflow in the hospital.

2 Related Work

2.1 Multimodal Data Fusion in Disease Diagnosis Models

In oncology, multiple modalities such as medical imaging, histopathology, genomic profiling, and electronic health records, are routinely used to characterize a patient's condition. Studies demonstrate that multimodal AI approaches can effectively address key challenges including cancer subtyping, survival prediction, and personalized treatment recommendation, underscoring their potential for improving clinical decision-making. Medical pathological images contain rich phenotypic information. By converting these images into high-fidelity, high-throughput collections of exploitable pathological subvisual features, we can capture patterns indistinguishable to the human eye, quantify clinical experience and knowledge, and mine valuable information to enhance clinical decision-making [8]. The fusion of these pathological subvisual features with other electronic medical record features can provide more accurate diagnosis and prognosis prediction. For instance, Popovici et al. [9] presented a novel approach for a joint analysis of histopathology images and gene expression data to find patterns in the integrated data. The clustering results identify patient categories with distinct imaging and genetic characteristics. Electronic medical records can provide support for multimodal data, and the clinical information extracted is low dimensional, usually based on the professional knowledge and long-term experience of doctors, which helps to provide richer guidance for diagnosis. Yan et al. [10] used structured electronic health records (EHR) data to improve the accuracy of pathological image classification, combining high-dimensional abstract features of the original pathological images with EMR, and extracting richer multi-level features through multiple convolutional layers to preserve local cell texture and tissue structure information. Multimodal data fusion is conducive to predicting individual prognosis to assist clinical precision treatment. For example, Yang et al. [11] used H&E staining histopathological images for the first time to predict the prognosis of breast cancer and developed a prediction framework based on pathological images and clinical information to assess the risk of recurrence and metastasis of HER2 positive breast cancer patients.

Information fusion methods can be divided into three categories according to the level of integration: data-level(early) fusion, feature-level(intermediate) fusion, and decision-level(late) fusion [12]. Data-level fusion combines raw input, preserving information but requiring strict alignment and risking high dimensionality. Feature-level fusion, the most common approach, integrates processed features from modality-specific networks. This flexible strategy captures rich interactions between modalities without needing precise data alignment, making it highly effective for heterogeneous data. Decision-level fusion merges final predictions from independent models, offering robustness and modularity at the cost of losing low-level feature interactions. Barros et al. [13] developed an artificial intelligence model using mammography imaging data and electronic medical record data to identify subtypes of breast lesions. The image features are extracted from the CNN model and connected to the selected clinical data features to construct a fusion model in the Extreme Gradient Boosting Tree model. This process belongs to deep feature-level fusion after model representation. Generally, the smaller the information loss of each modality before fusion is, the more sufficient the information fusion is, and the better the final fusion result is. From existing research, the correctness of this view is also proved, especially that feature-level fusion is better than decision-level fusion [14]. Feature-level fusion allows specialized architectures (e.g., CNNs for images, Transformers for text) to first capture modality-specific patterns before combining them via concatenation, summation, or attention mechanisms. Its key strength lies in capturing rich, complementary interactions between modalities without requiring strict low-level data alignment. Although designing an effective fusion architecture remains non-trivial, its flexibility and capacity for modeling cross-modal dependencies make it the prevailing paradigm in tasks such as medical diagnosis, where leveraging structured and heterogeneous data is critical. It is crucial to design or select appropriate feature extraction networks for each modality and design effective feature fusion mechanisms.

2.2 Knowledge Augmented Disease Diagnosis

Medicine is a discipline that heavily relies on knowledge. Diagnostic models obtained solely from data models are often not recognized by doctors and require the support of knowledge in the field of healthcare [15]. Knowledge graph, as a carrier of multi-source heterogeneous knowledge, has been widely used in medical research due to its structure, semantic, interpretable and other characteristics. In the field of assisting disease diagnosis and prediction, previous research has mainly applied knowledge graphs to clinical feature representation and disease diagnosis pathway inference.

Existing ML studies mainly leverage medical knowledge to learn efficient representations of medical concepts, they can improve the performance of downstream tasks, e.g., disease risk prediction. Common medical knowledge graphs include ICD, UMLS, SNOMED CT, etc. The hierarchical structure in the knowledge graph is used as internal knowledge to enrich disease representations by utilizing node information, thereby modeling patient representations more accurately. For example, Choi et al. [16] proposed GRAM, which utilizes the hierarchical structure of the international classification of disease (ICD) encoding system and attention mechanism to learn the representations of disease concepts and then apply the learned representations in the disease progression prediction task. The experimental results of three independent studies demonstrated that this method could significantly improve the performance in predicting the onset of rare diseases [16–18]. Zhang et al. [19] utilized the TransE and graph attention network to learn representations of medical concepts from a KG named KnowLife, and they applied the learned representations in predicting the onset of heart failure [20, 21]. Xing et al. [22] introduced multi-omics graph knowledge representation to predict in-hospital outcomes for pneumonia patients, graph convolutional network (GCN) was employed to determine omics similarity.

Knowledge graph provides a general point of view for the entity and relationship in the medical field, light on hidden patterns and information that might not be readily discernible from clinical notes. To minimize the implicit knowledge in clinical data and provide interpretable disease prediction pathways, previous studies proposed interpretable and knowledge-guided deep models to address these challenges [21]. Sun et al. [23] built a KG to record relationships between diseases and risk factors according to validated medical knowledge, then formulated disease prediction as a random walk on KGs, where a reinforcement learning (RL) agent navigates from patient-specific nodes (e.g., symptoms) to disease entities, generating interpretable trajectories. Experimental results validate the proposed model in interpretably evaluating and optimizing disease prediction. Yang et al. [24] proposed a Knowledge Guided Interpretable Disease Prediction method (KGxDP) via path reasoning over medical knowledge graphs and admission history, generated patient subgraphs using patient characteristics and medical knowledge graph, and updated subgraphs through graph inference using graph attention network (GAT) specified by node type and edge type.

Reflecting on previous research findings, both multimodal fusion and knowledge enhancement methods have been validated as effective approaches for improving diagnostic disease performance. Based on this, our study attempts to integrate these two methods, aiming to leverage the heterogeneous features from multimodal data while simultaneously utilizing knowledge to enhance and constrain these features.

3 Methods

In this section, we describe our proposed richer fusion network for breast cancer classification in detail. For the sake of clarity, we first introduce the overall framework of our method, as shown in Fig. 2. Then, we introduce our method from three sections: pathological image feature representation, knowledge-augmented patient representation, and multimodal data fusion.

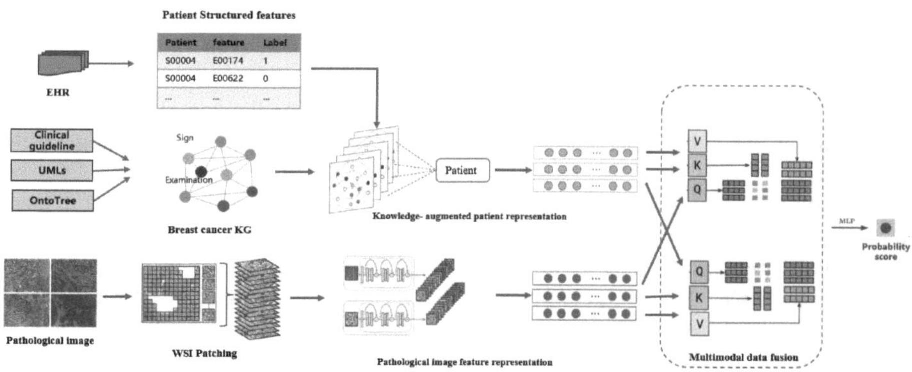

Fig. 2. A framework of knowledge-augmented multimodal learning for breast cancer diagnosis.

3.1 The Overall Framework

In terms of pathological image, Our approach involves identifying diagnostically relevant regions with CLAM and extracting deep features from the patches using a pre-trained ResNet50. These patch-level features are then aggregated into a single patient-level feature vector. (2) In terms of EHR data, we first use PubMedBERT to obtain semantic embeddings of medical entities and then apply a Graph Attention Network (GAT) to integrate structural knowledge from the graph, ultimately creating a knowledge-augmented patient representation. (3) During the feature fusion stage, a cross-modal attention mechanism is employed to integrate the high-dimensional feature vectors from both the knowledge-augmented data and the pathological images for each patient. The resulting fused features are ultimately used to predict the probability of breast cancer.

3.2 Pathological Image Feature Representation

The pathological manifestations of breast cancer are complex and diverse, and there are heterogeneity in clinical characteristics, histomorphology and gene changes [20]. It is necessary to use advanced digital pathological image analysis techniques to effectively distinguish them [25]. At present, More and more experts are using convolutional neural networks that fuse multi-scale features, the powerful feature capture capabilities of deep learning models such as CNN and Transformer are used to solve the above problems and better meet clinical needs [26]. Alqahtani et al. [27] proposed the Multiscale Squeeze and Excitation ResNet, which is based on ResNet and uses different max pooling layers to collect multi-scale features. The channel weights learned at each scale are fused to achieve an accuracy of 88.87% on the test set, ensuring the robustness of the classification model on different multiples of pathological images.

Whole slice image (WSI) technology allows pathologists to view and analyze the entire pathological section digitally, which not only significantly improves diagnostic efficiency but also enhances image accessibility and analysis accuracy. On this basis, image patch processing technology provides a more detailed and targeted analysis method, allowing pathologists to concentrate on analyzing image parts containing key diagnostic information. This method not only optimizes the use of computing resources, but also improves processing speed and diagnostic accuracy, especially when applying deep learning models for lesion classification and subtyping. For example, Huang et al. [28] proposed a breast pathology image classification method based on multi view patch embedding. This method extracts multi-scale features by constructing patches of different scales and converting them into embedding vectors. These patch embeddings are integrated through cross scale fusion modules, optimizing the complementarity and contextual relevance between features, significantly enhancing the classification ability of the model.

For patient image data, a pre-trained deep learning model is used to capture both local and global features of lesion regions. For example, WSI in pathological data often exhibit exceptionally high resolutions. To augment the data, a weakly supervised computational pathology tool, CLAM [29], is applied to identify diagnostically relevant regions and extract a set of image patches. Then, a pre-trained ResNet50 model [30] (without the classification layer) is employed to extract deep features from each image patch, through feature dimensionality reduction and attention-weighted aggregation, the multi-patch features are fused into a unified patient-level feature vector. The patch-level features from each WSI are aggregated by an attention-weighted average pooling to form a slide-level feature vector. If a patient has multiple WSIs, we average the slide-level features to obtain a patient-level feature vector.

Given a patient $\boldsymbol{P}$ has whole slide images $\{\boldsymbol{WSI}_1, \boldsymbol{WSI}_2, \ldots, \boldsymbol{WSI}_i\}$, $\boldsymbol{F_P}$ is the representation of the final patient-level feature vector. The feature extraction process can be formulated as:

$$\boldsymbol{F_P} = \frac{1}{i}\sum_{j=1}^{i} \boldsymbol{\Phi}_{agg}\left(\sum_{k=1}^{K} a_{j,k} \cdot \left(\boldsymbol{\Phi}_{resnet}\left(\boldsymbol{WSI}_{j,k}\right)\right)\right) \tag{1}$$

where $\boldsymbol{WSI}_{j,k}$ denotes the $\boldsymbol{k}$-th patch identified by CLAM from the $\boldsymbol{j}$-th WSI. $\boldsymbol{\Phi}_{resnet}$ represents the ResNet50 feature extraction function, which outputs a 1024-dimensional feature vector. $\boldsymbol{a}_{j,k}$ denotes the attention weight computed by CLAM. $\boldsymbol{\Phi}_{agg}$ is the feature aggregation function.

3.3 Knowledge-Augmented Patient Representation

Graph Attention Network (GAT) is a novel neural network model that operates on graph-structured data and uses attention mechanisms to achieve state-of-the-art results on both inductive and transudative learning tasks [31]. In the context of knowledge embedding, GAT plays a crucial role in injecting the rich structural information of a knowledge graph into entity representations. By propagating and aggregating information from a node's local neighborhood, GAT refines initial entity features. Xiao et al. [32] established a patient-disease bipartite graph, projects it onto a weighted patient network, employs GCN and GAT for feature extraction and node representation, and utilizes these representations for disease prediction. Based on previous research, we employ GAT to create a knowledge-augmented representation of patient features. This approach integrates structured medical knowledge (e.g., from a knowledge graph) with patient specific data to generate comprehensive patient feature vectors. Unlike traditional methods that rely solely on raw clinical data, our paradigm enriches the patient model by leveraging the rich semantic relationships and hierarchical structures encoded within biomedical knowledge bases. The typical pipeline involves two stages:

(1) Knowledge Graph Entity Embedding Learning. This stage aims to learn high-quality vector representations (entity embeddings) for each medical entity in the knowledge graph.

First, We define a knowledge graph $G = (V, E), E = \{(h, r, t)|h, t \in V, r \in R\}, |\mathcal{E}|, |\mathcal{E}| = m, |\mathcal{R}| = n$, where h represents the head entity, t represents the tail entity, and r signifies the relationship between them, for example, "ductal carcinoma in situ" (h)—"clinical features" (r)—"proliferative changes" (t).

Subsequently, the semantic embeddings generated by PubMedBERT [33] are used as the initial node features $h_v^{(0)}$ and fed into a two-layer Graph Attention Network (GAT). The GAT incorporates structural information from the knowledge graph into the entity representations by aggregating information from each node's neighbors via an attention mechanism. Each layer of the GAT operates according to Eqs. (2) and (3). Specifically, for each node, the GAT first computes a normalized attention weight α_{ij} for each of its neighbors. This weight determines the importance of neighbor j to the central node i during information aggregation. The updated representation of the node is then the weighted sum of the linearly transformed features of all its neighbors.

$$h_{kg}^{(l)} = \sigma\left(\sum_{j \in \mathrm{N}_i} \alpha_{ij}^{(l)} w^{(l)} h_j^{(l-1)}\right) \tag{2}$$

$$\alpha_{ij}^{(l)} = \frac{\exp(LeakyReLU(a^{(l)T}[W^{(l)} h_i^{(l-1)} || W^{(l)} h_j^{(l-1)}]))}{\sum_{\kappa \in \mathrm{N}_i} \exp(LeakyReLU(a^{(l)T}[W^{(l)} h_i^{(l-1)} || W^{(l)} h_j^{(l-1)}]))} \tag{3}$$

$h_i^{(l)}$ donates the embedding representation of node i at the $l - th$ layer. N_i is the set of neighboring nodes for node i (includes a self-loop), $W^{(l)}$ is the trainable weight matrix for the $l - th$ layer, used for feature transformation. σ donates a non-linear activation function (e.g., ELU).

By stacking two such GAT layers, the final representation $h_{kg}^{(2)}$ for each entity encodes not only its own textual semantics but also the structural graph information within its two-hop neighborhood.

(2) Patient Feature Embedding Aggregation. This stage aims to generate a single embedding representation for each patient, based on all medical entities associated with that patient.

First, a mapping table links each patient (identified by a patient_id) with one or more medical entities (e.g., diagnosed diseases, medications taken), $E_P = \{e_1, e_2, ..., e_i, .., e_N\}$. For instance, patient P001 might be associated with the features ['Age > 40', 'Bad activity', 'Not Smooth Surface']. Second, for each entity e associated with a patient, its corresponding graph embedding vector $h_{kg}(e_i)$ is retrieved from the embedding obtained in Stage 1. Finally, the retrieved entity embeddings are aggregated via average pooling to produce a comprehensive embedding vector representing the patient. Average pooling serves as a simple yet effective method for condensing all the patient's feature information into a fixed-dimensional vector. The final embedding vector V_P for patient P is computed as:

$$V_P = \frac{1}{N} \sum_{e \in E_P} h_{kg}(e_i) \tag{4}$$

3.4 Multimodal Data Fusion

During the fusion stage of features from various modalities, a dynamic fusion module for multimodal features is constructed. A cross-modal attention mechanism is used to fuse the high-dimensional feature vectors of knowledge-augmented feature and Pathological image feature of each patient. The cross-attention mechanism enables dynamic interaction between two distinct sequences by computing attention scores across them. Unlike self-attention, which operates within a single sequence, cross-attention uses one sequence as the query (Q) and another as the key (K) and value (V). This allows the model to focus on relevant parts of the second sequence while processing the first, effectively aligning and integrating heterogeneous information. Here, we employ a bidirectional cross-attention mechanism by implementing two distinct cross-attention modules that operate in opposite directions. Attention weights are generated to facilitate feature fusion. The fused features retain visual evidence from images and disease-associated logic from the knowledge graph. These are then input into a multilayer perception to generate a unified joint representation. The final classifier outputs probabilities for disease types, and a confidence score is computed based on the entropy of the probability distribution. High-confidence results reflect the model's certainty in the diagnosis, while low-confidence results indicate the need for manual review or additional examinations (Table 1).

Table 1. Algorithm of multimodal data fusion.

Algorithm: cross-modal attention mechanism
Input: Image features $\boldsymbol{F_P}$, Knowledge-augmented features $\boldsymbol{V_P}$
1. Q, K, V $\leftarrow$ LinearTransforms($\boldsymbol{F_P}$, $\boldsymbol{V_P}$)
2. *A_{F $\rightarrow$ V}, A_{V $\rightarrow$ F} $\leftarrow$ CrossAttention(Q, K, V)*
3. $\boldsymbol{F'_P}$, $\boldsymbol{V'_P}$ $\leftarrow$ FeatureInteraction($\boldsymbol{F_P}$, $\boldsymbol{V_P}$, A_{F $\rightarrow$ V}, A_{V $\rightarrow$ F})
4. $\boldsymbol{Z_P}$ $\leftarrow$ Concat($\boldsymbol{F'_P}$, $\boldsymbol{V'_P}$)
5. $\hat{y}$ $\leftarrow$ MLP($\boldsymbol{Z_P}$)
Output: Disease prediction $\hat{y}$

4 Experiments

4.1 Dataset

Pathological EMR Dataset [10]: this dataset contains medical records of 185 breast cancer patients, and for each patient, a total of 3764 high resolution(2048 × 1536 pixels) pathological images were collected. All pathological images were obtained using the same equipment at a 100 × or 200 × magnification. Each image is labeled as benign or malignant according to the main cancer type in each image. And they extracted 29 representative features which are used to describe the patients' condition from the EMR, include age, gender, family tumor history, tumor position, smooth surface, and the diagnosis, etc. (Fig. 3).

Number of medical records	185 (82 benign, 103 malignant)
Number of pathological images	3764 (1332 benign, 2432 malignant)
Size of pathological images	2048 × 1536 pixels
Color model of pathological images	R(ed)G(reen)B(lue)
Memory space of pathological images	3–20 MB
Number of features extracted from each case	29

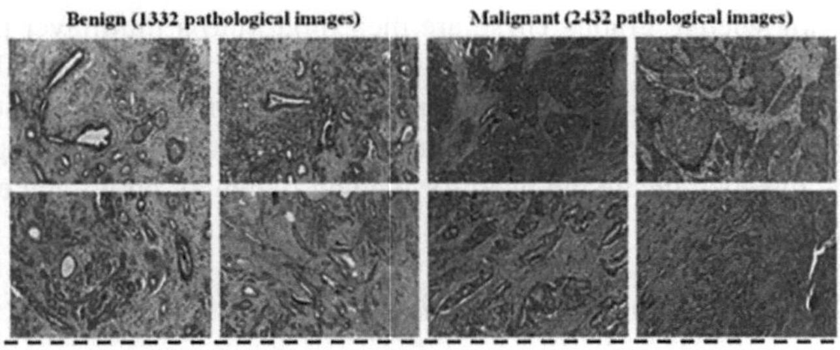

Fig. 3. Pathological EMR dataset.

Breast cancer knowledge graph: The main knowledge source of this study is the breast cancer Diagnosis and Treatment Guide (2022 Edition) [34] issued by the National Health Commission. The guide contains 7 topics, including breast cancer screening, diagnosis, histopathological diagnosis, differential diagnosis, treatment, diagnosis process and follow-up. Additionally, pathological knowledge from BI-RADS and OntoTree are used to enriched.Finally, we ultimately defined 10 primary concepts and 41 attribute relationships, contained 629 entities, 41 relations, 889 triplets. Since this study is mainly aimed at disease diagnosis of breast cancer, 350 triplets related to breast cancer diagnosis are selected for patient feature representation of knowledge enhancement, including breast cancer classification, risk factors, symptoms and signs etc. (Fig. 4).

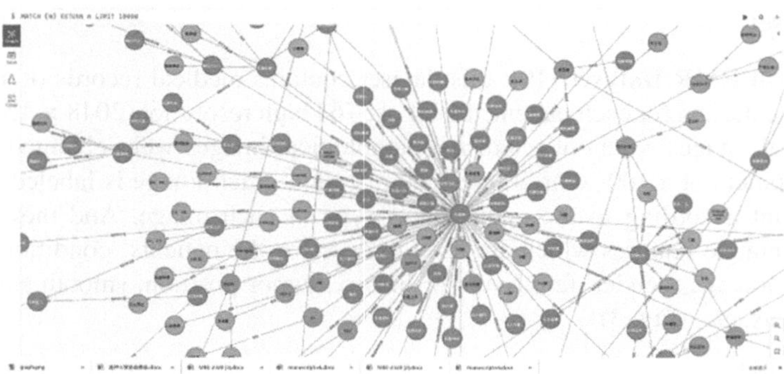

Fig. 4. Breast cancer knowledge graph.

4.2 Data Preprocessing

The goal of our study is to predict whether a patient's diagnosis is benign or malignant by integrating the patient's feature set, which is a binary classification task with labels

0 or 1. After filtering out duplicate patient IDs and image IDs that did not match patient IDs, a total of 183 patients and their related data were included in our study, including 81 benign and 102 malignant tumor patients. Randomly select 10 benign and 10 malignant patients as the test set, and the remaining 163 patients, 90% as the training set and 10% as the validation set.

In order to associate the clinical features of patients in the raw data with the nodes of the knowledge graph, we first convert the structured features in the raw data into text features based on range codes, such as converting "age: 1" to "age 20–40 years old" and "tumor border: 0" to "clear boundary". Subsequently, the transformed text features are matched with entities in the knowledge graph, and after automatic matching of text similarity and manual proofreading, the entity feature set of each patient *Ep* is obtained. *Ep* of 9 patients were ultimately empty due to missing clinical feature data, padding with zero vectors will be used in subsequent research (Table 2).

Table 2. The overall description of data.

	Basic data	Train	Validation	Test
Number of patients	183(81 benign, 102 malignant)	147	16	20(10benign, 10malignant)
Number of Pathological images	3693 (1302 benign, 2391 malignant)	135923 patches	15103 patches	16001 patches

4.3 Results

We mainly use the average Accuracy, Precision, Recall and F1 to evaluate the performance of our method. Furthermore, the performance of a classifier can be evaluated using the ROC curve and AUC.

In order to compare the effectiveness of cross modal feature fusion models, we combined three types of patient features: pathological image features, structured clinical features, and knowledge-augmented clinical features (KA data) in different combinations. The model results are shown in the table. Model A uses pathological image features alone and utilizes the Resnet50 model for feature extraction and classification prediction; Model B uses the patient's original structured electronic medical record features alone, and feature extraction uses the One hot method. The fusion of cross modal features in models D and E utilized the cross attention mechanism method mentioned in Section III. During the training process, the 1024 dimensional features extracted from pathological images are mapped to 512 dimensions through a feedforward neural network layer, and then cross fused with the 512 dimensional features represented by knowledge augmented patient features. The learning rate is 5e-4, dropout is 0.3, and the training batch size is 16. The model was trained under the following environment: an NVIDIA RTX 4090 24GB GPU, Python 3.12.4, CUDA 12.4, and PyTorch 2.4.0.

By comparison, it can be found that the effect of multimodal feature fusion is significantly better than that of single modality. The features augmented by knowledge can have a positive effect on classification performance, whether used alone or in combination with other modal features, achieving a classification effect of over 90%. In the test set, the combination of Pathological image and KA data achieved the best classification performance (99.63%) (Table 3).

Table 3. Results of different fusion of features.

Method	Accuracy (validation)	Accuracy (test)	P(test)		R(test)		F1(test)	
			B	M	B	M	B	M
A: Pathological image only	0.9095	0.7580	0.8069	0.7333	0.6060	0.8818	0.6920	0.8006
B: Structured data only	0.9925	0.85	1.0000	0.7692	0.7000	1.0000	0.8235	0.8696
C: KA data only	0.9667	0.95	1.0000	0.9091	0.9000	1.0000	0.9474	0.9524
D: Pathological image + Structured data	0.9993	0.9185	0.9842	0.8852	0.8367	0.9862	0.9012	0.9313
E: Pathological image + KA data	0.9957	0.9963	0.9987	0.9944	0.9931	0.9990	0.9959	0.9967

Evaluation of the ROC curves demonstrates that both Model E and Model D achieve Area Under the Curve (AUC) values approaching 1.00, indicating a highly discriminative and comparable ability to distinguish between positive and negative samples. However, a more nuanced analysis using the Precision-Recall Curve (PRC) reveals Model E 's superior performance in identifying positive cases (malignant patients). While both models exhibit curves that approach the upper-left corner in the ROC space, Model E attains a marginally higher AUC (0.9994 vs. 0.9931). This slight advantage is substantiated in the PRC analysis, where Model E not only achieves a higher Average Precision (AUPRC) (0.9997 vs. 0.9940) but also presents a curve closer to the ideal top-right corner. This signifies that Model E delivers exceptional precision (i.e. a minimal rate of false positives) while simultaneously maintaining a high recall (i.e., identifying nearly all true malignant cases). Such a balance is critical in breast cancer diagnosis to minimize both missed diagnoses and false alarms. In contrast, Model A's performance on both metrics (ROC-AUC = 0.8650; AUPRC = 0.8986) is substantially inferior, underscoring a significant gap in its diagnostic capability (Fig. 5).

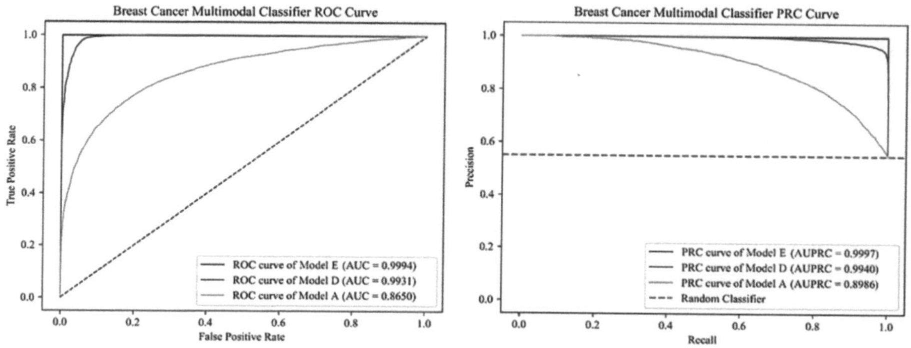

Fig. 5. ROC Curve and PRC Curve of different models.

In similar studies, Yang et al. [5] utilized a new and richer fusion network to integrate highly heterogeneous data to improve the accuracy of pathological image classification using structured EMR data, with the highest accuracy rate reaching 93.3%; Song [35] designed a multi-level fusion network for multimodal breast cancer diagnosis, with the highest accuracy of 93.62%. Compared with previous research results, our knowledge augmented multimodal breast cancer diagnosis system has better performance. However, it is worth noting that the way we partition the dataset is different, and the results may have some bias (Table 4).

Table 4. Comparison of accuracy with previous methods.

Method	Accuracy(validation)	Accuracy(test)
E: Pathological image + KA-data	0.9957	0.9963
Pathological image only (VGG16) [5]	0.845	0.836
Structured data only (29D) [5]	0.903	0.785
Stuctured data(29D*20) + Pathological image(FC-1280D)[5]	0.933	0.911
DenseNetGAT[30]	–	0.9362

5 Discussion

5.1 Comparison of Different Feature Fusion Methods

To investigate the impact of multi-feature integration on disease diagnosis and classification, we extended the baseline model by incorporating three distinct feature types: pathological images, knowledge-augmented (KA) data, and structured clinical data. Two fusion architectures were designed and evaluated: Model F first applies bidirectional cross-attention between pathological image features and KA data, followed by decision-level fusion with structured data; Model G instead fuses image features with structured data via bidirectional cross-attention, then combines the result with KA data at the decision level. Experimental results demonstrate that Model F significantly outperforms Model G (Table 5).

Table 5. Comparison of accuracy with different feature fusion methods.

Method	Accuracy(validation)	Accuracy(test)
F: Pathological image + KA-data + Structured data	0.9916	**0.9758**
G: Pathological image + Structured data + KA-data	0.9968	0.9148

We attribute this performance discrepancy to the stronger semantic complementarity between image features and knowledge-augmented representations. Pathological images provide visually grounded information—such as tumor morphology and tissue texture—while knowledge graphs encode structured medical knowledge, including disease relationships and pathological logic. Through bidirectional cross-attention, Model F achieves deep interaction between visual evidence and domain knowledge, enhancing the model's capacity to recognize clinically relevant patterns, for instance, by using ontological constraints to resolve ambiguities in visual findings or to highlight subtle anomalies indicative of malignancy.

In contrast, structured electronic health record often exhibit higher variability and contain episodic or descriptive elements that may not align robustly with image-derived features. Fusing them directly with image data in Model G may introduce noise or lead the model to rely on spurious correlations, thereby weakening feature learning. Moreover, since KA data embodies high-level medical reasoning, its influence is better preserved when incorporated at the decision level after robust vision–knowledge fusion, as in Model F. In Model G, however, the deep fusion of image and structured data may dilute the contribution of knowledge, and late-stage fusion with KA data offers limited capacity to recalibrate feature-level representations, ultimately reducing predictive accuracy.

5.2 Comparison of Different Knowledge Enhancement Methods

To further investigate the efficacy of different knowledge-augmented strategies for disease classification, we implemented and compared two distinct methods. The first Method (1), as detailed in Sect. 3.2, processes Knowledge Graph (KG) entities through a Graph Attention Network (GAT) and subsequently aggregates the resulting embeddings to construct a patient representation. The second Method (2) involves a structural augmentation of the original KG: we introduce dedicated patient nodes and create edges linking them to existing clinical entities. For instance, establishing a triple such as (Nipple Discharge, is_founded_in, Patient 001). This enriched graph is then processed by a GAT to directly learn a comprehensive embedding for each patient node, which serves as the final feature vector. The experimental results indicate that when using the augmented features alone for disease prediction, both Method (1) and Method (2) achieved comparable performance; however, Method (2) demonstrated better effectiveness on the validation set. In contrast, when combined with pathological image features, Method (1) yielded superior results (Table 6).

Table 6. Comparison of accuracy with different knowledge enhancement methods.

Method	Accuracy(validation)	Accuracy(test)
KA-data only (1)	0.9667	**0.95**
KA-data only (2)	**0.9911**	**0.95**
Pathological image + KA-data (1)	0.9957	**0.9963**
Pathological image + KA-data (2)	**0.9999**	0.9926

The patient node in Method (2) can indirectly observe patterns from similar patients (e.g., through shared symptoms or disease entities) via graph connections, thereby learning more discriminative representations. In contrast, the features of each patient in Method (1) are independently aggregated, lacking this direct global perspective. Meanwhile, during the message-passing process of the Graph Attention Network, the patient nodes directly interact with other patient nodes and medical entities, enabling the model to learn a more rational and smoother representation within the overall graph relational structure. This structural design reduces the risk of overfitting to the training set, resulting in more robust performance on the validation set. During the fusion stage, the features provided by Method (1) constitute a collection of fine-grained medical entity semantics, or "semantic labels." When fused with image features, these "labels" offer explicit contextual guidance and constraints for image understanding, facilitating more effective interaction.

5.3 Interpretability of Knowledge- Augmented

To explore how the GAT model leverages knowledge to augment patient feature representation, we visualized the process of patient node feature learning in Method (2). As shown in Fig. 6, the attention weight distributions across two GAT layers are displayed for five randomly selected malignant tumor patients. The upper section illustrates the first-layer attention weights, while the lower section corresponds to the second layer. This visualization reveals how the model hierarchically and selectively integrates information from the knowledge graph to construct patient representations.

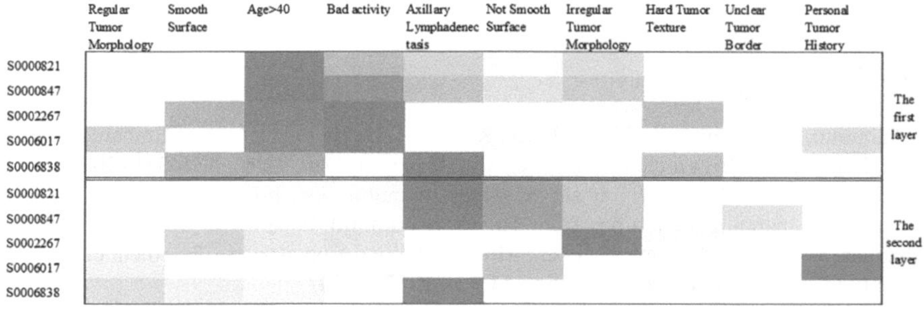

Fig. 6. The attention weight distributions across two GAT layers.

The first-layer attention, depicted in the upper part of the figure, is relatively concentrated, with primary emphasis on nodes such as "Age > 40" and "Bad activity". This reflects the model's initial strategy for information aggregation: it first prioritizes medically prevalent and highly relevant macroscopic risk factors. By rapidly identifying the most critical risk indicators shared across all patients, the model constructs a foundational feature representation for each patient node. The observed concentration suggests that, for these malignant tumor cases, the model attributes high and consistent discriminative value to these fundamental factors.

The second-layer attention, shown in the lower part of the figure, exhibits a more dispersed and diverse pattern. Different patient nodes attend to distinct combinations of features. For example: Patient S0000821 simultaneously focuses on "Irregular Tumor Morphology" and "Hard Tumor Texture", Patient S0000847 places greater emphasis on "Axillary Lymphadenectasis" and "Personal Tumor History". These indicate a more refined reasoning process at the higher layer. Building upon the foundational patient profile provided by the first layer, the second-layer GAT adaptively incorporates more specific information from the knowledge graph, tailored to each patient's unique context, to refine the diagnostic representation.

6 Conclusion

This study developed a novel knowledge-augmented multimodal learning framework for breast cancer diagnosis, which emulates the comprehensive diagnostic reasoning process of clinicians by effectively integrating pathological images, structured clinical features, and knowledge from medical guidelines. Through a series of experiments evaluating different feature combinations, we demonstrated the effectiveness and interpretability of knowledge augmentation and multimodal feature learning in breast cancer diagnosis. However, limited by the multimodal nature of the dataset, the findings of this study have yet to be extensively validated for diagnosing other diseases.

Acknowledgments. The publication of this paper is funded by the CAMS Innovation Fund for Medical Sciences (CIFMS) (Grant No. 2021-I2M-1-001).

Disclosure of Interests. The authors declare that they have no competing interests.

References

1. Giaquinto, A. N., Sung, H., Miller, K. D., Kramer, J. L., Newman, L. A., Minihan, A., Jemal, A., Siegel, R. L.: Breast cancer statistics. CA: Cancer J. Clin. **72**(6), 524–541 (2022)
2. Shaik, T., Tao, X.H., Li, L., et al.: A survey of multimodal information fusion for smart healthcare: mapping the journey from data to wisdom. Inf. Fusion **102**, 1020–1040 (2024)
3. Kumar, S., Rani, S., Sharma, S., et al.: Multimodality fusion aspects of medical diagnosis: a comprehensive review. Bioengineering **11**(12), 1233 (2024)
4. Zheng, Y., Conrad, R.D., Green, E.J., et al.: Graph attention-based fusion of pathology images and gene expression for prediction of cancer survival. IEEE Trans. Med. Imaging **43**(9), 3085–3097 (2024)

5. Teoh, J.R., Dong, J., Zuo, X.W., et al.: Advancing healthcare through multimodal data fusion: a comprehensive review of techniques and applications. Peer J Comput. Sci. **10**, e2298 (2024)
6. Lyu, W., Dong, X., Wong, R., et al.: A multimodal transformer: fusing clinical notes with structured EHR data for interpretable in-hospital mortality prediction. In: AMIA 2022 Annual Symposium Proceedings, pp. 719–728 (2023)
7. Mohamed, S.K., Nounu, A., Nováček, V.: Biological applications of knowledge graph embedding models. Brief. Bioinform. **22**(2), 1679–1693 (2021)
8. Lam, V.K., Byers, J.M., Robitaille, M.C.: A self-supervised learning approach for high throughput and high content cell segmentation. Commun Biol **8**, 780 (2025)
9. Popovici, V., et al.: Joint analysis of histopathology image features and gene expression in breast cancer. BMC Bioinform. **17**(1), 209 (2016)
10. Yan, R., Zhang, F., Rao, X.: Richer fusion network for breast cancer classification based on multimodal data. BMC Med. Inform. Decis. Mak. **21**(1), 1–15 (2021)
11. Yang, J., Ju, J., Guo, L.: Prediction of HER2-positive breast cancer recurrence and metastasis risk from histopathological images and clinical information via multimodal deep learning. Comput. Struct. Biotechnol. J. **20**, 333–342 (2022)
12. Khaleghi, B., Khamis, A., Karray, F.O., Razavi, S.N.: Multi sensor data fusion: a review of the state-of-the-art. Inf Fusion **14**(1), 28–44 (2013)
13. Barros, V., Tlusty, T., Barkan, E.: Virtual biopsy by using artificial intelligence-based multimodal modeling of binational mammography data. Radiology **306**(3), e220027 (2022)
14. Ramachandram, D., Taylor, G.W.: Deep multimodal learning: a survey on recent advances and trends. IEEE Signal Process. Mag. **34**(6), 96–108 (2017)
15. Warnat-Herresthal, S., Schultze, H., Shastry, K.L.: Swarm learning for decentralized and confidential clinical machine learning. Nature **594**(7862), 265–270 (2021)
16. Choi, E.: GRAM: graph-based attention model for healthcare representation learning. In: Proceedings of ACM SIGKDD International Conference on Knowledge Discovery and Data Mining, New York, NY, pp. 787–795 (2017)
17. Li, Y.: Knowledge guided diagnosis prediction via graph spatial temporal network. In: Proceedings SIAM International Conference Data Mining, Cincinnati, OH, pp. 19–27 (2020)
18. Ma, F.: KAME: Knowledge-based attention model for diagnosis prediction in healthcare. In: Proceedings of ACM International Conference on Information and Knowledge Manage, New York, NY, pp. 743–752 (2018)
19. Zhang, X., Qian, B., Li, Y., Yin, C., Wang, X., Zheng, Q.: KnowRisk: An interpretable knowledge-guided model for disease risk prediction. In: Proceedings of IEEE International Conference on Data Mining, Beijing, China, pp.1492–1497 (2019)
20. Knowlife: A versatile approach for constructing a large knowledge graph for biomedical sciences. BMC Bioinf. **16**(157), 157 (2015)
21. Yin, C.: Domain Knowledge guided deep learning with electronic health records. In: Proceedings of IEEE International Conference on Data Mining, Beijing, China, pp. 738–747 (2019)
22. Xing, W., et al.: Multi-omics graph knowledge representation for pneumonia prognostic prediction. IEEE J. Biomed. Health Inform. **29**(4), 3021–3034 (2025)
23. Sun, W., Dong, J., Shi, J., Huang, Z.: Interpretable disease progression prediction based on reinforcement reasoning over a knowledge graph. IEEE Trans. Syst., Man, Cybern.: Syst. **54**(3), 1948–1959 (2024)
24. Yang, Z., Lin, Y., Xu, Y., Hu, J., Dong, S.: Interpretable disease prediction via path reasoning over medical knowledge graphs and admission history. Knowl.-Based Syst. **281**, 111082 (2023)
25. Baxi, V., Edwards, R., Montalto, M.: Digital pathology and artificial intelligence in translational medicine and clinical practice. Mod. Pathol. **35**(1), 23–32 (2022)

26. Krithiga, R., Geetha, P.: Breast cancer detection, segmentation and classification on histopathology images analysis: a systematic review. Arch Computat Methods Eng **28**, 2607–2619 (2021)
27. Alqahtani, Y., Mandawkar, U., Sharma, A.: Breast cancer pathological image classification based on the multiscale CNN squeeze model. Comput. Intell. Neurosci. **2022**, 7075408 (2022)
28. Huang, S.K., Yu, Y.T., Huang, C.R.: Cross-scale fusion transformer for histopathological image classification. IEEE J. Biomed. Health Inform. **28**(1), 297–308 (2023)
29. Lu, M.Y., Williamson, D.F.K., Chen, T.Y.: Data-efficient and weakly supervised computational pathology on whole-slide images. Nat. Biomed. Eng. **5**, 555–570 (2021)
30. He, K., Zhang, X., Ren, S., Sun, J.: Deep residual learning for image recognition (2015). arXiv:1512.03385
31. Veličković, P., Cucurull, G., Casanova, A., Romero, A., Lio, P., Bengio, Y.: Graph attention networks (2017). arXiv:1710.10903
32. Xiao, C., Imel, E.A., Pham, N., Luo, X.: Patient-GAT: Sarcopenia prediction using multimodal data fusion and weighted graph attention networks. Proc. Symp. Appl. Comput. **2023**, 614–617 (2023)
33. Gu, Y., Tinn, R., Cheng, H., Lucas, M., Usuyama, N., Liu, X., Naumann, T., Gao, J., Poon, H.: Domain-specific language model pretraining for biomedical natural language processing (2020). arXiv:2007.15779
34. National Health Commission of the People's Republic of China. https://www.nhc.gov.cn/yzygj/c100068/202204/0c1f7d3aca0545abbeb02030ce255930.shtml. Last accessed 20 Sept 2024
35. Song, M.: Multimodal breast cancer diagnosis research and system based on multi-layer fusion network Yangzhou University (2023)

Retrieval-Augmented Relation Extraction for Medical Knowledge Graphs

Yu Song, Xinyang Li, Yunhao Li, Yunlong Li, Kejun Wu, Yuting Li, and Kunli Zhang(✉)

School of Computer Science and Artificial Intelligence, Zhengzhou University, Henan 450001, China
ieklzhang@zzu.edu.cn

Abstract. Medical entity relation extraction is crucial for building medical knowledge graphs and supporting clinical decision-making. Yet, current models struggle with scarce annotations and evolving domain knowledge. We propose Retrieval-Augmented Relation Extraction (RA-RE), a framework that combines static and dynamic retrieval mechanisms to enhance large language models. The core innovation lies in a Dynamic Semantic Confidence Evaluation (DSCE) module, which adaptively decides whether to retrieve external examples based on prediction reliability. This confidence-aware retrieval enables RA-RE to reduce annotation dependency while improving robustness and accuracy. The dynamic pipeline consists of zero-shot prediction, confidence evaluation, example retrieval, and final prediction, ensuring flexible and knowledge-driven relation extraction. Evaluations on multiple medical datasets and model scales show that RA-RE consistently outperforms strong baselines, highlighting the effectiveness of integrating confidence-aware retrieval into medical information extraction.

Keywords: Medical field · Relation extraction · Retrieval-Augmented generation · LLMs

1 Introduction

Entity-relationship extraction task, as one of the subtasks of information extraction, is one of the important research directions in natural language processing. Recently, major advances have been made in Large Language Models (LLMs), which have become the cornerstone models for studying Natural Language Processing (NLP) tasks. These LLMs [1] are usually continuously trained or fine-tuned on a natural corpus containing domain data to solve specific tasks.

Although the capabilities of the existing LLMs are already very robust, there are still some challenging issues. One of the most prominent challenges is that the model's performance is limited in a specific domain [2]. Another great challenge is the problem of updating knowledge [3]. To improve the performance and knowledge capacity of large models, increasing model parameters and efficient

Y. Zhang et al. (Eds.): CHIP 2025, CCIS 2884, pp. 347–361, 2026.
https://doi.org/10.1007/978-981-95-7299-1_20

fine-tuning are simple and effective methods. However, the marginal benefits diminish as the scale of model parameters increases and may be limited by factors such as computational resources and data quality [4]. Efficient fine-tuning, on the other hand, is suitable for injecting a small amount of domain knowledge and is not suitable for frequent execution. Another approach is Retrieval-Augmented Generation (RAG) [5], by adding an external knowledge base and inputting Query into the model together after retrieving relevant content in the knowledge base before model generation. RAG can effectively mitigate the problem of lack of specific knowledge and difficulty in updating the knowledge in models.

To address these challenges, this paper proposes a joint entity-relationship extraction method based on LLMs retrieval and generation, which combines LLMs with retrieval augments to retrieve similar information from external knowledge bases and combines the powerful generative capabilities of LLMs to improve entity relationship extraction.

Specifically, we constructed a local medical entity-relationship vector knowledge base as a retrieval repository. Fine-tuning and prediction experiments were performed using the WINGPT-14B-CHAT[1] model, which was pre-trained in the medical domain, and the generic model Llama3-Chinese-8B-Instruct.[2] The retrieval model and external knowledge vector embedding model are used with all-MiniLM-L6-v2.[3] Extensive experiments show that both in the model without fine-tuning and in the model with fine-tuning, the proposed method improves over the direct fine-tuning prediction method in terms of F1.

Our contribution can be summarized as follows:

- We propose static Retrieval-Augmented Entity Relationship Extraction (RA-RE), which includes: building a local entity-relationship medical knowledge base, constructing a RAG fine-tuning data, and RA-RE model.
- The retrieval mechanism is optimized on the basis of RA-RE, and the Dynamic Retrieval Enhanced Entity Relationship Extraction (DR-RE) method is proposed. The answer is retained if the model is more confident in the first prediction result, otherwise retrieval is performed.
- Extensive experiments demonstrate that our method improves the performance of entity-relationship tasks on different models and is cost-effective.

2 Related Work

Deep learning–based methods have achieved remarkable progress in relation extraction [6]. However, their performance often declines in real-world applications where data scarcity and long-tail distributions prevail [7]. Traditional models also face challenges in few-shot learning, which limits their adaptability

[1] https://hf-mirror.com/winninghealth/WiNGPT2-14B-Chat.
[2] https://modelscope.cn/models/FlagAlpha/Llama3-Chinese-8B-Instruct.
[3] https://modelscope.cn/models/bensonpeng/all-MiniLM-L6-v2.

to diverse scenarios. Recently, large language models (LLMs) have shown strong capabilities in relation extraction [8], and their ability to generalize in few-shot and zero-shot settings has attracted increasing attention [9].

Relation extraction approaches are typically categorized into pipeline-based and joint methods [10]. Pipeline methods perform entity recognition followed by relation classification [11]. Although simple to implement [12], they suffer from error propagation and a lack of task integration, which can reduce overall accuracy. Joint methods attempt to mitigate these issues by addressing both tasks simultaneously. In the medical domain, where labeled data is expensive and unevenly distributed, researchers have begun to explore the use of LLMs for automatic [13] annotation as a means to alleviate data scarcity [14].

Despite these advances, LLMs still face significant challenges. Hallucinations remain a critical issue, where models produce fluent but factually incorrect outputs [15]. Updating internal knowledge through retraining or fine-tuning is costly and inefficient [16]. Moreover, general-purpose LLMs often lack sufficient domain-specific knowledge [17], and training specialized models requires substantial resources.

To overcome these limitations, retrieval-augmented generation (RAG) has emerged as a promising paradigm. By integrating external knowledge bases into the generation process, RAG can mitigate hallucinations, simplify knowledge updating, and facilitate domain adaptation. Recent studies further demonstrate its potential for relation extraction. Xu et al. [18] highlighted the use of LLMs in generative relation extraction and suggested combining them with structured knowledge bases to enhance reasoning. Fan et al. [19] showed that RAG effectively improves the factual consistency of generated text while addressing knowledge obsolescence [20].

3 Methodology

In this section, We propose a joint extraction method for medical entity relationships based on augmented generation of external knowledge base retrieval. The proposed method can be subdivided into RA-RE and DR-RE. Static retrieval augment aims to directly input the similar example into the LLMs for prediction. Dynamic retrieval augment requires first input the Query into the LLMs for prediction, and then conduct a confidence assessment of the results. For those with a confidence level exceeding the threshold, a similarity search is performed; otherwise, the first prediction results are retained. Since dynamic retrieval adds a confidence assessment module on the basis of static retrieval, only the dynamic retrieval method needs to be displayed. The DR-RE can be divided into four parts: (1) Zero example prediction, (2) Dynamic Semantic Confidence Evaluation(DSCE), (3) Example retrieval and (4) Prediction. Figure 1 illustrates the overall framework of DR-RE method.

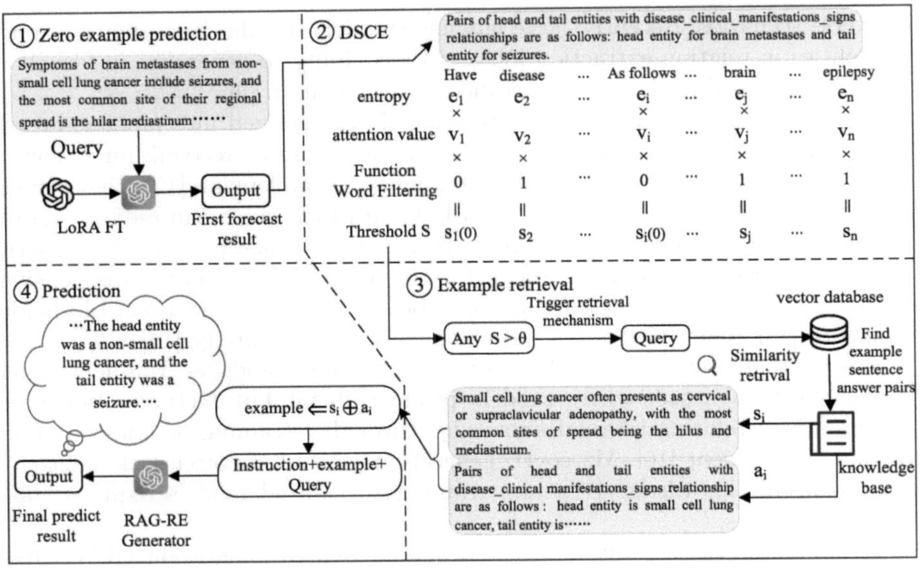

Fig. 1. DR-RE overall architecture

3.1 Zero Example Prediction

Zero-shot prediction refers to the capability of a large-scale model to perform predictions on unseen tasks or data without task-specific training. This capability relies on the broad knowledge and semantic understanding acquired during the model's pretraining phase, enabling it to handle novel tasks through reasoning and transfer learning. The user query is first fed into the LoRA-fine-tuned LLMs, which performs an initial inference step to generate a preliminary output. In this section, before making predictions, the general model is fine-tuned using the self-built RAG fine-tuning dataset to enhance the performance of the entity relationship extraction task, and the output is called the first prediction result.

3.2 Dynamic Semantic Confidence Evaluation

The retrieval module triggered by static predefined rules suffers from insufficient flexibility, as it cannot dynamically adjust retrieval strategies according to the context. However, the necessity of retrieval-augmented generation also depends on the importance of key tokens in the sequence, the semantics of these tokens, and their influence on subsequent tokens. The term confidence is generally used to represent the degree of trust in a particular result or prediction. Therefore, the Dynamic Semantic Confidence Evaluation (DSCE) module optimizes the retrieval activation process by assessing each token's uncertainty, semantic contribution, and contextual impact. The hidden states of the model are transformed through a linear layer, which maps the high-dimensional hidden representations to the vocabulary-sized dimension, thereby generating a score for each possible output token. These scores are then passed through the softmax function to obtain a probability distribution. The softmax function ensures that the probabilities of all possible tokens sum to one, making the distribution interpretable as the likelihood of generating each token given the context. Once this probability distribution is derived, the entropy of each token can be computed. Entropy serves as a measure of uncertainty in the probability distribution and reflects the model's confidence in predicting a specific token. A higher entropy indicates greater uncertainty about which token should appear at that position, whereas a lower entropy signifies stronger confidence in the prediction. By recording the entropy of the probability distributions of tokens within the model, we quantify the uncertainty of each token generated during the LLMs inference process.

Let a set of output sequences $T = \{t_1, t_2,...,t_n\}$ be generated by LLMs, where each t_i represents an individual token at position i in the sequence. For each t_i, the calculation formula of entropy E is shown as in Eq. 1.

$$E_i = -\sum_{w \in V} p_i(w) \log p_i(w) \tag{1}$$

where $p_i(w)$ is the probability that the model predicts token w to appear at position i given the list of tokens before t_i.

The self-attention mechanism inherent in the transformer-based LLMs is utilized to assign weights to tokens that represent the impact of the token on the subsequent context. For any given token t_i, its impact is quantified by recording the maximum attention value $a_{\max(i)}$ for each token in the attention score of the last Transformer layer of the LLMs, which records the maximum attention of all subsequent tokens. The attention value $A_{i,j}$ between two tokens is calculated as shown in Eq. 2.

$$A_{i,j} = \text{softmax}\left(\frac{Q_i K_j^T}{\sqrt{d_k}}\right) \tag{2}$$

where Q_i denotes the query vector of token t_i, K_j is the key vector of token t_j, and d_k denotes the dimension of the vector.

The maximum attention value of the token $a_{\max(i)}$ is determined by locating the highest $A_{i,j}$ for all $j > i$. $a_{\max(i)}$ is computed as shown in Eq. 3.

$$a_{\max(i)} = \max_{j>i} A_{i,j} \tag{3}$$

There are significant differences in the semantic contributions of different tokens, in which dummy words usually do not carry core semantic information. Therefore, by filtering dummy words, it is more effective to focus on tokens with important semantic value. Dummy word filtering is calculated as shown in Eq. 4.

$$s_i = \begin{cases} 0, & \text{if } t_i \in S, \\ 1, & \text{otherwise.} \end{cases} \tag{4}$$

where S is the set of deactivated words and s_i is the semantic contribution score of token t_i. The dummy words are filtered to ensure that only semantically valid tokens participate in the token uncertainty metric and retrieval decision process.

Combining the uncertainty, importance and semantics of the token, a final score is calculated for each token as shown in Eq. 5.

$$S_{\text{DSER}}\ (t_i) = E_i \cdot a_{\max(i)} \cdot s_i \tag{5}$$

The retrieval is activated when a token score s_i exceeds a predefined threshold θ in the output sequence $T = \{t_1, t_2, \ldots, t_n\}$ generated by LLMs.

3.3 Example Retrieval

The DSCE calculates the confidence level of the initial prediction result. If the confidence level exceeds the specified threshold, a retrieval is triggered. The text Query is mapped into a vector through the transformer encoder and then input into the vector database to perform similarity retrieval. The similar vector v_1 is returned and decoded into the text similar sentence s_i. Finally, find the corresponding answer a_i in the text knowledge base.

Example retrieval includes knowledge base construction and similarity example retrieval. The knowledge base is derived from CMeKG [21] and converts its structured triples into an instruction data format acceptable to the model. Each instruction data is in the form of a sentence answer pair, where the sentence is the medical text to be extracted entity relationship, and the answer is entity relationship sentence.

The entity-relation sentence knowledge base containing 63966 items was constructed as an external knowledge source for model retrieval. The cosine similarity algorithm is adopted in the retrieval process. Each Query vector is traversed through the vector database to calculate the cosine similarity with each data, and the top-1 similar sentences are retained as examples. The vector knowledge base only stores sentence vectors and does not vectorize answers.

In the similarity retrieval process, for the Query and the knowledge T_i in the knowledge base, whose corresponding vector representations are $\vec{q} = f(\text{Query})$ and $\vec{v}_i = f(T_i)$, respectively, the cosine similarity function $\cos(\vec{q}, \vec{v}_i)$ is used to compute the similarity, and the computational formula is shown in Eq. 6.

$$\cos(\vec{q}, \vec{v}_i) = \frac{\vec{q} \cdot \vec{v}_i}{|\vec{q}|\,|\vec{v}_i|} \tag{6}$$

where $\vec{q} \cdot \vec{v}_i = \sum_{i=1}^{384} q_i v_i, \quad |\vec{v}_i| = \sqrt{\sum_{i=1}^{384} v_i^2}$.

After calculating all the cosine similarities, a vector with the highest similarity is selected as the output in order of similarity values, i.e., the vector that is most similar to $\vec{q}$. The calculation is shown in Eq. 7.

$$v_1 = \arg\max_i \left(\cos(\vec{q}, \vec{v}_i)\right) \tag{7}$$

where v_1 denotes the vector with the highest cosine similarity.

3.4 Prediction

During the prediction phase, the task definition, similar examples, and the query are concatenated into a complete prompt, which is then fed into the LLMs to perform entity–relationship prediction. After constructing the similar examples, each example is formatted by concatenating the text and its corresponding answer into the form $s_i + a_i$. The user query is then appended after these examples and collectively input into the generator model to enhance prediction quality. After concatenating the similar examples, the complete prompt input to the model is shown in Fig. 2.

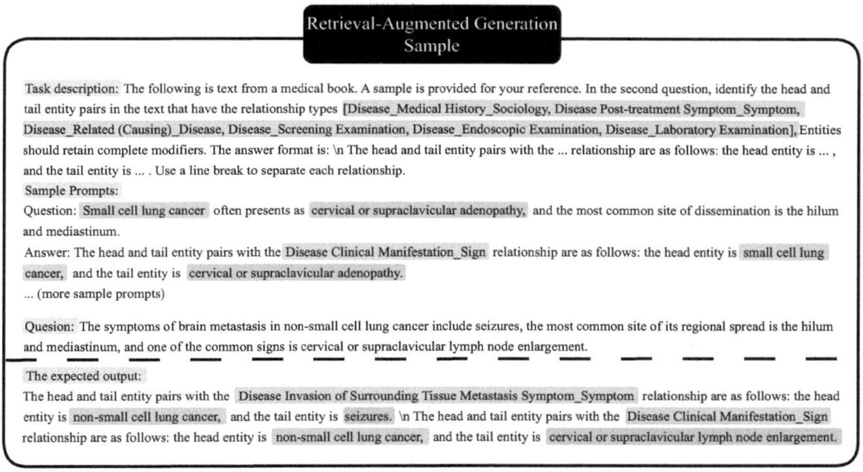

Fig. 2. Example of Retrieval-Augmented Data

In this section, WiNGPT2-14B-Chat and Llama3-Chinese-8B-Instruct, a large language model in the medical field, were selected for experiments. There were differences in the number of vertical domain data and parameters between the two models. WiNGPT2-14B-Chat model had a larger number of parameters and was pre-trained with vertical medical text, its performance was more stable than that of Llama3-Chinese-8B-Instruct. The setup of the generator model is divided into two settings, with and without fine-tuning, in which the examples are divided into top-1 similar examples and non-top-1 similar examples for experiments. The top-1 similarity examples represent the searched sentences in the vector knowledge base that are most similar to the user's query, while the non-top-1 similarity examples randomly select the sentences that are not most similar to the user's query as examples of the query examples.

3.5 Fine-Tuning Dataset Construction

The fine-tuning data of RA-RE and DR-RE are slightly different. Since both RA-RE methods add similar examples for prediction, there are no zero-shot prediction data in their fine-tuning data. However, the DR-RE method requires zero-shot prediction first. Therefore, 300 (30%) zero-shot fine-tuning data needs to be added to the fine-tuning data. Only the fine-tuned data distribution of DR-RE is presented below.

Based on the published Chinese Medical Information Extraction (CMeIE) dataset [22] and the Critical illness Entity and Relationship Corpus (CIC) [23], a training set suitable for RA-RE method was constructed and experiments were conducted. The test set is derived from the baseline KE-PromptRE method. Table 1 shows the statistics for the fine-tuned and test datasets. The triplet represents the medical entity relationship triplet.

Table 1. Training and test set statistics

Data	Name	Number	Triples
Fine-tuning the dataset	RA-RE_train	1000	1379
Test dataset	CIC	496	1157
	CMeIE	482	1098

The DR-RE fine-tuning data is to reconstruct the data distribution on the 1000 instruction fine-tuning data constructed in RA-RE, add 300 (30%) zero-shot medical entity relationship reasoning instruction fine-tuning data sets to ensure that the fine-tuned model has a certain zero-shot reasoning ability, and delete the corresponding number of non-entity relationship extraction data. The overall data volume remains consistent. The detailed distribution of individual tasks is shown in Table 2.

Table 2. DR-RE fine-tunes dataset distribution

Task name	Percentage (%)
Medical radio questions	5
Medical entity recognition	13
Semantic matching	4
Medical open question	12
Entity relationship joint extraction	50
Triplet language generation	5
Intent judgment	4
Code extraction triples	2
Relation selection	5

4 Experimental Setup

The experimental setup contains settings for the experimental environment as well as the model hyperparameters, details of which are shown in Table 3. M-H stands for Model hyperparameterization, F-T-H stands for Fine-tuning hyperparameter, H-C stands for hardware category. The GPU uses NVIDIA 4090-24GB, the environment uses Ubuntu 20.04.5 LTS, and the abbreviation g_a_steps stands for gradient_accumulation_steps.

Table 3. Experimental environment and hyperparameter setting

H-C	Version	M-H	size	F-T-H	size
Python	3.8.0	epochs	2.0	lora_rank	8
Transformers	4.37.2	batch_size	4	lora_trainable	c_attn
Pytorch	2.0.0	warmup_ratio	0.05	lora_alpha	16
Cuda	11.7	weight_decay	0.01	lora_dropout	0.0
Accelerate	0.21.0	learning_rate	5e-5	task_type	CAUSAL_LM
Peft	0.8.2	g_a_steps	2		

Metric. We used precision (p), recall (r) and F1-score (F_1) as evaluation indicators. The F_1 calculation formula is shown in Eq. 8:

$$F1 = \frac{2 * p * r}{p + r} \tag{8}$$

To explore the impact of different parameter sizes and different vertical domains on LLMs, we selected the WiNGPT2-14B-Chat model, which was fine-tuned in the medical domain, and the Llama3-Chinese-8B-Instruct model, which was a general-purpose model. All LLMs use the default hyperparameters settings.

5 Result and Discussion

5.1 Baseline Experiment

The baseline contrast experiment is from [24], The baseline experimental results are shown in Table 4, with the best performance highlighted in bold. These optimal results were achieved by a LoRA [25] instruction-tuned model trained on 400K entity-relation extraction data instances. The baseline method adopts the Few-Shot Learning setting, which is specifically divided into "5-way 0-shot" and "5-way 1-shot". "5-way 0-shot" means classifying test examples from 5 categories without providing any examples, while "5-way 1-shot" refers to classifying test examples from 5 categories, and providing 1 example for each category (that is, a total of 5 labeled examples).

Table 4. Way 0shot and 5way 1shot baseline comparison experiment. 'ft' stands for lora fine-tuning on the base model

Dataset	Model	Few-Shot (5w0s/5w1s)		
		P	R	F1
CMeIE	WINGPT-7B-CHAT	0.055/0.034	0.076/0.137	0.064/0.055
	WINGPT-14B-CHAT	0.269/0.349	0.168/0.288	0.207/0.315
	GPT-3.5	0.164/0.286	0.124/0.235	0.141/0.258
	GPT-4	0.313/0.372	0.262/0.393	0.285/0.382
	WINGPT-14B-CHAT-ft	**0.396/0.411**	**0.458/0.399**	**0.424/0.405**
CIC	WINGPT-7B-CHAT	0.123/0.118	0.071/0.082	0.090/0.097
	WINGPT-14B-CHAT	0.345/0.335	0.193/0.318	0.247/0.326
	GPT-3.5	0.159/0.290	0.113/0.253	0.132/0.270
	GPT-4	0.338/0.426	0.253/0.406	0.289/0.415
	WINGPT-14B-CHAT-ft	**0.505/0.545**	**0.553/0.479**	**0.528/0.510**

5.2 Experimental Results

In this section, we present the experimental results of our proposed methods. We first report the overall performance of RA-RE compared with baseline models. Then, we conduct ablation studies to investigate the impact of similarity filtering. Finally, we analyze the performance of DR-RE method under different threshold settings.

5.3 RA-RE Results

RA-RE augments model inputs by retrieving similar examples, with settings divided into fine-tuning and non-fine-tuning modes. Since fine-tuned models generally achieve superior performance, DR-RE is evaluated directly on the fine-tuned models.

The experiments were conducted on two large language models with different scales and domains: WINGPT-14B-CHAT and Llama3-Chinese-8B-Instruct. The results are reported in Tables 5 and 6, respectively.

We compared RA-RE with direct large model predictions, both with and without fine-tuning. The results show that RA-RE consistently outperforms the prompt-based baseline, demonstrating notable improvements on both the CMeIE and CIC datasets. Importantly, RA-RE achieves superior results even without fine-tuning, highlighting the effectiveness of incorporating retrieved examples. This improvement arises because retrieved examples are more likely to contain relevant entities and relations, thus guiding the model toward more accurate predictions.

Table 5. The main results of RA-RE method. Bold values are the optimal result. 'ft' stands for lora fine-tuning; 'w/o-ft' stands for lora-free fine-tuning; 'rs' stands for random sampling; 'simi' means that the similarity of example is top1; 'lack-re' means that the answer of the example lacks some entity relationship, that is, the answer is incomplete

Dataset	Base Model WINGPT-14B-CHAT	P	R	F1
CMeIE	RagRE-rs-w/o-ft	0.317	0.366	0.340
	RagRE-rs-ft	0.488	0.376	0.430
	RagRE-simi-w/o-ft	0.702	0.604	0.650
	RagRE-lack-re-ft	0.651	0.494	0.575
	RagRE-simi-re-ft	**0.823**	**0.753**	**0.786**
CIC	RagRE-rs-w/o-ft	0.337	0.375	0.355
	RagRE-rs-ft	0.374	0.409	0.391
	RagRE-simi-w/o-ft	0.616	0.529	0.569
	RagRE-lack-re-ft	0.661	0.546	0.598
	RagRE-simi-ft	**0.717**	**0.652**	**0.683**

Table 6. F1 scores of the base model Llama3-Chinese-8B-Instruct on CMeIE and CIC using the RA-RE method. Bold values are the optimal result

Dataset	Base Model Llama3-Chinese-8B-Instruct	P	R	F1
CMeIE	RA-RE-simi-lack-re-w/o-ft	0.419	0.331	0.370
	RA-RE-simi-lack-re-ft	0.624	0.474	0.539
	RA-RE-simi-w/o-ft	0.605	0.471	0.530
	RA-RE-same-re-ft	**0.757**	**0.723**	**0.740**
CIC	RA-RE-simi-lack-re-w/o-ft	0.372	0.229	0.283
	RA-RE-simi-lack-re-ft	0.606	0.396	0.479
	RA-RE-simi-w/o-ft	0.480	0.397	0.435
	RA-RE-simi-re-ft	**0.749**	**0.704**	**0.726**

5.4 Ablation Experiments

During retrieval, we observed that some test samples had a similarity score of 1 (simi1). This occurred because certain test queries also appeared in the training set, albeit with different target relations, leading to potential data leakage. Specifically, there were 223 such cases in CMeIE and 153 in CIC.

To eliminate this bias, we removed these simi1 samples and re-conducted the experiments. The results are summarized in Table 7. On both WINGPT-14B-CHAT and Llama3-Chinese-8B-Instruct (fine-tuned on 1000 samples), RA-RE consistently outperforms the KE-PromptRE baseline. Notably, RA-RE with fine-tuning achieves the highest F1 scores, confirming that our approach remains robust and effective even after filtering overlapping data.

Table 7. Comparison of KE-PromptRE and RA-RE methods without simil data on CMeIE and CIC datasets

Dataset	Model	Method	P	R	F1
CMeIE	WINGPT-14B-CHAT-ft	KE	0.436	0.482	0.458
		RA(w/o)	0.458	0.423	0.440
		RA-ft	**0.491**	**0.467**	**0.479**
	Llama3-8B-Instruct	RA(w/o)	0.294	0.250	0.270
		RA-ft	**0.400**	**0.428**	**0.413**
CIC	WINGPT-14B-CHAT-ft	KE	0.430	0.487	0.456
		RA(w/o)	0.422	0.400	0.411
		RA-ft	**0.502**	**0.445**	**0.472**
	Llama3-8B-Instruct	RA(w/o)	0.339	0.265	0.298
		RA-ft	**0.593**	**0.531**	**0.560**

KE = KE-PromptRE, RA(w/o) = RA-RE without fine-tuning, RA-ft = RA-RE with fine-tuning

5.5 DR-RE Results

We further evaluated DR-RE method. Table 8 reports the performance of the two models under different hallucination thresholds, where bolded numbers denote the best results.

Here, the retrieval number corresponds to the average number of retrieved examples per test instance. A threshold (TH) is applied to control retrieval, while "R-T" represents retrieval times. As the hallucination threshold increases, the number of retrieved examples decreases, leading to a gradual decline in F1 scores. This confirms that retrieved examples positively contribute to prediction accuracy.

Interestingly, the optimal threshold differs across models: WINGPT-14B-CHAT achieves its best performance at a lower threshold (0.2), while Llama3-Chinese-8B-Instruct performs best at 0.6. This suggests that the larger parameter size and richer pretraining knowledge of WINGPT-14B-CHAT enable it to maintain confidence and achieve better results with fewer retrieved examples.

6 Conclusion

This study addresses the challenges of outdated knowledge, hallucination, and high fine-tuning costs when LLMs are applied to medical entity-relationship extraction. We propose two retrieval-augmented generation methods: RA-RE

Table 8. The overall performance of the DR-RE method

Test	TH	R-T	Llama3-Chinese-8B-Instruct			TH	R-T	WINGPT-14B-CHAT		
			P	R	F1			P	R	F1
CMeIE	\	1	0.726	0.682	0.703	\	1	0.837	0.748	0.790
	0.6	0.995	**0.726**	**0.682**	**0.703**	**0.2**	0.985	**0.837**	**0.747**	**0.790**
	0.8	0.985	0.724	0.679	0.701	0.4	0.929	0.836	0.739	0.785
	1.0	0.967	0.730	0.671	0.699	0.6	0.818	0.828	0.708	0.763
	1.2	0.917	0.712	0.641	0.675	0.8	0.681	0.798	0.652	0.717
	1.4	0.862	0.700	0.618	0.656	1.0	0.528	0.762	0.750	0.655
CIC	\	1	0.699	0.589	0.639	\	1	0.774	0.648	0.705
	0.6	0.987	**0.699**	**0.589**	**0.639**	**0.2**	0.977	**0.759**	**0.656**	**0.705**
	0.8	0.962	0.667	0.586	0.624	0.4	0.798	0.771	0.630	0.694
	1.0	0.946	0.659	0.577	0.616	0.6	0.651	0.736	0.582	0.651
	1.2	0.892	0.642	0.556	0.596	0.8	0.678	0.743	0.592	0.659
	1.4	0.842	0.654	0.535	0.588	1.0	0.533	0.708	0.544	0.615

and DR-RE. By incorporating external medical knowledge bases, both methods reduce reliance on the model's internal parameters, significantly decreasing fine-tuning costs while improving generation quality. The RA-RE method uses only 1,000 instruction-tuning samples and constructs both text and vector knowledge bases to retrieve similar examples for prompt enhancement. Experimental results show that RA-RE outperforms the baseline method KE-PromptRE–which was trained on approximately 400k instructions–on both the CMeIE and CIC test sets, with maximum F1-score improvements of 0.362 and 0.155, respectively. The DR-RE method introduces a dynamic retrieval mechanism: it first performs zero-shot inference, then triggers retrieval only when tokens with confidence below a certain threshold are detected–indicating potential hallucinations. This strategy reduces unnecessary retrieval operations while maintaining high output quality. Experiments show that a 14B-parameter model fine-tuned with LoRA achieves higher F1-scores than RA-RE on both test sets, demonstrating a better trade-off between efficiency and accuracy.

In summary, the proposed static and dynamic retrieval-augmented methods effectively enhance the accuracy and reliability of medical entity-relationship extraction across different scenarios, offering a practical pathway for adapting LLMs to domain-specific tasks.

Acknowledgments. This work was supported by the National Science and Technology Major Project (2021ZD0111000).

References

1. Achiam, J., Adler, S., Agarwal, S., Ahmad, L., Akkaya, I., Aleman, F.L., Almeida, D., Altenschmidt, J., Altman, S., Anadkat, S., et al.: GPT-4 Technical Report (2023). arXiv:2303.08774
2. Li, Z., Dai, H., Li, P.: Generating diverse training samples for relation extraction with large language models (2025). arXiv:2505.23108
3. Wang, Q., Li, Y., Qiao, Q., Zhou, K., Li, Q.: Towards a more generalized approach in open relation extraction (2025). arXiv:2505.22801
4. Han, Z., Gao, C., Liu, J., Zhang, J., Zhang, S.Q.: Parameter-efficient fine-tuning for large models: A comprehensive survey (2024). arXiv:2403.14608
5. Wu, S., Xiong, Y., Cui, Y., Wu, H., Chen, C., Yuan, Y., Huang, L., Liu, X., Kuo, T.-W., Guan, N., et al.: Retrieval-augmented generation for natural language processing: a survey (2024). arXiv:2407.13193
6. Tang, W., Xu, B., Zhao, Y., Mao, Z., Liu, Y., Liao, Y., Xie, H.: UniRel: unified representation and interaction for joint relational triple extraction. In: Proceedings of the 2022 Conference on Empirical Methods in Natural Language Processing, pp. 7087–7099 (2022)
7. Wang, Q., Zhou, K., Qiao, Q., Li, Y., Li, Q.: Improving unsupervised relation extraction by augmenting diverse sentence pairs. In: Proceedings of the 2023 Conference on Empirical Methods in Natural Language Processing, pp. 12136–12147 (2023)
8. Duan, J., Liao, X., An, Y., Wang, J.: KeyEE: enhancing low-resource generative event extraction with auxiliary keyword sub-prompt. Big Data Min. Anal. **7**(2), 547–560 (2024)
9. Li, G., Wang, P., Liu, J., Guo, Y., Ji, K., Shang, Z., Xu, Z.: Meta in-context learning makes large language models better zero and few-shot relation extractors (2024). arXiv:2404.17807
10. Nguyen, T.H., Grishman, R.: Relation extraction: perspective from convolutional neural networks. In: Proceedings of the 1st Workshop on Vector Space Modeling for Natural Language Processing, pp. 39–48 (2015)
11. Socher, R., Huval, B., Manning, C.D., Ng, A.Y.: Semantic compositionality through recursive matrix-vector spaces. In: Proceedings of the 2012 Joint Conference on Empirical Methods in Natural Language Processing and Computational Natural Language Learning, pp. 1201–1211 (2012)
12. Zhong, Z., Chen, D.: A frustratingly easy approach for entity and relation extraction. In: Proceedings of the 2021 Conference of the North American Chapter of the Association for Computational Linguistics: Human Language Technologies, pp. 50–61 (2021)
13. Laskar, M.T.R., Jahan, I., Dolatabadi, E., Peng, C., Hoque, E., Huang, J.: Improving automatic evaluation of large language models (LLMs) in biomedical relation extraction via LLMs-as-the-judge (2025). arXiv:2506.00777
14. Labrak, Y., Rouvier, M., Dufour, R.: A zero-shot and few-shot study of instruction fine-tuned large language models applied to clinical and biomedical tasks. In: Proceedings of the 2024 Joint International Conference on Computational Linguistics, Language Resources and Evaluation (LREC-COLING 2024), pp. 2049–2066 (2024)
15. Dale, D., Voita, E., Barrault, L., et al.: Detecting and mitigating hallucinations in machine translation: model internal workings alone do well, sentence similarity even better. In: Proceedings of the 61st Annual Meeting of the Association for Computational Linguistics (ACL), pp. 36–50 (2023)

16. Zhang, N., Yao, Y., Tian, B., et al.: A comprehensive study of knowledge editing for large language models (2024). CoRR arXiv:2401.01286
17. Colombo, P., Pires, T.P., Boudiaf, M., et al.: SaulLM-7B: a pioneering large language model for law (2024). CoRR arXiv:2403.03883
18. Xu, D., Chen, W., Peng, W., et al.: Large language models for generative information extraction: a survey. Front. Comput. Sci. **18**(6), 186357 (2024)
19. Fan, W., Ding, Y., Ning, L., et al.: A survey on RAG meeting LLMs: Towards retrieval-augmented large language models. In: Proceedings of the 30th ACM SIGKDD Conference on Knowledge Discovery and Data Mining, pp. 6491–6501 (2024)
20. Zhong, Y., Gao, Y., Zhang, X., Wang, H.: ODDA: an OODA-driven diverse data augmentation framework for low-resource relation extraction. In: Findings of the Association for Computational Linguistics: ACL 2025, pp. 267–285 (2025)
21. Zhang, K., Ren, X., Zhuang, L., Zan, H., Zhang, W., Sui, Z.: Construction of Chinese medicine knowledge base. In: Proceedings of the Workshop on Chinese Lexical Semantics, pp. 665–675. Springer (2020)
22. Byambasuren, O., Yang, Y., Sui, Z., Dai, D., Chang, B., Li, S., Zan, H.: Preliminary study on the construction of Chinese medical knowledge graph. J. Chin. Inf. Process. **33**(10), 1–9 (2019)
23. Guan, T., Zan, H., Zhou, X., Xu, H., Zhang, K.: CMeIE: construction and evaluation of Chinese medical information extraction dataset. In: Proceedings of the CCF International Conference on Natural Language Processing and Chinese Computing, pp. 270–282. Springer (2020)
24. Zhang, K., Zhang, C., Zhang, W., Zan, H.: Corpus construction of critical illness entities and relationships. In: Proceedings of the Workshop on Chinese Lexical Semantics, pp. 61–75. Springer (2023)
25. Zhang, K., Li, Y., Wu, P., Li, Y., Zhang, C., Zan, H.: Knowledge enhancement with LLMs for few-shot medical relation extraction. In: Proceedings of the China Health Information Processing Conference, pp. 147–160. Springer (2024)

Cross-Type Biomedical Named Entity Recognition Method Based on Knowledge Distillation

Zhengyao Wang, JingYan Wang, Tingwei Geng, YanFang Wang, and Chi Yuan(✉)

School of Computer and Software, Hohai University, Nanjing, China
chiyuan1126@gmail.com

Abstract. Biomedical Named Entity Recognition (BioNER) is a key task in biomedical text processing and plays an important role in clinical decision support, drug research and development, and medical knowledge graph construction. Most traditional BioNERs use models trained for a single entity type. Although it performs well in a single specific field, it struggles to handle the complex task scenarios involving multi-entity type coexistence, uneven distribution of training data and heterogeneous labels. For this reason, we propose the KFC-Net framework that integrates knowledge distillation and cross-type entity recognition, which significantly improves the accuracy and deployment efficiency of the model in cross-type entity recognition tasks by adjusting the training strategy and lightweighting the model architecture. KFC-Net constructs a unified label space to solve the problem of predictive label conflicts in cross-type entity recognition, and applies a probabilistic aggregation strategy relying on the independence assumption to integrate the output distributions, ultimately training a student model with cross-type entity recognition capabilities. In the experimental validation of the three major tasks of diseases, chemical substances and genes, the F1-scores of KFC-Net ranked among the top, outperforming the traditional merging models and the mainstream baseline models. The framework effectively solves the label conflict problem in cross-type entity recognition and supports various lightweight student model architectures such as RoBERTa-base, DistilBERT, TinyBERT, etc. It can be flexibly selected according to the various hardware environment requirements to improve the feasibility of actual deployment.

Keywords: Biomedical named entity recognition · Knowledge distillation · Lightweight model

1 Introduction

With the continuous progress and deepening of medical research, researchers and clinicians have produced massive structured and unstructured data in the biomedical field. According to statistics, PubMed literature is increasing by millions every year, and the scale of text resources such as electronic health records, clinical trial reports, and drug instructions is expanding rapidly. These texts contain a wealth of medical knowledge

Y. Zhang et al. (Eds.): CHIP 2025, CCIS 2884, pp. 362–377, 2026.
https://doi.org/10.1007/978-981-95-7299-1_21

and are highly valuable for disease diagnosis, drug development and clinical decision support. However, manual processing and analyzing such massive amounts of text data cannot meet the actual needs. Therefore, Natural Language Processing (NLP) technology is used to automatically extract information from biomedical texts, serving as a key approach to advancing the development of precision medicine and intelligent medicine.

The term "Entity" was first proposed at the Sixth Message Understanding Conference (MUC-6) [1]. It mainly refers to phrases with special meaning or strong referentiality in the text, usually including proper nouns such as person names, place names, organization name, time, etc. Named Entity Recognition (NER) [2] aims to extract entities with specific meanings or strong referentiality from unstructured text, while Biomedical Named Entity Recognition (BioNER) is further specialized to identify and annotate professional terms such as genes, diseases, and drugs from raw text. BioNER is the foundation for building biomedical knowledge graphs and a key component of intelligent question answering, clinical decision support, and bioinformatics mining systems. However, there are notable differences from general-domain NER [3]: biomedical entity naming is complex, and traditional NLP methods have difficulty in accurately identifying terms such as "CDKN2A", which have both numbers and abbreviations. Cross-domain semantic ambiguity and the scarcity of labeled data seriously limit the performance of traditional supervised learning models.

Although the recent emergence of pre-trained language models, represented by Bidirectional Encoder Representations from Transformers (BERT), has effectively improved BioNER performance, most of the mainstream methods still use the type-specific modeling strategy, in which a separate model is trained for each entity type. This method has many limitations: different datasets have different labeling specifications and terminology systems, which limits the cross-type generalization ability of the model; Different types of entities coexist in medical texts, and type-specific models have difficulty effectively extracting and categorizing entities; Deploying multiple large models consume substantial resources, making it difficult to perform effective and timely entity recognition tasks in application scenarios with edge devices or low-resource environments.

In this paper, we propose a fusion-based multi-teacher knowledge distillation framework, which integrates the advantages of multiple type-specific teacher models to train a unified cross-type student model. This method retains the recognition ability of different entity types while avoiding the resource redundancy of deploying multiple separate models. Compared with the traditional scheme, the unified student model reduces the storage requirement by over 60%. Through the lightweight design of the student model, it can still run smoothly in low-resource computing environments such as edge devices, which provides a practical technical solution for edge computing scenarios such as mobile ward-round systems and wearable medical devices. The main contributions of this paper are as follows:

- We propose the KFC-Net framework for cross-type BioNER, which adopts a distillation-based cross-type entity recognition strategy to integrate the knowledge of multiple type-specific teacher models to produce a unified cross-type student model. In three mainstream BioNER tasks, namely diseases, chemicals, and genes, the F1-score of KFC-Net outperforms the traditional joint-training methods and existing baseline models, demonstrating strong transferability across tasks and accurate entity boundary recognition.

- The framework proposed in this paper has significant advantages in model lightweight. Through knowledge distillation technology, large teacher models such as RoBERTa-large can be distilled into student models of varying sizes. Moreover, since the proposed framework does not require additional modules, it is highly compatible with the original Transformer architecture and can be d directly integrated with existing model interpretation tools.
- To address the problem of negative knowledge transfer in cross-type entity recognition, the framework provides a general framework for cross-type knowledge fusion through its unique "teacher models specializing in individual types and student models learning accurate cross-type representations" model. Its probabilistic aggregation strategy and mixed loss function not only retain the high precision of type-specific model in specific fields, but also realize knowledge transfer in cross-type entity recognition, thereby providing a solution that can deal with the problems of complex labeling schemes and imbalanced data distributions in the biomedical field.

2 Related Work

In the field of BioNER, deep learning-based methods can achieve automatic feature extraction from raw text to abstract semantics by constructing multi-layer nonlinear neural networks, reducing reliance on manual feature engineering and better capturing complex semantic structures such as entity nesting and cross-sentence associations. Xu Li et al. [4] combined BERT with the BiLSTM-CRF model and achieved an average F1-score of 89.45% on biomedical datasets such as NCBI-disease [3] and BC5CDR-chem [5]. Lee et al. [6] used BioBERT and the Softmax function to achieve excellent performance on multiple datasets, demonstrating the benefits of automatic feature learning in neural networks.

Although the deep learning method significantly expands the performance upper limit of BioNER, it also introduces challenges such as large number of parameters, high training resource consumption and significant inference delay. Therefore, the current research focus has also shifted to how to achieve a balance between identification capabilities and operational efficiency and computational resource demands in actual deployment.

In this context, Knowledge Distillation (KD) technology [7] has garnered widespread attention because of its unique advantages [8–10]. Traditional knowledge distillation strategies often provide soft label guidance based on a single teacher model, but in multi-teacher distillation approach, by leveraging the diversity and complementary information across different model types, the generalization performance of learners can be enhanced more effectively, resulting in more effective model optimization. For example, Fukuda et al. [9] proposed the hypothesis that multiple teacher models can provide knowledge from different perspectives, which enhances the generalization ability of the student model in cross-dataset tasks. Xu Tan et al. [11] also proved the feasibility of multi-teacher distillation in the multilingual translation task.

3 Method

Aiming at the practical problems such as the coexistence of multiple types of entities, scattered training data and limited model deployment in BioNER, the core goal of the framework KFC-Net (Knowledge Fusion and Compression Network) proposed in this paper is to integrate the knowledge of multiple type-specific teacher models into a single student model by using knowledge distillation technology, to address the challenges of large model sizes, high inference costs, and limited adaptability in cross-type BioNER tasks. This section describes the training process of the framework, including data set aggregation, teacher model prediction, probability distribution aggregation and student model training.

3.1 Formalization of Problems

In the BioNER task, it is assumed that the set of entity types to be identified is $E = \{e_1, e_2, \cdots, e_{|E|}\}$, where e_i represents the type i entity. Each entity type corresponds to a labeled dataset $D_i = \{(x, y) \in X_i \times Y_i\}$, where X_i is a set of sentences, each sentence x is composed of a word sequence $\{\boldsymbol{x}_j\}_{j=1}^{H}$, and Y_i adopts the improved IOB2 annotation system [12]. The system contains three types of labels: entity start label *B*-e_i entity intermediate label *I*-e_i and non-entity label *O*. The objective of this paper is to build a unified cross-type entity recognition model, whose output label space is defined as:

$$y^{multi} = U_{i=1}^{|E|}\{B{-}e_i, B{-}e_i\}U\{O\} \tag{1}$$

For example, when $E = \{\text{disease, gene, drug}\}$, the set of labels that the model needs to predict is {*B*-disease, *I*-disease, *B*-gene, *I*-gene, *B*-drug, *I*-drug, *O*}. This formal definition solves the issue of label heterogeneity in cross-type entity recognition and provides a unified input-output framework for subsequent knowledge distillation.

3.2 KFC-Net Architecture

As a cross-type BioNER framework based on knowledge distillation, the overall training process of KFC-Net is shown in Fig. 1. It consists of four core stages: dataset aggregation, teacher model prediction, probability distribution aggregation and student model training, and realizes cross-task entity extraction and knowledge transfer, which collaboratively achieve cross-task entity extraction and knowledge transfer.

Datasets Aggregation. To build a unified training sample set, the sentences from multiple single-type datasets are concatenated and integrated into a joint training set:

$$D_S = \{(x, y) \in x_{S'} \times y_{S'}\}, x_{S'} = U_{i=1}^{|E|}X_i \tag{2}$$

where X_i is the set of sentences in the i type-specific dataset. In order to ensure the consistency and mutual exclusivity of the labels, the original labels set y_i is converted into a multi-type label space $y_{S'}$. The unlabeled entity type is uniformly marked as *O*, while the *B* and *I* labels are independently coded according to the entity category and the strategy in Sect. 3.1. This method not only maintains the integrity and consistency

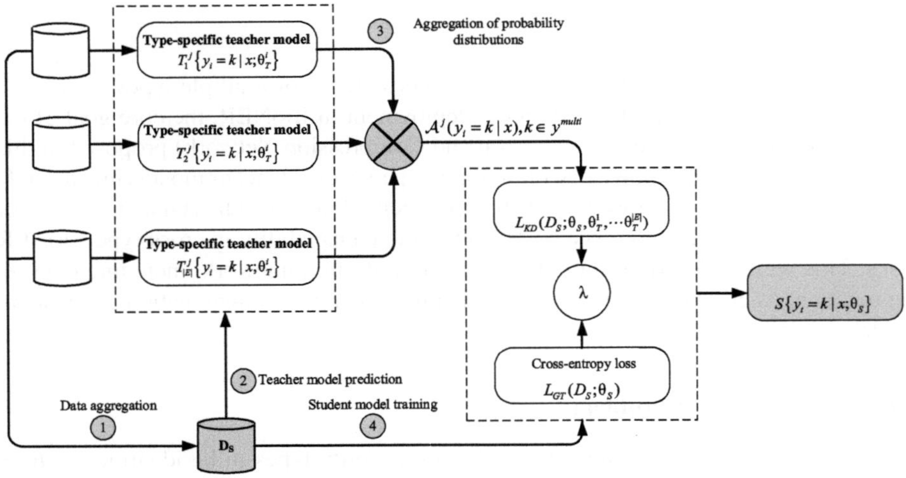

Fig. 1. Overall training process of KFC-net.

of the original annotations, but also provides systematic and diversified training data for the learning model.

Teacher Model Prediction. For each entity type e_i, an independent type-specific teacher model θ_T^i is trained. The teacher model is fine-tuned to convergence on the corresponding dataset $\boldsymbol{D_i}$ and outputs the label probability distribution for each word $\boldsymbol{x_j}$:

$$\boldsymbol{T}_i^j\left\{\boldsymbol{y_i} = k|x;\, \theta_{\boldsymbol{T}}^i\right\},\, k \in \{B, I, O\} \tag{3}$$

The distribution only covers the entity types that teachers focus on, and all other types of entities are treated as non-entities.

Probability Distribution Aggregation. The key to knowledge distillation is to integrate the heterogeneous knowledge of multiple type-specific teacher models and integrate them into a unified cross-type student model. Since each teacher only focuses on a single entity type, its prediction distribution has obvious task-specific characteristics. In order to realize multi-label collaborative learning, this paper proposes a probabilistic aggregation strategy based on independence assumption:

Probability of Entity Start Label (B-e $_i$*).* A token is assigned the label B-e_i only when teacher T_i predicts B while all other teachers T_j (J $\neq$ i) do not. The corresponding probability is computed as follows:

$$\mathcal{A}^j(B{-}e_i|x) = p_B^i \cdot \prod_{j \neq i}\left(P_I^j + P_O^j\right) \tag{4}$$

where p_B^i represents the probability that teacher T_i predicts B, and the product term $\prod_{j \neq i}\left(P_I^j + P_O^j\right)$ ensures that other teachers do not label the current token as the start position of the entity.

Probability of Internal Label (I-e$_i$*).* A token is assigned the label I-e_i only when teacher T_i predicts I and all other teachers T_j (J $\neq$ i) do not. The corresponding probability is computed as follows:

$$\mathcal{A}^j(I-e_i|x) = p_I^i \cdot \prod_{j \neq i} \left(P_B^j + P_O^j\right) \tag{5}$$

where p_I^i represents the probability that teacher T_i predicts I, and the product term $\prod_{j \neq i} \left(P_B^j + P_O^j\right)$ ensures that other teachers do not label the current token as the internal position of the entity.

Probability of non-entity Label (O). When all teachers predict O, the token is classified as a non-entity:

$$\mathcal{A}^j(O|x) = \prod_{i=1}^{|E|} p_O^j \tag{6}$$

Example. Taking the entity type set E = {disease, gene, drug} as an example, assume that predicted probability distributions of the three teacher models are as follows:

$$T_{disease}^j = [0.8, 0.1, 0.1] \tag{7}$$

$$T_{gene}^j = [0.05, 0.05, 0.9] \tag{8}$$

$$T_{drug}^j = [0.1, 0.1, 0.8] \tag{9}$$

According to the aggregation formula, the probability corresponding to the label *B*-disease is computed as follows:

$$\mathcal{A}^j(B-disease|x) = 0.8 \times (0.05 + 0.9) \times (0.1 + 0.8) = 0.684 \tag{10}$$

Similarly, the probabilities of the remaining labels are computed sequentially to obtain the complete aggregate distribution:

$$\mathcal{A}^j = [0.684, 0.0855, 0.009, 0.0405, 0.019, 0.0855, 0.072] \tag{11}$$

The label sequence {*B*-diseases, *I*-diseases, *B*-gene, *I*-gene, *B*-drug, *I*- drug, *O*}. This strategy solves prediction conflicts among teacher models through mathematical modeling, ensures the mutual exclusivity and consistency of multi-label, and mitigates noise interference caused by unlabeled entities in single- label datasets.

Student Model Training. The training process enables collaborative learning between knowledge transfer and annotation supervision by optimizing the hybrid loss function.

$$\mathcal{L} = \lambda \mathcal{L}_{KD} + (1 - \lambda)\mathcal{L}_{GT} \tag{12}$$

The loss function is designed to jointly optimize two objectives: probability distribution alignment and true label supervision. Its mathematical formulation is presented as follows:

Knowledge Distillation Loss ($\mathcal{L}_{KD}$). Kullback-Leibler (KL) divergence, a classical metric for measuring the difference between probability distribution, plays a fundamental role in knowledge distillation. Xu Tan et al. [11] demonstrated in their 2019 study on multilingual machine translation that when the teacher model produces sufficiently smooth soft labels, minimizing cross-entropy loss implicitly optimizes KL divergence. Chebotar et al. [8] further proved mathematically in the field of speech recognition that minimizing KL divergence is equivalent to optimizing cross-entropy loss. Therefore, the knowledge distillation loss function proposed in this study is defined as follows:

$$\mathcal{L}_{KD} = -\sum_{(x,y)\in D_S}\sum_{t=1}^{H}\sum\nolimits_{k\in y^{multi}} \mathcal{A}^j(k|x)\log S(y_t = k|x;\theta_S) \tag{13}$$

where $S(y_t = k|x;\theta_s)$ is the predicted probability of the student model.

True label loss ($\mathcal{L}_{GT}$). To ensure the fitting ability of the student model to the labeled data, the standard cross-entropy loss is introduced as a strong supervision signal:

$$\mathcal{L}_{GT} = -\sum_{(x,y)\in D_S}\sum_{t=1}^{H} 1\{y_t = k\}\log S(y_t = k|x;\theta_S) \tag{14}$$

where $1\{\cdot\}$ represents the one-hot label in the real annotation.

Hyperparameters Λ. The hyperparameter Λ determines the weight of the two, balancing knowledge transfer and direct learning from annotated data. Through joint optimization, the student model can simultaneously leverage the domain knowledge of the teacher model and the ground-truth of the labeled data to enable efficient cross-type entity recognition.

3.3 Inference Procedure

In the biomedical entity recognition task, the inference phase of this framework follows the standard inference process of the PyTorch framework, and integrates a pre-trained language model for cross-type entity recognition. The inference process mainly consists of three stages: text preprocessing, model forward propagation and label decoding, entity reconstruction, and result output. The detailed process is illustrated in Fig. 2:

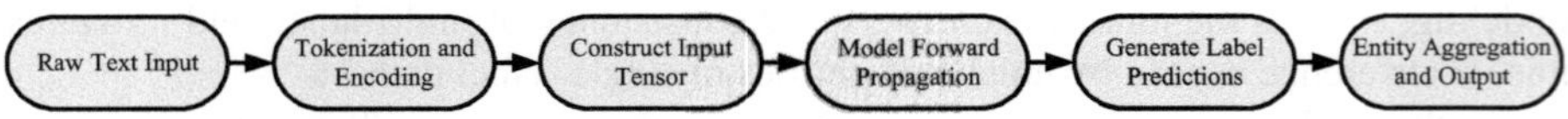

Fig. 2. Inference process.

Input Text Preprocessing. The first step in the inference phase is to apply domain-specific normalization preprocessing on the input text to solve the special challenges of biomedical text:

Word Segmentation and sub-word Optimization. The input sequence is processed by the special segmentation mechanism of the pre training language model. In view of the complex characteristics of terms in the biomedical field, the framework uses the byte-pair encoding algorithm of RoBERTa to split biomedical terms such as gene names and drug com-pounds into manageable sub-word units. For example, "Gefitinib" can be split as "Ge" and "##Fitinib".

Sequence Normalization. The system uses a dynamic sliding window to adjust the length of the input sequence, it applies context-aware truncation to long texts exceeding 128 tokens, while it adds '[PAD]' for shorter sequences to keep the input dimension consistent, so as to adapt to the batch input structure. Insert special tags, such as '[CLS]' and '[SEP]', at Both ends of the sequence to adapt to the input format of the transformer architecture.

Tensor Construction. The encoded token sequence, the corresponding attention masks and token type information are converted into tensor format as the input data of the model.

Model Forward Propagation and Label Prediction. After preprocessing, the input tensor is fed into the trained student model for inference. To improve resource utilization efficiency during the inference phase, the system disables backpropagation in this process and retains only the forward propagation path, thereby eliminating the additional computational cost of gradient calculations.

Hierarchical Feature Coding. The model first extracts the contextual semantic representations of each token in the sentence through the embedding layer and the multi-layer transformer encoder. These representations are then fed into a shared linear transformation layer to map features into a unified multi-label space. The output is the label scores for each token, that is, a unnormalized logits distribution.

Label Probability Generation. During label prediction, the model normalizes these logits to produce probability distributions over labels. The system selects the label with the maximum probability as the token's final predicted label.

Post-processing and Result Output. To ensure that the prediction results are practically useful, the system needs to restore the token-level label sequence to the entity boundaries and category information in the original text. The process primarily consists of the following steps:

Sub-word Aggregation. Based on the position mapping matrix generated by the tokenizer, the framework projects the sub-word prediction results onto the original text coordinates, and merges consecutive sub-words using a greedy algorithm to restore the complete entity boundary. For example, the segments "Ge" and "##Fitinib" are aggregated into "Gefitinib", and the mean probability of each sub-word is retained as the final predicted probability.

Noise Filtering. In order to improve the stability of the output results, a dynamic threshold mechanism is introduced. The average confidence of each identified entity is calculated, and if it is lower than the set threshold, it is eliminated to suppress the noise interference of the model in the uncertain boundary region.

Structured Output. The final output is presented in a structured format, including multi-dimensional information such as entity text, start and end positions, entity type label, and prediction confidence. The system can generate visual charts to assist with result analysis and decision-making. For example, the prediction radar chart for "Gefitinib" is shown in Fig. 3.

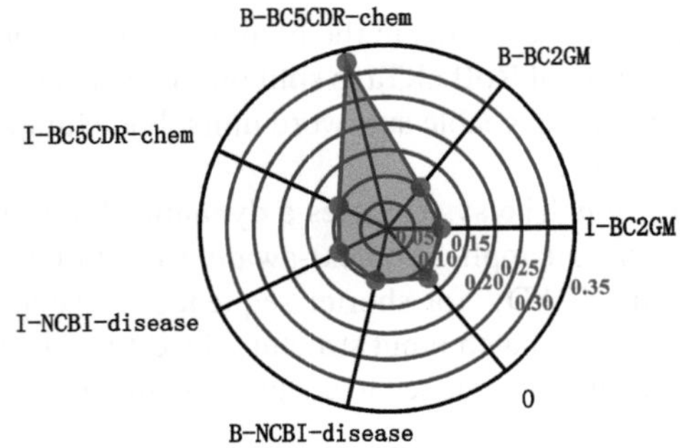

Fig. 3. Radar schematic diagram of prediction results

4 Experimental Results and Analysis

This chapter verifies the effectiveness and practicality of the KFC-Net cross-type BioNER framework in biomedical text processing on three authoritative benchmark datasets. These three datasets contain three key biomedical entity information: diseases, chemicals, and genes. The performance of KFC-Net is evaluated using traditional metrics such as precision, recall rate, and F1. From the perspective of lightweight deployment of models, this paper explores the balance between computational efficiency and resource occupation of student models of different scales. All the experiments are done in the same software and hardware environment, and we compare KFC-Net with various baseline models to objectively demonstrate the technical advantages of KFC-Net in cross-type entity recognition.

4.1 Introduction of Experimental Datasets

In this paper, we select three datasets: NCBI-disease [3], BC5CDR-chem [5] and BC2GM [13], which cover the typical and challenging entity categories in current biomedical information extraction research, and are widely used and representative. NCBI-disease, consisting of 793 PubMed medical abstracts, with a total of 6,892 annotated disease entities. It features rich text content and complex language structure, making it an important benchmark for disease entity recognition; BC5CDR-chem contains 1,500 papers, labeling 15,935 chemicals and 12,852 disease entities. It serves as an important test benchmark for chemical entity recognition; BC2GM focuses on gene name recognition, consisting of 20,510 sentences and 24,583 entity annotations, involving various naming methods and abbreviations. It serves as an important test benchmark in the field of gene recognition.

For all datasets, we adopt the same partitioning method as BioBERT [6]. The scheme has been validated in numerous international studies, effectively ensuring the fairness of model evaluation. Specifically, for NCBI-disease and BC5CDR- chem, the two classic corpora, we directly follow the partitioning methods provided by their original sources. For the BC2GM dataset, since it does not provide a development set, we use the stratified sampling method to extract 2,500 sentences from the original training set as the development set.

4.2 Experimental Setups

In the process of model training, reasonable parameter settings are crucial to improve the final performance. In this paper, we draw on numerous experiments and existing results, and systematically optimize the training parameters. The optimizer used is Adam with effective convergence in natural language processing tasks. The specific parameter settings are as follows: The initial learning rate is 5 × 10-5, the momentum parameters β_1 and β_2 are set to 0.9 and 0.999 respectively, and the stability coefficient is set to 1×10^{-8} to prevent numerical overflow. Considering GPU memory size and training efficiency, the batch size is set to 32, and the maximum sequence length is limited to 128 tokens.

After several rounds of testing, we found that, although the model has showed some improvement in earlier training rounds, the performance peaked after approximately 20 training rounds. This finding is consistent with the results of Lee et al. [6], suggesting that biomedical text processing tasks often require number of training rounds to effectively learn domain features.

In the field of machine learning and deep learning, PyTorch has become the framework of choice for many developers and researchers because of its flexibility and ease of use. In this paper, PyTorch is also employed for both training and prediction.

4.3 Experimental Results

Performance Analysis of the Teacher Model. Under the framework of knowledge distillation, the upper limit of the student model's performance depends on the quality of the teacher model. To construct a high-performance teacher model, we train the ner model individually on each dataset. The training process strictly follows the unified optimization strategy to ensure that the model achieves the optimal state for each respective task. The specific model parameters are presented in Table 1.

Table 1. Entity recognition performance evaluation of type-specific teacher models

Datasets	Entity types	Precision	Recall	F1
NCBI-disease	Disease	87.83	90.94	89.36
BC5CDR-chem	Chemical compounds	93.56	93.73	93.65
BC2GM	Genetic information	83.45	84.61	84.03

Cross-Type Model Comparison Experiment. To verify the practical effectiveness of the framework proposed in this study for cross-type entity recognition, we design and select four mainstream baseline models for comparison, covering a range of strategies from simple fusion to complex shared structures:

1. MERGED: The unified RoBERTa-large model is trained by directly merging individual entity datasets, reflecting the most direct implementation of cross-type entity recognition.

2. MTM-CW [14]: Based on the BiLSTM-CRF architecture, this model introduces a context-aware layer to achieve cross-type modeling, representing a fusion approach under the traditional neural network structure.
3. CollaboNET [15]: As a collaborative multi-model framework, it effectively addresses the type-conflict problem by integrating the prediction results of multiple type-specific models as additional input.
4. MT-BioNER [16]: Based on the Transformer structure, it enables information transfer between types by sharing part of the network layer between different tasks, which is a representative method in biomedical text processing in recent years.

All experiments were conducted on a cloud computing platform equipped with an NVIDIA RTX 4090D GPU, using precision, recall, and F1 of strict entity-level matching as evaluation metrics.

The experimental results are presented in Table 2. As can be seen, KFC-Net achieves the best F1-scores in all three datasets, demonstrating its strong cross-task generalization ability.

Table 2. Entity recognition performance evaluation of cross-type student models.

Datasets	Performance metrics	Merged	MTM-CW [14]	CollaboNET [15]	MT-BioNER [16]	KFC-Net
NCBI-disease	P	83.37	85.86	85.48	86.73	**86.87**
	R	85.52	86.42	87.27	89.70	**89.86**
	F1	84.43	86.14	86.36	88.10	**88.34**
BC5CDR-chem	P	94.36	89.10	94.26	88.46	**94.48**
	R	82.76	88.47	92.38	90.52	**92.77**
	F1	88.18	88.78	93.31	89.50	**93.62**
BC2GM	P	83.15	82.10	80.49	82.01	**83.29**
	R	80.75	79.42	78.99	84.04	**84.40**
	F1	81.93	80.74	79.73	83.01	**83.84**

In the disease recognition task, given the semantic complexity and long-tail distribution of disease entity names, the F1-score of KFC-Net is 88.34%, slightly surpassing that of MT-BioNER. The precision and recall of KFC-Net are 86.87% and 89.86%, respectively, demonstrating the strong adaptability of the proposed framework in accurately delineating entity boundaries.

In the chemical entity recognition task, KFC-Net achieves the F1-score of 93.62%, surpassing CollaboNET(93.31%), and significantly outperforming the MERGED model (88.18%). The precision and recall of KFC-Net are 94.48% and 92.77%, respectively, ranking highest among all comparison models. Moreover, KFC-Net also achieves the highest precision and recall of 94.48% and 92.77%, respectively, among all compared models.

In the gene identification task, despite challenges such as nested and abbreviated gene names, KFC-Net attains an F1-score of 83.84% and a recall of 84.40%, indicating its robust ability to recognize low-frequency entities.

Compared to the baseline model, CollaboNet performs similarly to the framework proposed in this study in chemical identification tasks. However, its multi-model collaboration requires loading multiple independent models simultaneously at runtime, consuming a significant amount of memory and computing resources which makes it unsuitable for deployment on lightweight devices with high-performance requirements. Although MT-BioNER achieves cross-type entity recognition through parameter sharing, its accuracy in disease identification is lower than KFC-Net. This also demonstrates that the knowledge distillation employed by KFC-Net can significantly reduce the mutual interference between different tasks.

Effect Analysis of Lightweight Model. To further enhance the deployability of the proposed framework in practical applications, this paper uses the knowledge distillation method to compress the large teacher model into multiple student models of varying sizes, systematically evaluating its performance in accuracy and efficiency. In this study, we use Roberta-large and RoBERTa-base of Lewis et al. [17], DistilRoBERTa introduced by Sanh et al. [18] and TinyBERT introduced by Jiao et al. [19] as fine-tuning models.

Regarding the loss function design, we combine two different loss functions. The knowledge distillation loss $\mathcal{L}_{KD}$ is implemented using KLDivLoss provided by the PyTorch framework, which extracts knowledge from teacher model; Additionally, NLL-Loss is used to compute the true label loss $\mathcal{L}_{GT}$, ensuring the model's ability to learn from labeled data.

We evaluated the recognition performance of each student model on three datasets, and the results are summarized in Table 3. As the most powerful teacher model, RoERTa-large achieved F1-scores of 88.34%, 93.62% and 83.84% for disease, chemical and gene recognition, respectively. However, its model size reached 1346.8MB and the inference speed was limited to 1524 sample/s. which constrains its deployment in real-time processing or mobile applications. In contrast, the RoBERTa-base model exhibited only a marginal decrease of approximately 2% in average F1-score, while the model size was reduced to 473.28 MB, and the inference speed was increased to 3950 samples/s, with overall performance being better. The further compressed models, DistilRoBERTa (253MB) and TinyBERT (54MB) sacrificed a certain degree of accuracy—declining to 75.25% and 68.26% respectively in gene tasks, but improved inference speed to 6728 samples/s and 7200 samples/s, which greatly enhances their practicality for edge computing devices and embedded applications. Notably, TinyBRET still maintains an F1-score of 83.82% in chemical recognition, making it particularly suitable for low-power, high-frequency text processing tasks.

Table 3. Entity recognition performance evaluation of lightweight models

Models	Training speed (Sample/s)	Training speed (Sample/s)	Volume (MB)	F1 (NCBI-disease)	F1 (BC5CDR-chem)	F1 (BC2GM)
RoBERTa-large [17]	118	1524	1,346.80	88.34	88.34	83.84
RoBERTa-base [17]	346	3950	473.28	86.15	86.15	81.62
DistilRoBERTa [18]	618	6728	253.19	82.52	82.52	75.25
TinyBERT [19]	1053	7200	54.39	77.39	77.39	68.26

4.4 Ablation Experiments

This section analyzes the impact of the hyperparameter λ in the mixed loss function on the performance of the student model. The loss function defined in Eq. (12) integrates the knowledge distillation loss and ground-truth supervision, where λ balances their relative contributions, reflecting the trade-off between soft labels and hard labels.

To systematically analyze the regulatory effect of λ, we trained student models with different λ values on NCBI-disease, BC5CDR-chem, and BC2GM, respectively, using the F1-score as the primary evaluation metric. The experimental results are presented in Table 4.

The experimental results demonstrate that the hyperparameter λ plays a crucial regulatory role in the entity recognition performance of the student model, especially within the lower value range. As shown by the experimental results, when $\lambda = 0$—meaning that only the true label loss is used—the F1-scores on all three datasets are lower than 5%, indicating that relying solely on limited labeled data is insufficient to support effective model training. This finding also confirms the label sparsity commonly observed in BioNER task. The suboptimal performance may arise from the difficulty of learning diverse and potentially conflicting labeling patterns within a unified cross-type label space, which complicates optimization and impedes model convergence. In contrast, the "MERGED" baseline in Sect. 4.2 demonstrates relatively better performance, likely due to its independent optimization, with training procedures and parameters specifically tuned for the mixed dataset. In our framework, however, the $\lambda = 0$ setting adheres to a unified training configuration, which more clearly highlights the inherent challenges associated with directly learning from mixed labels.

As the value of λ increases, the growing weight of knowledge distillation loss significantly enhances the model's performance. For instance, when λ increases from 0.2 to 0.4, the F1-score on the NCBI-disease dataset rises from 42.46% to 58.10%, while that on the BC5DR-chem dataset increases from 64.23% to 73.19%, illustrating the pivotal role of soft labels provided by the teacher model in facilitating knowledge transfer.

Table 4. Experimental results under different λ values.

F1 λ	NCBI-disease	BC5CDR-chem	BC2GM
0.0	1.11	3.60	0.81
0.2	42.46	64.23	43.80
0.4	58.10	73.19	56.36
0.6	67.20	78.41	65.29
0.8	77.52	84.64	73.25
0.85	79.54	86.44	74.78
0.9	81.14	88.26	76.84
0.95	84.62	91.04	80.20
0.99	88.34	93.62	83.84
1.0	82.40	92.51	82.39

Notably, when λ reaches 0.99, the model achieves optimal performance across all data sets (NCBI-disease: 88.34%, BC5DR-chem: 93.62%, BC2GM: 83.84%). This suggests that, under these conditions, the knowledge distillation loss and true label loss establish an ideal, mutually reinforcing relationship, reaching optimal coordination. The observation suggests that the teacher model effectively conveys the interrelationship between categories via soft labels, helping mitigate both overfitting and underfitting caused by the limited amount of labeled data. At the same time, although the weight of the true label loss is only 1%, the hard constraints provided by it can still effectively correct the possible distribution offset in the knowledge distillation process and ensure the accuracy and stability of the model learning process.

When $\lambda = 1$, completely disregarding the true labels and relying solely on the distillation signal, the F1-scores of the model across all datasets decline to varying extents, highlighting the necessity of true label supervision during the training process. Even with an extremely low weight, the model's generalization ability can still be enhanced through gradient correction.

To verify the reliability of the performance improvement when $\lambda = 0.99$ in the ablation experiment, an independent sample t-test was conducted to analyze the statistical significance of the key parameters. Ten independent experiments were conducted for $\lambda = 0.99$ and $\lambda = 0.95$ configurations respectively, with F1-scores recorded of each experiment. The specific analysis is presented in Table 5.

The statistical results show that the soft label contribution of the teacher model plays a key role in cross-type entity knowledge transfer, and the parameter configuration can significantly improve the recognition accuracy of the model for biomedical entities, which provides a reliable statistical basis for the parameter optimization of the framework proposed in this paper. In the case of limited labeled data, it should be given priority to increase the weight $\lambda \geq 0.9$ of the teacher model, and moderately retain a small amount of true label information. It ensures that the model can not only effectively learn prior knowledge, but also maintain the accuracy of the specific fields.

Table 5. Statistical results analysis

Datasets	λ	Sample size	Mean F1	Standard deviation	T-value	Significance
NCBI-disease	0.99	10	89.97	0.15	21.40	High
	0.95	10	85.82	0.28		
	0.99	10	93.50	0.11		
BC5CDR-chem	0.95	10	91.22	0.18	34.18	High
	0.99	10	84.14	0.21		
BC2GM	0.95	10	80.52	0.14	45.36	High

5 Conclusion

This paper presents KFC-Net framework for cross-type BioNER. The KFC-Net successfully demonstrates the synergistic value of knowledge distillation and cross-type entity recognition. It enhances the performance of cross-type BioNER, and offers a versatile framework for integrating multi-type entity knowledge. As technologies like dynamic distillation mechanisms and multimodal fusion continue to evolve, KFC-Net has the potential to bridge laboratory research and clinical practical applications, promoting the implementation of intelligent medical systems in the scenes of precision diagnosis, drug research and development.

Acknowledgments. This study is supported by National Natural Science Foundation of China (62302151).

References

1. Grishman, R., Sundheim, B.: Message understanding conference-6: a brief history. In: Proceedings of the 16th International Conference on Computational Linguistics (COLING 1996), Copenhagen, Denmark, pp. 466–471. ACL (1996)
2. Li, J., Sun, A., Han, J., Li, C.: A survey on deep learning for named entity recognition. IEEE Trans. Knowl. Data Eng. **34**(1), 50–70 (2022)
3. Zhao, S., Liu, T., Zhao, S., Wang, F.: A neural multi-task learning framework to jointly model medical named entity recognition and normalization (2018). arXiv:1812.09502
4. Xu, L., Li, J.: Biomedical named entity recognition based on BERT and BiLSTM-CRF. Comput. Eng. Sci. **43**(10), 1873–1879 (2021) (in Chinese)
5. Li, J., Sun, Y., Johnson, R.J., Sciaky, D., Wei, C.H., Leaman, R., Davis, A.P., Mattingly, C.J., Wiegers, T.C., Lu, Z.: BioCreative V CDR task corpus: a resource for chemical disease relation extraction. Database 2016, baw068 (2016)
6. Lee, J., et al.: BioBERT: a pre-trained biomedical language representation model for biomedical text mining. Bioinformatics **36**(4), 1234–1240 (2020)
7. Hinton, G., Vinyals, O., Dean, J.: Distilling the knowledge in a neural network (2015). arXiv: 1503.02531

8. Chebotar, Y., Waters, A.: Distilling knowledge from ensembles of neural networks for speech recognition. In: Proceedings of Interspeech 2016, pp. 3439–3443. ISCA, San Francisco (2016)
9. Fukuda, T., Suzuki, M., Kurata, G., Thomas, S., Cui, J., Ramabhadran, B.: Efficient knowledge distillation from an ensemble of teachers. In: Proceedings of Interspeech 2017, pp. 3697–3701. ISCA, Stockholm (2017)
10. Liu, Y., Zhang, W., Wang, J.: Adaptive multi-teacher multi-level knowledge distillation. Neurocomputing **415**, 106–113 (2020)
11. Tan, X., Ren, Y., He, D., Qin, T., Zhao, Z., Liu, T.-Y.: Multilingual neural machine translation with knowledge distillation (2019). arXiv:1904.08194
12. Sang, E.F.T.K., Veenstra, J.: Representing text chunks (1999). arXiv:cs/9907006
13. Smith, L., Tanabe, L.K., Ando, R.J.N.: Overview of BioCreative II gene mention recognition. Genome Biol. **9**(S2), S2 (2008)
14. Mehmood, T., Gerevini, A., Lavelli, A., Serina, I., et al.: Multi-task learning applied to biomedical named entity recognition task. In: CLiC-it, pp. 362–371 (2019)
15. Yoon, W., So, C.H., Lee, J., Kang, J.: CollaboNet: collaboration of deep neural networks for biomedical named entity recognition. BMC Bioinform. **20**(S10), 249 (2019)
16. Khan, M.R., Ziyadi, M., AbdelHady, M.: MT-BioNER: multi-task learning for biomedical named entity recognition using deep bidirectional transformers (2020). arXiv:2001.08904
17. Lewis, P., Ott, M., Du, J., Stoyanov, V.: Pretrained language models for biomedical and clinical tasks: understanding and extending the state-of-the-art. In: Proceedings of the 3rd Clinical Natural Language Processing Workshop, pp. 146–157. ACL, Online (2020)
18. Sanh, V., Debut, L., Chaumond, J., Wolf, T.: DistilBERT, a distilled version of BERT: smaller, faster, cheaper and lighter (2020). arXiv:1910.01108
19. Jiao, X., Yin, Y., Shang, L., Jiang, X., Chen, X., Li, L., Wang, F., Liu, Q.: TinyBERT: distilling BERT for natural language understanding (2020). arXiv:1909.10351

Shared Task 1

Overview of the Content Quality Control Task for Admission Records in Inpatient Electronic Medical Records in CHIP 2025

Lu Xiang[1(✉)], Sikai Liu[2], Weiyu Zhang[3], Jing Wang[2], Guoqiang Chen[4], Ying Lian[4], Zhiyang He[2], Gengyao Li[5], Yangyang Ou[2], and Wenpeng Lu[3]

[1] State Key Laboratory of Multimodal Artificial Intelligence Systems, Institute of Automation, CAS, Beijing, China
lu.xiang@nlpr.ia.ac.cn

[2] Xunfei Healthcare Technology Co., Ltd., Hefei, China
{skliu10,jingwang81,zyhe,yyou3}@iflytek.com

[3] Key Laboratory of Computing Power Network and Information Security, Ministry of Education, Shandong Computer Science Center (National Supercomputer Center in Jinan), Qilu University of Technology (Shandong Academy of Sciences), Jinan, China
{zwy,wenpeng.lu}@qlu.edu.cn

[4] Shandong Key Laboratory of Digital Diagnosis and Treatment of Thoracic Tumor, Shandong Engineering Research Center of Intelligent Surgery, The First Affiliated Hospital of Shandong First Medical University & Shandong Provincial Qianfoshan, Jinan, China

[5] Fanyu AI Research, Zhongke Fanyu Technology Co., Ltd, Beijing, China

Abstract. Content quality control (QC) of clinical records is a critical task for ensuring patient safety. However, systematically assessing narrative admission notes for information completeness, diagnostic consistency, and logical coherence remains a significant challenge, and public benchmarks are lacking. To address this need, we organized the *Content Quality Control Task for Admission Records in Inpatient Electronic Medical Records*. This task aims to evaluate the deep reasoning capabilities of Large Language Models (LLMs) on Electronic Medical Record (EMR) samples. The evaluation was structured into two distinct tracks: a *No-Finetuning Track* (Track A) and a *Finetuning Track* (Track B). The shared task attracted 283 teams from industry and academia, with the top-performing teams achieving overall scores of 0.7023 (Track A) and 0.7311 (Track B). This paper provides a comprehensive overview of the task design, the datasets, the evaluation metrics, and a summary of the innovative methods employed by the top-ranking teams.

Keywords: Medical quality control · Electronic medical record · Large language model

Y. Zhang et al. (Eds.): CHIP 2025, CCIS 2884, pp. 381–394, 2026.
https://doi.org/10.1007/978-981-95-7299-1_22

1 Introduction

Inpatient admission records are foundational documents in Electronic Medical Records (EMRs), capturing the critical patient history, physical examination findings, and initial diagnoses [10]. The quality of this initial record is paramount. Inaccuracies, incompleteness, or logical inconsistencies can lead to diagnostic errors and compromise patient safety. However, manual quality control (QC) of these narrative documents remains a laborious, time-consuming, and resource-intensive process, often subject to human variability and oversight [15]. Consequently, there is an urgent need for automated and intelligent methods that can rigorously assess the in-depth content quality of clinical narratives.

Existing automated quality control (QC) methodologies in healthcare primarily focus on structured data validation or apply rule-based algorithms to verify compliance with specific clinical guidelines [8,18,22,23]. While valuable, these approaches often fall short in evaluating the nuanced, semantic, and logical coherence of free-text clinical narratives. Recent large language models (LLMs) like GPT-4 [1] and Med-PaLM 2 [16] have demonstrated promising capabilities across diagnostic reasoning [4], clinical note generation [21], and automated clinical assessment [6]. However, to our knowledge, no public benchmark assesses an LLM's ability to perform comprehensive quality control on narrative medical records by *localizing* field-level defects, *attributing* them to specific quality rules, and *explaining* the judgment within admission notes.

To address this gap and benchmark the capabilities of LLMs on this task, we organized the **Content Quality Control Task for Admission Records in Inpatient Electronic Medical Records** in the 2025 China Health Information Processing Conference, with the help of the conference committees (http://cips-chip.org.cn/2025/eval1). The objective of this task is to develop and evaluate automated approaches for performing deep, content-based quality control on narrative EMRs. The evaluation is structured into two distinct tracks to investigate different technical settings.

Track A, the No-Finetuning Track, investigates the in-context learning (ICL) [13] and zero-shot reasoning capabilities of LLMs. In this track, participants were prohibited from finetuning model parameters but were permitted to use techniques like prompt engineering, ICL, and retrieval-augmented generation (RAG) [5]. Model parameters were restricted to 70B.

Track B, the Finetuning Track, investigates the performance of models when permitted to adapt to the specific task data. This track permitted participants to explore parameter-efficient fine-tuning (PEFT) methods [9,24] or full finetuning to maximize performance. To ensure a comparable evaluation basis with Track A, model parameters in this track were also restricted to 70B. This represents a scenario where a dedicated, local model is being developed for the QC task.

The shared task has attracted significant attention from both academia and industry, attracting 283 participating teams. This paper provides a comprehensive overview of the task, including the dataset construction and evaluation metrics, the winning teams and their methodologies, and a discussion of potential directions for future research.

2 Related Work

2.1 Quality Control in Clinical Texts

The evaluation of clinical text quality has evolved significantly, moving from simple, explicit rule-based checks to complex, semantic-level reasoning. This progression can be broadly categorized into three paradigms: rule-based systems, information extraction-based approaches, and methods leveraging LLMs.

Rule-based QC. Early approaches to EMR quality control were dominated by rule-based and statistical methods [20]. These systems typically involved manually crafted rules, regular expressions, or keyword matching to identify predefined errors. While effective for simple, explicit, and pre-defined errors, these methods are brittle, difficult to scale, and fundamentally incapable of understanding the semantic context or logical flow of narrative text.

Information Extraction-based QC. The second paradigm is centered on Information Extraction (IE). This approach utilizes models like BERT [3] to perform structured data extraction from free text. Many shared tasks in medical NLP, such as the i2b2/n2c2 challenges [7,17], fall into this category. While powerful, IE-based approaches to QC are *elemental* rather than *holistic*. They can verify the presence of information but struggle to evaluate its *quality*, *coherence*, or *consistency* against other parts of the record.

QC with LLMs. The evolution from domain-specific pre-trained models like BioBERT [12] to instruction-tuned, large-scale models like Med-PaLM 2 [16] has shifted the research focus from simple extraction to deep clinical reasoning. This line of inquiry focuses on using LLMs to evaluate and correct text. This includes foundational research on mitigating factual inconsistencies [19] and detecting documentation errors [2]. In parallel with this academic research, the practical feasibility of LLMs for QC is now being validated in real-world clinical deployments. Recent studies report significant gains in efficiency and dramatic improvements in record quality, with defect rates falling from a 7 to 10% baseline to below 2% in some cases [14]. Other implementations have achieved a near-perfect rate of Grade A records and slashed review times from hours to seconds [18]. While these real-world studies confirm the immense practical value of LLMs for clinical QC, they describe proprietary, in-house systems. A critical gap remains: the lack of a **public, standardized benchmark** to allow for reproducible research and transparent model comparison.

2.2 Related EMR Tasks

Beyond direct quality control, other public benchmarks have emerged to evaluate LLMs in related and complex EMR tasks. These benchmarks, however, do not focus on the end-to-end QC of narrative admission records. For instance, the EHRCon benchmark was developed to evaluate a model's ability to detect consistency between unstructured clinical notes and structured tables (note-table consistency) [11]. This is a crucial, but specific, aspect of logical consistency. Similarly, [23] propose CMQCIC-Bench, a benchmark where LLMs must answer

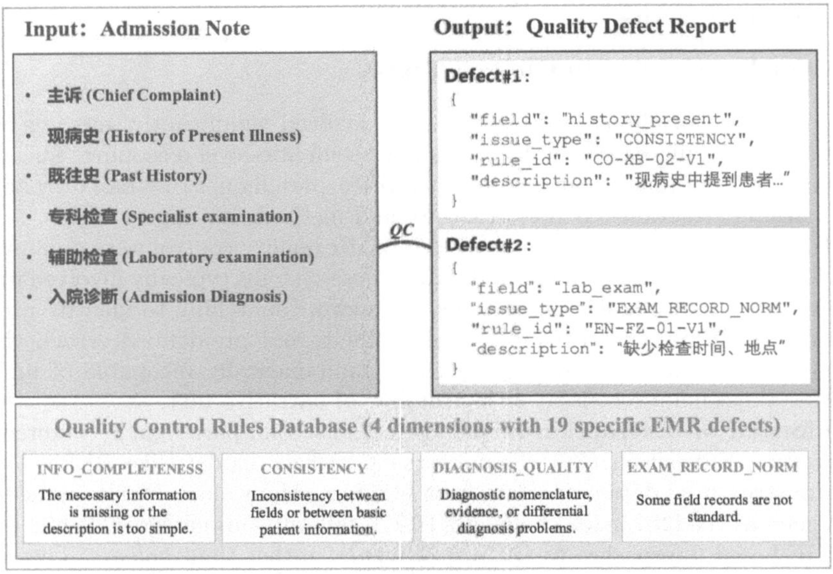

Fig. 1. An illustration of the Content Quality Control task for admission record. The model receives an admission record as input and processes it against a Quality Control Rules Database. The required output is a structured Quality Defect Report that lists each identified defect, specifying its corresponding field, issue_type, rule_id, and a textual description.

whether a patient satisfies a set of predefined quality indicators, such as stroke prevention or ICH improvement rate. While clinically relevant, these tasks operate at the document or multi-document level, without identifying specific fields or providing localized explanations.

Our shared task is designed to fill the gap left by these other works. It is designed to require models to perform a comprehensive, multi-dimensional QC assessment on narrative admission records, compelling them to not only identify issues but also to (1) *localize* defects at the field level, (2) *attribute* these defects to specific quality dimensions (e.g., completeness, consistency), and (3) *explain* the judgment, all within a unified, public evaluation framework.

3 Task Overview

3.1 Task Definition

This shared task focuses on Content Quality Control for narrative medical documents. The objective is to evaluate a model's ability to understand, reason, and identify defects within a common inpatient document based on a predefined set of clinical quality control rules. The task focuses on the admission record, and a conceptual overview is provided in Fig. 1.

The input for the task is a single admission record document. This document comprises several key text fields, such as chief complaint, history of present illness, past history, specialist examination, laboratory examination, admission diagnosis, and preliminary diagnosis. The task requires models to process the input text and generate a structured list of identified quality control defects. Each defect must be represented as an object with four mandatory fields:

- **field**: Denotes the specific EMR field (e.g., history_present) where the defect was identified.
- **issue_type**: Specifies the category of the defect, selected from four predefined types.
- **rule_id**: The identifier for the specific quality control rule that was violated.
- **description**: A brief, free-text explanation in Chinese ($\leq$100 characters) justifying the identified defect.

While the model's primary output is the structured list of individual defects, the task's evaluation also includes an assessment of the overall case compliance. A key design choice of this task is that models do not directly output this compliance status (e.g., compliant or non-compliant). Instead, as detailed in Sect. 3.5, the overall compliance judgment is subsequently calculated by the evaluators, based on a defect-driven scoring mechanism applied to the model's generated defect list.

3.2 Data Source and Preprocessing

The dataset for intrinsic quality control evaluation was primarily derived from a tertiary hospital, comprising a total of 1,600 admission records. To ensure clinical diversity and mitigate the risk of single-center bias, data were collected from multiple departments including cardiology, respiratory medicine, pediatrics, etc. This multi-department sampling strategy enhances the generalizability of the dataset, establishing it as a challenging benchmark capable of effectively evaluating model robustness.

Among 1600 records, 700 records were given without annotation. The remaining 900 annotated records were systematically partitioned into a training set, an A-leaderboard test set, and a B-leaderboard test set, with each subset containing 300 records. Prior to data annotation, the records underwent a two-step preprocessing phase:

- **De-identification:** We removed all direct identifiers (e.g., patient name, ID number, phone number) and replaced them with anonymous placeholders to comply with privacy protection regulations.
- **Data Cleaning:** We corrected common typographical errors using a medical terminology dictionary, removed non-informative symbols, and handled missing values or obvious outliers.

3.3 Data Annotation Process

We first defined the criteria for EMR content quality. The task is based on **4 core dimensions** and a total of **19 specific EMR defects**, which are aligned with national clinical standards (China's Electronic Medical Record Application Management Specification, 2023[1]). Each dimension was decomposed into specific, operable QC indicators. To ensure the reliability and accuracy of the labels, we adopted a rigorous three-stage double-blind verification process, similar to the multi-step procedures used in other medical benchmarks:

(1) **Preliminary Labeling and Guideline Creation:** A team of 10 annotators (5 attending physicians with ≥5 years of EMR management experience and 5 medical informatics experts familiar with QC standards) independently labeled 900 EMR samples. This initial phase was used to calibrate annotation criteria. Disagreements were resolved through group discussion to formulate a unified Annotation Guide.
(2) **Formal Annotation:** The annotators were divided into 5 pairs. Each pair labeled the same subset of EMRs using a custom-built annotation tool.
(3) **Consistency Verification:** A senior expert group (3 chief physicians and 2 associate professors in medical informatics) randomly sampled 15% of the fully labeled data to verify consistency. The Fleiss' Kappa coefficient for inter-annotator agreement was 0.89, confirming the high reliability of the final labels.

3.4 Data Distribution

The dataset provides broad coverage across seven key clinical departments. As shown in Fig. 2a, the 1,600 records are distributed across Oncology (17.4%), Cardiology (17.3%), Endocrinology (16.1%), Gynecology (14.9%), Orthopedics (12.6%), Pediatrics (12.6%), and Respiratory (9.1%). This multi-departmental composition ensures a wide representation of medical disciplines and mitigates evaluation bias that could arise from a dataset dominated by a single specialty. Furthermore, the distribution of annotated defects per record was analyzed, as depicted in Fig. 2b. This chart illustrates the frequency of defect counts, spanning from defect-free records (0 defects) to complex records with numerous issues (up to 9 defects).

A key strength of the dataset design is the high consistency in this distribution across the training (train), validation (testA), and test (testB) splits. As Fig. 2b illustrates, all three partitions exhibit a very similar distributional shape. The vast majority of records contain between 1 and 4 defects, with a pronounced peak in the 2–3 defect range. The dataset also includes a long tail of more complex cases (5 or more defects), as well as a small but important number of defect-free (0 defects) records. This distributional alignment ensures

[1] https://www.nhc.gov.cn/wjw/gfxwj/200205/8348500efb5b490c8db6519e818e96e3.shtml.

that the test sets are representative of the training data, allowing for a fair and robust evaluation of model generalization. This tiered and varied distribution requires models to be robust in handling records with varying defect densities while also being discriminative enough to correctly identify the (rare) defect-free cases, thereby preventing false positives.

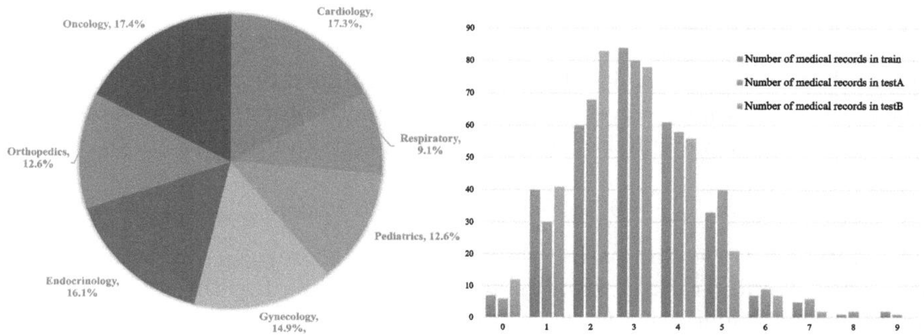

(a) Department Distribution (b) Defects Distribution

Fig. 2. Data distribution of the benchmark. (a) Department distribution of the 1,600 admission records, showing coverage across seven clinical specialties. (b) Distribution of the number of defects per record, shown separately for the training (train), validation (testA), and test (testB) sets.

3.5 Evaluation Metrics

The evaluation framework is designed to be comprehensive, assessing performance from two critical perspectives.

(1) Problem Extraction Ability. This dimension measures the model's accuracy in identifying and describing individual defects. A predicted defect is considered a True Positive (TP) only if the (field, issue_type, rule_id) triplet exactly matches a ground-truth annotation. Based on this, we calculate precision (P), recall (R), and F1-score. The quality of the generated description is evaluated using ROUGE-L. The final extraction score is a weighted sum:

$$\text{Score}_{extract} = 0.4 * F1 + 0.25 * P + 0.15 * R + 0.2 * ROUGE - L \quad (1)$$

(2) Overall Case Compliance Judgment. This dimension simulates the real-world task of making a final compliance judgment on the entire record. This is determined via a defect-driven scoring system: (i) Each record starts with a perfect score of 100; (ii) For each recognized defect, a predefined penalty score is deducted. Specifically, each of the 19 quality rules is assigned a penalty ranging from 1 to 3 points based on clinical severity, where 3 denotes the most critical violation; (iii) A record is classified as non-compliant if its final score falls below a threshold. Here, we define the threshold as 95, based on the hospital's strict quality assurance standards for Grade-A records.

The model's performance on this binary classification task (compliant vs. non-compliant) is then evaluated using a weighted F1-score. A TP here is a correctly identified non-compliant case. The compliance score is calculated as:

$$\text{Score}_{compliant} = 0.5 * F1 + 0.25 * P + 0.25 * R \tag{2}$$

(3) Final Overall Score. The two scores are combined to produce a single comprehensive score, which serves as the primary metric for the final leaderboard. The final score is a weighted average of $\text{Score}_{extract}$ and $\text{Score}_{compliant}$:

$$\text{Score}_{final} = 0.7 * \text{Score}_{extract} + 0.3 * \text{Score}_{compliant} \tag{3}$$

Comprehensive leaderboards, ranked by this Score_{final}, are published for both Track-A and Track-B. Awards are granted to the top three teams on the comprehensive leaderboard for each track.

4 Participating Teams and Methods

4.1 Participating Teams

This shared task is held in CHIP-2025 Conference as Shared Task 1. We held this shared task with the help of the Tianchi Team, and all the logistics are handled by the Tianchi platform[2]. The task attracted significant interest from both industry and academia, with a total of 283 teams registering for the competition. During the evaluation phase, 76 teams submitted active results to Leaderboard A (validation set). These submissions were evenly distributed between the two tracks, with 38 teams participating in the No-Finetuning track and 38 in the Finetuning track. For the final Leaderboard B (test set), 42 teams submitted predictions. This final group consisted of 26 teams in the No-Finetuning track and 16 teams in the Finetuning track.

4.2 Winning Teams

For both tracks, teams were ranked based on the final overall score (Score_{final}), as detailed in Sect. 3.5. In accordance with the regulations of the shared tasks in CHIP-2025, the top-3 teams from each track are eligible for awards and certificates issued by the CHIP-2025 committee. These teams were also invited to submit papers to share their techniques and experiences with the community.

Table 1 lists the top-3 performing teams from Track A (No-Finetuning) and Track B (Finetuning). The results show a clear performance gap between the two tracks, with the top score in the Finetuning track (0.7311) being higher than the top score in the No-Finetuning track (0.7023). This indicates that

[2] https://tianchi.aliyun.com/competition/entrance/532413.

while advanced non-finetuning methods are capable of achieving strong results, parameter-efficient finetuning on a small, labeled dataset (300 samples) provides a distinct performance advantage for this complex clinical QC.

Table 1. Top-3 teams and their results in the No-Finetuning and Finetuning tracks.

Team	Rank	Institution	$Score_{final}$	$Score_{extract}$	$Score_{compliant}$
Winners of No-Finetuning Track					
随机种子	1	(1) School of Computer Science and Technology, Xi'an Jiaotong University (2) The Second Affiliated Hospital of Xi'an Jiaotong University (Xibei Hospital)	0.7023	0.7125	0.6786
露露最强队	2	AthenaEyes CO.,LTD.	0.6644	0.6556	0.6850
地下小队	3	Central South University	0.6485	0.6420	0.6636
Winners of Finetuning Track					
Seeking Your Roots	1	Artificial Intelligence Research Institute on Education, Qilu Normal University	0.7311	0.7496	0.6881
leaf2025	2	(1) School of Computer Science and Technology, Xi'an Jiaotong University (2) The Second Affiliated Hospital of Xi'an Jiaotong University (Xibei Hospital)	0.7078	0.7166	0.6873
地下小队	3	Central South University	0.6918	0.6842	0.7095

4.3 Top-Ranked Solutions of the No-Finetuning Track

In the No-Finetuning track, participants were restricted from updating model parameters. Consequently, the top solutions focused on identifying the optimal way to guide frozen LLMs through advanced prompt engineering, agentic workflows, and the injection of external knowledge.

1st Place: 随机种子

The winning team introduced **MedShard**, a multi-agent framework designed to optimize the performance of local LLMs (specifically Qwen3-32B) without the need for training. Their core strategy, named *per-rule sharding*, employs four specialized agents to decompose the task. The **Cleaning Agent** filters the admission note to retain only the text segments strictly relevant to the specific rule being evaluated. Following this, the **QC Agent** executes an initial high-recall sweep using simplified logic to flag potential issues. A **Reflection**

Agent is then invoked specifically for items flagged as non-compliant to perform a secondary confirmation, effectively reducing false positives. Finally, an **Output Agent** standardizes the decisions and rewrites the rationales to match the required format and length constraints.

2nd Place: 露露最强战队

The second-ranked team developed a dual-enhancement framework that combines **Precision In-Context Learning (ICL)** with **Chain-of-Thought (CoT)** reasoning, utilizing the Qwen3-30B-A3B-thinking model. Their approach emphasizes strict data control and structured logic simulation. To implement Precision ICL, the team segments admission records into semi-structured components, such as the history of present illness. They utilize rule-specific configuration files to ensure that the model receives only the context necessary for the specific rule. To guide the inference process, they designed progressive prompts based on CoT logic. This mechanism leads the LLM through a human-like analytical process by starting with basic validity checks and advancing to complex logic matching before parsing the final output into a structured defect list.

3rd Place: 地下小队

The third-place solution adopted a hybrid architecture that synergizes deterministic rule-based checks with **Retrieval-Augmented Generation (RAG)**. For quality rules defined by objective criteria, the system bypasses the LLM and applies direct rule-based verification to conserve resources. For defects requiring semantic understanding, the system deploys a Qwen-32B model enhanced by RAG. A key innovation of their approach is the three-stage construction of their external knowledge base. It aggregates the official training set, high-value samples filtered from unlabeled medical records, and synthetic non-compliant examples generated by an LLM to simulate realistic defect patterns. During inference, the system retrieves the top-K most similar examples from this enriched knowledge base to provide the model with rich contextual references.

4.4 Top-Ranked Solutions of the Finetuning Track

In the Finetuning track, participants were permitted to update model parameters using the provided training data. The leading solutions demonstrated that combining parameter-efficient tuning with specialized data strategies is essential for maximizing performance on clinical tasks with limited annotated data.

1st Place: Seeking Your Roots

The winning team proposed a systematic framework based on **Phased Training** and **Multi-Granularity Prompting**. To address the scarcity of high-quality data, they devised a two-stage training curriculum. First, the Qwen2.5-32B base model underwent foundational concept learning using the pseudo-labeled samples generated via the DeepSeek API to establish a broad cognitive framework. This was followed by a knowledge refinement phase where the model was fine-tuned exclusively on the 300 high-quality human annotations to align with precise clinical standards. This strategy was further augmented by a hierarchical prompt design termed *single-rule judgment*, which decomposed the task into independent binary classification problems. Additionally, an 8x oversampling strategy was implemented to mitigate class imbalance.

2nd Place: leaf2025

The second-place solution introduced **M3-MedQC**, a framework featuring a **Multi-head**, **Multi-rule**, and **Multi-granularity** architecture built upon Qwen3-32B. Their primary innovation lay in the structural modification of the fine-tuning process itself. To accommodate the diverse nature of QC rules, they constructed two distinct classifier heads on top of the model encoder: a *Four-Group Head* that clustered rules by semantic frequency to enhance learning for sparse categories, and a *Top-10 Rule Head* that provided dedicated classifiers for the most frequent, high-impact rules. This architecture was implemented using Low-Rank Adaptation (LoRA) during training. Additionally, the inference mechanism incorporated rule-specific learnable thresholds to optimize the precision-recall balance across varying defect distributions.

3rd Place: 地下小队

The third-place team proposed a robust framework that integrates **Q-LoRA fine-tuning** with a **collaborative model-rule workflow**. To implement this, they fine-tuned the Qwen3-32B model on a dataset constructed via task decomposition, where each record and rule pair was treated as an independent training instance. This method prioritizes the synergy between deep semantic learning and deterministic logic by utilizing iteratively optimized instructions to guide the model through these focused single-rule checks. A key feature of their approach is a two-stage post-processing module: a correction step utilizing keyword lists to filter out hallucinations, and a completion step applying rigid rules to identify unambiguous errors, such as empty fields, that the model might overlook. This hybrid approach achieved the highest compliance score on the leaderboard.

4.5 Analysis of Top Team Solutions

A comparative analysis of the methodologies and results presented in Table 1 reveals several critical insights regarding the application of LLMs to medical quality control.

Parameter Updates Benefit Granular Extraction. A comparative analysis of $\text{Score}_{extract}$ reveals a notable performance advantage for finetuning methods. The top-performing team in the Finetuning track (Seeking Your Roots) achieved an extraction score of 0.7496, surpassing the best result in the No-Finetuning track (0.7125). This suggests that while prompt engineering can effectively guide reasoning logic, parameter updates are necessary for models to adapt to the specific, structured requirements for precise defect localization and description.

The Efficacy of Hybrid Architectures for Compliance Judgment. The $\text{Score}_{compliant}$ metric reflects the model's judgmental capability, measuring how accurately its extracted defects align with the overall compliance status of the record via a penalty mechanism. Achieving a high score requires judicious extraction, balancing the precision needed to avoid false penalties with the recall required to find the critical defects that determine non-compliance. The absolute highest score in this crucial dimension, 0.7095, was attained by the Finetuning team 地下小队. This superior result validates the efficacy of hybrid architectures, as their methodology explicitly integrates a rule-based post-processing module to handle deterministic errors (e.g., missing mandatory fields). This finding underscores that for clinical QC task, it is necessary to combine the semantic understanding of LLMs with rigid, deterministic rules.

Efficacy of Task Decomposition. A consistent trend among top-ranking solutions in both tracks is the adoption of task decomposition strategies. Whether through multi-agent sharding (随机种子) or single-rule training instances (Seeking Your Roots), successful teams decomposed the evaluation of 19 distinct quality rules into atomic sub-tasks. This consensus suggests that reducing the cognitive load and context complexity is a necessary prerequisite for achieving high accuracy in multi-dimensional medical QC tasks.

5 Conclusion

This paper provides an overview of the Content Quality Control Task for Admission Records, held as CHIP 2025 Shared Task 1, the first public, multi-dimensional benchmark evaluating LLMs for content quality control on narrative EMRs. The comprehensive evaluation revealed three critical insights: task decomposition was confirmed as a necessary prerequisite for high accuracy. Findings also confirmed a key performance trade-off: fine-tuning is necessary for precise, structured defect extraction, whereas pre-trained LLMs, when guided by advanced prompting, achieve comparable performance in overall compliance judgment. Additionally, the superior reliability of hybrid architectures, which combine LLM semantics with deterministic rule-based post-processing, was validated for clinical QC task.

Despite these advances, significant challenges remain in maintaining high precision (particularly in minimizing false-positive rates within deployed systems), ensuring generalizability across diverse institutional documentation styles, and accurately characterizing the complexity of rare, multi-defect cases. For future work, we intend to expand the dataset by incorporating records from additional clinical specialties, further refine multi-dimensional evaluation metrics to more effectively capture model behavior, and focus on translating these proven methodologies into reliable clinical applications that support standardized practices and enhance patient safety within hospital workflows.

Acknowledgments. This work is supported by the National Natural Science Foundation of China (No. 62376130), the Pilot Project for Integrated Innovation of Science, Education, and Industry of Qilu University of Technology (Shandong Academy of Sciences) (No.2025ZDZX01), and the Open Project of the Key Laboratory of Computing Power Network and Information Security, Ministry of Education (No. 25ZD017).

References

1. Achiam, J., Adler, S., Agarwal, S., Ahmad, L., Akkaya, I., Aleman, F.L., Almeida, D., Altenschmidt, J., Altman, S., Anadkat, S., et al.: Gpt-4 technical report (2023). arXiv:2303.08774
2. Ben Abacha, A., Yim, W.w., Fu, Y., Sun, Z., Yetisgen, M., Xia, F., Lin, T.: MEDEC: A benchmark for medical error detection and correction in clinical notes. In: Findings of the Association for Computational Linguistics: ACL 2025, pp. 22539–22550 (2025)
3. Devlin, J., Chang, M.W., Lee, K., Toutanova, K.: BERT: Pre-training of deep bidirectional transformers for language understanding. In: Proceedings of the 2019 Conference of the North American Chapter of the Association for Computational Linguistics: Human Language Technologies, vol. 1 (Long and Short Papers), pp. 4171–4186 (2019)
4. Dou, C., Zhang, Y., Jin, Z., Jiao, W., Zhao, H., Zhao, Y., Tao, Z.: Integrating physician diagnostic logic into large language models: Preference learning from process feedback. In: Findings of the Association for Computational Linguistics ACL 2024, pp. 2453–2473 (2024)
5. Gao, Y., Xiong, Y., Gao, X., Jia, K., Pan, J., Bi, Y., Dai, Y., Sun, J., Wang, M., Wang, H.: Retrieval-Augmented Generation for Large Language Models: A Survey (2023). arXiv:2312.10997
6. GU, Z., Jia, W., Piccardi, M., Yu, P.: Empowering large language models for automated clinical assessment with generation-augmented retrieval and hierarchical chain-of-thought. Available at SSRN 4835586 (2024)
7. Henry, S., Buchan, K., Filannino, M., Stubbs, A., Uzuner, O.: 2018 n2c2 shared task on adverse drug events and medication extraction in electronic health records. J. Am. Med. Inform. Assoc. **27**(1), 3–12 (2020)
8. Hsu, W., Han, S.X., Arnold, C.W., Bui, A.A., Enzmann, D.R.: A data-driven approach for quality assessment of radiologic interpretations. J. Am. Med. Inform. Assoc. **23**(e1), e152–e156 (2016)
9. Hu, E.J., yelong shen, Wallis, P., Allen-Zhu, Z., Li, Y., Wang, S., Wang, L., Chen, W.: LoRA: low-rank adaptation of large language models. In: International Conference on Learning Representations (2022)
10. Johnson, A.E., Bulgarelli, L., Shen, L., Gayles, A., Shammout, A., Horng, S., Pollard, T.J., Hao, S., Moody, B., Gow, B., et al.: Mimic-iv, a freely accessible electronic health record dataset. Scientific Data **10**(1), 1 (2023)
11. Kwon, Y., Kim, J., Lee, G., Bae, S., Kyung, D., Cha, W., Pollard, T., Johnson, A., Choi, E.: Ehrcon: dataset for checking consistency between unstructured notes and structured tables in electronic health records. In: Advances in Neural Information Processing Systems, vol. 37, pp. 89334–89345 (2024)
12. Lee, J., Yoon, W., Kim, S., Kim, D., Kim, S., So, C.H., Kang, J.: Biobert: a pre-trained biomedical language representation model for biomedical text mining. Bioinformatics **36**(4), 1234–1240 (2019)
13. Li, X., Lv, K., Yan, H., Lin, T., Zhu, W., Ni, Y., Xie, G., Wang, X., Qiu, X.: Unified demonstration retriever for in-context learning. In: Proceedings of the 61st Annual Meeting of the Association for Computational Linguistics (Volume 1: Long Papers), pp. 4644–4668 (2023)
14. Lv, J., Xu, Y., Jiang, M., Lv, Y., Sun, J., Lu, J., Wang, L., Wang, H.: A deepseek-powered locally deployed closed-loop system for enhancing quality control in electronic nursing documentation: development and clinical validation. J. Amer. Med. Inf. Assoc. **32**(10), 1526–1532 (2025)

15. Perkins, S.W., Muste, J.C., Alam, T., Singh, R.P.: Improving clinical documentation with artificial intelligence: a systematic review. Perspect. Health Inf. Manag. **21**(2), 1d (2024)
16. Singhal, K., Tu, T., Gottweis, J., Sayres, R., Wulczyn, E., Hou, L., Clark, K., Pfohl, S., Cole-Lewis, H., Neal, D., Schaekermann, M., Wang, A., Amin, M., Lachgar, S., Mansfield, P., Prakash, S., Green, B., Dominowska, E., Aguera y Arcas, B., Tomasev, N., Liu, Y., Wong, R., Semturs, C., Mahdavi, S.S., Barral, J., Webster, D., Corrado, G.S., Matias, Y., Azizi, S., Karthikesalingam, A., Natarajan, V.: Towards Expert-Level Medical Question Answering with Large Language Models (2023). arXiv:2305.09617
17. Stubbs, A., Kotfila, C., Uzuner, Ö.: Automated systems for the de-identification of longitudinal clinical narratives: overview of 2014 i2b2/uthealth shared task track 1. J. Biomed. Inform. **58**, S11–S19 (2015)
18. Tamang, S., Patel, M.I., Blayney, D.W., Kuznetsov, J., Finlayson, S.G., Vetteth, Y., Shah, N.: Detecting unplanned care from clinician notes in electronic health records. J. Oncol. Pract. **11**(3), e313–e319 (2015)
19. Tang, L., Sun, Z., Idnay, B., Nestor, J.G., Soroush, A., Elias, P.A., Xu, Z., Ding, Y., Durrett, G., Rousseau, J.F., et al.: Evaluating large language models on medical evidence summarization. NPJ Dig. Med. **6**(1), 158 (2023)
20. Wang, Z., Talburt, J.R., Wu, N., Dagtas, S., Zozus, M.N.: A rule-based data quality assessment system for electronic health record data. Appl. Clin. Inform. **11**(04), 622–634 (2020)
21. Yang, R., Tan, T.F., Lu, W., Thirunavukarasu, A.J., Ting, D.S.W., Liu, N.: Large language models in health care: development, applications, and challenges. Health Care Sci. **2**(4), 255–263 (2023)
22. Ye, Q., Yu, G., Liu, J., Chen, E., Dong, C., Lin, X., Liu, Z., Yu, H., Ruan, T.: Imqc: a large language model platform for medical quality control. In: Proceedings of the AAAI Conference on Artificial Intelligence, vol. 39, pp. 28810–28818 (2025)
23. Yu, G., Li, Y., Jiang, Z., Jin, Y., Dai, L., Lin, Y., Hou, R., Zhang, W., Fan, Y., Ye, Q., Liu, J., Ruan, T.: CMQCIC-bench: a Chinese benchmark for evaluating large language models in medical quality control indicator calculation. In: Findings of the Association for Computational Linguistics: ACL 2025, pp. 609–626 (2025)
24. Zhao, W.X., Zhou, K., Li, J., Tang, T., Wang, X., Hou, Y., Min, Y., Zhang, B., Zhang, J., Dong, Z., Du, Y., Yang, C., Chen, Y., Chen, Z., Jiang, J., Ren, R., Li, Y., Tang, X., Liu, Z., Liu, P., Nie, J.Y., Wen, J.R.: A Survey of Large Language Models (2023). arXiv:2303.18223

MedShard: Privacy-Preserving EMR QC with Rule Sharding and Multi-agent Collaboration

Sizhe Dang[1], Xin Lai[1](✉), Yifei Li[1], Penggang Chen[2], and Huqing Wang[2]

[1] School of Computer Science and Technology, Xi'an Jiaotong University, Xi'an, China
{darknight1118,Lyf331}@stu.xjtu.edu.cn, laixin@xjtu.edu.cn
[2] The Second Affiliated Hospital of Xi'an Jiaotong University (Xibei Hospital), Xi'an, China
{mickchen,huqingwang}@mail.xjtu.edu.cn

Abstract. Electronic medical records (EMRs) are widely digitized, yet their utility depends on data quality that is complete, correct, and temporally and semantically consistent. Relying on closed large models for automated quality control (QC) is costly and raises privacy concerns because clinical text contains protected information. Local small models are attractive but they have weaker long-context handling, more limited reasoning, and narrower knowledge coverage. We present *MedShard*, a training-free, privacy-preserving pipeline that configures locally deployable LLMs to perform EMR QC effectively. The method reduces context length through rule-aware sharding, simplifies complex rule logic with explicit templates, and injects lightweight domain knowledge using curated few-shot exemplars, all without updating model weights. The system coordinates four agents–Cleaning, QC, Reflection, and Output–to deliver high recall with precise final decisions and structured rationales. *MedShard* runs on a single on-premises A100 GPU with a vLLM backend. On the CHIP 2025 benchmark, it achieves rank 1 with an overall score of 70.23, while reducing text token usage and rule token cost by *89.18%* and *90.96%* compared with naive long-context prompting. Ablation studies indicate additive gains from rule sharding, regex gating, and reflection. We release prompts, rule schemas, and deployment scripts to support reproducibility and regional adaptation.

Keywords: EMRs · Multi-agent · Rule sharding

1 Introduction

Health systems worldwide are transitioning from paper to electronic medical records (EMRs) to enhance care quality, reduce errors and costs, and enable secondary uses. Evidence from comprehensive reviews indicates that these benefits become more pronounced when the quality of electronic records is higher

Y. Zhang et al. (Eds.): CHIP 2025, CCIS 2884, pp. 395–409, 2026.
https://doi.org/10.1007/978-981-95-7299-1_23

[4,10]. Accordingly, rigorous quality control (QC) of EMRs is essential to ensure that records are complete, correct, and temporally and semantically consistent for both clinical care and secondary use [3,24].

Traditionally, hospitals rely on trained clinicians to perform chart review and record quality auditing. However, when the volume of EMRs across an institution becomes very large, the workload requires substantial time and personnel resources [13,27]. Recent advances in large language models, including stronger handling of long clinical narratives, have led to growing expectations to use LLMs for automating EMR quality control or assisting clinicians [7,9,28,30]. Closed commercial models with extended context windows price inference by tokens, so long inputs keep costs high (see Fig. 1 for the token and cost illustration). More importantly, EMRs contain protected health information, and sending records to external services introduces regulatory obligations and privacy risk. Therefore, many institutions prefer local, on-premises deployment of smaller LLMs for routine quality control [8,9,32].

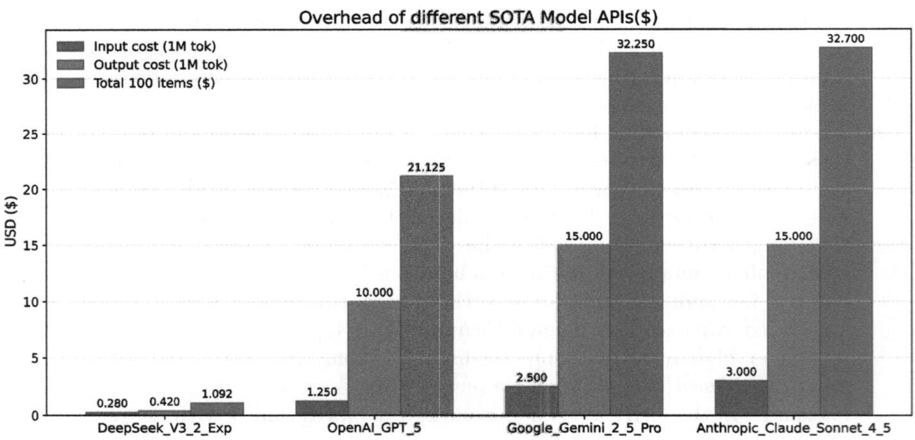

Fig. 1. The cost of inputting, outputting, and processing 100 QC samples using different SOTA models. Each QC sample has approximately 9k input tokens and approximately 20k output tokens (think content is included in the output tokens)

A natural implementation idea is to directly apply strategies designed for frontier closed models to smaller, locally deployable LLMs ($\leq$32B, deployable on a single A100), but in practice this often performs poorly. As Table 1 shows, because local models have far fewer parameters than SOTA systems, they typically exhibit weaker long-context handling, more limited reasoning ability, and narrower knowledge coverage. Therefore, local models require specialized optimization. Training-free, inference-side methods are often more practical than training-based approaches in resource-constrained hospital settings (for example, training commonly needs an order of magnitude more GPU memory than inference [6,37]). This leads to a practical question: **How can small, locally deployable LLMs be optimized in a training-free manner to perform EMR QC with outputs that closely match those from SOTA models and human annotations?**

Table 1. Comparison of model scale, context length, and training data

Model	Context length (tokens)	Parameters	Training data (tokens)
OPT-350M	2,048	0.35B	~180B
Llama 3 8B	8,192	8B	15T+
Qwen3-32B	32,768	32.8B	≈36T
DeepSeek-V3 (MoE)	128K	671B	14.8T
GPT-5 Pro (closed)	400K	–	–

To address these challenges, we propose *MedShard*, a training-free multi-agent pipeline that aims to maximize the utility of local LLMs by shrinking context length, decomposing complex rule logic, and lightly injecting domain knowledge via curated exemplars. Rather than judging all nineteen QC rules over the full note, MedShard performs per-rule sharding and item-level adjudication, which simplifies control flow and reduces token usage. A Cleaning agent segments the note and, for each rule, extracts the most relevant portions to shorten the context. A QC agent then conducts a high-recall first pass using the simplified logic. A Reflection agent revisits flagged items, injecting lightweight domain knowledge via targeted few-shot exemplars to refine borderline cases and reduce false positives without parameter updates. Finally, an Output agent assembles standardized decisions and concise rationales with explicit evidence spans to support interpretability. The pipeline is readily deployable on a single on-premises A100 GPU. Our contributions are summarized as follows:

- **Pipeline.** We introduce *MedShard*, a training-free, privacy-preserving EMR QC pipeline that handles each of the 19 rules as an independent decision path, thereby reducing token usage (Fig. 2).
- **Agents.** We design four agents that combines local LLMs and lightweight regular expressions: *Cleaning*, *QC*, *Reflection*, and *Output*. These agents shortens context through targeted extraction, simplifies complex rule logic with explicit templates, and compensates for knowledge gaps by injecting compact few-shot exemplars, while keeping the model weights fixed and supporting interpretability.
- **Reproducibility and results.** We provide complete prompts, evaluation scripts, and a vLLM-based local deployment that runs on a single A100 GPU. On the CHIP 2025 benchmark, our method achieves rank 1 with an overall score of 70.23.

Section 2 reviews related work on long-context modeling, multi-agent LLMs and EMR data quality. Section 3 details MedShard's formalization and agents. Section 4 presents experiments, ablations, and cost analyses. Section 5 summarizes the advantages and limitations of the method, as well as future prospects.

2 Related Work

2.1 Long-Context Large Language Models

Large Language Models have rapidly expanded their context window lengths in recent years, yet effectively utilizing very long inputs remains challenging. For instance, even models capable of 8K+ tokens often struggle to retain or utilize information in the middle portions of long documents [1,36]. Studies have found that model performance tends to degrade when crucial content is neither at the beginning nor end of the context, a phenomenon dubbed "lost in the middle" [20]. In particular, Liu et al. (2024) showed that current LLMs do not robustly use information from the middle of lengthy inputs, performing best when relevant text is at the start or end of the prompt [20]. Simply increasing the context window (e.g., from 4K tokens to 16K or more) also incurs significant computational cost for example, GPT-4 with a 32K window is roughly twice as expensive as its 8K version [34]; alternative strategies such as positional interpolation expand usable context with minimal changes [5]. This motivates research into more efficient long-text handling strategies. One approach is **retrieval augmentation**, where the model only attends to snippets retrieved as relevant, instead of the entire long document. Xu et al. (2024) demonstrate that a 4K-context model augmented with a retriever can match the performance of a 16K-context model on long-document tasks while using much less computation [34]; more broadly, RAG-style methods and large-scale retrieval (e.g., RETRO) support long-text reasoning without quadratic attention costs [2,17]. Another line of work focuses on architecture modifications for efficient long-text processing. Transformer variants like Longformer and BigBird introduced sparse or local attention to reduce quadratic complexity, enabling handling of documents thousands of tokens long [1,36]. However, implementing or fine-tuning these solutions can be resource-intensive. In practice, an attractive alternative–especially for resource-constrained settings–is to **split** or preprocess long inputs into smaller, relevant chunks that a standard LLM can manage, possibly using domain knowledge or rules to guide this segmentation [17]. Our work adopts this pragmatic strategy of breaking a lengthy medical record into focused sections, aided by preprocessing heuristics, instead of relying on a single monolithic long-context model.

2.2 LLM-Based Multi-Agent Systems

Rather than using a single large model to perform a complex task, an emerging paradigm is to employ multiple LLM-driven agents that collaborate or specialize. Multi-agent frameworks leverage the idea that different agents can handle subtasks or roles and then communicate to achieve an overall goal, akin to a team of specialists. This approach has shown promise in complex problem-solving and simulations [14,29,35]. For example, the CAMEL framework (Li et al., 2023) uses two cooperative agents in a role-playing setup (e.g., a "user" agent and an "assistant" agent) to autonomously drive a conversation and solve tasks without human intervention [18]. By guiding each agent with specific role prompts, CAMEL demonstrated improved capability in generating solutions through agent-agent dialogues. Similarly, MetaGPT (Hong et al., 2023) organizes multiple LLM agents to mimic a software engineering team (with roles like project manager, developer, etc.), which communicate via a shared message board to plan and implement software projects [11]. This structured coordination yields more coherent and thorough outputs than a single agent working alone. Another notable system is AutoGen (Wu et al., 2023), an open-source framework that enables developers to create multi-agent conversations where agents can be LLMs, tools, or humans. AutoGen allows flexible agent behaviors and has been applied to domains like math problem solving, coding, and decision-making [33]. These works illustrate that multi-agent collaboration can overcome some limitations of individual models by dividing labor and allowing iterative refinement through agent interactions. In addition to multi-agent collaboration, researchers have explored an agent's ability to self-reflect and refine its outputs. For instance, Shinn et al. (2023) propose **Reflexion**, where a single LLM agent uses feedback to verbally reflect on its mistakes and stores these reflections in memory to improve subsequent attempts [31]; related self-refinement loops have also been shown effective [23]. Overall, the use of multiple LLM agents whether in parallel or through internal self-dialogue is a powerful strategy to boost reasoning, planning, and accuracy. Our proposed method is inspired by this paradigm: we design a pipeline of collaborative agents (for cleaning, preliminary checking, reflecting, and final decision), each focusing on a specific stage of the quality control task. This modular design aims to maximize the strengths of a smaller local model via specialization and iterative improvement, much like multi-agent frameworks reported in the literature.

2.3 Automated Clinical Text Quality Control and Lightweight Models

Applying NLP to electronic medical records (EMRs) has long been seen as a way to improve documentation quality and patient safety. Prior studies have used rule-based or machine learning methods to automatically detect errors, inconsistencies, or omissions in clinical notes. For example, Li et al. (2014) developed algorithms to flag adverse events and medical errors in neonatal intensive care unit notes using structured rules and text processing [19]. As clinical free-text data grew, researchers also built specialized language models for the medical domain to achieve better accuracy on healthcare tasks without resorting to extremely large generic models. A prominent example is BioBERT, a BERT model pre-trained on biomedical corpora to improve biomedical text mining performance [16]; generative and task-adaptive variants such as BioGPT and ClinicalT5 further improve biomedical and clinical text generation and understanding [21,22]. In the era of generative LLMs, there is increasing interest in using these models for clinical text quality control for instance, to have an LLM review a patient note and identify missing or non-compliant entries. However, deploying API-based large models (e.g., GPT-4 or other proprietary LLMs) in healthcare settings raises serious **privacy and security** concerns, as patient records often contain sensitive personal health information. Regulatory guidelines such as HIPAA and GDPR limit how such data can be transmitted or processed externally. Recent commentary has stressed the importance of privacy-preserving strategies when using LLMs on EHR data, including the use of locally deployed models that keep data on-premises [15]. Running LLMs locally mitigates the risk of data leakage but introduces another challenge: computational resource limits typically force the use of much smaller models (e.g., 7B–13B parameters) in place of 100B+ parameter state-of-the-art models. These smaller local models often suffer in reasoning ability, knowledge breadth, and especially context length. To address this, researchers have looked at preprocessing and knowledge injection techniques to boost small models on medical tasks, as well as **parameter-efficient adaptation** and compression (e.g., DistilBERT and LoRA) [12,26]. Qu et al. (2024) recently proposed a compact local LLM approach for clinical note analysis that incorporates a preprocessing step using **regular expressions** and keyword filters to highlight critical information before feeding text into a 7B model [25]. Our work is aligned with this direction of optimizing smaller models for medical applications. We focus on **automated quality control of EMR text** under high privacy constraints, meaning our solution cannot rely on a large cloud-based model and must instead make the most of a moderate-sized local LLM. We draw on ideas from prior art: we use rule-guided preprocessing (similar to Qu et al.) to segment the medical record into the minimal units needed for each check, and we employ multiple passes or "agents" to mimic a more powerful model's reasoning first casting a wide net to catch potential issues (high recall), then iteratively refining and explaining the results. This approach bridges gaps identified in related work: it addresses the context length issue by decomposition, and compensates for the smaller model's limited inference capacity through structured, step-by-step agent collaboration [12,21,22,26]. In summary, our method brings together trends in long-text LLM processing, multi-agent collaboration, and privacy-preserving clinical NLP to enable efficient automatic quality control on medical records with a lean local model.

3 Method

3.1 Problem Definition

Let $\mathcal{P}_t$ denote the space of long-form EMR narratives (free text) and let $\mathcal{P}_r$ be the set of QC rules, $\mathcal{R} = r_1, \ldots, r_{19} \subseteq \mathcal{P}_r$. For a given record $x \in \mathcal{P}_t$, each rule $r \in \mathcal{R}$ is associated with a ground-truth judgment $y_r^\star \in$ OK, NOK, a textual rationale $D_r^\star$. We deploy a fixed, locally hosted LLM f_θ (weights frozen) and a *training-free* workflow W that orchestrates f_θ across modules (cleaning, QC, reflection, output). For each rule r, the workflow returns

$$\Phi_r(x) = \big(W(x; f_\theta)\big)_r = \big(\hat{y}_r, \hat{D}_r\big),$$

where $\hat{y}_r$ is the predicted judgment and $\hat{D}_r$ is the rationale.

Rule-conditioned microcontext (inside the workflow). Within W, the cleaning module performs *rule-conditioned extraction* to produce a compact context $c_r = \text{Clean}_W(x, r) \subseteq x$ that contains text most relevant to r. No protected health information is transmitted externally; all computation remains on premises. This selector must also satisfy a per-rule token budget:

$$\text{tokens}(c_r) \leq B, \qquad \forall r \in \mathcal{R}.$$

Objective. Given references $\mathcal{Y}^\star = (y_r^\star, D_r^\star), \quad r \in \mathcal{R}$, we seek a training-free workflow W that, using the fixed f_θ, minimizes task loss under resource and privacy constraints:

$$\min_{W \in \mathcal{W}_{\text{tf}}} \sum_{r \in \mathcal{R}} \left[\mathcal{L}_{\text{cls}}(\hat{y}_r, y_r^\star) + \alpha \mathcal{L}_{\text{expl}}(\hat{D}_r, D_r^\star) \right] \tag{1}$$

Here $\mathcal{L}_{\text{cls}}$ measures decision accuracy (e.g., F1), $\mathcal{L}_{\text{expl}}$ measures explanation adequacy (e.g., ROUGE-L). The feasible set $\mathcal{W}_{\text{tf}}$ consists of *training-free* workflows that differ only in prompts, rule templates, regex gates, and module wiring–not in model parameters.

Goal. Under this formulation, finding $(\mathcal{P}_{tk}, \mathcal{P}_{rk}) \subseteq (\mathcal{P}_t, \mathcal{P}_r)$ is *implicitly* realized by the internal cleaner $\text{Clean}_W(\cdot)$ that produces c_r for each rule r. The remaining modules use c_r to generate $\Phi_r(x)$ so as to minimize (1), thereby aligning predictions and rationales with references while respecting privacy and token budgets.

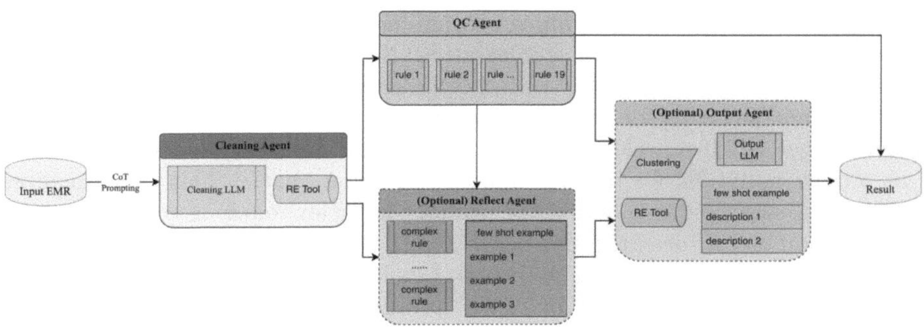

Fig. 2. MedShard workflow overview

3.2 Workflow Overview

Given an EMR note x and the rule set $\mathcal{R} = r_1, \ldots, r_{19}$, the pipeline produces, for each rule r, a decision $\hat{y}_r \in \text{OK}, \text{NOK}$ and a short rationale $\hat{D}_r$. The workflow follows a splitrecallreflectexplain pattern (Fig. 2).

Rule-aware sharding and packing. The system creates a compact, rule-conditioned context c_r by extracting passages in x that are most relevant to r. Lightweight regex gates and section cues act as a token budgeter and router. When multiple snippets match, a packer ranks and concatenates them until a per-rule budget B_r is met.

High-recall first pass. For each r, the QC template queries the local LLM over c_r to propose a provisional label $\tilde{y}_r$ and candidate rationale $\tilde{D}_r$. Prompts are conservative and favor recall to avoid early false negatives.

Targeted reflection. Items flagged as NOK are re-examined by a reflection routine that injects compact, curated exemplars and performs targeted self-checks. The goal is to resolve borderline cases and reduce false positives without parameter updates.

Standardized reporting. Final decisions $(\hat{y}_r, \hat{D}_r)$ are rendered into a normalized schema. Conflicts are resolved with simple policies (e.g., rule precedence), and all intermediate artifacts are logged for audit and error analysis.

The entire pipeline is training-free. It operates with frozen model weights, modifies only prompts and rule templates, and runs locally with vLLM batching and caching. Privacy is preserved by keeping all computation on premises and by restricting contexts to the minimum needed for each rule.

3.3 Four Agents

We implement the workflow with four lightweight agents. Each agent exposes clear inputs, outputs and prompts so that the pipeline can be composed, debugged, and extended.

Cleaning agent (rule-conditioned extraction). Input: EMR note x and rule r. *Output:* Compact context $c_r \subseteq x$. *Operation:* Normalize sections, align common fields, split sentences, and apply rule-specific cues and regex filters to collect the most relevant passages for r. Rank candidates and pack them under a per-rule token budget B_r. If no relevant text is found, emit an empty context and mark r as provisionally OK for downstream confirmation. *Notes:* This agent realizes the internal selection step and is the primary lever for reducing context length.

QC agent (recall-oriented first pass). Input: (c_r, r). *Output:* Provisional label $\tilde{y}_r$ and candidate rationale $\tilde{D}_r$. *Operation:* Invoke a per-rule prompt that encodes a simplified decision template for r. The prompt requests an explicit label and minimal evidence text. When confidence is low and context is not empty, the agent defers to reflection. *Policy:* Bias toward recall to minimize false negatives in the first stage.

Reflection agent (precision-focused refinement). Input: $(\tilde{y}_r, \tilde{D}_r, c_r, r)$. *Output:* Refined $(\hat{y}_r, \tilde{D}_r)$. *Operation:* This agent is invoked *only if* $\tilde{y}_r = \text{NOK}$. It issues a brief confirmation query over c_r to obtain a secondary decision $\bar{y}_r \in \text{OK}, \text{NOK}$. The final output is

$$(\hat{y}_r, \hat{D}_r) = \begin{cases} (\text{NOK}, \tilde{D}_r), & \text{if } \tilde{y}_r = \text{NOK}; \\ (\text{OK}, \epsilon), & \text{if } \tilde{y}_r = \text{OK}, \end{cases}$$

where ϵ denotes an empty rationale. If $\tilde{y}_r = \text{OK}$, this agent is skipped.

Output agent (standardization). Input: $(\hat{y}_r, \tilde{D}_r), r \in \mathcal{R}$. *Output:* $(\hat{y}_r, \hat{D}_r)$, $r \in \mathcal{R}$ and a compact case-level summary. *Operation:* Process each pair $(\hat{y}_r, \tilde{D}_r)$ independently. For $\hat{y}_r = \text{OK}$, emit (OK, ϵ), where ϵ denotes an empty rationale. For $\hat{y}_r = \text{NOK}$, rewrite $\tilde{D}_r$ using a rule-specific output template populated by pre-collected style exemplars (controlled vocabulary, phrasing patterns, and length limits), yielding $\hat{D}_r$ that matches annotator style as closely as possible (e.g., ≤ 100 characters, concise evidence cue, normalized terminology).

Implementation notes. All agents are training-free. They differ only in prompt templates, routing rules, and light regex filters. The system uses vLLM for batched inference and caching, applies a per-rule token budget B_r, and never transmits protected content outside the local environment.

4 Experiments

4.1 Experimental Setup

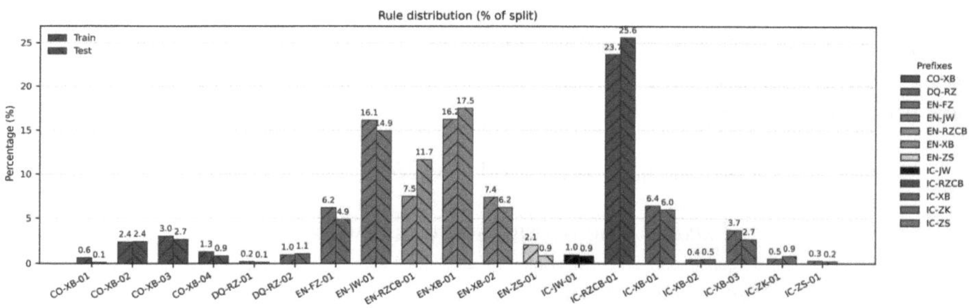

Fig. 3. Rule distribution on Train(924 total) and Test(823 total)

Task. We evaluate MedShard on the CHIP 2025 EMR QC benchmark, which targets *intrinsic* quality control for admission notes. The input is a single EMR document of type ADM_NOTE containing common sections (e.g., *chief_complaint*, *history_present*, *history_past*, *special_exam*, *lab_exam*, *admission_diagnosis*, *initial_diagnosis*). The system must output a set of QC findings for that record.

Dataset. The dataset is divided into a training set and a test set. The training set contains 1000 data points, of which 300 are labeled. The test set contains 300 data points.

Output schema. Each finding is an object with four required fields:

- **field** (String): the violated section;
- **issue_type** (String): one of `INFO_COMPLETENESS`, `CONSISTENCY`, `DIAGNOSIS_QUALITY`, `EXAM_RECORD_NORM`;

- **rule_id** (String): the rule identifier;
- **description** (String, $\leq$ 100 Chinese characters): concise rationale with evidence.

Tracks and resource constraints. Two tracks share the same test sets and metrics but differ in allowed methods. **Track-A (no fine-tuning)** forbids parameter updates; in-context learning and retrieval augmentation are allowed (external KBs must be declared). **Track-B (fine-tuning)** permits fine-tuning on the official data and RAG. Both tracks cap model size at $\leq$ 70B parameters.

Metrics. Evaluation comprises two dimensions: (i) *problem extraction* at the finding level and (ii) *case-level compliance.*
(1) Problem extraction. A predicted finding counts as true positive (TP) only if (`field`, `issue_type`, `rule_id`) exactly matches the reference. Otherwise it is a false positive (FP); missed references are false negatives (FN). Let $P, R, F1$ be precision, recall, and F1 at the finding level, and let ROUGE $-$ L be computed over `description`. The composite score is:

$$\text{Score}_{\text{extract}} = 0.4 \cdot F1 + 0.25 \cdot P + 0.15 \cdot R + 0.2 \cdot \text{ROUGE} - L.$$

(2) Case-level compliance. A case starts at 100 points; only exact-match findings (as above) are eligible for predefined rule-based deductions. After deductions, a score < 95 marks the case *non-compliant.* Using the resulting case labels, we compute $P, R, F1$ and report:

$$\text{Score}_{\text{compliant}} = 0.5 \cdot F1 + 0.25 \cdot P + 0.25 \cdot R.$$

(3) Final leaderboard score. The overall score is a weighted sum:

$$\text{Final} = 0.7 \cdot \text{Score}_{\text{extract}} + 0.3 \cdot \text{Score}_{\text{compliant}}.$$

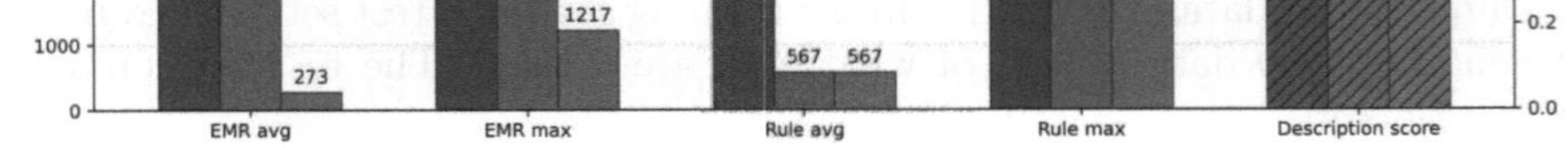

Fig. 4. Tokens saving and description score

4.2 Main Results

Rule distribution and token savings. Figure 3 summarizes per-rule frequencies on Train and Test. Figure 4 reports token footprints for three configurations: *Naive Long-Context* (no sharding, no regex), *LLM-only (Rule-by-Rule)* (per-rule prompts without regex), and *MedShard (ours)*. MedShard consistently reduces average tokens per decision on both Train and Test, with the largest relative savings on cross-section consistency rules.

Table 2. Results of the top five methods

Method	Final	extract	E-F1	E-P	E-R	Expl	Compl	C-F1	C-P	C-R
Ours	0.702	0.713	0.775	0.723	0.835	0.483	0.679	0.673	0.597	0.772
Method 2	0.670	0.673	0.727	0.670	0.795	0.475	0.665	0.650	0.535	0.826
Method 3	0.669	0.665	0.704	0.701	0.707	0.512	0.677	0.677	0.670	0.685
Method 4	0.664	0.656	0.712	0.625	0.826	0.454	0.685	0.670	0.553	0.848
Method 5	0.648	0.642	0.706	0.649	0.774	0.405	0.664	0.655	0.563	0.783

Overall performance. Table 2 presents the primary metrics on the Test set. MedShard attains the highest *Final* score while maintaining strong problem-extraction quality and case-level compliance, together with markedly fewer tokens and lower latency. The LLM we used throughout the process was Qwen3-32B, which had only half the required number of parameters(70B) and did not use any external knowledge bases of the RAG class.

Table 3. Ablation on MedShard components (IC-XB-01)

Method	P	R	F1	ROUGE-L
Full (MedShard)	0.389	0.746	0.512	0.499
– Cleaning agent	0.305	0.864	0.451	0.419
– QC agent	0.323	0.169	0.222	0.405
– Reflect agent	0.311	0.932	0.466	0.481
– Output agent	0.389	0.746	0.512	0.284

4.3 Ablation Studies

Agent-level ablation (Train). We remove one component at a time from MedShard while keeping others unchanged. Table 3 shows that removing *Cleaning* (no sharding/packing) increases tokens and hurts recall, especially for dispersed-evidence rules; disabling *QC* leds to a significant decrease in recalls;removing *Reflection* raises false positives; and skipping *Output* standardization yields unstable rationale length and span alignment.

Engineering ablation (test). To isolate the effect of lightweight regex routing, we compare *LLM-only (Rule-by-Rule)* against *LLM+Regex (Rule-by-Rule)* under identical prompts and budgets. Figure 4 shows consistent token and latency reductions with small but steady gains in accuracy.

Takeaways. Sharding and packing mitigate long-context dilution while reducing token usage; reflection improves precision on borderline cases without weight updates; and regex routing offers tangible efficiency gains with minor accuracy benefits.

5 Conclusion

We introduced *MedShard*, a rule-sharded, multi-agent pipeline that shortens context, simplifies decision logic, and compensates for knowledge gaps with compact exemplars. Experiments on CHIP 2025 show rank 1 performance with an overall score of 70.23, just using 32B Qwen model.
Limitations. The approach relies on hand-crafted rule schemas and regex gates, so portability across institutions may require retuning extraction patterns and prompts. Domain drift and heterogeneous documentation styles can affect recall, and curated few-shot exemplars introduce maintenance overhead. The evaluation metrics are sensitive to annotator habits, and using ROUGE-L for descriptive rationales can be overly mechanical, penalizing valid paraphrases.
Future work. We will explore combining the training-free inference pipeline with lightweight, reasoning-oriented fine-tuning when feasible, and develop a more objective QC benchmark with multi-rater consensus and semantic grading metrics.

Acknowledgments. This work is supported by grants from the National Natural Science Foundation of China (NSFC), grant numbers [72274152, 62402376, 62572389].

References

1. Beltagy, I., Peters, M.E., Cohan, A.: Longformer: The long-document transformer. arXiv preprint arXiv:2004.05150 (2020)
2. Borgeaud, S., Mensch, A., Hoffmann, J., Cai, T., Rutherford, E., Millican, K., Van Den Driessche, G.B., Lespiau, J.B., Damoc, B., Clark, A., et al.: Improving language models by retrieving from trillions of tokens. In: International Conference on Machine Learning, pp. 2206–2240. PMLR (2022)
3. Campanella, P., Lovato, E., Marone, C., Fallacara, L., Mancuso, A., Ricciardi, W., Specchia, M.L.: The impact of electronic health records on healthcare quality: a systematic review and meta-analysis. Eur. J. Public Health **26**(1), 60–64 (2016)

4. Chaudhry, B., Wang, J., Wu, S., Maglione, M., Mojica, W., Roth, E., Morton, S.C., Shekelle, P.G.: Systematic review: impact of health information technology on quality, efficiency, and costs of medical care. Ann. Intern. Med. **144**(10), 742–752 (2006)
5. Chen, S., Wong, S., Chen, L., Tian, Y.: Extending context window of large language models via positional interpolation (2023). arXiv:2306.15595
6. Dang, S., Guo, Y., Zhao, Y., Ye, H., Zheng, X., Dai, G., Tsang, I.: Fzoo: Fast zeroth-order optimizer for fine-tuning large language models towards adam-scale speed (2025). arXiv:2506.09034
7. Ge, J., Li, M., Delk, M.B., Lai, J.C.: A comparison of a large language model vs manual chart review for the extraction of data elements from the electronic health record. Gastroenterology **166**(4), 707–709 (2024)
8. Griot, M., Vanderdonckt, J., Yuksel, D.: Implementation of large language models in electronic health records (2025)
9. Heilmeyer, F., Böhringer, D., Reinhard, T., Arens, S., Lyssenko, L., Haverkamp, C.: Viability of open large language models for clinical documentation in german health care: real-world model evaluation study. JMIR Med. Inform. **12**, e59617 (2024)
10. Holly, L., Smith, R.D., Ndili, N., Franz, C., Stevens, E.A.G.: A review of digital health strategies in 10 countries with young populations: do they serve the health and wellbeing of children and youth in a digital age? Front. Digital Health **4**, 817810 (2022)
11. Hong, S., Zhuge, M., Chen, J., Zheng, X., Cheng, Y., Wang, J., Zhang, C., Wang, Z., Yau, S.K.S., Lin, Z., et al.: Metagpt: Meta programming for a multi-agent collaborative framework. In: The Twelfth International Conference on Learning Representations (2023)
12. Hu, E.J., Shen, Y., Wallis, P., Allen-Zhu, Z., Li, Y., Wang, S., Wang, L., Chen, W., et al.: Lora: Low-rank adaptation of large language models. ICLR **1**(2), 3 (2022)
13. Hu, Z., Melton, G.B., Moeller, N.D., Arsoniadis, E.G., Wang, Y., Kwaan, M.R., Jensen, E.H., Simon, G.J.: Accelerating chart review using automated methods on electronic health record data for postoperative complications. In: AMIA Annual Symposium Proceedings, vol. 2016, p. 1822 (2017)
14. Irving, G., Christiano, P., Amodei, D.: Ai safety via debate (2018). arXiv preprint arXiv:1805.00899
15. Jonnagaddala, J., Wong, Z.S.Y.: Privacy preserving strategies for electronic health records in the era of large language models. npj Digital Med. **8**(1), 34 (2025)
16. Lee, J., Yoon, W., Kim, S., Kim, D., Kim, S., So, C.H., Kang, J.: Biobert: a pre-trained biomedical language representation model for biomedical text mining. Bioinformatics **36**(4), 1234–1240 (2020)
17. Retrieval-augmented generation for knowledge-intensive nlp tasks: Lewis, P., Perez, E., Piktus, A., Petroni, F., Karpukhin, V., Goyal, N., Küttler, H., Lewis, M., Yih, W.t., Rocktäschel, T., et al. Adv. Neural. Inf. Process. Syst. **33**, 9459–9474 (2020)
18. Li, G., Hammoud, H., Itani, H., Khizbullin, D., Ghanem, B.: Camel: Communicative agents for" mind" exploration of large language model society. Adv. Neural. Inf. Process. Syst. **36**, 51991–52008 (2023)
19. Li, Q., Melton, K., Lingren, T., Kirkendall, E.S., Hall, E., Zhai, H., Ni, Y., Kaiser, M., Stoutenborough, L., Solti, I.: Phenotyping for patient safety: algorithm development for electronic health record based automated adverse event and medical error detection in neonatal intensive care. J. Am. Med. Inform. Assoc. **21**(5), 776–784 (2014)

20. Liu, N.F., Lin, K., Hewitt, J., Paranjape, A., Bevilacqua, M., Petroni, F., Liang, P.: Lost in the middle: How language models use long contexts. Trans. Assoc. Comput. Linguist. **12**, 157–173 (2024)
21. Lu, Q., Dou, D., Nguyen, T.: Clinicalt5: A generative language model for clinical text. In: Findings of the Association for Computational Linguistics: EMNLP 2022. pp. 5436–5443 (2022)
22. Luo, R., Sun, L., Xia, Y., Qin, T., Zhang, S., Poon, H., Liu, T.Y.: Biogpt: generative pre-trained transformer for biomedical text generation and mining. Brief. Bioinf. **23**(6), bbac409 (2022)
23. Madaan, A., Tandon, N., Gupta, P., Hallinan, S., Gao, L., Wiegreffe, S., Alon, U., Dziri, N., Prabhumoye, S., Yang, Y., et al.: Self-refine: Iterative refinement with self-feedback. Adv. Neural. Inf. Process. Syst. **36**, 46534–46594 (2023)
24. Middel, B.: The impact of electronic health records on time efficiency of physicians and nurses: a systematic review1. Nederlands Tijdschrift voor Evidence Based Practice **6**(1), 14–16 (2008)
25. Qu, Y., Dai, Y., Yu, S., Tanikella, P., Schrank, T., Hackman, T., Li, D., Wu, D.: A novel compact llm framework for local, high-privacy ehr data applications (2024). arXiv:2412.02868
26. Sanh, V., Debut, L., Chaumond, J., Wolf, T.: Distilbert, a distilled version of bert: smaller, faster, cheaper and lighter (2019). arXiv:1910.01108
27. Sarkar, S., Seshadri, D.: Conducting record review studies in clinical practice. J. Clin. Diagnost. Res.: JCDR **8**(9), JG01 (2014)
28. Schaye, V., DiTullio, D., Guzman, B.V., Vennemeyer, S., Shih, H., Reinstein, I., Weber, D.E., Goodman, A., Wu, D.T., Sartori, D.J., et al.: Large language model-based assessment of clinical reasoning documentation in the electronic health record across two institutions: Development and validation study. J. Med. Internet Res. **27**, e67967 (2025)
29. Schick, T., Dwivedi-Yu, J., Dessì, R., Raileanu, R., Lomeli, M., Hambro, E., Zettlemoyer, L., Cancedda, N., Scialom, T.: Toolformer: Language models can teach themselves to use tools. Adv. Neural. Inf. Process. Syst. **36**, 68539–68551 (2023)
30. Schuemie, M.J., Ostropolets, A., Zhuk, A., Korsik, U., Seo, S.I., Suchard, M.A., Hripcsak, G., Ryan, P.B.: Standardized patient profile review using large language models for case adjudication in observational research. npj Digital Med. **8**(1), 18 (2025)
31. Shinn, N., Cassano, F., Gopinath, A., Narasimhan, K., Yao, S.: Reflexion: Language agents with verbal reinforcement learning. Adv. Neural. Inf. Process. Syst. **36**, 8634–8652 (2023)
32. Vaid, A., Landi, I., Nadkarni, G., Nabeel, I.: Using fine-tuned large language models to parse clinical notes in musculoskeletal pain disorders. The Lancet Digital Health **5**(12), e855–e858 (2023)
33. Wu, Q., Bansal, G., Zhang, J., Wu, Y., Li, B., Zhu, E., Jiang, L., Zhang, X., Zhang, S., Liu, J., et al.: Autogen: Enabling next-gen llm applications via multi-agent conversations. In: First Conference on Language Modeling (2024)
34. Xu, P., Ping, W., Wu, X., McAfee, L., Zhu, C., Liu, Z., Subramanian, S., Bakhturina, E., Shoeybi, M., Catanzaro, B.: Retrieval meets long context large language models (2023). arXiv:2310.03025
35. Yao, S., Zhao, J., Yu, D., Du, N., Shafran, I., Narasimhan, K.R., Cao, Y.: React: Synergizing reasoning and acting in language models. In: The Eleventh International Conference on Learning Representations (2022)

36. Zaheer, M., Guruganesh, G., Dubey, K.A., Ainslie, J., Alberti, C., Ontanon, S., Pham, P., Ravula, A., Wang, Q., Yang, L., et al.: Big bird: Transformers for longer sequences. Adv. Neural. Inf. Process. Syst. **33**, 17283–17297 (2020)
37. Zhao, Y., Dang, S., Ye, H., Dai, G., Qian, Y., Tsang, I.: Second-order fine-tuning without pain for llms: A hessian informed zeroth-order optimizer. In: The Thirteenth International Conference on Learning Representations

Dual Enhancement with In-Context Learning and Chain-of-Thought: Large Language Model-Driven Intelligent Connotation Quality Control of Medical Records

Xiduo Lu, Weihua Jing, Qiu Jin, Gang Hao, Wen Chao Deng, Yupeng Chen, Yi Li, Xin Wei(✉), and Dong Wang(✉)

Athena Eyes CO., LTD, Beijing, China
{luxiduo,jingweihua,jinqiu,haogang,dengwenchao,chenyupeng,liyi, weixin,wangdong}@email.com,
{luxiduo,jingweihua,jinqiu,haogang,dengwenchao,chenyupeng,liyi, weixin,wangdong}@a-eye.cn

Abstract. This study focuses on the "Connotative Quality Control of Admission Records in Medical Records by Large Language Models" task at the China Health Information Processing Conference (CHIP) 2025, under the non-fine-tuning track. The task involves predicting connotative quality control defects using 300 unannotated admission records each for validation and testing. We employ the Qwen3-30B-A3B-Thinking-2507 model without fine-tuning and propose a dual-enhancement framework integrating precision in-context learning and Chain-of-Thought (CoT) reasoning. The framework first applies semi-structured segmentation to extract rule-relevant content from medical records, reducing irrelevant information. It then introduces a stepwise judgment mechanism based on CoT to decompose abstract quality control logic into executable reasoning steps. Results are output in structured JSON format to ensure interpretability. Experimental results show that our method achieved 2nd place on the test set (final ranking) with a comprehensive score of 0.6644. This work demonstrates the feasibility of applying non-fine-tuned LLMs enhanced by precision in-context learning and CoT reasoning to medical record connotative quality control, offering a practical and referential approach for intelligent medical record quality assurance.

Keywords: Large Language Model · In-Context Learning · Chain-of-Thought Reasoning

1 Introduction

Medical records refer to the documents created by healthcare professionals during clinical activities, utilizing various formats such as text, symbols, charts, and images. They serve as a systematic compilation of critical medical information.

Y. Zhang et al. (Eds.): CHIP 2025, CCIS 2884, pp. 410–422, 2026.
https://doi.org/10.1007/978-981-95-7299-1_24

Implementing robust quality control (QC) in medical documentation is crucial, as it enhances patient safety, mitigates doctor-patient disputes, and elevates the overall standard of healthcare delivery. However, relying solely on manual efforts to perform quality control for hundreds or even thousands of QC rules across multiple types of medical documents is extremely labor-intensive and virtually impossible to accomplish comprehensively.

In recent years, Large Language Models (LLMs) have advanced rapidly. With their strong capabilities in natural language processing (NLP) and knowledge reasoning, they have shown transformative potential in the healthcare field [1–3]. Approximately 80%of healthcare data consists of unstructured data, such as electronic health records and imaging reports. LLMs can efficiently analyze such data, significantly reducing the documentation burden on healthcare professionals and supporting the allocation of medical resources toward core diagnostic and treatment activities. LLMs have demonstrated considerable advantages in areas such as clinical decision support [4,5] and drug research and development [6], among others.

The China Health Information Processing Conference (CHIP) 2025 has established a dedicated track for the task of "Connotative Quality Control of Medical Admission Records Using Large Language Models." This task centers on employing LLMs to perform connotative quality control on admission records and to construct a comprehensive evaluation framework, with a specific focus on information integrity, diagnostic standardization, and logical consistency. The project aims to assess the capabilities of LLMs in comprehending and reasoning with medical texts, thereby paving the way for their deeper integration into AI-assisted medical record quality control.

However, despite these promising prospects, key challenges remain when applying LLMs to the connotative QC of medical records:

(1) **High complexity of medical documents**: Patient information is scattered across numerous documents with non-standardized expressions, requiring cross-document resolution. This demands strong long-context understanding and semantic analysis from models.
(2) **Dependence on and limitations of medical knowledge**: LLMs face timeliness constraints and hallucination risks, potentially yielding non-compliant conclusions. While Retrieval-Augmented Generation (RAG) can alleviate these issues, its efficacy relies heavily on retrieval accuracy.
(3) **Difficulty in clinical reasoning and analysis**: Connotative QC rules often involve complex and abstract logic, making it highly challenging to translate these rules into precise, executable instructions for LLMs.
(4) **Isolation of hospital intranet environments and insufficient server resources**: These constraints significantly limit the scale of LLMs that can be deployed in clinical settings.

To address the aforementioned challenges, this study proposes a dedicated LLM-based solution for the connotative QC of medical records. Its core innovations lie in a systematic approach to overcoming application bottlenecks through a three-in-one strategy encompassing "precision In-context learning", "chain-of-thought reasoning enhancement", and "lightweight model deployment".

To address the complexity of medical documents, this study abandons the extensive input mode of feeding entire medical record documents into the model, and innovatively designs a mechanism for semi-structured medical record processing and precise in-context input. Specifically, the system pre-parses and integrates scattered multi-source documents, identifies and extracts paragraphs and fields strongly related to specific QC rules, and only inputs key evidence chain fragments into the LLMs (instead of the entire medical records). This approach significantly reduces irrelevant information and noise, lowers the model's cognitive load in long-text processing, and ensures the accuracy of semantic understanding and logical analysis.

To tackle the dual challenges of reliance on medical knowledge and complex reasoning, this study constructs a "rule-knowledge-reasoning" three-layer enhancement framework. On one hand, an executable judgment logic chain is developed for each connotative QC rule, decomposing abstract clinical rules into a series of specific subtask steps that the LLMs can execute. On the other hand, in chain-of-thought prompting, the LLMs is forced to sequentially present the retrieved evidence, the relied-on rule clauses, and the step-by-step reasoning process before outputting the final QC conclusion. This not only significantly mitigates the model's "hallucination" issue but also makes the decision-making process transparent and traceable, meeting the requirements for clinical interpretability.

In response to the limited resource situation of hospital intranets, this solution selects a model with 30B (30 billion) parameters for targeted optimization and deployment after evaluation. A model of this scale can meet the needs of complex task processing, while its computing and storage costs are much lower than those of 100-billion-parameter models. It enables private deployment on conventional hospital server clusters, which not only ensures the security requirement that medical data does not leave the hospital but also controls the costs of deployment and operation.

In summary, to address the multiple core challenges faced by LLMs in the scenario of connotative QC of medical records, this study proposes a systematic solution integrating "precision in-context learning" and "chain-of-thought reasoning enhancement". By implementing semi-structured processing on complex medical record texts, accurately extracting key information chains for input into the model, and simultaneously combining with the chain-of-thought prompting technology custom-designed for each QC rule, this solution ensures the traceability of the clinical decision-making process and the interpretability of QC conclusions. On this basis, it provides a practical technical pathway for the safe implementation and efficient application of LLMs in real-world medical environments, and also offers innovative practical references for solving key issues such as the complexity of medical documents, the reliability of model reasoning, and the adaptability to clinical scenarios.

2 Related Work

2.1 Quality Control of Medical Records by LLMs

In recent years, LLMs in medical documents have become a hotspot for smart healthcare research, and relevant practices have initially confirmed its technical feasibility and value.

Lv et al. [7] proposed a locally deployed, DeepSeek-driven closed-loop quality control system for electronic nursing records, employing a multi-dimensional QC strategy described as "real-time + final + vertical". Their results demonstrated that the LLMs integration reduced the defect rate in medical records from 710% to 02%, shortened QC time by 3.2 times, and significantly improved both the accuracy of documentation and process efficiency. Similarly, Liu et al. [8] developed an AI-powered medical record QC system capable of real-time record review, cutting the average review time per record from 4200 s to just 2 s. The proportion of Grade A records increased from 89.43%to 99.21%, indicating a notable reduction in recording errors and improved completeness and accuracy of medical content. Furthermore, several Chinese tertiary Grade A hospitals have adopted DeepSeek-based intelligent electronic medical record management systems [9,10], which facilitate real-time quality analysis and documentation support, further validating the practical feasibility and significant benefits of LLMs in this application scenario.

2.2 Precision In-Context Learning

In the field of NLP, particularly in LLM-based applications, precision in-context learning is a core element for enhancing task performance [11,12]. Existing research has primarily focused on context enhancement methods, which aim to construct precise contexts through optimized information retrieval and representation.

For longitudinal information processing in clinical settings, the TIMER [13] method employs time-aware instruction tuning, associating each instruction response pair with a specific timestamp. This enables the model to accurately match cross-temporal medical events during reasoning, effectively improving its ability to interpret patient timelines. The E-CARP framework [14], on the other hand, utilizes parameterized memory networks and dynamic relational reasoning mechanisms to dynamically activate keyword semantics from input text. It achieves precise in-context perception while maintaining classification accuracy and significantly improving reasoning efficiency. In long-text processing, the VisInContext approach [15] renders lengthy texts into images and processes them with visual encoders, thereby reducing the number of text tokens fed into the model. This helps the model focus on core content and demonstrates potential in document-based question-answering tasks. Conversely, when the context contains a large amount of irrelevant information–termed "imprecise context"–key information can be diluted. For example, in conventional long medical record processing, feeding the full text directly may cause information overload, making it difficult for the model to capture the evidence chains required by QC rules, ultimately compromising judgment accuracy. In high-stakes fields such as healthcare, precision in-context learning is also closely tied to model safety and interpretability. For instance, the CLIN-LLM framework [4] uses RAG to accurately retrieve evidence corresponding to a patient's condition from large-scale medical knowledge bases and supplies it as context to the model. This not only improves diagnostic and recommendation accuracy but also enhances the trustworthiness of outcomes by providing transparent decision bases.

2.3 Chain-of-Thought Reasoning

Traditional prompting methods, which require models to generate final answers directly, exhibit limitations in complex reasoning tasks. Without guidance through intermediate reasoning steps, models often miss the gradual thought process, leading to incorrect conclusions–particularly in multi-step analytical tasks involving arithmetic, commonsense, or logical reasoning. Chain-of-Thought (CoT) reasoning directly addresses these limitations by guiding models to generate sequential intermediate reasoning steps, simulating human-like progressive problem-solving. Its core advantages are as follows:

- **Interpretability and error diagnosis**: CoT externalizes the model's reasoning process, making it transparent. Researchers and users can pinpoint the exact stages where errors occur by examining intermediate steps, enabling targeted corrections and model improvement.
- **Overcoming architectural depth constraints**: The Transformer architecture has inherent limitations in supporting deep, continuous reasoning internally. CoT extends reasoning into the external textual space by explicitly generating intermediate steps as text, thereby breaking the "fixed-depth" computation barrier and enabling handling of more complex problems.
- **Flexible enhancement and extensibility**: Building on the basic chain structure, researchers have developed various enhancements. For example, the Self-Consistency method [16] samples multiple reasoning paths and uses majority voting to improve answer accuracy and robustness. Furthermore, CoT structures have evolved from linear chains to tree [17] and graph-based [18] forms, allowing the exploration of multiple reasoning paths and strengthening performance in complex planning tasks.

Notably, Zero-Shot CoT significantly lowers the application barrier: simply appending the prompt "Let's think step by step" [19] after a question can effectively trigger the model's reasoning capability, which produce reasonable reasoning chains without task-specific examples, and has been shown to yield significant performance gains across diverse reasoning benchmarks.

3 Dataset

The data used in this study originate from the dataset for the connotative QC task of medical admission records, released by the organizers of CHIP2025. The dataset includes a training set, a validation set, and a test set. Specifically, the training set contains 1,000 admission records, of which only 300 are annotated; both the validation and test sets contain 300 admission records each, all of which are unannotated. Each admission record represents an independent case and covers sections such as chief complaint, history of present illness, past medical history, specialist examinations, auxiliary examinations, admission diagnosis, and preliminary diagnosis. Sensitive patient information–including certain time points, result values, and textual content–has been artificially desensitized.

For the connotative QC task, the organizers have defined 19 rules. Each rule specifies the relevant section, problem type, problem name, rule ID, and connotative logic. These rules primarily assess the admission records along dimensions such as information completeness, documentation standardization, and logical consistency. For instance, checking for missing diagnostic information, overly verbose chief complaint descriptions, or inconsistencies between the chief complaint and the history of present illness. For each of the 19 rules, a determination must be made as to whether corresponding defects exist in a given admission record. If defects are identified, a defect list should be generated, where each defect entry includes the relevant section, problem type, rule ID, defect description, and basis for judgment; if no defects are found, the list remains empty. Examples of the data, annotation specifications, and QC rules are provided in Fig. 1.

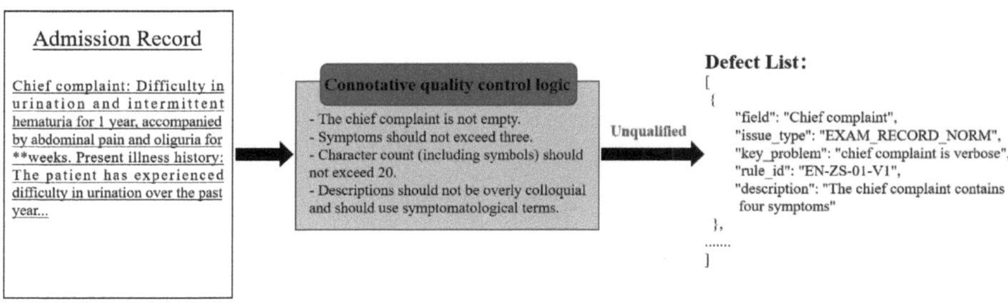

Fig. 1. The rule-driven workflow for connotative quality control of admission records. The process begins with inputting the admission record, applies specific QC logic (e.g., symptom count and character length limits) to components such as the chief complaint, and outputs a structured defect list if the record is deemed unqualified

4 Method

For the connotative medical record QC task based on LLMs, this study proposes a dual-enhancement framework that integrates precision in-context learning and CoT reasoning. The framework is implemented entirely via model API without fine-tuning or reliance on external databases, as illustrated in Fig. 2.

To achieve precision in-context learning, admission records first undergo semi-structured segmentation, with each document systematically decomposed into key sections–such as chief complaint and history of present illness. Subsequently, section-specific configuration files are constructed for each QC rule, ensuring that only rule-relevant content is delivered to the model while irrelevant information is rigorously excluded. In terms of prompt design, a stepwise judgment guidance mechanism based on CoT logic is introduced, leading the model through reasoning from basic to complex steps and simulating human-like progressive analysis. Finally, for each individual rule, the prompt and corresponding document segments are integrated into an input sequence, which is processed by the LLMs. The output is then parsed structurally to extract the QC result and a concise explanatory basis.

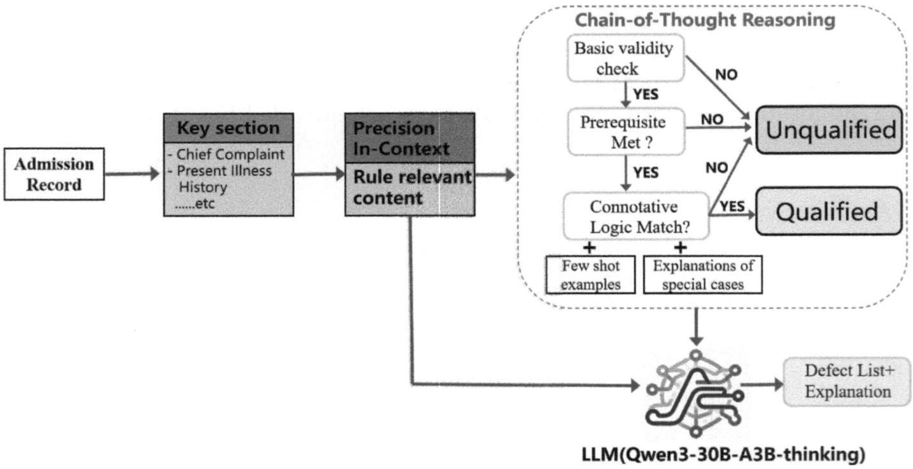

Fig. 2. The proposed connotative medical record quality control workflow integrating precision in-context learning and CoT reasoning. Key sections are first extracted from the admission record and filtered for rule relevance. This precision context, along with few-shot examples, is input to the LLM (Qwen3-30B-A3B-thinking), which executes a multi-step reasoning chain (validity check → prerequisite evaluation → logic matching) to determine a qualification status and produce a structured defect list with explanations

4.1 Precision In-Context Learning

The construction of precision in-context learning is essential for enabling efficient and accurate quality control in medical record analysis. We employ a semi-structured segmentation strategy to systematically decompose each admission record into fixed semantic sections–such as chief complaint, history of present illness, and past medical history–enabling modular organization of the document content. This approach is feasible because admission records are typically completed in standardized sections rather than in free-form narratives.

For each connotative QC rule, we construct a dedicated section configuration file that specifies which document modules are relevant to the rule. This ensures that only content strongly associated with the rule is input into the LLMs, effectively filtering out irrelevant information. For instance, the rule assessing "inconsistency between chief complaint and history of present illness" only requires the chief complaint and present illness sections as input. In contrast, the rule evaluating "missing diagnosis" necessitates the full admission record to comprehensively assess the patient's condition.

This strategy offers two key advantages. First, the combination of semi-structured segmentation and rule-specific configuration significantly reduces textual redundancy in LLMs inputs, mitigating reasoning deviations caused by information overload. Second, the resulting modular precision context provides a semantically focused information foundation for subsequent Chain-of-Thought reasoning, enabling the model to concentrate on the core logical elements pertinent to each rule. This input-layer optimization ensures both the accuracy and efficiency of QC judgments.

4.2 Chain-of-Thought Reasoning

Given the complexity and multi-constraint nature of connotative medical record QC rules, this study develops a stepwise judgment guidance framework based on the Chain-of-Thought reasoning logic of "from shallow to deep, from easy to difficult.". This framework simulates the analytical process of clinical QC experts through a hierarchical and progressive reasoning chain. It decomposes the QC judgment into multi-stage tasks: first, performing basic validity verification; after passing this step, verifying the prerequisite conditions for rule application; then conducting an in-depth analysis of the alignment between document semantics and rule criteria; and finally, rendering a qualitative conclusion of "qualified" or "unqualified" in accordance with rule specifications, supplemented by explanations for special cases and precautions.

To enhance the model's rule comprehension and execution consistency, a small number of high-quality few-shot examples are incorporated into the framework. The model is explicitly instructed to output structured results in JSON format, including a mandatory reasoning basis to ensure traceability.

As an example, consider the rule: "consistency of the longest onset time of the same clinical manifestations in the chief complaint and present illness history." The CoT-guided reasoning process unfolds as follows:

- Stage 1: Check whether the chief complaint and present illness history contain valid content. If the present illness history is recorded as an empty string (e.g., "Present illness history:" " "), the record is directly deemed unqualified (excluding information masking cases).
- Stage 2: Identify core clinical manifestations in the chief complaint (e.g., "headache and vomiting") and match them with symptom descriptions of the same type in the present illness history.
- Stage 3: Extract all onset times of the matched manifestations from both sections, taking the longest duration as the core judgment criterion.
- Stage 4: Compare the longest onset times between the two sections, handling special cases such as masked time information (e.g., "1 months ago" vs. "8 months ago" is clearly inconsistent → unqualified; "* weeks" or "-9-*1" is unjudgeable → qualified; "1 months ago" vs. "4 weeks ago" is consistent → qualified).
- Output: Generate a structured JSON result containing the relevant section, rule ID, conclusion, and basis (e.g., "The onset time of headache and vomiting in the chief complaint is 4 days, while the longest in the present illness history is 10 days; the two are inconsistent → unqualified").

The advantages of this CoT reasoning framework are threefold:

(1) Progressive reasoning: The step-by-step task decomposition avoids reasoning leaps and misjudgments that may occur when the model directly attempts complex judgments, thereby improving accuracy.
(2) Enhanced robustness: Integration of few-shot examples and special-case handling standardizes the model's understanding of rule boundaries, particularly under scenarios like information masking or partial data absence.
(3) Interpretable and reusable outputs: Structured JSON results with mandatory reasoning bases ensure interpretability and support review and error tracing, meeting both academic and clinical needs.

5 Experiment and Results

5.1 Parameter Settings

Our experiments utilized the Qwen3-30B-A3B-Thinking-2507 large language model in deep thinking mode, accessed via application programming interface (API) through Alibaba's Bailian platform. No model fine-tuning, external knowledge bases, or additional resources were employed. To ensure reproducibility and minimize randomness, key inference parameters were fixed as follows: temperature = 0, top p = 1, top k = 1, and a fixed random seed (seed = 12345), ensuring deterministic outputs for identical inputs.

5.2 Evaluation Metrics

Evaluation was conducted along two dimensions:

(1) Problem Extraction Ability: Assessed using F1 score, precision, and recall to measure defect identification performance (reflecting control over false positives and missed detections), along with ROUGE-L to evaluate the accuracy of defect explanations.
(2) Case Overall Compliance Determination: Evaluated using F1 score, precision, and recall to gauge the model's capability in judging whether a case meets quality control standards (reflecting control over misjudgments and omissions).

The final comprehensive score was computed as a weighted sum: problem extraction ability contributed 70% and overall compliance determination contributed 30%.

5.3 Results

As shown in Table 1, Our method achieved competitive performance in the non-fine-tuning track of the CHIP 2025 task, ranking first on the validation set and second on the final test set. This section presents a detailed analysis of the results from both model comparison and metric perspectives. The comprehensive scores on the validation set and test set are 0.6669 and 0.6644, respectively, showing highly consistent results. This indicates that our method maintains well-maintained stability across different data distributions. The close alignment of key metrics between the validation and test sets further confirms the strong generalization capability and robustness of the proposed framework. The detailed results are available on the official CHIP 2025 website (cips-chip.org.cn).

Model Comparison We conducted comparative experiments using three model variants: Qwen3-14B, Qwen3-32B, and Qwen3-30B-A3B-Thinking-2507. As summarized in Table 1, Qwen3-30B-A3B-Thinking-2507 demonstrated superior performance across nearly all evaluation metrics. Specifically, it achieved a overall score of 0.6644, surpassing Qwen3-14B and Qwen3-32B by 1.96% and 0.10%, respectively. In overall compliance score, it reached 0.6850, exceeding the other two models by 5.70% and 2.50%. The model also attained the highest explanation text quality score and the highest overall compliance recall. This performance advantage can be attributed to its enhanced reasoning capability and deep thinking mode, which are particularly beneficial for handling the complex logic and multi-step judgments required in connotative quality control tasks.

Metric Analysis An analysis of the metric breakdown reveals that recall values generally exceed precision across both problem extraction and overall compliance evaluations. For instance, the best results of test set, in triple extraction, the recall rate reached 0.8262, significantly higher than the precision of 0.6250.

Similarly, in overall compliance judgment, recall (0.8478) surpassed precision (0.5532). This pattern indicates that our method is more inclined to identify potential defects–even at the risk of including some false positives–rather than overlooking true issues. This characteristic is desirable in medical quality control settings, where missing a true defect (low recall) is typically considered more critical than issuing a false alert.

Table 1. Comparison results of different models

Model	Qwen3-30B	Qwen3-14B	Qwen3-32B	Qwen3-30B
Dataset	Validation set	Test set	Test set	Test set
Overall score	0.6669	0.6448	0.6633	**0.6644**
Defect extraction score	0.6478	0.6521	0.6648	0.6556
Triple extraction F1	0.7169	0.7146	0.7233	0.7117
Triple extraction precision	0.6503	0.6360	0.6425	0.6250
Triple extraction recall	0.7987	0.8153	0.8275	0.8262
Explanation text quality	0.3935	0.4247	0.4535	0.4537
Overall compliance score	0.7114	0.6280	0.6600	0.6850
Overall compliance F1	0.7014	0.6147	0.6489	0.6695
Overall compliance precision	0.6012	0.5108	0.5489	0.5532
Overall compliance recall	0.8417	0.7717	0.7935	0.8478

6 Conclusion

This study addresses the "Connotative Quality Control of Admission Records" task at CHIP 2025–a shared task focused on applying large language models to connotative medical record quality control. We propose a non-fine-tuning approach that leverages the Qwen3-30B-A3B-Thinking-2507 model within a dual-enhancement framework combining precision context and Chain-of-Thought reasoning. This design effectively mitigates challenges posed by the high complexity of medical texts and intricate connotative logic. In the non-fine-tuning track, our method achieved second place in the final test set ranking. These results demonstrate the feasibility of using non-fine-tuned LLMs–augmented by precision in-context learning and CoT reasoning–for connotative medical record QC. The proposed framework offers a reference methodology for future research on intelligent medical record analysis and quality assurance.

References

1. Yu, E., Chu, X., Zhang, W., Meng, X., Yang, Y., Ji, X., Wu, C.: Large language models in medicine: applications, challenges, and future directions. Int. J. Med. Sci. **22**(11), 2792–2801 (2025). https://doi.org/10.7150/ijms.111780
2. AlSaad, R., Abd-Alrazaq, A., Boughorbel, S., Ahmed, A., Renault, M.A., Damseh, R., Sheikh, J.: Multimodal large language models in health care: applications, challenges, and future outlook. J. Med. Internet Res. **25**(26), e59505 (2024). https://doi.org/10.2196/59505
3. Zhang, K., Meng, X., Yan, X., Ji, J., Liu, J., Xu, H., Zhang, H., Liu, D., Wang, J., Wang, X., Gao, J., Wang, Y.G., Shao, C., Wang, W., Li, J., Zheng, M.Q., Yang, Y., Tang, Y.D.: Revolutionizing health care: the transformative impact of large language models in medicine. J. Med. Internet Res. **7**(27), e59069 (2025). https://doi.org/10.2196/59069
4. Hasan, M.M., Mostafiz, R., Hossain, M.A., Paul, B.K.: CLIN-LLM: a safety-constrained hybrid framework for clinical diagnosis and treatment generation (2025)
5. Peng Jun, X., Kan, S.X., Jin, J., Zhang, Z.J., Ya Xin, G., Zhang, B., Zhou, Y.L.: Multimodal large language models in medical research and clinical practice: development, applications, challenges and future. Neurocomputing **660**, 131817 (2026). ISSN 0925–2312. https://doi.org/10.1016/j.neucom.2025.131817
6. Shin, E., Bhat, A.G., Ramanathan, M.: Large language models for clinical trial protocol assessments. Clin. Pharmacol. Ther. (2025). https://doi.org/10.1002/cpt.70096
7. Lv, J., Xu, Y., Jiang, M., Lv, Y., Sun, J., Lu, J., Wang, L., Wang, H.: A DeepSeek-powered locally deployed closed-loop system for enhancing quality control in electronic nursing documentation: development and clinical validation. J. Am. Med. Inform. Assoc. **32**(10), 1526–1532 (2025). https://doi.org/10.1093/jamia/ocaf109
8. Liu, H., Li, Z., Song, Z.: Comprehensive lifecycle quality control of medical data—automated monitoring and feedback mechanisms based on artificial intelligence. Technol. Health Care **33**(5), 2125–2135 (2025). https://doi.org/10.1177/09287329251330222
9. Case study. https://chima.org.cn/Html/News/Articles/17248.html. Accessed 26 Feb 2025
10. Case study. https://wjhospital.com.cn/Html/News/Articles/20005710.html. Accessed 21 Mar 2025
11. Qiao, S., Ou, Y., Zhang, N., Chen, X., Yao, Y., Deng, S., Tan, C., Huang, F., Chen, H.: Reasoning with language model prompting: a survey (2022). arXiv:2212.09597
12. Wei, J., Wang, X., Schuurmans, D., Bosma, M., Ichter, B., Xia, F., Chi, E.H., Le, Q.V., Zhou, D.: Chain-of-thought prompting elicits reasoning in large language models. In: Proceedings of the 36th International Conference on Neural Information Processing Systems (NIPS '22), pp. 24824–24837. Curran Associates Inc., Red Hook, NY, USA (2022). Article 1800
13. Wu, J., Wang, H., et al.: TIMER: temporal instruction modeling and evaluation for longitudinal clinical records. npj Digit. Med. **8**, 577 (2025). https://doi.org/10.1038/s41746-025-01965-9
14. Zhang, Y., Wang, S., Ding, Q.: E-CARP: an enhanced context-aware reasoning framework for interpretable text classification. ChinaXiv (2025). https://doi.org/10.12074/202508.00132

15. Wang, A.J., Li, L., Lin, Y., Li, M., Wang, L., Shou, M.Z.: Leveraging visual tokens for extended text contexts in multi-modal learning. In: Proceedings of the 38th International Conference on Neural Information Processing Systems (NIPS '24), vol. 37, pp. 14325–14348. Curran Associates Inc., Red Hook, NY, USA (2025). Article 457
16. Wang, X., Wei, J., Schuurmans, D., Le, Q., Chi, E.H., Zhou, D.: Self-consistency improves chain of thought reasoning in language models (2022). arXiv:2203.11171
17. Yao, S., Yu, D., Zhao, J., Shafran, I., Griffiths, T.L., Cao, Y., Narasimhan, K.: Tree of thoughts: deliberate problem solving with large language models. In: Oh, A., Neumann, T., Globerson, A., Saenko, K., Hardt, M., Levine, S. (eds.) Advances in Neural Information Processing Systems 36–37th Conference on Neural Information Processing Systems, NeurIPS 2023, vol. 36. Neural Information Processing Systems Foundation (2023)
18. Besta, M., Blach, N., Kubíček, A., Gerstenberger, R., Gianinazzi, L., Gajda, J., Lehmann, T., Podstawski, M., Niewiadomski, H., Nyczyk, P., Hoefler, T.: Graph of thoughts: solving elaborate problems with large language models. In: AAAI Conference on Artificial Intelligence (2023)
19. Kojima, T., Gu, S.S., Reid, M., Matsuo, Y., Iwasawa, Y.: Large language models are zero-shot reasoners (2022). arXiv:2205.11916

Semantic Quality Control of EMR Admission Notes: Integrating Rule Guidance, Prompt Optimization, and RAG

Yuxin Liu, Yitong Pan, Wusi Zhen, and Junwen Duan(✉)

Hunan Provincial Key Lab on Bioinformatic, School of Computer Science and Engineering, Central South University, Changsha, China
{liuyuxin,panyitong,zhenwusi,jwduan}@csu.edu.cn

Abstract. This paper presents a system for Shared Task 1 of the 11th China Health Information Processing Conference (CHIP 2025): Semantic Quality Control for Inpatient Electronic Medical Records (EMRs). Our framework integrates rule-guided strategies, Retrieval-Augmented Generation (RAG), and iterative prompt optimization within a Natural Language Processing (NLP) paradigm to improve semantic-level quality control. The system decomposes complex multi-rule tasks into single-rule subtasks and applies feedback-based prompt refinement for higher logical accuracy. To mitigate limited data, a Large Language Model (LLM) is used for data augmentation. In evaluation, rule-based judgments handle simple cases, while LLM-based reasoning addresses complex ones. The proposed approach achieved a comprehensive score of 0.6484 on the no-fine-tuning track, demonstrating its effectiveness.

Keywords: Semantic Quality Control · Electronic Medical Records (EMRs) · Retrieval-Augmented Generation (RAG) · Large Language Models (LLMs) · Natural Language Processing (NLP)

1 Introduction

As the primary vehicle for medical information, the EMR plays a pivotal role in clinical diagnosis, scientific research, and health management. The accuracy, standardization, and structure of EMR are directly linked to the safety and quality of patient care and provide a reliable data foundation for medical data governance and intelligent decision-making [24]. With the rapid growth of medical data and an increasing demand for quality control, developing high-precision, interpretable, and automated quality control systems for EMRs has become a key research challenge in medical Artificial Intelligence [8].

Traditionally, medical quality control has relied on rule-based frameworks and supervised deep learning models. While rule-based systems offer standardization and controllability, their effectiveness is often limited by the scope of

Y. Zhang et al. (Eds.): CHIP 2025, CCIS 2884, pp. 423–433, 2026.
https://doi.org/10.1007/978-981-95-7299-1_25

expert knowledge, making them difficult to adapt to diverse medical texts. Supervised models, despite their automation and generalization capabilities, are frequently constrained by shifts in data distribution and a scarcity of annotated data [22], leading to suboptimal performance in semantic understanding and cross-domain robustness. In recent years, research has shifted towards intelligent quality control solutions that leverage LLMs. By incorporating mechanisms such as RAG [13], knowledge injection, and human-in-the-loop feedback, these advanced systems can perform multi-level semantic reasoning and factual verification, enabling them to make interpretable judgments on medical records and significantly improving their generalization and clinical utility.

Task 1 of the 11th China Health Information Processing Conference (CHIP 2025), titled "Semantic Quality Control for Inpatient EMRs," focuses on advancing the automated quality control of electronic medical records. The task challenges participants to develop systems that automatically detect violations within structured inpatient records, which contain fields such as the Chief Complaint and History of Present Illness. For each identified issue, these systems must generate a structured annotation specifying the field, issue type, the violated rule's ID, and a detailed description. The evaluation is governed by a comprehensive set of 19 rules spanning four key dimensions: INFO COMPLETENESS (IC), CONSISTENCY (CO), DIAGNOSIS QUALITY (DQ), and EXAM RECORD NORM (EN). This setup requires solutions that integrate deep semantic comprehension with complex medical knowledge, aiming to systematically assess the practical value of intelligent quality control systems in a clinical context.

To address the challenges outlined above, this paper proposes an intelligent quality control method that integrates a rule-driven strategy with RAG, prompt optimization, and LLM collaboration. Our approach transforms complex, multi-rule quality control into a series of manageable, single-rule sub-problems through data segmentation. We then utilize iterative feedback and RAG to enhance the LLM's adaptability to domain-specific tasks, augmenting its performance with contextual information from medical knowledge bases. On Leaderboard B of the CHIP 2025 no-fine-tuning track, our method achieved a comprehensive score of 0.6484, validating its accuracy, generalization, and practical potential for inpatient EMR quality control.

2 Related Work

2.1 LLMs

LLMs, primarily built upon the Transformer architecture [21], have become a cornerstone in NLP. Through pre-training on large-scale corpora and subsequent fine-tuning, these models exhibit robust capabilities in semantic understanding, reasoning, and generation. Recent LLMs, including the GPT series [16], BERT [5], T5 [17], Baichuan [25], and Qwen [2], have achieved state-of-the-art performance on both general and domain-specific tasks. Within the medical domain, specialized models like BioBERT [11] and ClinicalBERT [1] have undergone pre-training on clinical texts, proving effective in applications such as medical record summarization and automated interpretation. As their parameter scales and data diversity have increased, LLMs are increasingly being applied to tasks such as parsing structured medical texts, question answering, summarization, and reasoning.

2.2 Prompt Engineering

Prompt Engineering is the practice of designing and optimizing input prompts to guide an LLM toward performing specific downstream tasks more accurately and controllably. In recent years, it has become a key technique for adapting LLMs to domain-specific challenges. Various strategies, including automated prompt discovery with AutoPrompt [19], the Prompt Tuning fine-tuning method [12], and techniques like Few-Shot [3] and Chain-of-Thought (CoT) prompting [23], have proven effective in scenarios such as medical question answering and entity recognition. Studies have shown that through iterative optimization and task decomposition, prompt engineering can significantly improve the performance and robustness of LLMs [15], reduce the need for extensive fine-tuning, and enhance adaptability to domain-specific knowledge.

2.3 RAG

RAG is an emerging paradigm that integrates information retrieval with generative models. By augmenting LLMs with external knowledge bases, RAG significantly enhances a model's ability to handle knowledge-intensive tasks and scenarios with dynamic facts. This approach dynamically retrieves relevant documents to serve as context for text generation, thereby improving the factual consistency and interpretability of the output. RAG methodologies, such as REALM [7], FiD [9], and KAT [6], have been widely applied in domains including medical literature retrieval, knowledge-based question answering, and anomaly detection.

2.4 Integration of EMR Quality Control and LLMs

Traditional methods for EMR quality control have relied on manual, rule-based systems; however, the integration of LLMs represents a promising new direction [20]. By utilizing pre-trained models as a foundation, the application of prompt engineering and rule fusion to the automated quality control of structured medical records improves both violation detection and the generation of detailed problem descriptions. Intelligent systems, such as MedGPT and various BERT-based auditing models, have achieved notable success in the automated review of clinical data. These systems effectively alleviate the manual quality control burden and establish a technical foundation for medical intelligence. Particularly in scenarios involving large-scale, real-world hospital data, LLM-driven automated quality control has demonstrated significant practical value.

3 Methodology

Our methodology for automated EMR quality control is an LLM-based framework, depicted in Fig. 1. It integrates meticulous data preprocessing with advanced techniques—RAG and iterative prompt engineering—to steer the model's complex reasoning and validation process.

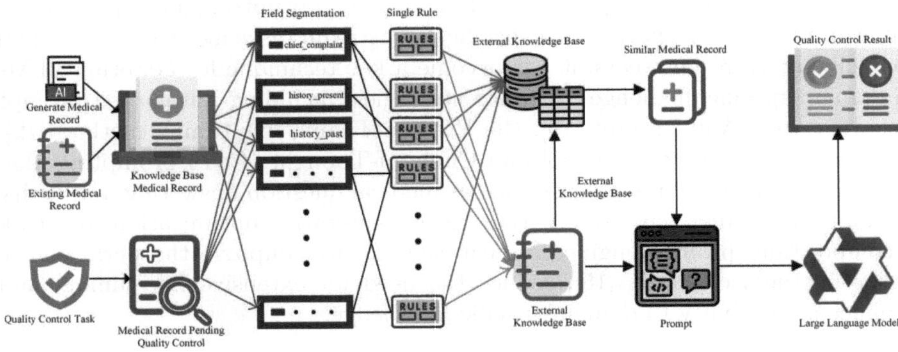

Fig. 1. LLM-based prompt generation workflow.

3.1 Data Preprocessing

The data preprocessing stage transforms raw medical record data and quality control rules into a structured, standardized format, preparing it for subsequent stages.

Rule Structuring. We first converted the Excel file of quality control rules into a structured JSON format. Each rule was transformed into a distinct JSON object containing its key information. This structured rule set serves as the foundational reference for prompt generation and quality control judgments, ensuring all operations adhere to the official definitions.

EMR Content Parsing. The raw EMR data contains a single `emr_content` field concatenating multiple sections. Observing that each quality control rule typically targets only a few specific fields, we parsed this long-form text into a structured dictionary. We used regular expression matching based on key field names (e.g., "Chief Complaint:", "History of Present Illness:") to map each section to a key-value pair. For unlabeled data with a different format, a more robust regex pattern with boundary detection was implemented. This decomposition simplifies the complex multi-rule quality control task into a series of manageable single-rule sub-tasks and reduces noise by providing the LLM with only the necessary fields for each check.

Sub-task Data Grouping. To support RAG and in-context learning for these single-rule sub-tasks, we further processed the parsed training data. For each quality control rule, we extracted the required input fields from all training records. If a record did not violate that specific rule, its output was labeled as compliant; otherwise, it was labeled as non-compliant, accompanied by an explanation. This grouping facilitates efficient data retrieval and simplifies compliance determination during the quality control and prompt optimization phases.

3.2 Prompt Engineering

Our prompt engineering process was designed to systematically improve the LLM's quality control accuracy through multi-turn iteration and automated optimization.

Initial Prompt Generation. We began by constructing a meta-prompt that consolidated meta-information, including quality control rule definitions, data analysis insights, and the distribution characteristics of non-compliant samples. This meta-prompt, which encapsulated rule logic and common deficiencies, was fed to an LLM to automatically generate an initial set of professionally-focused and task-specific prompts.

Automated Iterative Optimization. Following initial generation, we employed an automated optimization framework for multi-turn iterative refinement. We established an evaluation metric that calculated a matching score between predicted outcomes and ground-truth annotations. In each iteration, the optimizer prompted the LLM to perform an error analysis on the current prompt and generate an improved version. By cumulatively collecting failed samples, a feedback loop continuously refined the prompt's phrasing, example selection, and logical emphasis. Over 10 iterations, this process progressively improved the matching score from an initial value of approximately 0.5 to over 0.95.

Targeted Refinement. To validate the optimized prompts, we conducted a full quality control pass on the training set. For the few prompts that still yielded suboptimal performance, we repeated the iterative optimization process using a more powerful LLM. Each underperforming prompt underwent 5 additional iterations, and we selected the version that yielded results most consistent with the ground truth.

Manual Refinement for Edge Cases. Despite the automated optimization, certain challenges persisted. Text de-identification obscured critical information, making temporal consistency difficult to assess. Additionally, uncommon and meaningless character strings sometimes misled the LLM into incorrectly perceiving fields as non-empty. We therefore performed final manual refinements to make the prompts more tolerant of de-identified temporal expressions and better able to discern genuinely empty fields.

3.3 RAG

The RAG component retrieves relevant, high-quality reference samples during the quality control process, enabling the LLM to leverage compliant and non-compliant cases for its judgments.

Knowledge Base Construction. A high-quality external knowledge base is crucial for RAG. Our knowledge base was constructed in three stages. First, the pre-grouped training set served as the initial component ("train"). Second, we performed quality control on 700 unlabeled medical records, filtered them to retain only high-value samples (excluding simple missing-field cases), and merged them with the initial set ("train+unlabeled"). Finally, to obtain more non-compliant examples, we augmented the dataset by prompting an LLM to convert compliant samples from the training set into non-compliant ones, emulating patterns observed in true non-compliant data. These generated samples were added to form the complete knowledge base ("train+unlabeled+generated").

Retrieval Mechanism. During quality control, we used a sentence transformer based Chinese embedding model [18] to vectorize the content of all samples in the knowledge base. The input for vectorization was a concatenation of the field name and its corresponding value. For each new medical record, its relevant fields were vectorized using the same process. We then employed cosine similarity [4] to retrieve the K most similar reference samples (typically K = 3–4). These retrieved examples provide the LLM with potent in-context learning material.

Efficiency Optimization. To enhance computational efficiency, all generated vector embeddings were cached locally. During quality control, the system first checks the cache for existing embeddings. If found, they are loaded directly; otherwise, they are generated and then cached for future use. This design ensures both high system throughput and vector space consistency.

3.4 Medical Record Quality Control

Our quality control workflow integrates efficient, rule-based preliminary checks with the nuanced analytical power of a LLM. This hybrid approach ensures both the rapid identification of straightforward deficiencies and the accurate detection of complex, latent issues, optimizing for both speed and thoroughness.

Preliminary Checks. For each medical record under review, an empty `problems` array is initialized to store any identified violations. For a subset of rules where non-compliance is determined by an empty or invalid field, the system first performs a direct check. If a field meets these criteria, the corresponding quality control issue is immediately logged in the `problems` array without invoking the LLM. This strategy conserves significant time and computational resources.

LLM-driven Deep Analysis. In all other cases, the system utilizes the Qwen-32B LLM to perform a deep-level semantic analysis. The system extracts the fields required by a given rule, vectorizes their content, and retrieves the K most similar samples from the external knowledge base via RAG. The fields under review, the retrieved samples, and the corresponding optimized prompt are then passed to an LLM orchestration framework. The model returns a JSON object indicating compliance and, if non-compliant, a generated description of the issue. This information is then formatted into a complete problem object and appended to the record's `problems` array, concluding one cycle of single-rule quality control.

4 Experiments

4.1 Dataset

The dataset used in this study is the official test set of CHIP 2025 Shared Task 1, containing 300 inpatient electronic medical records. An example of the preprocessed structured data format is shown in Fig. 2.


```
[
  {
    "record_id": "MED_QC_ADM_0001_testB",
    "record_type": "ADM_NOTE",
    "emr_content": {
      "主诉": "反复发热*周",
      "现病史": "患者于*周前出现头昏，反复恶心呕吐，晨起呕吐胃液，泡沫尿，尿量减少，白天体温升高，波动在*.6~*.8℃，夜间可自行
      "既往史": "患者平素体质良好。有肺Ca病史，手术+化疗+靶向药治疗，目前口服埃克替尼治疗。高血压、高血脂病史。按国家计划免疫
      "体格检查": "T*6.*℃, P6*次/分, R15次/分, BP1*/8*mmHg\n一般状况发育正常，营养一般，神志清晰，体位自主，面容与表情安静，
      "专科检查": "None",
      "辅助检查": "1*-*外院CT左肺上叶改变，术后？较我院*-*1-16结节增大。右肺上叶磨玻璃病灶，右肺微小结节，较前片变化不大。右
      "入院诊断": "['发热,血管炎(?),肾功能不全,蛋白尿,高血压,高脂血症,肺恶性肿瘤\\r\\r,*日\\r']",
      "初步诊断": "['发热,血管炎(?),肾功能不全,蛋白尿,高血压,高脂血症,肺恶性肿瘤\\r\\r,*日\\r']",
      "入院主诊断": "None",
      "修正主诊断": "None",
      "初步主诊断": "None",
      "病史陈述者": "患者本人"
    },
    "problems": []
  },
```


Fig. 2. An example of a structured data sample from the official dataset.

4.2 Evaluation Metrics

The evaluation metrics strictly adhere to the official standards of the CHIP 2025 Shared Task 1. The primary evaluation criterion is a Comprehensive Score, which is a weighted average of two sub-scores: an issue extraction score ($\text{Score}_{\text{extract}}$) and an overall compliance score ($\text{Score}_{\text{compliant}}$).

The final Comprehensive Score is calculated as:

$$\text{Score}_{\text{final}} = 0.7 \times \text{Score}_{\text{extract}} + 0.3 \times \text{Score}_{\text{compliant}} \tag{1}$$

The issue extraction score, $\text{Score}_{\text{extract}}$, which evaluates the accuracy of identifying and describing specific non-compliance issues, is defined as:

$$\text{Score}_{\text{extract}} = 0.4 \times \text{F1} + 0.25 \times \text{P} + 0.15 \times \text{R} + 0.2 \times \text{ROUGE-L} \tag{2}$$

The ROUGE-L metric, used for evaluating the quality of the generated issue descriptions, is based on the work of Lin [14].

The overall compliance score, $\text{Score}_{\text{compliant}}$, which assesses the binary classification accuracy for each record's compliance status, is defined as:

$$\text{Score}_{\text{compliant}} = 0.5 \times \text{F1} + 0.25 \times \text{P} + 0.25 \times \text{R} \tag{3}$$

4.3 Experimental Setup

For our experiments, we selected three prominent LLMs: Baichuan-M2-32B, Qwen3-32B, and QwQ-32B. All models were loaded using their official pre-trained weights without any additional fine-tuning. The models were deployed on high-performance servers and invoked for batch inference via their respective APIs.

To ensure a fair and controlled comparison, a consistent experimental environment was maintained across all models. This included identical data inputs, output processing pipelines, and prompt templates. Each model was integrated with our multi-stage optimized prompts and our RAG pipeline, which was built using the DSPy framework [10], to assess the performance gains attributable to our proposed methodology.

4.4 Results and Analysis

The experiments systematically evaluated the quality control performance of different LLMs when paired with various knowledge base configurations. The comprehensive scores for both Track A and Track B are detailed in Table 1.

Table 1. Scores of different model and external knowledge base combinations

Model	Knowledge base	Score_A	Score_B
Baichuan-M2-32B	Train	0.6257	–
Baichuan-M2-32B	Train+unlabeled	0.6511	–
QwQ-32B	Train+unlabeled	0.6667	0.6418
Qwen3-32B	Train+unlabeled+generated	–	0.6308
QwQ-32B	Train+unlabeled+generated	–	0.6484

Effectiveness of an Enriched Knowledge Base. The experimental results highlight the significant impact of an enriched knowledge base. For instance, the Baichuan-M2-32B model's performance on Track A improved from 0.6257 to 0.6511 after its knowledge base was augmented with unlabeled data ('train+unlabeled'). This relative increase of 4.1% demonstrates that exposing the model to a greater diversity of EMR examples enhances its ability to generalize and apply quality control rules accurately.

Comparison of Base LLM Performance. The choice of the base LLM also proved to be a critical factor. Under identical 'train+unlabeled' settings, QwQ-32B achieved a score of 0.6667 on Track A, outperforming Baichuan-M2-32B and suggesting a stronger inherent capability for medical text comprehension. This superiority was further confirmed when using the most extensive knowledge base ('train+unlabeled+generated'), where QwQ-32B scored 0.6484 on Track B, higher than the 0.6308 achieved by Qwen3-32B under the same conditions.

Benefit of Synthetic Data Augmentation. Furthermore, the inclusion of synthetically generated non-compliant samples provided an additional performance lift. For the QwQ-32B model, expanding the knowledge base from 'train+unlabeled' to 'train+unlabeled+generated' elevated its Track B score from 0.6418 to 0.6484. This improvement indicates that targeted augmentation with synthetic negative examples helps the model recognize more subtle and diverse violation patterns, thereby improving its robustness on challenging cases.

Summary of Findings. In summary, QwQ-32B consistently demonstrated the most robust performance, particularly when supported by a comprehensive, multi-source knowledge base. The results affirm that the synergy between a capable base model, a richly augmented knowledge base, and high-quality prompt engineering is an effective strategy for enhancing EMR quality control. This validates our proposed method's adaptability and practical value for this task.

5 Conclusion

This paper presents a medical quality control framework for the CHIP 2025 Shared Task 1, which integrates rule-based guidance with advanced LLM techniques. By combining RAG with an automated prompt optimization pipeline, our approach effectively steers LLM judgments using structured domain knowledge. This synergy of data, prompts, and rules enabled our system to achieve a comprehensive score of 0.6484 in the official evaluation, demonstrating that LLMs can perform high-accuracy, rule-compliant tasks when properly constrained.

Future work will focus on three key areas: enhancing scalability through an automated field extraction system, expanding the external knowledge base with higher-quality data sources and refined generation methods, and improving transparency for medical professionals by integrating a more interpretable decision-making framework.

Acknowledgement. This work was supported in part by National Natural Science Foundation of China (No. 62576363), the Natural Science Foundation of Hunan Province (No. 2025JJ50342) and Changsha Municipal Natural Science Foundation Project (No. kq2502144). This work was carried out in part using computing resources at the High-Performance Computing Center of Central South University.

References

1. Alsentzer, E., Murphy, J., Boag, W., Weng, W.H., Jindi, D., Naumann, T., McDermott, M.: Publicly available clinical BERT embeddings. In: Proceedings of the 2nd Clinical Natural Language Processing Workshop, pp. 72–78 (2019)
2. Bai, J., Bai, S., Chu, Y., Cui, Z., Dang, K., Deng, X., Fan, Y., Ge, W., Han, Y., Huang, F., et al.: Qwen technical report (2023). arXiv:2309.16609

3. Brown, T., Mann, B., Ryder, N., Subbiah, M., Kaplan, J.D., Dhariwal, P., Neelakantan, A., Shyam, P., Sastry, G., Askell, A., et al.: Language models are few-shot learners. Adv. Neural Inf. Process. Syst. **33**, 1877–1901 (2020)
4. Chowdhury, G.G.: Introduction to Modern Information Retrieval. Facet Publishing (2010)
5. Devlin, J., Chang, M.W., Lee, K., Toutanova, K.: Bert: Pre-training of deep bidirectional transformers for language understanding. In: Proceedings of the 2019 Conference of the North American Chapter of the Association for Computational Linguistics: Human Language Technologies, Volume 1 (Long and Short Papers), pp. 4171–4186 (2019)
6. Gui, L., Wang, B., Huang, Q., Hauptmann, A.G., Bisk, Y., Gao, J.: Kat: a knowledge augmented transformer for vision-and-language. In: Proceedings of the 2022 Conference of the North American Chapter of the Association for Computational Linguistics: Human Language Technologies, pp. 956–968 (2022)
7. Guu, K., Lee, K., Tung, Z., Pasupat, P., Chang, M.: Retrieval augmented language model pre-training. In: International Conference on Machine Learning, pp. 3929–3938. PMLR (2020)
8. Hripcsak, G., Albers, D.J.: Next-generation phenotyping of electronic health records. J. Am. Med. Inform. Assoc. **20**(1), 117–121 (2013)
9. Izacard, G., Grave, E.: Leveraging passage retrieval with generative models for open domain question answering. In: Proceedings of the 16th Conference of the European Chapter of the Association for Computational Linguistics: Main Volume, pp. 874–880 (2021)
10. Khattab, O., Singhvi, A., Maheshwari, P., Zhang, Z., Santhanam, K., Vardhamanan, S., Haq, S., Sharma, A., Joshi, T.T., Moazam, H., et al.: Dspy: compiling declarative language model calls into self-improving pipelines (2023). arXiv:2310.03714
11. Lee, J., Yoon, W., Kim, S., Kim, D., Kim, S., So, C.H., Kang, J.: Biobert: a pre-trained biomedical language representation model for biomedical text mining. Bioinformatics **36**(4), 1234–1240 (2020)
12. Lester, B., Al-Rfou, R., Constant, N.: The power of scale for parameter-efficient prompt tuning (2021). arXiv:2104.08691
13. Lewis, P., Perez, E., Piktus, A., Petroni, F., Karpukhin, V., Goyal, N., Küttler, H., Lewis, M., Yih, W.t., Rocktäschel, T., et al.: Retrieval-augmented generation for knowledge-intensive nlp tasks. Adv. Neural Inf. Process. Syst. **33**, 9459–9474 (2020)
14. Lin, C.Y.: Rouge: a package for automatic evaluation of summaries. In: Text Summarization Branches Out, pp. 74–81 (2004)
15. Ouyang, L., Wu, J., Jiang, X., Almeida, D., Wainwright, C., Mishkin, P., Zhang, C., Agarwal, S., Slama, K., Ray, A., et al.: Training language models to follow instructions with human feedback. Adv. Neural Inf. Process. Syst. **35**, 27730–27744 (2022)
16. Radford, A., Narasimhan, K., Salimans, T., Sutskever, I., et al.: Improving language understanding by generative pre-training (2018)
17. Raffel, C., Shazeer, N., Roberts, A., Lee, K., Narang, S., Matena, M., Zhou, Y., Li, W., Liu, P.J.: Exploring the limits of transfer learning with a unified text-to-text transformer. J. Mach. Learn. Res. **21**(140), 1–67 (2020)
18. Reimers, N., Gurevych, I.: Sentence-bert: sentence embeddings using siamese bert-networks (2019). arXiv:1908.10084

19. Shin, T., Razeghi, Y., Logan IV, R.L., Wallace, E., Singh, S.: Autoprompt: eliciting knowledge from language models with automatically generated prompts (2020). arXiv:2010.15980
20. Thirunavukarasu, A.J., Ting, D.S.J., Elangovan, K., Gutierrez, L., Tan, T.W., Teo, Z.L.: Large language models in medicine. Nat. Med. **29**(8), 1930–1940 (2023)
21. Vaswani, A., Shazeer, N., Parmar, N., Uszkoreit, J., Jones, L., Gomez, A.N., Kaiser, Ł., Polosukhin, I.: Attention is all you need. Adv. Neural Inf. Process. Syst. **30**, (2017)
22. Wang, Y., Wang, L., Rastegar-Mojarad, M., Moon, S., Shen, F., Afzal, N., Liu, S., Zeng, Y., Mehrabi, S., Sohn, S., et al.: Clinical information extraction applications: a literature review. J. Biomed. Inform. **77**, 34–49 (2018)
23. Wei, J., Wang, X., Schuurmans, D., Bosma, M., Xia, F., Chi, E., Le, Q.V., Zhou, D., et al.: Chain-of-thought prompting elicits reasoning in large language models. Adv. Neural Inf. Process. Syst. **35**, 24824–24837 (2022)
24. Weiskopf, N.G., Weng, C.: Methods and dimensions of electronic health record data quality assessment: enabling reuse for clinical research. J. Am. Med. Inform. Assoc. **20**(1), 144–151 (2013)
25. Yang, A., Xiao, B., Wang, B., Zhang, B., Bian, C., Yin, C., Lv, C., Pan, D., Wang, D., Yan, D., et al.: Baichuan 2: open large-scale language models (2023). arXiv:2309.10305

Leveraging Phased Training and Multi-granularity Prompting with Large Language Models for Few-Shot Quality Control of Electronic Medical Records

Chengfei Li[1(✉)], Chunyu Wang[2], Bin Liu[1], Yunjie Zhang[1], Liwei Cai[1], and Bei Zhao[1]

[1] Artificial Intelligence Research Institute on Education, Qilu Normal University, Jinan, Shandong 250200, People's Republic of China
{lichengfei,liubin}@qlnu.edu.cn, 1337843804@qq.com, 3202086896@qq.com, 2059301725@qq.com

[2] School of Geography and Tourism, Qilu Normal University, Jinan, Shandong 250200, People's Republic of China
cywang@qlnu.edu.cn

Abstract. The scarcity of high-quality annotated data hinders content quality control (QC) for clinical electronic medical records (EMRs). Addressing the CHIP-2025 shared task with only 300 annotated samples, we propose an integrated solution featuring a novel phased training strategy. Our approach combines systematic data preprocessing and multi-granularity prompt engineering, where the most effective "single-rule judgment" method decomposes the complex QC task into 19 independent binary classifications. The two-phase training strategy first learns from 700 pseudo-labeled samples generated via the DeepSeek API, then refines knowledge using the 300 human annotations, with $8 \times$ oversampling to mitigate class imbalance. Our method achieved a score of 0.73 on the Test-B dataset, with phased training as the key contributor, providing a reproducible framework for LLM application in low-resource clinical QC.

Keywords: Large language models · Clinical content quality control · Phased training strategy · Prompt engineering · Curriculum learning

1 Introduction

Electronic Medical Records (EMRs) are central to modern healthcare [1], with content quality being critical for clinical decisions and patient safety [2]. Unlike traditional quality control (QC) focusing on formal aspects, content QC evaluates the intrinsic logic and completeness of clinical narratives—a more complex task. While large language models (LLMs) offer automation potential [3], their medical use is limited by scarce high-quality annotated data [4]. This study addresses the CHIP-2025 task on inpatient record QC under the constraint of only 300 annotated samples.

Conventional fine-tuning tends to overfit in low-resource settings [5], and prompt-based methods alone are inadequate for handling 19 distinct QC rules. We propose

Y. Zhang et al. (Eds.): CHIP 2025, CCIS 2884, pp. 434–448, 2026.
https://doi.org/10.1007/978-981-95-7299-1_26

an integrated approach featuring a novel phased training strategy inspired by curriculum learning [6]: initial concept learning on 700 pseudo-labeled samples, followed by refinement on 300 high-quality annotations. This maximizes learning efficiency and generalization.

Our framework combines systematic data engineering, multi-granularity prompts, and phased training. Key components include data cleaning, a single-rule judgment prompt decomposing the task into 19 binary classifications, and 8 $\times$ oversampling for class imbalance. Evaluation shows a score of 0.73 on Test-B, with phased training as the main contributor, providing a reproducible framework for low-resource clinical QC.

2 Related Work

2.1 LLMs in Clinical Quality Control

LLMs are increasingly applied to clinical quality control. Yan et al. proposed LLM-DQR, an automated method for generating electronic health record data quality rules, achieving coverage rates of 97.1% (PIC dataset) and 99.6% (MIMIC-IV dataset) [7]. Zhao et al. developed EMRModel, integrating LoRA-based fine-tuning with code-style prompts to convert medical dialogues into structured records, improving the F1 score by 49.5% over standard models [8].

2.2 Prompt Engineering in Medical Applications

Prompt engineering significantly enhances LLM performance in medical tasks. Hu et al. designed task-specific prompts for clinical named entity recognition, improving the extraction of medical problems, treatments, and tests [9]. Wang et al. showed that tailored prompts increase precision in standardizing obstetric diagnosis text [10]. Chen et al. introduced EMPOWER, a framework using medical terminology attention and multi-dimensional evaluation to reduce factual errors by 24.7% and improve specificity by 19.6% [11]. Long et al. proposed Multi-expert Prompting, which aggregates responses from simulated experts to boost truthfulness and informativeness [12].

2.3 Phased Training and Curriculum Learning Strategies

Phased training, inspired by curriculum learning, organizes training from simple to complex examples to improve low-resource learning [6]. Hein et al. applied iterative prompt refinement for clinical information extraction, demonstrating that phased training enhances model accuracy and reliability [13].

2.4 Data Engineering and Class Imbalance in Clinical NLP

Data preprocessing and class imbalance mitigation are critical for clinical NLP. Shah et al. emphasized that systematic data cleaning and oversampling improve model accuracy [14]. Matos et al. developed EHR-monize, showing that GPT-4o with 10-shot prompting achieves high accuracy in medical concept abstraction when supported by rigorous data preprocessing [15].

3 Methods

3.1 Data Preprocessing and Engineering

High-quality data serves as the fundamental prerequisite for effective model learning. In few-shot scenarios where annotated data is extremely limited, the importance of data quality becomes particularly critical. To ensure maximum utility from limited data resources, this study performed systematic cleaning, standardization, and structuring of the raw data. The complete data processing workflow is illustrated in Fig. 1.

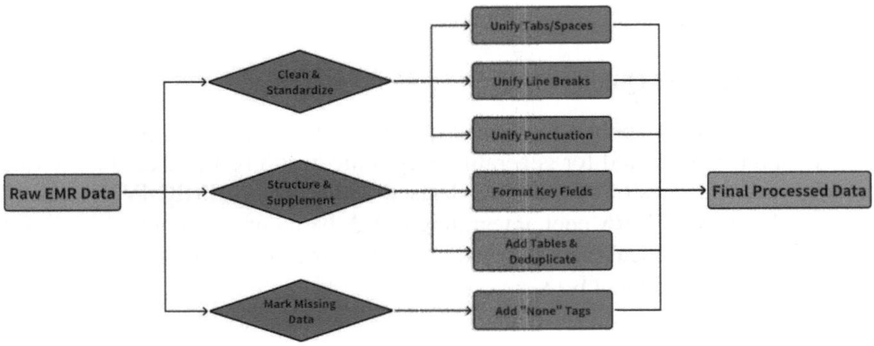

Fig. 1. Workflow of the core data preprocessing steps, including text cleaning and standardization, structured medical text processing, and normalized representation of missing fields.

Text Cleaning and Standardization. EMR data, sourced from diverse hospital systems and clinical staff, often contains inconsistencies in formatting, characters, and punctuation. These variations introduce noise that hinders model comprehension. We applied rigorous cleaning: unifying tabs and multiple spaces into single spaces, removing carriage returns, and simplifying line breaks. English punctuation was converted to Chinese equivalents, aligning with medical writing conventions. Extra spaces around quotation marks and periods were removed, and irregular symbol combinations were corrected.

Structured Medical Text Processing. The 700 unannotated records were initially in separate fields. To form coherent text for LLM processing while retaining structure, we inserted line breaks before 11 key field types to mark boundaries. Where field content was split from table data, we merged them into complete descriptions and removed redundant fields, ensuring each record became a well-structured textual unit.

Normalized Representation of Missing Fields. In real-world data, some fields were entirely absent—a state distinct from being present but empty. To prevent misattribution and semantic ambiguity during concatenation, we explicitly marked missing fields with a "None" identifier during structuring. This clarification helps the model accurately distinguish between non-existent and empty fields.

3.2 Multi-granularity Prompt Engineering and Task Decomposition

Accurately conveying the complex and specialized task of medical content quality control to the model is crucial, and prompt design plays a key role. Prompts define the task's input/output format and embody its fundamental objective, specific criteria, and underlying logic. This study constructed a multi-granularity prompt system, guiding the model to understand the task from multiple angles through prompts at different abstraction levels. The overall design of the prompt system is illustrated in Fig. 2.

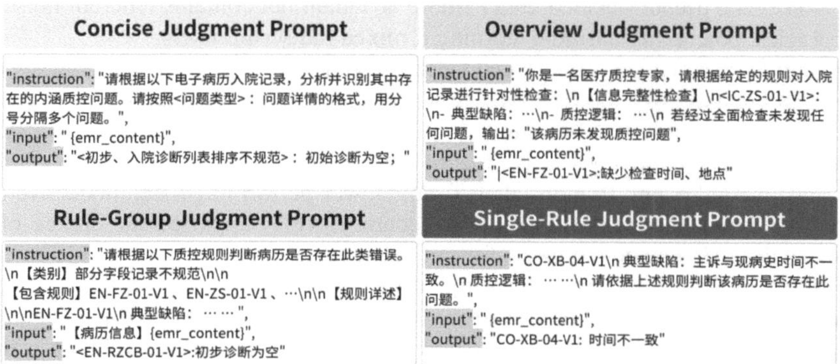

Fig. 2. Overview of the multi-granularity prompt engineering framework, including concise judgment, overview judgment, single-rule judgment, and rule-group judgment prompts, each designed for specific task decomposition and reasoning granularity.

Concise Judgment Prompt. A minimalist baseline providing only the core task description. The model receives the full record and outputs identified problems or a no-problem statement. This tests the model's inherent capability with minimal guidance.

Overview Judgment Prompt. Requires the model to evaluate the entire record against all 19 QC rules at once. The prompt defines the role, task, and provides full rule details. Outputs problems in a structured format. While designed for holistic analysis, it often led to missed or imprecise rule application.

Single-Rule Judgment Prompt. The core innovation decomposes the multi-label task into 19 independent binary judgments. Each prompt targets one rule, providing its ID, Description, and Logic. The Model Evaluates the Full Text Against Only that Rule, Significantly Simplifying the Learning Objective.

Rule-Group Judgment Prompt. A balanced approach grouping the 19 rules into 4 related categories. Separate prompts are used for each group, requiring category-level judgment. Performance was intermediate between the overview and single-rule methods.

3.3 Phased Training Strategy

The core methodological contribution of this work is the proposal and systematic validation of a phased training strategy designed for heterogeneous-quality data. Inspired by curriculum learning principles, this strategy addresses the central challenge in few-shot scenarios by defining a two-phase training process that effectively leverages both limited high-quality annotated data and larger volumes of lower-quality pseudo-labeled data. It was identified as the primary factor behind the final performance achieved.

Problem Analysis and Strategic Motivation. The available data consisted of 300 high-quality, meticulously human-annotated samples and 700 pseudo-labeled samples generated via the DeepSeek API. These datasets exhibit significant quality differences. The high-quality data offers accuracy and consistency but is scarce, risking overfitting if used alone. The pseudo-labeled data is more abundant but contains inherent noise and inaccuracies, potentially harming learning if mixed indiscriminately.

A quantitative analysis highlighted these differences: the gold-standard dataset contained 924 issues across 300 records (average ~3.08 per record), with 97.7% of records containing at least one issue. In contrast, pseudo-labels generated by the DeepSeek-V3.2-Exp API identified over 10 issues per record on average, suggesting a stricter, potentially over-sensitive judgment. Pseudo-labels from a lower-performing local model averaged closer to 3 issues/record but with lower accuracy. This supported the choice of the higher-quality API-generated labels for initial training.

Guided by insights from human cognitive development, we hypothesized that a model's learning process should mirror a progressive approach: establishing a general understanding before refining precise knowledge. The complete phased training workflow is illustrated in Fig. 3.

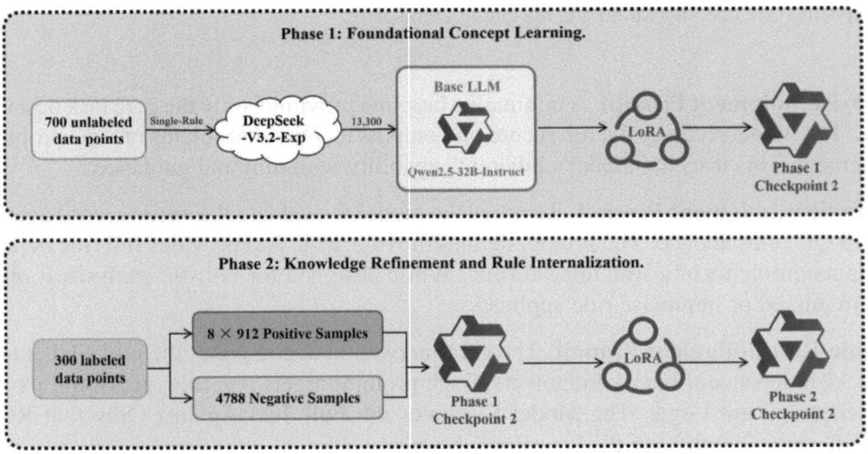

Fig. 3. Workflow of the two-phase training strategy. Phase 1 uses a large-scale pseudo-labeled dataset to establish a general task understanding. Phase 2 fine-tunes the Phase 1 checkpoint using a smaller, high-quality, human-annotated dataset with oversampling to refine precise knowledge.

Phase 1: Foundational Concept Learning. The first phase is termed the "Foundational Concept Learning" phase. The core objective of this phase is to allow the model to conduct extensive preliminary study, thereby establishing a basic cognitive framework for the task. In this phase, we train the base model using the 700 pseudo-labeled data points. The specific API call parameters were configured as shown in Table 1.

Table 1. API parameters for pseudo-labeling.

Parameter	Value
API version	DeepSeek-V3.2-Exp
Temperature	0.1
top_p	0.95
max_tokens	512
Prompt strategy	Single-rule judgment prompt

From a mathematical formalism perspective, let the parameters of the original base model be θ_0. The pseudo-labeled dataset used in the first phase is denoted as $D_{\text{pseudo}} = \{(\mathbf{x}_i^p, y_i^p)\}_{i=1}^{N_p}$, where $\mathbf{x}_i^p$ represents the i-th medical record text and y_i^p represents the corresponding pseudo-label. It is particularly important to note that, combined with the single-rule judgment prompt strategy mentioned earlier, each medical record is expanded into 19 independent training samples (corresponding to the 19 quality control rules). Therefore, the actual training sample size for the first phase is $N_p = 700 \times 19 = 13{,}300$.

The optimization objective for this phase is to minimize the empirical risk over the pseudo-labeled dataset:

$$\theta_1^* = argmin_\theta \mathcal{L}_1(\theta; D_{pseudo}) = argmin_\theta \frac{1}{N_p} \sum\nolimits_{i=1}^{N_p} \ell\left(f_\theta\left(x_i^p\right), y_i^p\right) \tag{1}$$

where ℓ represents the cross-entropy loss function and f_θ denotes the language model's prediction function parameterized by θ.

For training efficiency, we used LoRA(Low-Rank Adaptation) [16]. This method approximates parameter updates via low-rank decomposition. For a pretrained weight matrix $W_0 \in R^{d \times k}$, LoRA introduces trainable matrices $A \in R^{d \times r}$ and $B \in R^{r \times k}$ (where rank $r \ll min(d, k)$), resulting in the updated weights $W = W_0 + \alpha \cdot BA$, where α is a scaling factor. The original weights W_0 remain frozen, drastically reducing the number of trainable parameters.

A cosine annealing learning rate schedule was applied, defined by:

$$\eta_t = \eta_{min} + \frac{1}{2}(\eta_{max} - \eta_{min})\left(1 + cos\left(\frac{T_{cur}}{T_{max}}\pi\right)\right) \tag{2}$$

with initial learning rate $\eta_{max} = 1 \times 10^{-4}$, minimum learning rate $\eta_{min} = 0$, current step T_{cur}, and total steps T_{max}. Training proceeded for 3 epochs.

The primary value of Phase 1 is building task-specific prior knowledge. Despite noise, the large dataset exposes the model to diverse record structures, task formats, and the general scope of the QC rules—akin to a "preview" stage.

Phase 2: Knowledge Refinement and Rule Internalization. The primary objective of the second phase, "Knowledge Refinement and Rule Internalization," was to calibrate the model's judgment using high-quality annotations, transitioning from the broad familiarity gained in Phase 1 to precise task execution. The model was initialized with the optimal checkpoint from Phase 1, θ_1^{best}, and fine-tuned exclusively on the set of 300 high-quality, human-annotated samples.

Let the high-quality annotated dataset be defined as $D_{gold} = \left\{\left(x_j^g, y_j^g\right)\right\}_{j=1}^{N_g}$. Consistent with the methodology in Phase 1, the single-rule judgment prompt strategy was applied, decomposing each medical record into 19 distinct training instances. To address the significant class imbalance inherent in the expanded dataset, an 8 × oversampling strategy was applied to the positive samples (those flagged with quality control issues). Defining the positive and negative sample sets as S_{pos} and S_{neg} respectively, the final, balanced training set for Phase 2 is formally constructed as:

$$D_{stage2} = S_{neg} \cup \left(S_{pos} \times 8\right) \tag{3}$$

This balancing procedure adjusted the positive-to-negative ratio from an initial ~1:5.3 to a more equitable ~1.5:1, thereby directing greater optimization pressure towards the correct identification of the critical, yet scarce, positive cases.

The formal optimization objective for this phase was to minimize the loss on this balanced dataset:

$$\theta_2^* = argmin_\theta \mathcal{L}_2\left(\theta; D_{stage2}\right) \tag{4}$$

The second phase serves to inject high-fidelity supervisory signals, refining the model's understanding and correcting potential biases or inaccuracies learned from the noisier pseudo-labels of Phase 1. With a foundational task framework already established, Phase 2 operates as a precision-tuning stage. A Bayesian interpretation views this as updating the prior distribution $p\left(\theta \mid D_{pseudo}\right)$ from Phase 1 with the likelihood of the high-quality data, yielding a superior posterior distribution $p\left(\theta \mid D_{gold}, D_{pseudo}\right)$.

To isolate the effect of the data and phased strategy, all hyperparameters were kept consistent with Phase 1. The Epoch 2 checkpoint was selected as optimal, since the model achieves effective generalization within the first two epochs on small high-quality data, while further training risks overfitting the 300 samples. The complete phased training workflow is formally defined as follows:

$$\theta_0 \xrightarrow[\text{Stage 1:}\mathcal{D}_{\text{pseudo}}]{\text{Epoch 2 checkpoint}} \theta_1^* \xrightarrow[\text{Stage 2:}\mathcal{D}_{\text{pseudo}}]{\text{Epoch 2 checkpoint}} \theta_2^* = \theta_{\text{final}} \tag{5}$$

where:

- θ_0 represents the parameters of the original base model (Qwen2.5-32B-Instruct).
- D_{pseudo} denotes the dataset of 700 pseudo-labeled records (expanded to 13300 training instances).
- θ_1^* is the checkpoint from the second training epoch of Phase 1.
- $D_{balanced}$ is the balanced, high-quality training set derived from the 300 annotated samples after applying 8 × oversampling to the positive instances.
- θ_2^* is the checkpoint from the second training epoch of Phase 2.
- θ_{final} denotes the final model parameters used for evaluation.

4 Experiments

4.1 Task Definition

This study addresses the CHIP-2025 task on quality control for inpatient admission records. The task requires analyzing a single record to identify content issues, outputting structured results for each issue comprising four fields: the record field, the issue_type(e.g., Information Completeness), the violated rule_id, and a concise Chinese description. The core challenges involve comprehending clinical narratives, assessing compliance against 19 QC rules, and generating precise descriptions.

4.2 Dataset

The dataset used in this study was provided by the organizers of the CHIP-2025 shared task. Its composition is summarized in Table 2.

Table 2. Composition and annotation status of the CHIP-2025 dataset.

Dataset	Number of records	Annotation status
Train	1000	300 records are annotated
Test-A	300	Annotated (for evaluation)
Test-B	300	Annotated (for evaluation)

The 300 annotated records in the training set were meticulously labeled by medical experts with extensive clinical experience, with each record undergoing strict review against the QC rules. While of high quality, this annotated portion is limited in size. The remaining 700 records in the training set are unannotated raw admission records.

4.3 Evaluation Metrics

Issue extraction is evaluated by defect identification performance (*Precision, Recall, F1*) and explanation quality (*ROUGE-L*). *TP* requires exact match on the (field, issue_type, rule_id) triple; *FP* represents incorrect detections; *FN* represents missed defects. The extraction score is computed as:

$$Score_{extract} = 0.4 \times F1 + 0.25 \times P + 0.15 \times R + 0.2 \times ROUGE - L \quad (6)$$

Overall compliance uses a defect-driven penalty mechanism: detected defects only incur penalties if their (field, issue_type, rule_id) exactly matches a rule in the rule base. Starting from 100 points, penalties are subtracted and records scoring below 95 are deemed non-compliant. Binary classification performance is evaluated using *F1*, *Precision*, and *Recall* with weights of 50%, 25%, and 25% respectively. The final leaderboard score combines both dimensions:

$$Score_{final} = 0.7 \times Score_{extract} + 0.3 \times Score_{compliant} \quad (7)$$

4.4 Experimental Records and Result Analysis

This section details the ablation studies. Experiments for Tables 1, 2 and 3 used Test-A; Tables 4, 5 and 6 used Test-B.

Ablation on Data Replication Strategy. We tested the data replication strategy using Qwen2.5-7B-Instruct, replicating the 300 annotated samples to 300, 900, and 3000 instances. results on Test-A are in Table 3.

Table 3. Ablation Study on Data Replication (Qwen2.5-7B-Instruct)

Samples	Final score	Issue extract	Compl. Judg	Explan. qual
300	0.458356	0.469333	0.432743	0.372150
900	0.478264	0.508983	0.406584	0.439111
3000	0.479427	0.516447	0.393045	0.420952
300	0.458356	0.469333	0.432743	0.372150

Scaling from 300 to 900 samples improved the Final Score by ~ 0.02 (4.4% relative gain), confirming the benefit of increased data volume in few-shot settings. Further scaling to 3000 led to saturation (~0.001 gain), showing diminishing returns. Thus, 900 samples were used subsequently.

Ablation on Data Cleaning Strategy. We evaluated the data preprocessing efficacy by comparing performance with/without cleaning across different data scales. Results on Test-A are in Table 4.

Table 4. Ablation study on data cleaning (Qwen2.5-7B-Instruct)

Samples	Cleaning status	Final score	Issue extract	Compl. Judg	Explan. qual
300	Raw data	0.458356	0.469333	0.432743	0.372150
300	Cleaned data	0.467581	0.478825	0.441345	0.429255
900	Raw data	0.478264	0.508983	0.406584	0.439111
900	Cleaned datadata	0.503875	0.495248	0.524003	0.469253
3000	Raw data	0.479427	0.516447	0.393045	0.420952
3000	Cleaned data	0.508376	0.496191	0.536809	0.458006

Data cleaning provided stable gains across all scales (+0.009 to + 0.029 Final Score). The Compliance Judgment score improved most significantly, indicating standardized formatting aids accurate judgment. Explanation Quality also notably increased, validating cleaning's positive impact.

Ablation Study on Phased Training Strategy. To validate the effectiveness of the phased training strategy, we compared the impact of different data sources for phase 1.

"Fine-tuned Model Inference" Refers to using pseudo-labels generated by a locally fine-tuned, lower-performance model. "DeepSeek-V3.2-Exp Inference" Refers to pseudo-labels generated by calling the high-quality commercial API. The data volume Format is "Phase 1 + Phase 2". Results on Test-A are in Table 5.

Table 5. Ablation study on Phased training with different Phase 1 data sources (Qwen2.5-7B-Instruct)

Phase 1 data source	Data volume	Final score	Issue extract	Compl. Judg	Explan. qual
Fine-tuned model (Test-A 0.6)	700 + 300	0.514968	0.535669	0.466667	0.469636
Fine-tuned model (Test-A 0.6)	700 + 900	0.540476	0.543984	0.532292	0.470912
DeepSeek-V3.2-Exp API	700 + 300	0.547804	0.542192	0.560899	0.469979
DeepSeek-V3.2-Exp API	**700 + 900**	**0.554282**	**0.547983**	**0.568979**	**0.475623**

The phased training strategy significantly outperformed single-stage training (0.504). Using high-quality pseudo-labels from the DeepSeek API in Phase 1 (0.554) clearly surpassed using lower-quality labels (0.540) by 0.014, underscoring the importance of initial data quality. Furthermore, increasing the volume of high-quality annotated data in Phase 2 (from 300 to 900 samples) yielded consistent gains (0.007 to 0.025), demonstrating its crucial role within this framework.

Ablation Study on Prompt Strategies. Starting from this experiment, we switched to the Qwen2.5-32B-Instruct model and the Test-B dataset. This experiment systematically compared four prompt strategies of varying granularity within the phased training framework. Results on Test-B are in Table 6.

Table 6. Ablation study on prompt strategies in phased training (Qwen2.5-32B-Instruct)

Prompt strategy	Effective samples	Final score	Issue extract	Compl. Judg	Explan. qual
Concise judgment	700 + 300	0.580193	0.582363	0.575130	0.507523
Overview judgment	700 + 300	0.605103	0.601933	0.612500	0.495937
Single-rule judgment	**19 x 700 + 19 x 300**	**0.656030**	**0.67912**	**0.602150**	**0.477797**
Rule-group judgment	4 × 700 + 4 × 300	0.636652	0.654637	0.594687	0.475699

The Single-Rule Judgment strategy achieved the best performance (Final Score: 0.656), surpassing the next best (Rule-Group) by 0.019. Its superiority was most evident in Issue Extraction (0.679 vs. 0.655), underscoring that decomposing the task into 19 independent binary classifications significantly reduces complexity. Although Overview Judgment scored higher in Explanation Quality (0.496), likely due to a holistic view aiding description comprehensiveness, this advantage was outweighed by lower accuracy.

Ablation Study on Oversampling Strategy. Building upon the optimal single-rule judgment prompt strategy, we further investigated the impact of different sample balancing schemes. Since the single-rule approach expands each record into 19 training samples, it introduces a severe class imbalance issue (positive/negative ratio ~1:5.3). Experiments compared the effects of different oversampling strategies, results on Test-B are in Table 7.

Table 7. Ablation study on oversampling (OS) strategy in phased training (Qwen2.5-32B-Instruct)

Phase 2 Data (P/N ratio)	Sample count	Final score	Issue extract	Compl. Judg	Explan. qual	Compl. recall
Errors Only × 3	912 × 3	0.456807	0.379697	0.636731	0.323366	1.000000
6 × OS	912 × 6 + 4788	0.713683	0.738455	0.655881	0.497155	0.630435
6 × OS × 2	10260 × 2	0.697438	0.734946	0.609922	0.494882	0.554348
8 x OS	**912 x 8 + 4788**	**0.731139**	**0.74959**	**0.68807**	**0.500689**	**0.706522**

The sample balancing strategy significantly impacted performance. While the "Learn Errors Only" approach achieved perfect compliance recall, it led to an extremely low Issue Extraction score (0.380) and a Final Score of 0.457, confirming the need for balanced learning. Progressively increasing the oversampling ratio from 6 × to 8 × steadily improved the Final Score (0.714 to 0.731), boosting both the Issue Extraction and Compliance Judgment scores. The 8 × ratio was identified as optimal, achieving the best metric balance with a compliance recall of 0.707 and high precision, beyond which the risk of overfitting from excessive repetition increases.

Other Exploratory Work. Beyond the core strategies, we explored several other techniques, results on Test-B are in Table 8.

- Data Rewriting Augmentation: Correct input fields were replaced with errors to generate 250 × 19 synthetic samples. The resulting Final Score (0.695) was 0.036 lower than the 8 × oversampling baseline (0.731), indicating that simplistic field substitution may introduce noise by failing to mimic real-world complexity.

Table 8. Ablation study on other explorations (Qwen2.5-32B-Instruct)

Exploration	Final score	Issue extract	Compl. Judg	Explan. qual
Data rewriting augmentation	0.695351	0.718391	0.641590	0.499703
Input redundancy removal	0.694071	0.713813	0.648006	0.483235
Self-consistency verification	0.721322	0.749971	0.654473	0.503573
Comprehensive strategy integration	0.696453	0.736696	0.602554	0.501215

- Input Redundancy Removal: Only quality-control-related fields were retained. When applied to the 8 × oversampling setup, the score dropped to 0.694, demonstrating that full clinical context aids model understanding even for indirect rules.
- Self-Consistency Verification: Voting was applied to 10 outputs from a lower-scoring model (0.71) and 6 from a higher-scoring model (0.73). The result (0.721) was slightly below the baseline, suggesting that for this deterministic task, consistency is more critical than stochastic exploration.
- Comprehensive Strategy Integration: Combining all above techniques led to a significant performance drop (0.696), highlighting that their blind integration causes negative interactions and increased complexity.
- These explorations yielded key insights: 1) The task prioritizes data quality and deterministic judgment over diversity; 2) Full context is superior to aggressive feature selection; 3) Technique combinations require careful, task-specific validation.

Optimal Configuration and Final Performance. Based on the systematic ablation studies, the optimal configuration was determined as follows:

- Base Model: Qwen2.5-32B-Instruct
- Data Preprocessing: Full text cleaning and structured processing pipeline
- Prompt Strategy: 19 Single-Rule Judgment prompts
- Training Strategy: Phased Training
  - Phase 1: 700 × 19 pseudo-labels from DeepSeek API; 3 epochs, checkpoint at Epoch 2.
  - Phase 2: 300 × 19 high-quality annotated samples (900 × 19 total), 8 × oversampling on positive samples; 3 epochs, checkpoint at Epoch 2.
- Training Config: LoRA fine-tuning, learning rate 1e-4, cosine learning rate scheduler.

5 Results and Discussion

5.1 Core Findings and Validation

The proposed framework achieved a final score of 0.731 on the CHIP-2025 task. The effectiveness of three core strategies was conclusively validated:

- Phased Training was the paramount contributor, yielding a decisive ~10% improvement (0.554 vs. 0.504) over single-stage training. This "broad-then-precise" paradigm effectively leverages heterogeneous-quality data.
- Single-Rule Prompting proved superior, outperforming the next best prompt strategy by 0.019. Decomposing the task into 19 binary judgments significantly reduced complexity, most notably improving issue extraction.
- Sample Balancing identified 8 × oversampling as optimal, which boosted compliance recall by 12%. The failure of the "Learn Errors Only" strategy (score: 0.457) underscored the necessity of balanced learning.

5.2 Additional Insights and Limitations

Exploratory work revealed that techniques like data rewriting augmentation or strategy integration caused performance degradation, indicating that the core model judgments were highly accurate and complex combinations needed caution. A rule-based post-processing engine was implemented but rarely triggered. The main limitations include room for improvement in high-level compliance judgment, a 19x increase in computational cost, and the need for further generalizability validation. The framework's engineering-oriented approach demonstrates applicability to other data-sensitive professional domains.

6 Conclusion and Future Work

6.1 Research Contributions and Summary

This study established a complete, systematic technical pathway for few-shot medical text quality control, achieving a competitive score with only 300 annotated samples.The primary contributions are threefold:

1. Phased Training Strategy: Innovatively resolved the data efficiency-generalization conflict in few-shot learning.
2. Task Decomposition via Prompting: Significantly reduced task complexity and enhanced data utilization efficiency.
3. Practical Engineering Insights: Provided a rich set of validated strategies and "negative results" as a valuable reference for applied LLM research in special-ized domains.

6.2 Future Directions

Future work will focus on two key trajectories:

Methodology Enhancement: Deepening the core phased training approach through dynamic hyperparameter configuration and multi-stage progressive learning; optimizing pseudo-label quality via model ensembles and active learning; and enhancing medical reasoning through structured knowledge integration (e.g., RAG).

Practical Deployment: Addressing computational efficiency via model lightweighting and dynamic rule selection to reduce overhead; and improving system explainability and human-in-the-loop interactive interfaces for real-world clinical integration and continuous optimization.

Acknowledgments. The authors sincerely thank the organizers of the CHIP 2025 evaluation task for providing the dataset and competition platform via Tianchi. We are especially grateful to Ms. Lu Xiang from the Institute of Automation, Chinese Academy of Sciences, for her invaluable guidance and detailed feedback during the manuscript revision process. Her expertise greatly improved the quality of this work. This study received no external funding.

References

1. Jha, A.K., DesRoches, C.M., Campbell, E.G., Donelan, K., Rao, S.R., Ferris, T.G., Shields, A., Rosenbaum, S., Blumenthal, D.: Use of electronic health records in U.S. hospitals. N. Engl. J. Med. **360**(16):1628–38 (2009). https://doi.org/10.1056/NEJMsa0900592. Epub 2009 Mar 25. PMID: 19321858
2. Cebul, R.D., Love, T.E., Jain, A.K., Hebert, C.J.: Electronic health records and quality of diabetes care. N. Engl. J. Med. **365**(9), 825–833 (2011). https://doi.org/10.1056/NEJMsa1102519. PMID: 21879900
3. Brown, T.B., Mann, B., Ryder, N., Subbiah, M., Kaplan, J., Dhariwal, P., Neelakantan, A., Shyam, P., Sastry, G., Askell, A., Agarwal, S., Herbert-Voss, A., Krueger, G., Henighan, T.J., Child, R., Ramesh, A., Ziegler, D.M., Wu, J., Winter, C., Hesse, C., Chen, M., Sigler, E., Litwin, M., Gray, S., Chess, B., Clark, J., Berner, C., McCandlish, S., Radford, A., Sutskever, I., Amodei, D.: Language Models are Few-Shot Learners. ArXiv, abs/2005.14165 (2020)
4. Rajkomar, A., Dean, J., Kohane, I.: Machine learning in medicine. N. Engl. J. Med. **380**(14), 1347–1358 (2019). https://doi.org/10.1056/NEJMra1814259. PMID: 30943338
5. Devlin, J., Chang, M., Lee, K., Toutanova, K.: BERT: Pre-training of Deep Bidirectional Transformers for Language Understanding. North American Chapter of the Association for Computational Linguistics (2019)
6. Bengio, Y., Louradour, J., Collobert, R., Weston, J.: Curriculum learning. Proceedings of the 26th Annual International Conference on Machine Learning, 41–48 (2009). https://doi.org/10.1145/1553374.1553380
7. Xie, S., Cai, H., Sun, Y., Lv, X.: LLM-DQR: LARGE language model-based automated generation of data quality rules for electronic health records. J. Biomed. Inform. **172**, 104951 (2025). https://doi.org/10.1016/j.jbi.2025.104951. Epub ahead of print. PMID: 41205689
8. Zhao, S., Feng, Q., He, Z., Sun, P., Wang, Y., Tao, X., Lu, X., Cheng, M., Wu, X., Wang, Y., Liang, W.: EMRModel: A Large Language Model for Extracting Medical Consultation Dialogues into Structured Medical Records (2025). ArXiv, abs/2504.16448
9. Hu, Y., Chen, Q., Du, J., Peng, X., Keloth, V.K., Zuo, X., Zhou, Y., Li, Z., Jiang, X., Lu, Z., Roberts, K.E., Xu, H.: Improving Large Language Models for Clinical Named Entity Recognition via Prompt Engineering (2023). ArXiv
10. Wang, L., Bi, W., Zhao, S., Li, Y., Zhang, Y., Wang, Y.: Investigating the impact of prompt engineering on the performance of large language models for standardizing obstetric diagnosis text: comparative study. JMIR Formative Res. **8**, e53216 (2024). https://doi.org/10.2196/53216
11. Chen, Y., He, Y., Yang, J., Zhang, D., Yuan, Z., Khan, M. A., Baili, J., Yee, P.L.: EMPOWER: Evolutionary Medical Prompt Optimization With Reinforcement Learning (2025). arXiv preprint arXiv:2508.17703
12. Long, D., Yen, D.N., Luu, A.T., Kawaguchi, K., Kan, M., Chen, N.F.: Multi-expert Prompting Improves Reliability, Safety and Usefulness of Large Language Models (2024). ArXiv, abs/2411.00492

13. Hein, D., Christie, A., Holcomb, M., Obafemi-Ajayi, T.: Prompts to Table: Specification and Iterative Refinement for Clinical Information Extraction with Large Language Models (2025). medRxiv. https://doi.org/10.1101/2025.02.11.25322107
14. Shah, K., et al.: Large language model prompting techniques for advancement in clinical medicine. J. Clin. Med. **13**(17), 5101 (2024). https://doi.org/10.3390/jcm13175101
15. Matos, J., Gallifant, J., Pei, J., Wong, A.I.: EHRmonize: A Framework for Medical Concept Abstraction from Electronic Health Records using Large Language Models (2024). arXiv preprint arXiv:2407.00242
16. Hu, J.E., Shen, Y., Wallis, P., Allen-Zhu, Z., Li, Y., Wang, S., Chen, W.: LoRA: Low-Rank Adaptation of Large Language Models (2021). ArXiv, abs/2106.09685

M3-MedQC: A Method for Inherent Quality Control of Electronic Medical Records Based on Large Language Models and Multi-granularity Evaluation

Tianxiang Xu[1], Xiaoyan Zhu[1(✉)], Hangyu Cheng[1], Peizhuo Yao[2], and Haoran Duan[1]

[1] School of Computer Science and Technology, Xi'an Jiaotong University, Xi'an 710049, China
tianxiangxu@stu.xjtu.edu.cn, zhu.xy@xjtu.edu.cn, 1191702980@qq.com

[2] The Second Affiliated Hospital of Xi'an Jiaotong University, Xi'an 710049, China
2541098693@qq.com

Abstract. Inherent quality control (IQC) of electronic medical records (EMRs) is a critical component in improving healthcare quality and patient safety. However, traditional manual quality control is inefficient and lacks standardized criteria. Although large language models (LLMs) have demonstrated remarkable potential in natural language processing tasks, their application to EMR quality control—where fine-grained structured output and complex logical reasoning are required—remains challenging. To address this issue, we propose M3-MedQC, a novel automated IQC framework. Specifically, we train the model based on the Qwen3 LLM using the Low-Rank Adaptation (LoRA) technique and design a multi-head classification architecture to handle multi-rule and multi-dimensional issue detection. More importantly, M3-MedQC incorporates a multi-granularity evaluation system, which not only assesses the model's ability to identify problems at the triplet level, but also evaluates its overall compliance judgment at the record level. In the China Health Information Processing Conference (CHIP) 2025 shared task, our approach achieved second place with a final score of 70.78, providing an effective technical framework and evaluation system for future research on automated medical quality control.

Keywords: Electronic medical record · Inherent quality control · Large language model · Multi-granularity evaluation

1 Introduction

The quality of inpatient care lies at the heart of healthcare service systems, directly affecting patient safety and treatment outcomes [1]. Among the various components, the inpatient electronic medical record (EMR), particularly the admission note that thoroughly documents the diagnostic and therapeutic process, serves as a fundamental source for clinical decision support, quality assessment, and medical research [2, 3]. In clinical practice, admission notes are primarily narrative texts integrating critical medical

Y. Zhang et al. (Eds.): CHIP 2025, CCIS 2884, pp. 449–462, 2026.
https://doi.org/10.1007/978-981-95-7299-1_27

information such as chief complaint, present illness, past history, physical examination, auxiliary tests, preliminary diagnosis, and treatment plan. The completeness, logical consistency, and normativity of these contents are key indicators of intrinsic document quality—collectively referred to as inherent quality control (IQC) [4].

However, in real-world clinical environments, factors such as physicians' heavy workloads, heterogeneous writing habits, and potential cognitive biases frequently lead to quality-related issues, including missing information, insufficient diagnostic reasoning, timeline inconsistencies, and irregular documentation [5]. Most healthcare institutions still rely heavily on formal quality control such as checking completion deadlines, signatures, or manually auditing random samples [6]. Such traditional approaches are inefficient, low in coverage, and highly subjective, making it difficult to establish standardized and reproducible quality management systems [7]. Hence, developing automated and intelligent IQC methods capable of understanding complex clinical logic is of great significance for improving care quality, ensuring patient safety, and optimizing clinical workflows.

Recent advances in artificial intelligence (AI) have shown promise for the automated analysis of medical texts [8, 9]. From early rule-based and statistical learning models [10, 11] to deep learning methods based on BERT [12] and its variants [13], researchers have made continuous progress in applying AI to quality control tasks. Nevertheless, these approaches suffer from limited generalization and poor understanding of complex semantics.

Large language models (LLMs), with their extensive world knowledge and deep semantic understanding, offer a new avenue to address these limitations [14]. In the medical domain, models such as Med-PaLM 2 [15] and HuatuoGPT [16] have demonstrated near-expert performance in medical question answering. However, applying LLMs to EMR quality control remains challenging in three main aspects:

- Task alignment. IQC requires models to produce fine-grained structured outputs—accurately identifying the field, issue type, and corresponding rule, and generating precise textual descriptions. This is fundamentally different from standard free-text generation or single-label classification tasks.
- Domain adaptation. Although general-domain LLMs possess broad knowledge, they still require domain-specific fine-tuning to master dozens of detailed QC rules. However, the vast parameter size of LLMs makes full-parameter fine-tuning prohibitively expensive in resource-limited settings.
- Evaluation framework. Existing studies mostly adopt instance-level metrics such as accuracy or F1-score, lacking a comprehensive evaluation system that reflects real-world QC performance [17]. The ultimate goal of QC is not merely to detect all issues but to determine the overall compliance of an EMR—a dimension often overlooked in prior work.

To foster research in this area, the China Health Information Processing Conference (CHIP) 2025[1] established an Inherent Quality Control Task targeting admission notes in inpatient EMRs, providing high-quality, multi-department, multi-disease datasets. The

[1] http://www.cips-chip.org.cn/.

task requires models to perform multi-dimensional analysis on each record and output precise structured QC results, offering a valuable benchmark for related studies.

To tackle the above challenges, we explore the application of parameter-efficient fine-tuning (PEFT) of LLMs to EMR quality control and propose M3-MedQC, an innovative Multi-head, Multi-rule, and Multi-granularity framework. Our main contributions are as follows:

- An efficient IQC framework. We propose M3-MedQC, built upon Qwen3-32B and fine-tuned using Low-Rank Adaptation (LoRA) for parameter efficiency. A multi-head classification architecture is designed to achieve high-precision detection of multiple QC rules with minimal trainable parameters.
- A novel multi-granularity evaluation system. We design a two-dimensional evaluation framework that breaks through the limitations of conventional single-metric approaches: (a) Problem extraction capability, evaluating the model's precision, recall, F1-score, and text quality at the triplet level; (b) Record-level compliance judgment, simulating real-world deduction mechanisms to assess whether a record is compliant as a whole, thereby better reflecting clinical applicability.
- Comprehensive experiments and analysis. We conduct extensive experiments, including ablation studies, to validate the effectiveness of each module. In the CHIP 2025 evaluation, our method achieved an overall score of 70.78, ranking second and outperforming most existing systems, thereby establishing a strong benchmark for future research.

2 Related Word

2.1 Automated Quality Control Techniques for EMRs

The development of automated quality control techniques for EMRs has generally undergone three stages: rule-based methods, statistical machine learning, and deep learning approaches. Early research was dominated by rule-based methods, which relied on manually constructed knowledge bases and logical rules developed by medical experts to perform pattern matching and consistency checking on EMR texts. For instance, Serhani et al. [18] developed an adaptive expert system for detecting logical conflicts between diagnostic statements and test results. Such methods are highly interpretable but suffer from poor generalization and high maintenance costs for rule bases, making them ill-suited for the diverse linguistic expressions and complex medical scenarios in clinical practice.

With the rise of machine learning, statistical approaches gradually gained traction. Researchers began using models such as Support Vector Machines (SVMs) and Conditional Random Fields (CRFs) to automatically learn QC patterns from annotated data, thereby reducing dependence on manual rules. For example, Wang et al. [19] integrated both structured and unstructured features from EMRs and applied ensemble learning to automatically classify record completeness. However, these methods still required extensive feature engineering and lacked the ability to capture deep semantic representations or perform cross-field logical reasoning.

In recent years, end-to-end deep learning models, particularly pre-trained language models such as BERT [12] and RoBERTa [20], have achieved major breakthroughs by learning powerful linguistic representations from large-scale corpora. Models such as BioBERT [21] and ClinicalBERT [13], which are further pre-trained on biomedical or clinical texts, have demonstrated significant improvements in tasks such as medical entity recognition and relation extraction. Nevertheless, directly applying these models to IQC—a task that requires deep understanding, multi-label classification, and precise structured outputs—remains challenging. These models often lack sufficient domain-specific knowledge and transparent reasoning chains.

It is also noteworthy that most prior studies, whether rule-based or deep learning-based, have evaluated model performance solely at the instance level using metrics such as precision, recall, and F1-score. Few have considered how models perform within the real-world clinical QC workflow. To address this critical gap, our study proposes a multi-granularity evaluation framework that comprehensively assesses both problem-level and record-level QC performance.

2.2 Applications of LLMs in the Medical Domain

The application of LLMs in the medical domain has evolved from general capability validation to domain-specific adaptation [22]. Early studies primarily explored the zero-shot or few-shot capabilities of general-purpose LLMs (e.g., the GPT series) in medical question answering, revealing their potential to encode broad medical knowledge [23]. In recent years, research has increasingly shifted toward the development of domain-specialized medical LLMs, which are further trained or fine-tuned on large-scale biomedical and clinical datasets to achieve substantial gains in professional competence [24]. For example, Med-PaLM 2 [15] has achieved near-expert physician-level performance on simplified medical question answering tasks, while HuatuoGPT [16], which integrates medical knowledge graphs with dialogue data, demonstrates strong reasoning and diagnostic capabilities.

In the context of EMRs, LLMs have been applied to tasks such as clinical note generation [24, 25] and diagnostic reasoning [26, 27]. However, applying LLMs to EMR quality control, which demands complex logical reasoning and structured output, remains at an early stage. The challenges outlined in Sect. 1—task alignment, domain adaptation, and evaluation design—are the main barriers. Our study directly addresses these challenges by designing a novel fine-tuning strategy and model architecture to fully explore the potential of LLMs in IQC tasks.

2.3 Parameter-Efficient Fine-Tuning Techniques

Due to the massive number of parameters in LLMs, full-parameter fine-tuning requires prohibitive computational and storage costs. To mitigate this, researchers have developed PEFT techniques, which adapt models to new tasks by updating only a small subset of parameters or introducing lightweight trainable modules, while preserving the general knowledge encoded in the pre-trained model [28]. Among PEFT methods, LoRA [29] is one of the most widely adopted for LLMs. LoRA injects two low-rank matrices (A and B) in parallel to existing weight matrices to approximate parameter updates. During inference, these updates can be merged with the original weights, introducing no additional latency.

In the medical domain, PEFT techniques are increasingly applied to address challenges such as data sensitivity, annotation scarcity, and limited computational resources [30, 31]. For example, Shi et al. [32] proposed MedAdapter, achieving performance comparable to full fine-tuning in clinical text classification tasks. However, for tasks like inherent quality control, which are multi-label, multi-dimensional, and precision-sensitive, it remains unclear how to design the most effective PEFT strategy—particularly regarding task-specific components such as classification heads.

In this study, we adopt the LoRA approach and further propose an innovative module-preserving strategy, ensuring that while fine-tuning the Qwen3 backbone, the task-critical multi-head classifier is also adequately optimized. This design achieves an excellent balance between training efficiency and model performance in complex QC scenarios.

3 Methodology

3.1 Task Definition

To enhance the automation and accuracy of EMR quality control, we formalize the problem as a multi-rule textual compliance detection task. Given an admission record D composed of multiple structured text fields:

$$D = \{f_1 : s_1, f_2 : s_2, \ldots, f_N : s_N\} \tag{1}$$

where f_i denotes the field name (e.g., chief complaint, present illness), and s_i represents its textual content.

The model is required to detect all violations in D with respect to a predefined rule base $R = \{r_1, r_2, \ldots, r_m\}$ and output a structured set of detected issues $P = \{p_1, p_2, \ldots, p_k\}$. Each issue p_k is precisely represented as a quadruple:

$$p_k = (\mathit{field}_k, \mathit{issue\ type}_k, \mathit{rule\ id}_k, \mathit{description}_k) \tag{2}$$

where $\mathit{field}_k \in \{f_1, f_2, \ldots, f_N\}$ specifies the field in which the issue occurs; $\mathit{issue\ type}_k$ denotes the problem category, including *Info Completeness, Exam Record Norm, Consistency,* and *Diagnosis Quality*; $\mathit{rule\ id}_k \in R$ identifies the violated rule in the knowledge base; and $\mathit{description}_k$ provides a natural language explanation of the violation.

The core challenges of this task lie in (1) the semantic interdependence among multiple fields, (2) the complex logical structure of quality control rules, and (3) the severe imbalance across rule samples. To address these challenges, we propose M3-MedQC, whose overall framework is illustrated in Fig. 1. It consists of four key modules: data preprocessing and prompt engineering, multi-head parameter-efficient fine-tuning, multi-rule inference and detection, and multi-granularity evaluation.

3.2 Data Preprocessing and Prompt Engineering Module

The data preprocessing and prompt engineering module transforms raw EMR data into model-processable training samples. For each quality control rule r_i, we identify a corresponding set of related fields F_{r_i}. Based on this, we design an evidence extraction mechanism as follows:

1. Traverse each field $f \in F_{r_i}$ in order of priority and retrieve its textual content s_f.
2. Segment s_f into individual sentences and select the first m sentences (with $m = 3$ in M3-MedQC) as field-level evidence.
3. If no valid evidence is found in the key fields, the first sentence from the global summary field is used as a fallback.
4. All selected evidence snippets are concatenated into a unified evidence string.

To standardize model input, we design a fixed instruction template inspired by the instruction-tuning paradigm. This template explicitly separates rule conditions from evidence content, guiding the model to focus on rule–evidence relationships and mitigating task ambiguity, while also improving instruction comprehension and transferability across rule types.

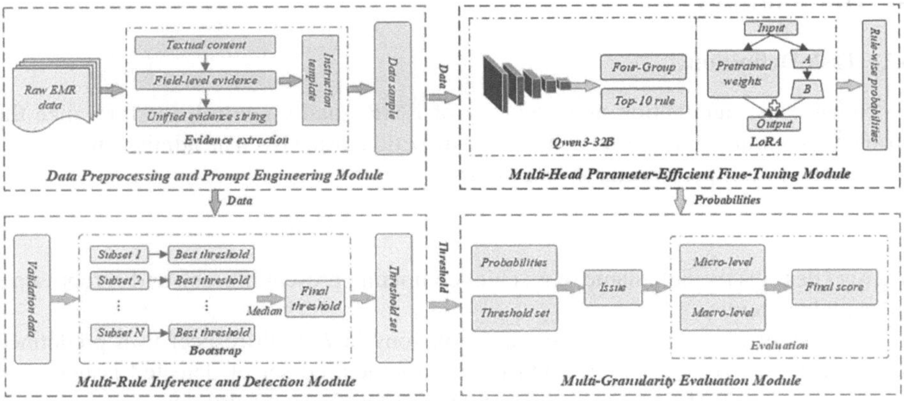

Fig. 1. Overview of the M3-MedQC framework.

3.3 Multi-head Parameter-Efficient Fine-Tuning Module

The parameter-efficient fine-tuning module comprises two major components: a multi-head classification architecture and a LoRA-based fine-tuning strategy. To address the multi-rule detection challenge inherent to medical quality control, we build upon the Qwen3-32B base model [33] and introduce two complementary multi-head classifier designs on top of its encoder layer:

- Four-Group Head Architecture. All rules are grouped into four semantic–frequency-based clusters *G1, G2, G3, G4*, each sharing an independent binary classification head $Head_g$. This design facilitates better learning for low-frequency and semantically sparse rules.
- Top-10 Rule Head Architecture. For the ten most frequent rules, each rule r_j is assigned a dedicated binary head $Head_j$, enabling specialized detection of high-impact rules.

During training, the model encodes the preprocessed sequence and performs mean pooling over the last hidden states to obtain a sequence-level representation $h_{pooled} \in$

$\mathbb{R}^h$, which is then fed into the corresponding classification head to produce rule-wise probabilities.

To achieve efficient and scalable adaptation, we apply LoRA [29] fine-tuning to Qwen3-32B. For a linear layer with base weight $W_0 \in \mathbb{R}^{d\times k}$, the forward propagation is modified as:

$$H = W_0 x + \Delta W x = W_0 x + B \cdot A x \tag{3}$$

where $A \in \mathbb{R}^{r\times k}$ and $B \in \mathbb{R}^{d\times r}$ are low-rank matrices with rank $r = \min(d, k)$. In our configuration, $r = 16$ and the scaling factor α=32. LoRA is applied to the linear projection layers *q_proj, k_proj, v_proj,* and *o_proj*, while the *modules_to_save* mechanism ensures the classification heads are fully updated during fine-tuning.

3.4 Multi-rule Inference and Detection Module

Due to the substantial differences in sample distribution and semantic complexity across rules, assigning a dedicated learnable threshold to each rule can better balance precision and recall. Thus, the multi-rule inference and detection module utilizes the fine-tuned model from the previous stage to perform either parallel or sequential scanning over all rules and outputs violation probabilities for each rule.

For each rule r_i, we determine an optimal threshold θ_i that maximizes its validation performance. To mitigate overfitting, we employ a bootstrap-based robust estimation: we resample $B = 200$ bootstrap subsets from dataset, and for each subset *b*, we conduct a grid search (step = 0.01) to find the best $\theta_i^{(b)}$.

The final threshold is the median of all $\theta_i^{(b)}$, clipped to the interval *[0.05, 0.95]* to avoid extreme values. For rules with fewer than three samples, the default threshold is fixed at 0.5. During inference, a record is deemed to violate rule r_i only if its predicted probability $p_i > \theta_i$. The corresponding descriptive information is then generated to construct the complete issue quadruple p_k.

3.5 Multi-Granularity Evaluation Module

To comprehensively evaluate the performance of medical quality control systems, we design a multi-granularity evaluation framework following the official CHIP competition standards. The evaluation comprises two complementary dimensions:

Micro-level Issue Extraction Evaluation. This dimension assesses the model's ability to extract fine-grained issues. We treat each triple (*field*, *issue type*, *rule id*) as a single unit for calculating precision (*P*), recall (*R*) and F1 score. A true positive (TP) indicates that a predicted triple exactly matches the annotated one, false positives (FP) represent predicted triples not present in annotations, and false negatives (FN) denote missed annotated triples. Additionally, the *ROUGE-L* metric is used to measure textual similarity between generated and reference descriptions. The final micro-level score is computed as:

$$Score_{extract} = 0.4 \times F1 + 0.25 \times P + 0.15 \times R + 0.2 \times ROUGE - L \tag{4}$$

Macro-level Record Compliance Evaluation. This dimension simulates real-world quality control scenarios by assessing record-level compliance decisions. Each record starts with 100 points; for every valid issue (a correctly matched TP), the score is reduced according to the predefined rule base. If the remaining score falls below 95, the record is deemed non-compliant; otherwise, it is compliant. Based on this binary classification, we again compute precision, recall, and F1, yielding the macro-level score:

$$Score_{compliant} = 0.5 \times F1 + 0.25 \times P + 0.25 \times R \tag{5}$$

The overall quality control performance is then obtained by a weighted combination of the two dimensions:

$$Score_{final} = 0.7 \times Score_{extract} + 0.3 \times Score_{compliant} \tag{6}$$

which jointly reflects the system's accuracy in fine-grained issue detection and its effectiveness in holistic compliance assessment.

In summary, M3-MedQC integrates modular system design and multi-level optimization to achieve an end-to-end QC pipeline, encompassing data construction, model training, rule-based inference, and multi-granularity evaluation.

4 Experiments

4.1 Dataset

The dataset used in this study was provided by the official CHIP2025 evaluation. Detailed statistics are presented in Table 1. The dataset contains a total of 1,000 EMRs, among which 300 records include fine-grained annotations. To meet the requirements of model training, we randomly split the dataset into training and validation sets with a 9:1 ratio. In addition, CHIP2025 provides two official test sets (A and B), each containing 300 annotated EMRs. All primary experiments in this study are evaluated on Test Set B, while ablation experiments are conducted on the validation set. The evaluation metrics follow the multi-granularity evaluation framework introduced in Sect. 3.5.

Table 1. Dataset statistics.

Dataset	# Records	# Fine-grained annotated records	# Rule instances	Positive ratio
Training	900	270	5130	~16.0%
Validation	100	30	570	~16.3%
Test A	300	300	–	–
Test B	300	300	–	–

4.2 Experimental Settings

All experiments were conducted on Ubuntu OS with Python 3.10 and PyTorch 2.5.1. All pretrained model weights were obtained from Hugging Face Models [34]. Fine-tuning and evaluation were performed on eight NVIDIA A100 GPUs (80 GB each). The AdamW [35] optimizer was adopted for all models, trained for 50 epochs, with the cross-entropy loss used as the objective function. Detailed hyperparameter configurations are summarized in Table 2.

Table 2. Hyperparameter settings.

Hyperparameter	Value	Hyperparameter	Value
Optimizer	AdamW	Learning rate	1e-4
Loss function	Cross-entropy	Batch size	8
Max sequence length	4096	LoRA rank	16
Weight decay	0.01	LoRA α	32
Warmup ratio	0.05	LoRA dropout	0.05
Gradient accumulation steps	16	LoRA target modules	q_proj, k_proj, v_proj, o_proj

4.3 Results

To comprehensively evaluate the effectiveness of the proposed method, we compared it against several representative baselines, including BERT-FT [12] (a fully fine-tuned BERT-base model) and Qwen3 zero-shot [33] (direct inference using prompt engineering without fine-tuning).

Table 3 presents the overall performance on Test Set B (only a subset of clinically relevant metrics is shown due to space limitations). As can be seen, the proposed M3-MedQC achieves the best results. For example, it attains a $Score_{final}$ of 0.7078, substantially outperforming both Qwen3 zero-shot and BERT-FT, demonstrating the overall superiority of our approach.

At the micro level, M3-MedQC achieves the highest $Score_{extract}$ (0.7166) and exhibits an exceptionally high recall (0.8250), which is crucial for QC scenarios where minimizing missed detections is more important than precision. At the macro level, M3-MedQC also delivers the best overall performance, again showing a high recall (0.7717), indicating that the model tends to classify records as non-compliant more conservatively—consistent with the clinical principle of "erring on the side of caution".

Regarding the generated explanation texts, M3-MedQC achieves a *ROUGE-L* score of 0.4836, outperforming other methods but still leaving room for improvement. We attribute this to the fact that fine-tuning encourages the model to focus on triplet classification accuracy, potentially at the expense of generation diversity and fluency, which explains the gap between model outputs and physician-annotated references.

Table 3. Overall performance comparison.

Method	ROUGE-L	$Score_{extract}$	$Score_{compliant}$	$Score_{final}$
BERT-FT	0.4359	0.6808	0.5629	0.6454
Qwen3-32B zero-shot	0.4251	0.6272	0.5614	0.6075
M3-MedQC	0.4836	0.7166	0.6873	0.7078

To further understand the behavior of M3-MedQC, we analyzed its performance on ten representative rules under the multi-head rule classification architecture. As shown in Table 4, model performance correlates positively with rule frequency. Specifically, high-frequency rules (e.g., IC-RZCB-01-V1, EN-XB-01-V1) exhibit substantially higher scores than low-frequency rules (e.g., CO-XB-03-V1), suggesting that model performance is heavily dependent on training data size. Moreover, rules concerning logical consistency perform worse on average (around 0.55), likely due to their need for cross-field reasoning, which poses a greater challenge.

Table 4. Detailed performance of ten representative rules.

Rule ID	Issue Type	Frequency (%)	P	R	F1	Score
IC-RZCB-01-V1	Info completeness	73	0.8527	0.9052	0.8782	0.8786
EN-XB-01-V1	Exam record norm	50	0.8079	0.8472	0.8271	0.8274
EN-JW-01-V1	Exam record norm	49.7	0.6685	0.9675	0.7907	0.8044
EN-RZCB-01-V1	Exam record norm	23	0.7706	0.8750	0.8195	0.8212
EN-XB-02-V1	Exam record norm	22.7	0.7000	0.8235	0.7568	0.7593
IC-XB-01-V1	Info completeness	19.7	0.4500	0.3673	0.4045	0.4066
EN-FZ-01-V1	Exam record norm	19	0.7273	0.8000	0.7619	0.7628
CO-XB-03-V1	Consistency	9.3	0.6667	0.4545	0.5405	0.5506
IC-XB-03-V1	Info completeness	7.3	0.9524	0.9091	0.9302	0.9305
CO-XB-02-V1	Consistency	7.3	0.3400	0.8500	0.4857	0.5404

4.4 Ablation Study

Due to the privacy and proprietary nature of the CHIP competition dataset, ablation studies were conducted on the validation set to verify the contribution of each component in M3-MedQC. As shown in Table 5, removing LoRA fine-tuning and performing full-parameter fine-tuning instead leads to similar performance but with significantly higher computational cost and resource consumption. When a unified threshold (0.5) is applied, performance drops notably, highlighting the importance of rule-specific threshold configuration. Similarly, using a single classification head for all rules results in substantial degradation. We attribute this to imbalanced data distributions across rules, which negatively affect model learning.

Table 5. Ablation results.

Method	P	R	F1	Score
M3-MedQC	0.6667	0.8000	0.7273	0.7303
– w/o LoRA	0.9333	0.5600	0.7000	0.7233
– Unified threshold	0.6250	0.7143	0.6667	0.6682
– Single rule head	0.8000	0.5714	0.6667	0.6762

These findings validate the effectiveness of our multi-group four-class heads and ten-rule heads, and further demonstrate that specialized modeling for high-frequency core rules yields substantial gains in medical QC tasks.

5 Discussion

The experimental results comprehensively validate the effectiveness of the proposed M3-MedQC, while the multi-granularity evaluation framework reveals the model's performance characteristics at different levels. For instance, at the micro level, M3-MedQC functions as a high-recall detector for identifying potential problems in medical records; at the macro level, it behaves as a strict quality gatekeeper that tends to make conservative compliance judgments. These characteristics make M3-MedQC particularly suitable for clinical QC scenarios, where a low tolerance for missed detections is of critical importance.

Nevertheless, the results also expose certain limitations of M3-MedQC in handling complex logical reasoning and natural language generation. This may largely stem from the limited size of the training data. In future work, we plan to enhance these capabilities by (1) expanding the training dataset, (2) incorporating external medical knowledge graphs to provide structured domain knowledge, and (3) improving the training objectives—such as treating explanatory text generation as an independent learning task—to further improve the fluency and diversity of generated descriptions.

6 Conclusion

This study systematically explores an LLM-based automated solution for quality control of EMRs—a task of great clinical significance. To address the challenges posed by diverse QC rules and structured output requirements, we propose a comprehensive framework named M3-MedQC. First, by leveraging LoRA, we efficiently adapt the general-purpose Qwen3-32B model to the specialized medical QC domain, fine-tuning only approximately 0.26% of parameters while achieving a strong balance between performance and efficiency. Second, we design a multi-head classifier architecture, where high-frequency rules are equipped with dedicated classification heads, significantly improving the model's accuracy in rule-level detection.

More importantly, we go beyond conventional single-level evaluation schemes by introducing a multi-granularity evaluation framework. This framework assesses not only the model's micro-level recognition ability (i.e., identifying rule violations within medical records) but also its macro-level judgment capability, simulating real-world QC workflows that assess the overall compliance of an entire EMR. This provides a more comprehensive and clinically grounded perspective for evaluating model performance in IQC tasks.

Acknowledgments. This work was supported by the National Natural Science Foundation of China under Grant Nos. 72274152, 62402376, and 62572389.

References

1. Bates, D.W., et al.: The safety of inpatient health care. N. Engl. J. Med. **388**, 142–153 (2023)
2. Romano, M.J., Stafford, R.S.: Electronic health records and clinical decision support systems: impact on national ambulatory care quality. Arch. Intern. Med. **171**, 897–903 (2011)
3. Park, Y.-T., Kim, Y.S., Yi, B.-K., Kim, S.M.: Clinical decision support functions and digitalization of clinical documents of electronic medical record systems. Healthc. Inform. Res. **25**, 115–123 (2019)
4. Zhang, S., Quan, Y.Y., Chen, J.: Construction and application of an ICU nursing electronic medical record quality control system in a Chinese tertiary hospital: a prospective controlled trial. BMC Nurs. **23**, 493 (2024)
5. Wright, A., et al.: Analysis of clinical decision support system malfunctions: a case series and survey. J. Am. Med. Inform. Assoc. **23**, 1068–1076 (2016)
6. Xie, P., et al.: Application and research of closed loop quality control management system for electronic nursing documents. Chin. J. Nurs. **53**, 806–809 (2018)
7. Wang, L.-R., Wang, Y., Lou, Y., Li, Y., Zhang, X.-G.: The role of quality control circles in sustained improvement of medical quality. SpringerPlus **2**, 141 (2013)
8. Ostherr, K.: Artificial intelligence and medical humanities. J. Med. Human. **43**, 211–232 (2022)
9. Ahmad, Z., Rahim, S., Zubair, M., Abdul-Ghafar, J.: Artificial intelligence (AI) in medicine, current applications and future role with special emphasis on its potential and promise in pathology: present and future impact, obstacles including costs and acceptance among pathologists, practical and philosophical considerations. A comprehensive review. Diagnostic Pathol. **16**, 24 (2021)

10. Wang, Y., et al.: A clinical text classification paradigm using weak supervision and deep representation. BMC Med. Inform. Decis. Mak. **19**, 1 (2019)
11. Liu, S. et al.: Implementation of a cohort retrieval system for clinical data repositories using the observational medical outcomes partnership common data model: proof-of-concept system validation. JMIR Med. Inf. 8 (2020)
12. Devlin, J., Chang, M.-W., Lee, K., Toutanova, K.: BERT: Pre-training of deep bidirectional transformers for language understanding. In: Proceedings of the 2019 Conference of the North American Chapter of the Association for Computational Linguistics: Human Language Technologies, Volume 1 (Long and Short Papers), pp. 4171–4186. Association for Computational Linguistics (2019)
13. Alsentzer, E., et al.: Publicly available clinical BERT embeddings. In: Proceedings of the 2nd Clinical Natural Language Processing Workshop, pp. 72–78. Association for Computational Linguistics (2019)
14. Touvron, H. et al.: Llama: Open and efficient foundation language models. arXiv preprint arXiv:2302.13971 (2023)
15. Singhal, K., et al.: Toward expert-level medical question answering with large language models. Nat. Med. **31**, 943–950 (2025)
16. Zhang, H. et al.: HuatuoGPT, Towards taming language model to be a doctor. In: Findings of the Association for Computational Linguistics: EMNLP 2023, pp. 10859–10885. Association for Computational Linguistics, (2023)
17. Liu, H., Li, Z., Song, Z.: Comprehensive lifecycle quality control of medical data - automated monitoring and feedback mechanisms based on artificial intelligence. Technol. Health Care **33**, 2125–2135 (2025)
18. Serhani, M.A., Benharref, A., Nujum, A.R.: An adaptive expert system for automated advices generation-based semi-continuous M-health monitoring. In: Brain Informatics and Health, pp. 388–399. Springer International Publishing (2014)
19. Wang, M., Wei, Z., Jia, M., Chen, L., Ji, H.: Deep learning model for multi-classification of infectious diseases from unstructured electronic medical records. BMC Med. Inform. Decis. Mak. **22**, 41 (2022)
20. Liu, Y. et al.: RoBERTa: A Robustly Optimized BERT Pretraining Approach. ArXiv abs/1907.11692, (2019)
21. Lee, J., et al.: BioBERT: a pre-trained biomedical language representation model for biomedical text mining. Bioinformatics (Oxford, England) **36**, 1234–1240 (2019)
22. Wang, D., Zhang, S.: Large language models in medical and healthcare fields: applications, advances, and challenges. Artif. Intell. Rev. **57**, 299 (2024)
23. Liévin, V., Hother, C.E., Motzfeldt, A.G., Winther, O.: Can large language models reason about medical questions? Patterns 5 (2024)
24. Kumichev, G., et al.: MedSyn: LLM-based synthetic medical text generation framework. In: ECML PKDD 2024, pp. 215–230. Springer Nature Switzerland (2024)
25. Zhang, X., et al.: Data augmented large language models for medical record generation. Appl. Intell. **55**, 88 (2024)
26. Kang, L. et al.: LLM-driven medical document analysis: enhancing trustworthy pathology and differential diagnosis. In: International Conference on Document Analysis and Recognition, pp. 613–628. Springer Nature Switzerland (2025)
27. Xu, R., Shi, W., Wang, J., Zhou, J., Yang, C.: MedAssist: LLM-empowered medical assistant for assisting the scrutinization and comprehension of electronic health records. Companion Proceedings of the ACM on Web Conference 2025, pp. 2931–2934. Association for Computing Machinery, Sydney NSW, Australia (2025)
28. Han, Z., Gao, C., Liu, J., Zhang, J., Zhang, S.Q.: Parameter-efficient fine-tuning for large models: a comprehensive survey. arXiv preprint arXiv:2403.14608 (2024)

29. Hu, E.J., et al.: Lora: Low-rank adaptation of large language models. ICLR **1**, 3 (2022)
30. Balne, C.C.S., Bhaduri, S., Roy, T., Jain, V., Chadha, A.: Parameter efficient fine tuning: a comprehensive analysis across applications. arXiv preprint arXiv:2404.13506 (2024)
31. Khan, W. et al.: A Comprehensive survey of foundation models in medicine. IEEE Reviews in Biomedical Engineering 1–22 (2025)
32. Shi, W. et al.: MedAdapter: efficient test-time adaptation of large language models towards medical reasoning. In: Proceedings of the 2024 Conference on Empirical Methods in Natural Language Processing, pp. 22294–22314. Association for Computational Linguistics (2024)
33. Yang, A. et al.: Qwen3 technical report. arXiv preprint arXiv:2505.09388 (2025)
34. Wolf, T. et al.: Transformers: state-of-the-art natural language processing. Proceedings of the 2020 Conference on Empirical Methods in Natural Language Processing: System Demonstrations, pp. 38–45. Association for Computational Linguistics, Online (2020)
35. Loshchilov, I., Hutter, F.: Decoupled weight decay regularization. arXiv preprint arXiv:1711.05101 (2017)

Quality Control of Electronic Medical Records Content Based on Q-LoRA Fine-Tuning and a Hybrid Model-Rule Approach

Wusi Zhen, Yitong Pan, Yuxin Liu, and Junwen Duan(✉)

Hunan Provincial Key Lab on Bioinformatics, School of Computer Science and Engineering, Central South University, Changsha, China
{zhenwusi,panyitong,liuyuxin,jwduan}@csu.edu.cn

Abstract. High-quality electronic medical records (EMRs) are fundamental for patient safety, clinical decision-making, and precision medicine. However, traditional manual quality control is inefficient, inconsistent, and inadequate for the growing complexity of clinical data. We introduce a large language model (LLM)-based framework that combines parameter-efficient Q-LoRA fine-tuning with task decomposition to enable automated, rule-specific validation of EMR content. This approach leverages iteratively optimized instruction prompts to guide the model through focused single-rule checks, thereby enhancing both accuracy and explainability. Evaluated on a curated dataset using the Qwen3-32B model, our method achieved a comprehensive score of 0.6918, demonstrating a substantial performance improvement over untuned baselines. By integrating intelligent instruction generation, modular task decomposition, and scalable fine-tuning, this framework provides a robust and adaptive solution for clinical data quality assurance. Our study underscores the potential of combining large-scale generative models with domain-specific adaptation to transform medical data governance and set new benchmarks for automated, high-fidelity clinical data evaluation.

Keywords: Electronic Medical Records · Quality Control · Prompt Engineering · Q-LoRA Fine-Tuning

1 Introduction

With the widespread digitalization of healthcare, EMRs have become the core data infrastructure in clinical practice. Narrative medical records, particularly those from a patient's initial hospitalization, are critical for subsequent diagnosis, treatment, and clinical research. The quality of these records—specifically their completeness, consistency, and standardization—directly impacts clinical outcomes. However, variations in physicians' documentation habits and the complexity of clinical scenarios often lead to information gaps, logical inconsistencies,

Y. Zhang et al. (Eds.): CHIP 2025, CCIS 2884, pp. 463–474, 2026.
https://doi.org/10.1007/978-981-95-7299-1_28

and non-standardized descriptions. Traditional quality control, which relies on manual review, is inefficient, costly, and prone to inconsistent standards and subjective bias.

The emergence of LLMs offers new avenues to address these challenges. LLMs based on the Transformer architecture acquire extensive linguistic knowledge and powerful reasoning capabilities through pretraining on massive text corpora [21]. Nevertheless, applying general-purpose LLMs to highly specialized, rule-driven tasks such as quality control of medical records presents two primary challenges. First, crafting high-quality, unambiguous instructions is critical to ensure that the model accurately comprehends the task. Second, medical record quality control is an inherently complex, multi-objective verification task. Tasking the model with identifying all potential violations across multiple rules in a single pass can impose an excessive cognitive load, leading to omissions or misjudgments.

To overcome these challenges, this paper introduces an end-to-end solution. We first employ the DeepSeek-V3 model to generate high-quality instruction prompts through an iterative optimization process, thereby replacing the cumbersome and subjective process of manual prompt design. Next, we adopt a task decomposition strategy, breaking down the complex multi-rule quality control task into 19 focused, independent sub-tasks. This allows the model to concentrate on one rule at a time during both training and inference. The Qwen3-32B model is then adapted to the medical domain by applying Q-LoRA parameter-efficient fine-tuning on the dataset constructed using this strategy. This paper provides a detailed account of the complete methodology—from automated prompt generation and specialized fine-tuning to serialized inference—and offers a practical technical framework for the application of LLMs in medical quality control.

2 Related Work

2.1 Large Language Models

In recent years, LLMs have demonstrated transformative progress in natural language processing. Pretrained on massive and diverse corpora, these models, often containing hundreds of billions of parameters, exhibit exceptional capabilities in tasks such as machine translation, sentiment analysis, and contextual text generation. Early pretrained language models like BERT [6] primarily focused on natural language understanding and relied on fine-tuning to adapt to specific downstream applications. Subsequent generative models, such as GPT-2, showcased strong multi-task capabilities without task-specific training [18]. The current generation of LLMs, exemplified by the GPT series [3] and LLaMA [20], has established a new technological paradigm. By leveraging autoregressive architectures and instruction fine-tuning [16], these models achieve remarkable performance in open-domain dialogue, complex reasoning, and instruction-following, even in few-shot or zero-shot scenarios.

The robust transfer learning and task adaptation capabilities of LLMs have spurred their adoption across various fields, including education, finance, and healthcare. In the medical domain, initial efforts centered on adapting BERT-style models to clinical text. Domain-specific pretraining on biomedical corpora, as exemplified by BioBERT [7], was a strategy that proved both common and effective. More recently, the paradigm has shifted toward large-scale generative models. Researchers have developed specialized LLMs like Med-PaLM [19], which are engineered to meet the stringent requirements of professionalism and reliability for tasks such as clinical text processing and knowledge-based question answering. However, training new medical LLMs from scratch demands substantial computational resources and vast amounts of medical data. Consequently, in practical hospital settings, directly deploying existing large models or applying lightweight adaptation techniques is often more feasible. For EMR quality control, traditional approaches rely heavily on manual review or shallow, rule-based pattern matching, rendering them incapable of effectively analyzing the complex semantic logic in free-text records or assessing consistency across multiple sections. In contrast, LLMs, with their powerful semantic understanding capabilities, can deeply parse medical texts to evaluate information completeness, diagnostic evidence sufficiency, and the logical consistency of narrative descriptions within EMRs—a capability already demonstrated in clinical information extraction tasks [1].

2.2 Prompt Engineering

The imperative to enhance the semantic and logical accuracy of clinical texts has driven the adoption of LLM-based approaches for medical document quality management. In this context, prompt engineering has emerged as a crucial discipline, facilitating the adaptation of general-purpose language models to specialized domains [15] and unlocking their zero-shot reasoning capabilities [12]. Techniques involving precise and directive prompts, such as Chain-of-Thought (CoT) reasoning [23], can effectively steer models toward generating outputs that adhere to clinical standards. The inclusion of representative examples or clearly defined quality control criteria within prompts can further improve model performance on free-text records. Moreover, crafting prompts with language that conforms to medical writing standards and aligns with clinical narrative logic can bolster the model's comprehension of medical terminology, diagnostic sequences, and causal relationships. Consequently, the continuous optimization of prompt templates and semantic guidance strategies is essential for enhancing the stability of LLMs in medical quality control tasks, offering a scalable pathway for automated EMR quality assessment.

2.3 Parameter-Efficient Fine-Tuning

Fine-tuning is a widely employed technique for adapting large-scale language models to new domains and tasks, a process that uses domain-specific data to specialize the model and improve task alignment. However, conventional full-parameter fine-tuning is often computationally prohibitive and can yield suboptimal results, particularly when the target domain diverges significantly from the pretraining corpus. These limitations have spurred the development of Parameter-Efficient Fine-Tuning (PEFT) methods. Early approaches like Adapter Tuning [8] introduced the concept of modifying only a small fraction of the model's parameters. Subsequent innovations such as Prefix-Tuning [14] and Prompt Tuning [13] further refined this principle.

PEFT methods achieve efficient domain adaptation by drastically reducing the number of trainable parameters. Low-Rank Adaptation (LoRA) [9], for instance, injects trainable low-rank matrices into the model's linear layers. This significantly curtails the number of adaptable parameters while maintaining or even enhancing performance in multi-task and cross-domain scenarios. Extending this technique, Q-LoRA [5] integrates low-rank adaptation with low-bit quantization. This combination further minimizes the memory footprint, making it feasible to fine-tune exceptionally large models on a single GPU or in other resource-constrained environments.

3 Methodology

3.1 Data Preprocessing

Rule Parsing, Field Extraction, and Data Partitioning. Firstly, the quality control rules, initially documented in tabular format, were converted into structured JSON objects. Each JSON object comprehensively encapsulated the problem type, definition, typical defects, relevant fields, and a unique rule identifier, providing a standardized reference for automated quality control. From these structured rules, we extracted and generated a master list of all required quality control fields, serving as a baseline for subsequent data processing. Subsequently, based on this master list, the EMR texts for both training and testing were partitioned. To ensure precise segmentation, this process employed field-based matching, thereby avoiding reliance on inconsistent delimiters such as line breaks or punctuation. The selection of these key fields was strictly guided by the Ministry of Health's "Basic Specifications for Medical Record Writing" and cross-validated against both the training and testing datasets to ensure their applicability and accuracy.

Data Structuring and Feature Extraction. For data structuring, each quality control rule was applied sequentially. The text corresponding to the rule's specified quality control fields was extracted, generating key-value pairs where the field name served as the key and the extracted text as the value. This structured format was crucial for creating rule-specific inputs for model training and inference, transforming unstructured textual data into features directly usable by the model.

Training Data Labeling and Test Set Construction. Finally, to prepare the training data, we implemented a labeling mechanism. For each rule, records that did not violate the rule were labeled "qualified." Records that did violate it were labeled "unqualified," and an explanation derived from the rule's description was appended. The test set was constructed similarly by filtering the data based on the quality control fields relevant to each individual rule, ensuring the accuracy and relevance of the test data.

3.2 LLM-Assisted Instruction Generation and Iterative Optimization

Our methodology for prompt engineering advanced beyond rule-based templates and manual example augmentation to a more refined, LLM-assisted workflow, drawing inspiration from automatic prompt engineering (APE) [26] and self-instruction tuning [22]. The process began by leveraging the Deepseek-V3 model to perform an in-depth analysis of our training data, identifying the frequency and primary causes of quality control failures for each rule. These data-driven insights were then integrated with the core quality control logic and a small set of seed prompts to guide Deepseek-V3 in generating an initial set of instruction prompts.

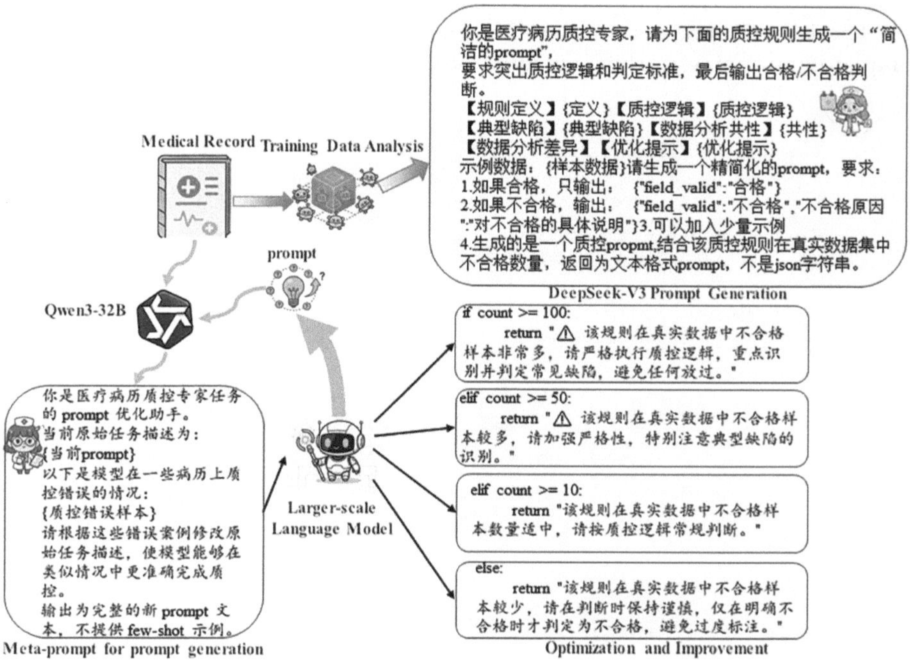

Fig. 1. LLM-based prompt generation workflow.

While these initial prompts provided a strong baseline, they required further refinement to address two key issues: the imbalanced distribution of “qualified” and “unqualified” samples across different rules, and potential biases inherent in some seed prompts. To overcome this, we designed and implemented an automated optimization loop, conceptually analogous to the DSPy framework [10], to programmatically enhance the prompts. In each iteration, the generated prompts were first validated using sub-70B parameter models (e.g., Qwen3-32B). Errors identified during this validation were collected and used as corrective feedback for the ultra-large Deepseek-V3 model, which then produced a refined prompt set. This cycle was repeated, selecting the best-performing prompts at each stage. To mitigate the risk of overfitting, the iterative process was terminated when validation accuracy reached 95%. Our experiments determined that 10 iterations yielded the optimal prompt set for our quality control tasks. The complete LLM-based prompt generation workflow is illustrated in Fig. 1.

3.3 Task Decomposition and Q-LoRA Fine-Tuning

We constructed our fine-tuning dataset based on the principle of task decomposition [11], wherein each (EMR, rule) pair was transformed into an independent training instance. The prompt for each instance contained instructions specifically crafted for the corresponding rule to maximize its relevance and utility. The Qwen3-32B model was then fine-tuned on this decomposed dataset. The complete fine-tuning workflow is illustrated in Fig. 2.

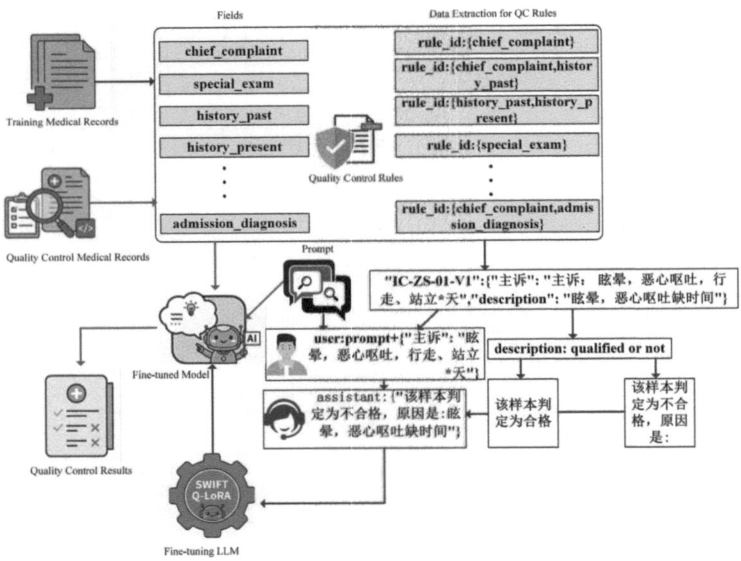

Fig. 2. Fine-tuning Workflow of the Qwen3-32B Model.

The fine-tuning process was implemented using the SWIFT framework with Q-LoRA. Model weights were loaded in 4-bit precision, and training was confined to the LoRA adapters (rank = 8) injected into all linear layers. To optimize training efficiency on a single NVIDIA A800 GPU (80GB), we also employed Flash Attention and sequence packing techniques, as proposed by Dao et al. [4].

LoRA, a lightweight fine-tuning method, is widely adopted for the parameter-efficient adaptation of large models. The method is based on the foundational insight that weight updates for adapting pre-trained models exhibit a low intrinsic rank. Therefore, instead of directly updating the original weight matrix $W \in \mathbb{R}^{m \times n}$, LoRA freezes the original weights and approximates the parameter increment ΔW using a pair of low-rank matrices, $A \in \mathbb{R}^{m \times r}$ and $B \in \mathbb{R}^{r \times n}$, where $r \ll \min(m, n)$

$$\Delta W = AB \tag{1}$$

Consequently, the model's forward pass is modified to:

$$h = Wx + \Delta Wx = Wx + ABx \tag{2}$$

During training, only matrices A and B are updated, while the original weights W remain unchanged. For inference, the effective weights W' are computed by merging the updates with the original weights:

$$W' = W + AB \tag{3}$$

By reducing the number of trainable parameters from $m \times n$ to $r(m + n)$, LoRA significantly decreases memory and computational overhead during training, while achieving performance comparable to that of full-parameter fine-tuning.

Q-LoRA extends this principle to further enhance resource efficiency, enabling the fine-tuning of exceptionally large models on a single GPU. Its core innovation is the quantization of the pretrained model weights into a 4-bit NormalFloat (NF4) format—an information-theoretically optimal data type that substantially reduces model size while preserving distributional fidelity. Specifically, the original weights W are quantized to $\hat{W}_{\text{NF4}}$ using a non-uniform quantization function $\mathcal{Q}_{\text{NF4}}(\cdot)$.

To mitigate performance degradation from quantization, Q-LoRA dynamically dequantizes these low-precision weights to a higher-precision format (e.g., bfloat16) during the forward and backward passes:

$$\tilde{W} = \mathcal{D}(\hat{W}_{\text{NF4}}) \tag{4}$$

Here, $\mathcal{D}(\cdot)$ represents the dequantization operation. Furthermore, Q-LoRA incorporates a double quantization strategy, where the quantization constants themselves are quantized to further reduce the memory footprint. When combined with other memory-saving techniques like Paged Attention and sequence packing, Q-LoRA provides a practical solution for adapting large models in resource-constrained environments.

3.4 Inference Workflow and Post-processing

Following a serialized inference process where the fine-tuned model evaluates each EMR against 19 distinct rules, the raw outputs undergo a two-stage, rule-based post-processing module to maximize accuracy. First, a correction step increases precision by filtering out known LLM false positives using a predefined list of keywords. Second, a completion step enhances recall by applying deterministic rules to the original EMR text. This second stage identifies unambiguous errors—such as empty mandatory fields or simple formatting violations—that the LLM may have missed. A new issue is added only if it was not previously detected by the model, ensuring the final output synergistically combines the LLM's deep semantic analysis with the reliability of hard-coded validation.

4 Experiments

4.1 Dataset and Evaluation Metrics

Our experiments were conducted on the official dataset from the 11th China Health Information Processing Conference (CHIP2025) shared task on admission record quality control. This dataset comprises 300 manually annotated training samples, which provided a robust foundation for model fine-tuning.

To evaluate model performance, we adopted the official Comprehensive Score as the primary metric. This composite metric is designed to assess both the model's accuracy in identifying specific quality issues and its correctness in making an overall compliance judgment for the entire medical record. By balancing precision and recall across these aspects, the Comprehensive Score offers a holistic evaluation of the model's practical effectiveness in the quality control task. It is calculated as follows:

$$\text{Score}_{\textbf{final}} = 0.7 \times \text{Score}_{\textbf{extract}} + 0.3 \times \text{Score}_{\textbf{compliant}} \tag{5}$$

The issue extraction score $\text{Score}_{\textbf{extract}}$ is defined as:

$$\text{Score}_{\textbf{extract}} = 0.4 \times F1 + 0.25 \times P + 0.15 \times R + 0.2 \times \text{ROUGE-L} \tag{6}$$

The overall compliance score $\text{Score}_{\textbf{compliant}}$ is defined as:

$$\text{Score}_{\textbf{compliant}} = 0.5 \times F1 + 0.25 \times P + 0.25 \times R \tag{7}$$

4.2 Experimental Setup

All experiments were conducted on a single NVIDIA A800 GPU equipped with 80GB of VRAM. Our software stack was built upon the SWIFT framework, leveraging PyTorch [17] as the core deep learning library. Key dependencies included the Transformers library [24] for model handling, bitsandbytes for quantization, and flash-attn for optimized attention mechanisms.

4.3 Fine-Tuning Implementation Details

We fine-tuned the Qwen3-32B base model [2] using Alibaba's open-source SWIFT framework [25]. Model weights were loaded in the NF4 data type to reduce memory footprint. LoRA modules were injected into all linear layers, with the lora_rank set to 8 and the scaling factor lora_alpha set to 32, to balance

Table 1. Hyperparameters for Q-LoRA Fine-tuning of Qwen3-32B.

Parameter	Value
Base Model	Qwen3-32B
Max Sequence Length	8192
Epochs	1
Batch Size (per device)	1
Gradient Accumulation Steps	8
Learning Rate	1e-4
Warmup Ratio	0.05
Quantization Bits	4
BNB Compute Dtype	bfloat16
BNB Double Quantization	True
LoRA Rank	8
LoRA Alpha	32
LoRA Target Modules	All linear layers
Attention Implementation	FlashAttention
Sequence Packing	True
Liger Kernel	True
Dataloader Workers	4

model performance and computational cost. Flash Attention and Packing optimizations were enabled during training to improve throughput and GPU memory utilization on a single A800 GPU. Leveraging the "Intelligent Instruction" and "Task Decomposition" strategies, the model learned and consolidated 19 professional judgment capabilities during fine-tuning, resulting in strong task-specific adaptability. During inference, a serialized verification workflow was adopted, consisting of 19 steps. Each step utilized dedicated prompts constructed according to the rules described in Sect. 3.3 for independent reasoning. After inference, results were cleaned and supplemented based on rules to ensure accuracy and consistency. This approach demonstrated strong adaptability and stability in single-rule judgment tasks, validating the feasibility of efficient fine-tuning for complex instruction-based tasks.

The fine-tuning of the Qwen3-32B base model [2] was conducted using the open-source SWIFT framework [25]. To optimize memory usage, the model's weights were loaded in the 4-bit NF4 data type. LoRA modules were injected into all linear layers to facilitate parameter-efficient adaptation. Training was further accelerated by enabling Flash Attention and sequence packing, which enhanced throughput and memory utilization on the A800 GPU. The specific hyperparameters for this Q-LoRA process, which were chosen to balance model capability and computational overhead, are detailed in Table 1.

Through this fine-tuning process, guided by our "Intelligent Instruction" and "Task Decomposition" strategies, the model was effectively trained to master 19 distinct quality control sub-tasks. This modular training strategy directly informed our inference process, for which we implemented a serialized verification workflow. Each EMR is evaluated sequentially across 19 steps, and in each step, the model performs an independent assessment against a single quality control rule using its specialized prompt (as detailed in Sect. 3.3). Following inference, a rule-based post-processing step was applied to clean and standardize the model's outputs. This decoupled approach demonstrated remarkable stability and validated the efficacy of using PEFT for complex, multi-faceted, instruction-based tasks.

4.4 Quality Control Results Analysis

To evaluate the efficacy of our proposed methods, we conducted a series of comparative experiments. We assessed the performance of different model sizes (Qwen3-8B and Qwen3-32B) and measured the impact of both our Q-LoRA fine-tuning process and a rule-based post-processing step. The results, benchmarked using the official Comprehensive Score, are summarized in Table 2.

Table 2. Comparative Results of Different Model Configurations.

Configuration	Comprehensive Score
Qwen3-8B + Fine-Tuned	0.5569
Qwen3-8B + Fine-Tuned + Post-Processed	0.5725
Qwen3-32B	0.5973
Qwen3-32B + Fine-Tuned	0.6906
Qwen3-32B + Fine-Tuned + Post-Processed	0.6918

The baseline performance, established by the un-tuned Qwen3-32B model, was a Comprehensive Score of 0.5973. Our full proposed pipeline—combining the larger Qwen3-32B model with Q-LoRA fine-tuning and post-processing—achieved the top score of 0.6918. This represents a relative performance gain of approximately 15.8% over the baseline, showcasing a significant enhancement in quality control capabilities.

5 Conclusion

In this study, we introduced an automated framework that overcomes the limitations of manual EMR quality control by synergizing a task decomposition strategy with LLM-powered instruction optimization. By applying Q-LoRA fine-tuning to the Qwen3-32B model, we achieved a 15.8% improvement in the Comprehensive Score, increasing it from 0.5973 to 0.6918. This result validates our hybrid approach, proving that parameter-efficient fine-tuning, guided by modular, rule-specific instructions, is a highly effective method for specializing LLMs for complex clinical validation tasks and provides a viable blueprint for their application in medical governance.

Looking ahead, we will extend this work by exploring multimodal data integration, parallel validation architectures for enhanced efficiency, direct integration with hospital information systems (HIS) for real-time feedback, and continuous learning mechanisms to ensure long-term model adaptation and reliability.

Acknowledgments. This work was supported in part by National Natural Science Foundation of China (No. 62576363), the Natural Science Foundation of Hunan Province (No. 2025JJ50342) and Changsha Municipal Natural Science Foundation Project (No. kq2502144). This work was carried out in part using computing resources at the High-Performance Computing Center of Central South University.

References

1. Agrawal, M., Hegselmann, S., Lang, H., Kim, Y., Sontag, D.: Large language models are few-shot clinical information extractors. arXiv preprint arXiv:2205.12689 (2022)
2. Bai, J., Bai, S., Chu, Y., Cui, Z., Dang, K., Deng, X., Fan, Y., Ge, W., Han, Y., Huang, F., et al.: Qwen technical report. arXiv preprint arXiv:2309.16609 (2023)
3. Brown, T., Mann, B., Ryder, N., Subbiah, M., Kaplan, J.D., Dhariwal, P., Neelakantan, A., Shyam, P., Sastry, G., Askell, A., et al.: Language models are few-shot learners. Adv. Neural. Inf. Process. Syst. **33**, 1877–1901 (2020)
4. Dao, T., Fu, D., Ermon, S., Rudra, A., Ré, C.: Flashattention: fast and memory-efficient exact attention with io-awareness. Adv. Neural. Inf. Process. Syst. **35**, 16344–16359 (2022)
5. Dettmers, T., Pagnoni, A., Holtzman, A., Zettlemoyer, L.: Qlora: efficient finetuning of quantized llms. Adv. Neural. Inf. Process. Syst. **36**, 10088–10115 (2023)
6. Devlin, J., Chang, M.W., Lee, K., Toutanova, K.: Bert: pre-training of deep bidirectional transformers for language understanding. In: Proceedings of the 2019 Conference of the North American Chapter of the Association for Computational Linguistics: Human Language Technologies, Volume 1 (Long and Short Papers), pp. 4171–4186 (2019)
7. Gu, Y., Tinn, R., Cheng, H., Lucas, M., Usuyama, N., Liu, X., Naumann, T., Gao, J., Poon, H.: Domain-specific language model pretraining for biomedical natural language processing. ACM Trans. Comput. Healthc. (HEALTH) **3**(1), 1–23 (2021)
8. Houlsby, N., Giurgiu, A., Jastrzebski, S., Morrone, B., De Laroussilhe, Q., Gesmundo, A., Attariyan, M., Gelly, S.: Parameter-efficient transfer learning for nlp. In: International Conference on Machine Learning, pp. 2790–2799. PMLR (2019)
9. Hu, E.J., Shen, Y., Wallis, P., Allen-Zhu, Z., Li, Y., Wang, S., Wang, L., Chen, W., et al.: Lora: low-rank adaptation of large language models. ICLR **1**(2), 3 (2022)
10. Khattab, O., Singhvi, A., Maheshwari, P., Zhang, Z., Santhanam, K., Vardhamanan, S., Haq, S., Sharma, A., Joshi, T.T., Moazam, H., et al.: Dspy: compiling declarative language model calls into self-improving pipelines. arXiv preprint arXiv:2310.03714 (2023)

11. Khot, T., Trivedi, H., Finlayson, M., Fu, Y., Richardson, K., Clark, P., Sabharwal, A.: Decomposed prompting: a modular approach for solving complex tasks. arXiv preprint arXiv:2210.02406 (2022)
12. Kojima, T., Gu, S.S., Reid, M., Matsuo, Y., Iwasawa, Y.: Large language models are zero-shot reasoners. Adv. Neural. Inf. Process. Syst. **35**, 22199–22213 (2022)
13. Lester, B., Al-Rfou, R., Constant, N.: The power of scale for parameter-efficient prompt tuning. arXiv preprint arXiv:2104.08691 (2021)
14. Li, X.L., Liang, P.: Prefix-tuning: optimizing continuous prompts for generation. arXiv preprint arXiv:2101.00190 (2021)
15. Liu, P., Yuan, W., Fu, J., Jiang, Z., Hayashi, H., Neubig, G.: Pre-train, prompt, and predict: a systematic survey of prompting methods in natural language processing. ACM Comput. Surv. **55**(9), 1–35 (2023)
16. Ouyang, L., Wu, J., Jiang, X., Almeida, D., Wainwright, C., Mishkin, P., Zhang, C., Agarwal, S., Slama, K., Ray, A., et al.: Training language models to follow instructions with human feedback. Adv. Neural. Inf. Process. Syst. **35**, 27730–27744 (2022)
17. Paszke, A., Gross, S., Massa, F., Lerer, A., Bradbury, J., Chanan, G., Killeen, T., Lin, Z., Gimelshein, N., Antiga, L., et al.: Pytorch: an imperative style, high-performance deep learning library. Adv. Neural Inf. Process. Syst. **32** (2019)
18. Radford, A., Wu, J., Child, R., Luan, D., Amodei, D., Sutskever, I., et al.: Language models are unsupervised multitask learners. OpenAI Blog **1**(8), 9 (2019)
19. Singhal, K., Azizi, S., Tu, T., Mahdavi, S.S., Wei, J., Chung, H.W., Scales, N., Tanwani, A., Cole-Lewis, H., Pfohl, S., et al.: Large language models encode clinical knowledge. Nature **620**(7972), 172–180 (2023)
20. Touvron, H., Martin, L., Stone, K., Albert, P., Almahairi, A., Babaei, Y., Bashlykov, N., Batra, S., Bhargava, P., Bhosale, S., et al.: Llama 2: open foundation and fine-tuned chat models. arXiv preprint arXiv:2307.09288 (2023)
21. Vaswani, A., Shazeer, N., Parmar, N., Uszkoreit, J., Jones, L., Gomez, A.N., Kaiser, Ł., Polosukhin, I.: Attention is all you need. Adv. Neural Inf. Process. Syst. **30** (2017)
22. Wang, Y., Kordi, Y., Mishra, S., Liu, A., Smith, N.A., Khashabi, D., Hajishirzi, H.: Self-instruct: aligning language models with self-generated instructions. In: Proceedings of the 61st Annual Meeting of the Association for Computational Linguistics (Volume 1: Long Papers), pp. 13484–13508 (2023)
23. Wei, J., Wang, X., Schuurmans, D., Bosma, M., Xia, F., Chi, E., Le, Q.V., Zhou, D., et al.: Chain-of-thought prompting elicits reasoning in large language models. Adv. Neural. Inf. Process. Syst. **35**, 24824–24837 (2022)
24. Wolf, T., Debut, L., Sanh, V., Chaumond, J., Delangue, C., Moi, A., Cistac, P., Rault, T., Louf, R., Funtowicz, M., et al.: Transformers: state-of-the-art natural language processing. In: Proceedings of the 2020 Conference on Empirical Methods in Natural Language Processing: System Demonstrations, pp. 38–45 (2020)
25. Zhao, Y., Huang, J., Hu, J., Wang, X., Mao, Y., Zhang, D., Jiang, Z., Wu, Z., Ai, B., Wang, A., et al.: Swift: a scalable lightweight infrastructure for fine-tuning. In: Proceedings of the AAAI Conference on Artificial Intelligence, vol. 39, pp. 29733–29735 (2025)
26. Zhou, Y., Muresanu, A.I., Han, Z., Paster, K., Pitis, S., Chan, H., Ba, J.: Large language models are human-level prompt engineers. In: The Eleventh International Conference on Learning Representations (2022)

Shared Task 2

Overview of CHIP 2025 Shared Task 2: Discharge Medication Recommendation for Metabolic Diseases Based on Chinese Electronic Health Records

Juntao Li[1], Haobin Yuan[1], Ling Luo[1(✉)], Tengxiao Lv[1], Yan Jiang[2], Fan Wang[2], Ping Zhang[2], Huiyi Lv[2], Jian Wang[1], Yuanyuan Sun[1], and Hongfei Lin[1]

[1] Dalian University of Technology, Dalian 116024, Liaoning, China
{juntaoli,tengxiaolv,yhhhb}@mail.dlut.edu.cn, {syuan,lingluo, wangjian,hflin}@dlut.edu.cn

[2] The Second Affiliated Hospital of Dalian Medical University, Dalian 116023, Liaoning, China
zping717@medmail.com.cn

Abstract. Discharge medication recommendation plays a critical role in ensuring treatment continuity, preventing readmission, and improving long-term management for patients with chronic metabolic diseases. This paper present an overview of the CHIP 2025 Shared Task 2 competition, which aimed to develop state-of-the-art approaches for automatically recommending appropriate discharge medications using real-world Chinese EHR data. For this task, we constructed CDrugRed, a high-quality dataset consisting of 5,894 de-identified hospitalization records from 3,190 patients in China. This task is challenging due to multi-label nature of medication recommendation, heterogeneous clinical text, and patient-specific variability in treatment plans. A total of 526 teams registered, with 167 and 95 teams submitting valid results to the Phase A and Phase B leaderboards, respectively. The top-performing team achieved the highest overall performance on the final test set, with a Jaccard score of 0.5102, F1 score of 0.6267, demonstrating the potential of advanced large language model (LLM)-based ensemble systems. These results highlight both the promise and remaining challenges of applying LLMs to medication recommendation in Chinese EHRs. The post-evaluation phase remains open at https://tianchi.aliyun.com/competition/entrance/532411/.

Keywords: Medication recommendation · Electronic health records · Large language models · Metabolic diseases

1 Introduction

With the global incidence of chronic metabolic diseases—such as diabetes, hypertension, and fatty liver disease—continuing to rise, their treatment and management have become increasingly complex. Patients with metabolic disorders often suffer from multiple comorbidities, require long-term pharmacological treatment, and exhibit significant individual variability. The selection of medications appropriate medications after

Y. Zhang et al. (Eds.): CHIP 2025, CCIS 2884, pp. 477–489, 2026.
https://doi.org/10.1007/978-981-95-7299-1_29

hospital discharge plays a critical role in ensuring long-term disease control, preventing readmission, and improving treatment safety. During hospitalization, rich diagnostic, laboratory, and treatment information is continuously recorded in electronic health records (EHRs). These records provide valuable real-world data for developing precise and intelligent discharge medication recommendation systems that can assist clinicians in optimizing personalized treatment strategies [1–3].

In recent years, drug recommendation has received increasing research attention, with most studies primarily focusing on English-language datasets such as MIMIC-III [4] and MIMIC-IV [5]. Despite the growing research interest, there remains a lack of standardized shared tasks for drug recommendation based on real-world EHR data. In particular, research and evaluation efforts based on Chinese clinical data are still in their early stages. Publicly available benchmark datasets and standardized evaluation criteria are essential to ensure fair comparisons across different approaches. Therefore, we organized the discharge medication recommendation task for metabolic diseases based on Chinese EHRs at the China Health Information Processing Conference (CHIP), aiming to promote research on intelligent medication recommendation in real-world Chinese healthcare settings [6]. As shown in Fig. 1, the task involves inputting de-identified inpatient Chinese EHR texts into the models to automatically recommend drugs selected from a predefined candidate list.

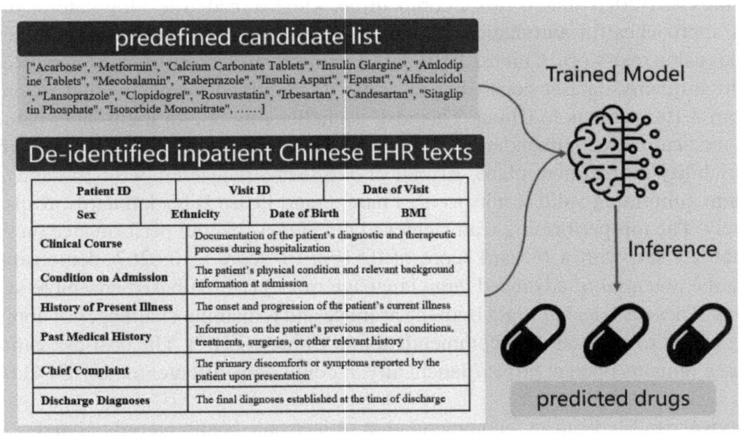

Fig. 1. Overview of the discharge medication recommendation task

The task's evaluation competition was hosted on the Tianchi platform (https://tianchi.aliyun.com/competition/entrance/532411/information) and consisted of two phases: Phase A (development set) for model training and Phase B (test set) for final evaluation. The competition attracted active participation from universities, enterprises, and research institutions. A total of 526 teams registered, among which 167 teams submitted results for the Phase A leaderboard, and 95 teams participated in the Phase B evaluation. The results revealed numerous promising approaches for Chinese EHR-based drug recommendation. The top-ranked team achieved the best performance, with a Jaccard score of 0.5102 and an F1 score of 0.6267, demonstrating the feasibility and potential of applying advanced machine learning and natural language processing methods to discharge medication recommendation tasks.

To further advance research in the field, a post-evaluation phase was launched after the competition to encourage continued exploration using the dataset. In this paper, the following sections first review related work, then provide a detailed description of the dataset construction, task definition and evaluation metric. Subsequently, we analyze the key methods adopted by the top-performing teams and their results, and finally present a summary and outlook for this evaluation.

2 Related Work

To promote the development of artificial intelligence technologies in the biomedical domain, a growing number of challenge evaluations have been organized, such as BioCreative (https://www.ncbi.nlm.nih.gov/research/bionlp/biocreative), China Conference on Knowledge Graph and Semantic Computing (CCKS) [7], China National Conference on Computational Linguistics (CCL), and CHIP. Although many of these evaluations are held annually and cover a wide range of biomedical topics, tasks specifically targeting medication recommendation remain relatively scarce. Recently, Task 9 of CCL25-Eval (https://tianchi.aliyun.com/competition/entrance/532301) has focused on the core challenges of syndrome differentiation and herbal prescription generation in Traditional Chinese Medicine. Given clinical symptom descriptions as input, participants are required to generate personalized herbal prescriptions. In contrast, our task centers on modern medicine, targeting discharge medication recommendation for metabolic diseases based on real electronic medical records. Moreover, our evaluation is supported by a larger, high-quality dataset, enabling more comprehensive benchmarking and facilitating the development of robust, data-driven medication recommendation models.

With the continuous development of large language models (LLMs) [8–12], their applications in the healthcare have expanded rapidly, leading to the emergence of numerous medical LLMs [13–15]. These models are typically trained on medical corpora and have achieved strong performance across various benchmark tasks [16–18]. For example, Med-PaLM 2 [19] integrates large-scale, high-quality medical data with multi-stage instruction fine-tuning to enhance capabilities in medical question answering, clinical reasoning, medical knowledge retrieval, and professional text generation. In the Chinese medical context, LLMs such as HuatuoGPT-o1 [20] have been developed for complex medical reasoning tasks. HuatuoGPT-o1 is trained on a dataset of 40,000 verifiable medical questions and employing a medical verifier to evaluate output quality, thereby enabling quantifiable optimization of reasoning pathways.

In recent years, a growing number of open-source medical datasets have also been released [21–24], most of which serve as benchmarks for evaluating the performance of medical LLMs. Research on discharge medication recommendation heavily relies on open EHR and clinical text data for model training and validation [25–27]. Among these datasets [4, 5, 28], the MIMIC series [4, 5] from Beth Israel Hospital is one of the most widely used, playing a crucial role in studies on diagnosis prediction, prognosis modeling, and medication recommendation. However, most existing datasets for drug recommendation are based on English-language data, and Chinese datasets remain scarce.

The DAILMED dataset [29], which adopts a dialogue-based paradigm for medication recommendation, is among of the few available Chinese datasets in this field. Therefore, we introduce CDrugRed [30], the Chinese discharge medication recommendation dataset focusing on metabolic diseases. This dataset provides a valuable foundation for developing and evaluating intelligent medication recommendation systems tailored to Chinese clinical practice.

3 Material and Methods

3.1 Task Definition

In this shared task, the systems of participating teams are required to predict a set of discharge medications for patients with metabolic diseases based on de-identified Chinese EHR texts. The recommended medications must be selected from a predefined candidate drug list. The input to the model consists of the patient's inpatient records, and the output is a patient-specific list of medications that would be appropriately prescribed at discharge. Participants were encouraged to explore diverse technical solutions, including traditional machine learning, deep learning, pretrained language models, or retrieval-augmented generation methods. To ensure fairness and reproducibility, the task imposed certain constraints: (1) The total model size was limited to 10 billion parameters; (2) The use of external resources or knowledge bases was permitted only if their sources were explicitly declared. These standardized requirements aimed to promote methodological innovation while maintaining the integrity and comparability of system performance across participating teams.

3.2 Dataset Description

The evaluation was conducted using the CDrugRed dataset [30], a new Chinese discharge medication recommendation dataset focused on metabolic diseases. This dataset was developed to facilitate research on intelligent and interpretable clinical medication recommendation. CDrugRed is constructed from real electronic medical records collected at a top-tier tertiary hospital in China, covering 5,894 de-identified hospitalization records from 3,190 patients spanning the years 2013 and 2023. The dataset includes 651 candidate drugs and provides rich clinical information, including basic demographic data, admission conditions, inpatient clinical course, laboratory and examination results, past medical history, discharge diagnoses, and actual discharge medications prescribed by physicians. An example is shown in Table 1. To protect patient privacy and ensure data quality, the dataset underwent a multi-stage processing pipeline involving large-model-assisted de-identification, standardized drug-name normalization, and manual review to ensure data security and consistency with clinical terminology.

For model training and evaluation, the dataset was divided into training, validation, and test sets at a ratio of 6:1:3 based on unique patient identifiers. This ensured that multiple visits from the same patient were confined to a single subset, thereby preserving data independence and avoiding information leakage. Detailed statistics are presented in Table 2.

Table 1. Example data format

Items	Example
Patient ID	2
Visit ID	"2-1"
Sex	"Female"
Date of birth	"1940-12"
Ethnicity	"Han Chinese"
BMI	27.3
Date of visit	"2015-03"
Clinical course	"Outpatient urine test: ketone bodies: + leukocytes: 250/μl; microscopic examination: 7–9/HP. Upon admission: urinalysis: leukocytes +++ urine leukocytes 62.25/HP (↑). After oral rehydration, repeat urinalysis showed leukocytes and ketones (−). Steamed bun meal test results reported: glycated hemoglobin……"
Condition on admission	"The patient was admitted with the chief complaint of polydipsia, polyuria, and polyphagia for 5 years, dysuria with poor glycemic control for 2 months. Key physical examination findings: T 36.6 °C, P 76 bpm, R 22 breaths/min, BP 160/80 mmHg……"
History of present illness	"Five years prior, the patient developed polydipsia, polyuria, and polyphagia without obvious precipitating factors, and presented to ** Hospital. Fasting blood glucose was 16.7 mmol/L. The patient was treated with metformin, repaglinide, and acarbose for glycemic control……"
Past medical history	"No history of coronary heart disease. Denies history of infectious diseases including hepatitis, tuberculosis, and malaria. No history of food or drug allergy. No history of trauma, surgery, or blood transfusion. Immunization history is unknown"
Chief complaint	"Polydipsia, polyuria, and polyphagia for 5 years; dysuria with poor glycemic control for 2 months"
Discharge diagnoses	["Type 2 Diabetes Mellitus", "Diabetic Ketosis", "Urinary Tract Infection", "Diabetic Macrovascular Complications",…]
Discharge medications	["Acarbose", "Repaglinide", "Rosuvastatin", "Telmisartan", "Amlodipine", "Calcium Carbonate Tablets"]

CDrugRed captures realistic disease progression patterns and comorbidity profiles of Chinese patients with metabolic diseases, offering a valuable benchmark for advancing data-driven clinical decision support and intelligent medication recommendation research in Chinese healthcare settings.

Table 2. Statistical summary of the CDrugRed dataset

Dataset	Number of Patients	Number of Visits
Train	1910	3602
Validation	320	570
Test	960	1722

3.3 Baseline System

To provide a reference for comparison with the participants' systems, we established an LLM-based baseline model. Specifically, we conducted supervised fine-tuning (SFT) based on the GLM4-9B-Chat model using the LoRA method. The fine-tuning hyperparameters are summarized in Table 3, and the corresponding instruction template is illustrated in Fig. 2. For the instruction training data construction, all patient information fields excluding discharge medications were concatenated to form the instruction input, while the corresponding discharge medication list was used as the output. This instruction-response formulation enables the model to learn the mapping between clinical context and medication recommendation, thereby establishing a large language model–based baseline for this task.

Table 3. LoRA fine-tuning hyperparameters for GLM4-9B-Chat

Hyperparameter	Value
Batch size	1
Gradient accumulation	4
Learning rate	1e-4
LoRA rank	8
LoRA alpha	16
Epoch	10

SFT Prompt Template (zh)	SFT Prompt Template (en)
你作为三甲医院主任医师，需根据患者完整病历和药物列表，严格遵循临床规范生成出院带药方案。病历如下： 【患者核心信息】 • 基础体征：{sex}/{age}岁（注意年龄相关剂量调整） • 过敏史：{allergy} • 生理指标：身高{height}cm 体重{weight}kg BMI{bmi} 【临床诊疗关键点】 ▶ 诊疗过程描述：{process} ▶ 入院情况：{admission} ▶ 主诉：{complaint} ▶ 现病史：{history now} ▶ 既往史：{history_past}（关注慢性病用药史） ▶ 出院诊断：{diagnosis}（核心依据） 【待选药物库】{drug_str} 【输出规范】 请从给定的药物列表中推荐该患者的“出院带药列表”，请仅输出以下格式："药物A,药物B,药物C,……" 严格按照格式回答，不要输出任何解释或额外内容。	You are a chief physician at a top-tier hospital. Based on the patient's complete medical record and medication list, you must strictly follow clinical guidelines to generate a discharge medication plan. The medical record is as follows: [Patient Core Information] • Basic vitals: {sex}/{age} years old (pay attention to age-related dose adjustments) • Allergy history: {allergy} • Physiological indicators: Height {height} cm, Weight {weight} kg, BMI {bmi} [Key Clinical Points] ▶ Description of treatment process: {process} ▶ Admission condition: {admission} ▶ Chief complaint: {complaint} ▶ Present illness history: {history_now} ▶ Past medical history: {history_past} (pay attention to chronic medication history) ▶ Discharge diagnosis: {diagnosis} (core basis) [Medication Library for Selection] {drug_str} [Output Specification] Please recommend this patient's "discharge medication list" from the given medication options. Only output in the following format: "DrugA, DrugB, DrugC, ..." Answer strictly in this format. Do not output any explanation or additional content.

Fig. 2. Instruction template used for baseline model training. (Note that the English prompt is not part of the input, it is the translation of the Chinese.)

3.4 Evaluation Metric

Since the discharge medications are restricted to a predefined set of 651 candidate drugs, this task can be treated as a multi-label classification problem. Accordingly, two commonly used metrics, i.e., Jaccard score and F1 score, are adopted to comprehensively evaluate system performance.

$$Jaccard = \frac{1}{N}\sum_{i=1}^{N}\frac{|y_i \cap \hat{y}_i|}{|y_i \cup \hat{y}_i|} \tag{1}$$

$$Precision(y_i, \hat{y}_i) = \frac{|y_i \cap \hat{y}_i|}{|\hat{y}_i|} \tag{2}$$

$$Recall(y_i, \hat{y}_i) = \frac{|y_i \cap \hat{y}_i|}{|y_i|} \tag{3}$$

$$f1(y_i, \hat{y}_i) = 2 \cdot \frac{Precision(y_i, \hat{y}_i) \cdot Recall(y_i, \hat{y}_i)}{Precision(y_i, \hat{y}_i) + Recall(y_i, \hat{y}_i)} \tag{4}$$

In the metrics, y denotes the set of ground-truth drugs, $\hat{y}$ denotes the set of drugs predicted by the model, and $|X|$ denotes the number of elements in set X.

To obtain overall system performance, macro-averaged precision, recall, and F1 scores are computed across all N patient records:

$$\text{AVG\_P} = \frac{1}{N}\sum_{i=1}^{N} Precision(y_i, \hat{y}_i) \tag{5}$$

$$\text{AVG\_R} = \frac{1}{N}\sum_{i=1}^{N} Recall(y_i, \hat{y}_i) \tag{6}$$

$$\text{F1} = \frac{1}{N}\sum_{i=1}^{N} f1(y_i, \hat{y}_i) \tag{7}$$

Finally, the overall ranking score used for leaderboard evaluation is defined as the average of the Jaccard and F1 scores, which balances the model's performance in terms of both label overlap and predictive accuracy:

$$\text{Score} = \frac{1}{2} \cdot (Jaccard + F1) \tag{8}$$

This composite metric ensures a fair and comprehensive assessment of system performance across all participating teams.

4 Results

A total of 526 teams registered for this shared task. Among them, 167 teams submitted valid results to the Phase A leaderboard, and 95 teams submitted results to the Phase B leaderboard. These teams are from a diverse range of organizations, including universities, enterprises, and research institutions. Each team was allowed to submit up to three runs per day, and the highest historical score was recorded as the team's final leaderboard result.

4.1 Evaluation Results

During Phase A, participants were evaluated on the validation set, while Phase B used the test set for the final leaderboard ranking. The best results achieved by the participants, along with the baseline performances in both phases, are summarized in Table 4.

Table 4. Best results and baseline performances on both leaderboards

Phase	Type	Jaccard	AVG_P	AVG_R	F1	Score
Leaderboard A	Best result	0.5025	0.6764	0.6077	0.6164	0.5594
	Baseline	0.4444	0.5751	0.5958	0.5621	0.5032
Leaderboard B	Best result	0.5102	0.6905	0.6121	0.6267	0.5685
	Baseline	0.4477	0.5864	0.5872	0.5648	0.5062

As shown in Table 4, the top-performing systems achieved notable improvements over the baseline, particularly in the Jaccard and F1 scores. The best-performing model in Phase A and B achieved final scores of 0.5594 and an F1 score of 0.5685, outperforming the baseline by 5.62% and 6.23%, respectively.

Table 5 further presents the results of the top ten teams on Leaderboard B. The first-ranked team, DeepDrug, achieved the highest overall score of 0.5685, establishing a clear lead over other teams. In contrast, the performance gap among the second to tenth teams is relatively small, with overall scores ranging from 0.5226 to 0.5453, suggesting a high degree of competitiveness in this range.

Table 5. The performance results of top 10 ranking teams.

Team	Rank	Jaccard	AVG_P	AVG_R	F1	Score
DeepDrug	1	0.5102	0.6905	0.6121	0.6267	0.5685
ZZUNLP	2	0.4876	0.6897	0.5735	0.6031	0.5453
suxiao818	3	0.4870	0.6740	0.5810	0.6014	0.5442
晚安东莞	4	0.4790	0.6333	0.6070	0.5965	0.5378
H-3-C	5	0.4732	0.6430	0.5857	0.5899	0.5316
对对队	6	0.4721	0.6194	0.6019	0.5883	0.5302
Med-LLM	7	0.4697	0.6317	0.5812	0.5851	0.5274
IIGROUP	8	0.4669	0.6345	0.5858	0.5850	0.5260
Seeking Your Roots	9	0.4644	0.6068	0.6036	0.5826	0.5235
熬夜美少女战士	10	0.4628	0.6276	0.5771	0.5824	0.5226
Baseline	28	0.4477	0.5864	0.5872	0.5648	0.5062

Overall, 27 teams outperformed the baseline on Leaderboard B. These results show that many participating teams effectively leveraged model fine-tuning, data augmentation, and ensemble strategies to substantially enhance predictive performance compared to the baseline. The consistent improvement across multiple teams underscores the potential of LLMs for clinical decision support tasks, particularly when combined with domain-specific data augmentation and prompt design strategies.

4.2 Descriptions of Top Five Teams

Team DeepDrug (Tencent Jarvis Lab)

The DeepDrug team proposed a generative recommendation framework integrating multi-dimensional feature enhancement and multi-scale model fusion. At the data representation level, they introduced drug category annotations, explicit patient meta-features, and disease–drug co-occurrence knowledge to enhance clinical semantic understanding. They also applied order perturbations to diagnostic and medication lists to improve model robustness and generalization. At the model level, they performed full supervised fine-tuning based on the Qwen-series LLMs and adopted differentiated training strategies for models of different parameter sizes to obtain complementary ensembles. During inference, a hierarchical weighted-voting fusion mechanism was introduced, assigning adaptive weights based on validation performance to balance bias and variance across model predictions.

Team ZZUNLP (Zhengzhou University)

The ZZUNLP team developed a systematic solution across the dimensions of data, model training, and inference. To address the domain specificity of medical text and the scarcity of labeled data, they designed prompt templates tailored for clinical medication reasoning and introduced a pseudo-labeling data-augmentation strategy. They used the cross-entropy loss of label sequences as a confidence indicator to filter high-quality pseudo-labeled samples. Multiple open-source LLMs were fine-tuned using LoRA and optimized with the liger-kernel cross-entropy loss for efficient memory utilization. For inference, they employed a two-stage hierarchical ensemble: in stage one, weighted voting was applied separately within model groups trained on original data and augmented data to obtain high-confidence predictions; in stage two, an adaptive fusion strategy based on differences in predicted list length and Jaccard similarity further improved final recommendation performance.

Team suxiao818 (MISUMI (China) Precision Machinery Trading Co., Ltd.)

The suxiao818 team implemented a fine-tuning and ensemble-based framework built upon multiple LLMs. They split the dataset (9:1) into training and validation subsets and selected the top-performing four models with LoRA fine-tuning for ensemble. To mitigate randomness in generative decoding, each model produced multiple predictions under different decoding temperatures, which were fused using majority voting. Candidate drugs appearing in more than half of the predictions were retained and ranked by frequency, with list length truncated to the average.

Team 晚安东莞 (South China Normal University)

This team fine-tuned Qwen2.5-7B-Instruct for discharge medication generation. In data preprocessing, they designed prompt strategies for electronic medical records, concatenating all fields of a case as model input to generate structured or natural-language-style drug lists. They then performed supervised fine-tuning via LoRA. At inference, they ran multiple temperature settings for models outputting the different styles, and selected the three best-performing configurations for ensemble. They further normalized drug names to improve consistency. The final ensemble used a voting rule: drugs appearing in at least two lists were retained; if there was no overlap, the union of all predictions was used to increase recall.

Team H-3-C (H3C Technologies Co., Limited)

The H-3-C team designed a data-centric approach emphasizing rare-drug oversampling and ensemble enhancement. Low-relevance fields (such as patient index, gender, BMI) were removed, and samples containing rare drugs were duplicated or triplicated based on frequency thresholds. To increase data diversity, they introduced order-shuffled samples and combined them with the oversampled set, resulting in 6,740 augmented samples. Five open-source LLMs were fine-tuned using LoRA on these datasets. During inference, fuzzy string matching normalized predicted drugs to the candidate list, supplemented by a manually curated alias mapping table. Final predictions were generated via majority voting (appearing in $\geq$3 models), with sequential backfilling from GLM4-9B-Chat and CareBot_Medical_multi-llama3-8b-instruct models for empty outputs.

4.3 Analysis of Top Team Solutions

Table 6 presents the performance of the top five teams on the Leaderboard B. Since all these teams adopted model ensemble strategies, we report both their best single-model (Single) results and their best ensembled results. The ensemble approaches generally led to consistent performance gains across all teams, highlighting the importance of model diversity and fusion in this multi-label clinical prediction task.

Table 6. Single and ensemble results of the top five ranking teams on the test set. Single refers to Best Single Model

Team	Rank	Method	Jaccard	AVG_P	AVG_R	F1	Score
DeepDrug	1	Single	–	–	–	–	–
		Ensemble	0.5102	0.6905	0.6121	0.6267	0.5685
ZZUNLP	2	Single	0.4480	0.5837	0.5902	0.5648	0.5064
		Ensemble	0.4876	0.6897	0.5735	0.6031	0.5453
suxiao818	3	Single	0.4700	0.6498	0.5750	0.5865	0.5283
		Ensemble	0.4870	0.6740	0.5810	0.6014	0.5442
晚安东莞	4	Single	0.4644	0.6044	0.6082	0.5821	0.5232
		Ensemble	0.4790	0.6333	0.6070	0.5965	0.5378
H-3-C	5	Single	0.4538	0.5965	0.5946	0.5715	0.5127
		Ensemble	0.4732	0.6430	0.5857	0.5899	0.5316

Notably, the second-place team (ZZUNLP) achieved the largest performance gain after ensemble fusion, with its score increasing from 0.5064 to 0.5453, underscoring the effectiveness and sophistication of its two-stage ensemble strategy. This approach combines intra-group weighted voting with inter-group adaptive fusion. It demonstrates that carefully designed hierarchical ensemble mechanisms can capture complementary model strengths more effectively than simple averaging or majority voting. Overall, these findings highlight that, while large language models provide strong baselines, ensemble-based optimization remains a crucial technique for improving the stability and accuracy of clinical drug recommendation systems.

5 Conclusion

In this paper, we established the first benchmark for discharge medication recommendation in metabolic diseases using Chinese EHR data through the CHIP 2025 Shared Task 2. The high level of participation and diverse system designs reflect strong community engagement and the growing interest in data-driven clinical decision support. The top-performing teams demonstrated that ensemble frameworks combining domain-specific fine-tuned LLMs can effectively leverage EHR information to improve discharge medication prediction. This shared task provides valuable insights into the practical application of NLP and machine learning for personalized medication management, contributing to the advancement of precision medicine in chronic metabolic care.

Despite these advances, challenges remain in addressing label imbalance, rare medication usage, and generalizing across institutions. For future work, we plan to expand the dataset with additional clinical contexts from multiple institutions, incorporating multi-modal data such as laboratory and medical imaging, and moving beyond drug name recommendation to generating complete medication regimens, including dosage and instructions. These efforts aim to promote explainable and trustworthy AI systems for clinical medication applications.

Acknowledgments. This research was supported by the Natural Science Foundation of China (No. 62302076, 62276043), the Fundamental Research Funds for the Central Universities (No. DUT25YG108), and the Research Project on High Quality Development of Hospital Pharmacy, National Institute of Hospital Administration, NHC, China (No. NIHAYSZX2525).

References

1. Zhang, Y., Chen, R., Tang, J., Stewart, W.F., Sun, J.: Leap: learning to prescribe effective and safe treatment combinations for multimorbidity. In: Proceedings of the 23rd ACM SIGKDD International Conference on Knowledge Discovery and Data Mining, pp. 1315–1324 (2017)
2. Shang, J., Xiao, C., Ma, T., Li, H., Sun, J.: Gamenet: graph augmented memory networks for recommending medication combination. In: Proceedings of the AAAI Conference on Artificial Intelligence. vol. 33, pp. 1126–1133 (2019)
3. Yang, C., Xiao, C., Ma, F., Glass, L., Sun, J.: Safedrug: dual molecular graph encoders for recommending effective and safe drug combinations. In: 30th International Joint Conference on Artificial Intelligence, IJCAI 2021, pp. 3735–3741. International Joint Conferences on Artificial Intelligence (2021)
4. Johnson, A.E., Pollard, T.J., Shen, L., Lehman, L.W.H., Feng, M., Ghassemi, M., Moody, B., Szolovits, P., Anthony Celi, L., Mark, R.G.: Mimic-iii, a freely accessible critical care database. Scientific Data **3**(1), 1–9 (2016)
5. Johnson, A.E., et al.: Mimic-iv, a freely accessible electronic health record dataset. Scientific Data **10**(1), 1 (2023)
6. Etemadi, M., et al.: A systematic review of healthcare recommender systems: open issues, challenges, and techniques. Expert Syst. Appl. **213**, 118823 (2023)
7. Li, J., Luo, L., Lv, T., Liu, C., Qi, J., Yang, Z., Wang, J., Lin, H.: Instruction fine-tuning of large language models for traditional Chinese medicine. In: China Conference on Knowledge Graph and Semantic Computing, pp. 419–430. Springer (2024)
8. Achiam, J., Adler, S., Agarwal, S., Ahmad, L., Akkaya, I., Aleman, F.L., Almeida, D., Altenschmidt, J., Altman, S., Anadkat, S. et al.: Gpt-4 technical report. arXiv preprint arXiv: 2303.08774 (2023)
9. Yang, A., Li, A., Yang, B., Zhang, B., Hui, B., Zheng, B., Yu, B., Gao, C., Huang, C., Lv, C., et al.: Qwen3 technical report. arXiv preprint arXiv:2505.09388 (2025)
10. GLM, T., Zeng, A., Xu, B., Wang, B., Zhang, C., Yin, D., Zhang, D., Rojas, D., Feng, G., Zhao, H. et al.: Chatglm: a family of large language models from glm-130b to glm-4 all tools. arXiv preprint arXiv:2406.12793 (2024)
11. Meta, A.: The llama 4 herd: The beginning of a new era of natively multimodal ai innovation. https://ai.meta.com/blog/llama-4-multimodal-intelligence/, checked on **4**(7), 2025 (2025)
12. Guo, D., Yang, D., Zhang, H., Song, J., Zhang, R., Xu, R., Zhu, Q., Ma, S., Wang, P., Bi, X. et al.: Deepseek-r1: Incentivizing reasoning capability in llms via reinforcement learning. arXiv preprint arXiv:2501.12948 (2025)

13. Luo, L., et al.: Taiyi: a bilingual fine-tuned large language model for diverse biomedical tasks. J. Am. Med. Inform. Assoc. **31**(9), 1865–1874 (2024)
14. Chen, J., Wang, X., Ji, K., Gao, A., Jiang, F., Chen, S., Zhang, H., Song, D., Xie, W., Kong, C. et al.: Huatuogpt-ii, one-stage training for medical adaption of llms. arXiv preprint arXiv: 2311.09774 (2023)
15. Xiong, H., Wang, S., Zhu, Y., Zhao, Z., Liu, Y., Huang, L., Wang, Q., Shen, D.: Doctorglm: Fine-tuning your Chinese doctor is not a herculean task. arXiv preprint arXiv:2304.01097 (2023)
16. Zhou, H., Liu, F., Wu, J., Zhang, W., Huang, G., Clifton, L., Eyre, D., Luo, H., Liu, F., Branson, K. et al.: A collaborative large language model for drug analysis. Nat. Biomed. Eng., 1–12 (2025)
17. Dou, C., Liu, C., Yang, F., Li, F., Jia, J., Chen, M., Ju, Q., Wang, S., Dang, S., Li, T. et al.: Baichuan-m2: Scaling medical capability with large verifier system. arXiv preprint arXiv: 2509.02208 (2025)
18. Wang, G., Gao, M., Yang, S., Zhang, Y., He, L., Huang, L., Xiao, H., Zhang, Y., Li, W., Chen, L. et al.: Citrus: Leveraging expert cognitive pathways in a medical language model for advanced medical decision support. arXiv preprint arXiv:2502.18274 (2025)
19. Singhal, K., et al.: Toward expert-level medical question answering with large language models. Nat. Med. **31**(3), 943–950 (2025)
20. Chen, J., Cai, Z., Ji, K., Wang, X., Liu, W., Wang, R., Hou, J., Wang, B.: Huatuogpt-o1, towards medical complex reasoning with llms. arXiv preprint arXiv:2412.18925 (2024)
21. Jin, D., Pan, E., Oufattole, N., Weng, W.H., Fang, H., Szolovits, P.: What disease does this patient have? a large-scale open domain question answering dataset from medical exams. Appl. Sci. **11**(14), 6421 (2021)
22. Jin, Q., Dhingra, B., Liu, Z., Cohen, W., Lu, X.: Pubmedqa: a dataset for biomedical research question answering. In: Proceedings of the 2019 Conference on Empirical Methods in Natural Language Processing and the 9th International Joint Conference on Natural Language Processing (EMNLP-IJCNLP), pp. 2567–2577 (2019)
23. Liu, J., et al.: Benchmarking large language models on cmexam-a comprehensive Chinese medical exam dataset. Adv. Neural. Inf. Process. Syst. **36**, 52430–52452 (2023)
24. Yue, W., Wang, X., Zhu, W., Guan, M., Zheng, H., Wang, P., Sun, C., Ma, X.: Tcmbench: a comprehensive benchmark for evaluating large language models in traditional chinese medicine. arXiv preprint arXiv:2406.01126 (2024)
25. Wu, R., Qiu, Z., Jiang, J., Qi, G., Wu, X.: Conditional generation net for medication recommendation. In: Proceedings of the ACM Web Conference 2022, pp. 935–945 (2022)
26. Zhao, Z., Jing, Y., Feng, F., Wu, J., Gao, C., He, X.: Leave no patient behind: Enhancing medication recommendation for rare disease patients. In: Proceedings of the 47th International ACM SIGIR Conference on Research and Development in Information Retrieval, pp. 533–542 (2024)
27. Zhao, Z., Fan, C., Gao, C., Feng, F., He, X.: Addressing overprescribing challenges: Fine-tuning large language models for medication recommendation tasks. arXiv preprint arXiv: 2503.03687 (2025)
28. Pollard, T.J., Johnson, A.E., Raffa, J.D., Celi, L.A., Mark, R.G., Badawi, O.: The eicu collaborative research database, a freely available multi-center database for critical care research. Scientific data **5**(1), 1–13 (2018)
29. He, Z., Han, Y., Ouyang, Z., Gao, W., Chen, H., Xu, G., Wu, J.: Dialmed: a dataset for dialogue-based medication recommendation. arXiv preprint arXiv:2203.07094 (2022)
30. Li, J., Yuan, H., Luo, L., Jiang, Y., Wang, F., Zhang, P., Lv, H., Wang, J., Sun, Y., Lin, H.: Cdrugred: a Chinese drug recommendation dataset for discharge medications in metabolic diseases. arXiv preprint arXiv:2510.21084 (2025)

Towards Discharge Medication Recommendation via Multi-scale Model Training and Multi-dimensional Feature Enhancement

Zhihong Zhu, Huimin Huang, and Xian Wu(✉)

Tencent Jarvis Lab, Shenzhen, China
{profzhu,huiminhuang,kevinxwu}@tencent.com

Abstract. Discharge medication recommendation is a critical task in clinical decision support, aiming to assist physicians in determining safe and personalized prescriptions based on inpatient electronic health records (EHRs). However, the complexity of multi-disease comorbidities, long-tail medication distributions, and the scarcity of annotated data pose significant challenges for existing methods. In this paper, we propose a framework that integrates multi-dimensional feature enhancement and multi-scale model training to improve model accuracy and generalization. At the data level, we construct a feature-augmented EHR representation by incorporating pharmacological categories, patient meta-features, and disease–drug statistical priors, coupled with structural perturbation strategies to alleviate data sparsity. At the model level, we adopt a multi-scale fine-tuning strategy using Qwen series language models of different parameter sizes, followed by a two-level hierarchical ensemble that fuses complementary knowledge across model scales and augmentation variants. Experiments on the CHIP 2025 Shared Task 2 (Discharge Medication Recommendation for Metabolic Diseases) dataset demonstrate that our approach achieves state-of-the-art performance, surpassing both the official baselines and all other participating systems.

Keywords: Large Language Models · Natural Language Processing · Discharge Drug Recommendation

1 Introduction

Metabolic diseases, such as diabetes and hypertension, represent a class of major chronic conditions characterized by complex pathological mechanisms and marked individual heterogeneity [24]. These diseases pose a serious threat to public health and socioeconomic development. In clinical practice, managing patients with multiple coexisting metabolic disorders remains particularly challenging, as treatment regimens often involve intricate drug combinations and long-term monitoring [26,32]. Thus, rational drug selection must account for multiple factors, including medical history, comorbidities, and potential drug–drug interactions. To address these challenges, recent studies [11,16] have emphasized the

Y. Zhang et al. (Eds.): CHIP 2025, CCIS 2884, pp. 490–502, 2026.
https://doi.org/10.1007/978-981-95-7299-1_30

need for intelligent medication management models that assist physicians and pharmacists in formulating precise [20], individualized treatment plans, thereby enhancing therapeutic efficacy and minimizing adverse drug reactions.

Building upon this motivation, this study focuses on Task 2 of the CHIP 2025 Shared Task: Intelligent Discharge Medication Recommendation Based on Inpatient Electronic Health Records (EHRs) [12,13]. Formally, given a segment of narrative text from a patient's hospitalization record (including chief complaint, present illness history, diagnosis, and treatment details), the model aims to recommend an appropriate list of medications to be prescribed at discharge [2]. The goal of this shared task is to automatically generate discharge medication plans through comprehensive analysis of inpatient EHRs, thereby promoting rational drug use and improving long-term management of metabolic diseases.

To address the challenges of improving task accuracy and overcoming the inherent limitations of single-model approaches, this study proposes an integrated framework that combines innovations at both the data and model levels. At the data level, we design a systematic feature-enhanced data augmentation pipeline to mitigate issues such as high annotation cost, limited sample size, and long-tail distribution involving rare diseases or complex medication regimens [30]. This strategy fully exploits the potential of existing data, thereby improving the model's generalizability and robustness. At the model level, we adopt a multi-scale learning paradigm instead of relying on a single end-to-end generative model, which often suffers from "black-box" opacity and low controllability in clinical decision-making. Specifically, we develop an ensemble learning [7] framework that integrates multiple models trained at different granularities and optimization scales, enabling complementary strengths across sub-tasks and yielding more reliable discharge medication recommendations.

Overall, the main contributions of this work are summarized as follows:

- We propose a multi-dimensional data augmentation framework to address medical data bottlenecks such as limited annotation and long-tail distribution.
- We develop a multi-stage ensemble learning framework that integrates multiple models trained at different granularities, leveraging their complementary strengths to improve decision accuracy and robustness.
- The proposed method achieved the highest accuracy in the CHIP 2025 Shared Task 2: Discharge Medication Recommendation for Metabolic Diseases from Chinese EHRs, demonstrating its effectiveness and generalizability.

2 Related Work

2.1 Large Language Models

Large language models (LLMs) have become the cornerstone of modern natural language processing (NLP), achieving strong comprehension, reasoning, and generation abilities through large-scale pre-training on diverse text corpora. Recent advances in model architecture and scaling have produced influential representatives such as GPT [1] and Gemini [6] in the commercial domain, as well as open-source counterparts like Qwen [17,23] and LLaMA [9,18], which demonstrate robust generalization and contextual understanding across a wide range of tasks [22,29]. Meanwhile, continuous progress in instruction tuning and alignment [31] has refined LLMs' reasoning capability [4] and strengthened their adaptability to complex, human-centered applications.

The healthcare domain has become a particularly promising area for LLM applications. Recent studies [11] have demonstrated that these models can interpret electronic health records (EHRs), summarize patient information, and provide contextual support for clinical diagnosis and treatment planning [21]. They also assist in medical education, literature retrieval, and doctor–patient communication, showing potential to improve both efficiency and accessibility of healthcare services [20]. Despite these advances, applying LLMs to clinical settings such as metabolic disease management remains highly challenging because medical texts contain domain-specific terminology, implicit reasoning, and high safety requirements [10]. Overcoming these challenges is crucial for building reliable and clinically aligned medical LLM systems that can truly assist healthcare professionals in complex decision-making processes.

2.2 Ensemble Learning

Ensemble learning has proven to be an effective strategy for improving model robustness and accuracy by aggregating the outputs of multiple learners. Instead of relying on a single model, ensemble frameworks exploit the diversity among models trained with different data distributions, parameter scales, or optimization strategies [15,19]. This diversity helps reduce both variance and bias, leading to better generalization across heterogeneous clinical data.

Classical ensemble paradigms can be broadly categorized into three types. Bagging (e.g., Random Forest [3]) trains base learners in parallel and aggregates their predictions through majority voting or averaging to stabilize results. Boosting (e.g., GBDT [8]) builds a sequence of weak models, where each subsequent learner focuses on correcting the residual errors of its predecessors. Stacking employs a meta-learner that integrates the predictions of multiple base models to capture higher-order dependencies among them.

In this study, we adopt a two-level hierarchical ensemble specifically designed for discharge medication recommendation. The first level aggregates models of different parameter scales and data augmentation variants to capture complementary knowledge across sub-tasks. The second level fuses the outputs of high-capacity models with the first-level ensemble to achieve a balanced trade-off between accuracy and stability.

3 Method

Task Definition. Formally, given a hospitalization record $X = \{x_1, x_2, \dots, x_n\}$ comprising narrative segments such as chief complaint, diagnosis, and treatment, the model aims to predict a *set* of discharge medications $Y = \{y_1, y_2, \dots, y_m\}$. The learning objective is to model the conditional probability distribution:

$$P(Y|X;\theta) = \prod_{y_i \in Y} P(y_i|X;\theta), \tag{1}$$

and infer the most probable medication set:

$$\hat{Y} = \{y_i \mid P(y_i|X;\theta) \geq \tau\}, \tag{2}$$

where τ is a decision threshold controlling the number of predicted drugs, and θ denotes model parameters (Fig. 1).

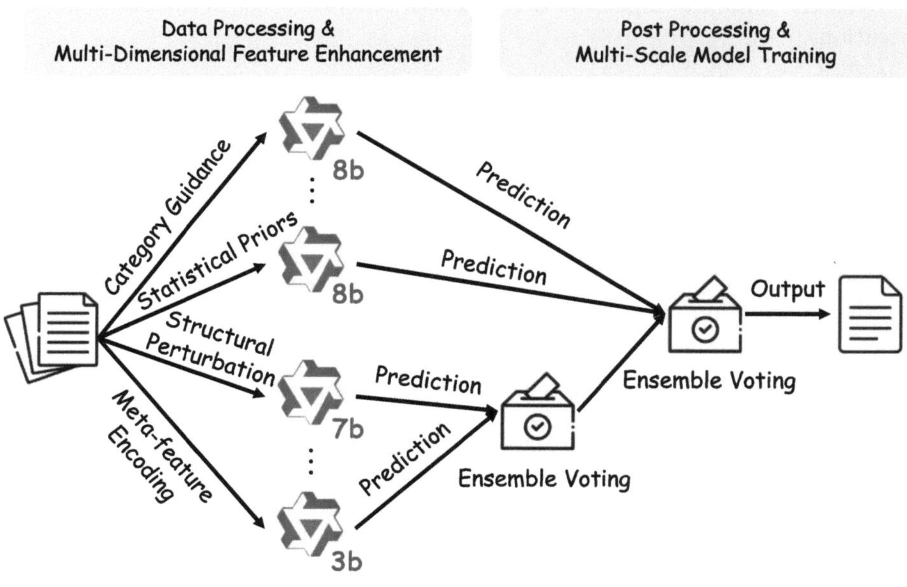

Fig. 1. Overview of our discharge medication recommendation framework.

3.1 Data Processing

Before model training, we first convert each inpatient record into an instruction–output format to better align with instruction-tuned large language models. Each sample consists of a structured EHR-based case description and a corresponding target medication list. The input text includes patient demographics, admission and discharge information, diagnostic descriptions, and detailed treatment records. All numeric indicators, laboratory results, and medication mentions were retained to preserve clinical reasoning cues.

Since the raw EHR records contain numerous nested elements, we conducted a series of preprocessing steps to improve input consistency and reduce noise. Specifically, we removed redundant punctuation, simplified nested brackets, and normalized medication names. In the output side, to make the prediction format more interpretable and model-friendly, we eliminated quotation marks and brackets from the medication lists—transforming the original structure, into a simplified textual sequence. This adjustment allows the model to focus on semantic decoding rather than JSON-style syntax generation.

Input–Output Format for Medication Recommendation

Prompt Example:
[Instruction]
Given the following inpatient EHR record, generate a list of discharge medications.
[Input]
Sex: Female, Age: 67, BMI: 27, Diagnosis: Diabetes, Hypertension, Fatty Liver Disease...
[Output]
Drug_1, Drug_2,...

An illustration of the constructed prompt template is shown above. The prompt follows a consistent structure during both training and inference, ensuring that instruction cues remain aligned across datasets.

3.2 Multi-dimensional Feature Enhancement

To address data sparsity in this medication recommendation task, we construct a multi-dimensional feature enhancement framework that augments the original hospitalization record with clinically meaningful information. Each record X is composed of different textual elements such as admission notes, medical history and laboratory descriptions: $X = \{x_{\text{chief}}, x_{\text{history}}, x_{\text{diagnosis}}, x_{\text{treatment}}, x_{\text{meta}}\}$. Here, x_{meta} includes structured fields (e.g., sex, age, BMI, visit time). The enhanced representation X' is defined as:

$$X' = f_{\text{enh}}(X) = X \cup \{K_{\text{cat}}, K_{\text{meta}}, K_{\text{stat}}, K_{\text{pert}}\}, \tag{3}$$

where $f_{\text{enh}}(\cdot)$ denotes the enhancement operator, and the added components are detailed below.

(1) Drug Category Guidance. Following the clinical reasoning logic (*disease → drug category → specific drug*), we inject pharmacological category information

as an intermediate semantic layer. For each drug y_i in the candidate medication list, we employ Gemini 2.5 Pro [6] to generate its corresponding category description:

$$c_i = g_{\text{cat}}(y_i), \tag{4}$$

where g_{cat} automatically assigns each drug to a clinically relevant class (e.g., *aspirin* → *antiplatelet drug*). The final input sequence is augmented with annotated tokens $\{y_i[c_i]\}$, providing the model with structured pharmacological semantics. The complete prompt used to query the LLM is presented below.

Pharmacological Category Generation Prompt

You are a medical and pharmaceutical expert. Your task is to assign an accurate pharmacological drug class to the given medication.

Drug Name: {Drug Name}

Task Requirements:

1. Assign a concise and accurate pharmacological category (in Chinese) to this drug.
2. The category should follow pharmacological classification.
3. If the drug name itself is a category (e.g., "BTK inhibitor"), use that category directly.
4. Prefer commonly used and authoritative pharmacological classifications.

Output format: Output only the category name (one short Chinese string), with no explanation.

(2) Patient Meta-feature Encoding. To capture patient-specific variability, we extract key demographic and physiological attributes from the EHR, including sex, age, BMI, and visit count. Age is derived from the birth date, BMI is discretized following Chinese clinical thresholds [25] (e.g., underweight, normal, overweight, obese), and visit count reflects disease chronicity. These normalized attributes are converted into concise textual tags and appended to the case description (e.g., "female [overweight], age group [60–80], third visit"), enabling the model to better perceive individual differences relevant to medication decisions.

(3) Statistical Disease–Drug Priors. To provide explicit prescribing knowledge, we analyze the empirical co-occurrence distribution between discharge diagnoses d and medications y from the entire training set. For each diagnosis, the conditional probability of prescribing a drug is computed as:

$$p(y|d) = \frac{\text{freq}(d, y)}{\sum_{y'} \text{freq}(d, y')}. \tag{5}$$

The top-k drugs with the highest $p(y|d)$ values (set to $k = 5$ in our experiments) are selected to form the prior knowledge set K_{stat}.

(4) Structural Perturbation Augmentation. To enhance model robustness and reduce order sensitivity [5], we design two complementary perturbation strategies applied independently to the diagnosis and medication sequences. For the diagnosis side, secondary diagnoses are randomly permuted while keeping the primary diagnosis fixed. For the medication side, the order of discharge drugs in Y is randomly shuffled. Formally, the augmented dataset is defined as:

$$\mathcal{D}' = \{(X'_r, Y'_r)\}_{r=1}^{R}, \quad X'_r = \pi_r^{(d)}(X),\ Y'_r = \pi_r^{(y)}(Y), \tag{6}$$

where $\pi_r^{(d)}(\cdot)$ and $\pi_r^{(y)}(\cdot)$ denote the diagnosis- and drug-level permutations, respectively, and R is the number of augmented variants.

3.3 Multi-scale Model Training

Building on the enhanced dataset $\mathcal{D}'$, we adopt a multi-scale model training paradigm to exploit the complementary strengths of language models with varying capacities. Specifically, multiple models from the Qwen series [17,23] (including 3B, 7B, and 8B scales) are fine-tuned under different data augmentation configurations, allowing each scale to learn distinct semantic and reasoning patterns. Rather than employing all variants across scales, we selectively utilize representative models to balance performance diversity and computational efficiency.

3.4 Post-processing

To ensure the clinical validity of generated results, we apply strict post-processing that constrains model outputs within the predefined candidate drug list. Given a model prediction $\hat{Y}_i = \{\hat{y}_1, \hat{y}_2, \ldots, \hat{y}_m\}$ and the official candidate set $\mathcal{C}$, each predicted drug $\hat{y}_j$ is matched to its closest entry in $\mathcal{C}$ using hierarchical matching rules—exact, base-name, and fuzzy similarity matching—implemented via string normalization and sequence alignment. Only valid candidates are retained:

$$\hat{Y}_i^* = \{\hat{y}_j \mid \mathrm{match}(\hat{y}_j, \mathcal{C}) \geq \tau\}, \tag{7}$$

where τ is the similarity threshold (empirically set to 0.8).

3.5 Hierarchical Ensemble Inference

After obtaining post-processed predictions from all fine-tuned models, we adopt a two-level hierarchical ensemble strategy to integrate complementary outputs across model scales and training variants. In the first stage, we aggregate the predictions of models M_5–M_9 (7B and 3B scales) to form an intermediate ensemble output $\hat{Y}^{(1)}$, capturing diverse knowledge from smaller and medium-scale models. The confidence score for each candidate drug $y \in \mathcal{C}$ is computed as:

$$S^{(1)}(y) = \sum_{i=5}^{9} w_i \cdot \mathbb{I}(y \in \hat{Y}_i^*), \tag{8}$$

and the first-level ensemble output is defined as:

$$\hat{Y}^{(1)} = \{y \mid S^{(1)}(y) \geq \tau_1\}, \tag{9}$$

where τ_1 denotes the first-level fusion threshold.

In the second stage, we merge $\hat{Y}^{(1)}$ with the predictions of models M_1–M_4 (8B scale) to obtain the final recommendation. The confidence is calculated as:

$$S^{(2)}(y) = \sum_{i=1}^{4} w_i \cdot \mathbb{I}(y \in \hat{Y}_i^*) + w^{(1)} \cdot \mathbb{I}(y \in \hat{Y}^{(1)}), \tag{10}$$

and the final ensemble output is given by:

$$\hat{Y}_{\text{final}} = \{y \mid S^{(2)}(y) \geq \tau_2\}, \tag{11}$$

where $w^{(1)}$ represents the weight of the first-level ensemble and τ_2 is the global fusion threshold optimized on the validation set.

4 Experiments

4.1 Datasets

We use the CDrugRed dataset [11] released in the CHIP 2025 Shared Task 2. The dataset contains de-identified Chinese inpatient records including diagnoses, medical history, clinical notes, and discharge prescriptions. Following the official split (3602/570/1722 for train/validation/test), we further performed a patient-level re-split, holding out 100 patients (204 visit records) from the official training set as an offline validation set for model tuning. Table 1 summarizes both the official and our experimental splits on the CDrugRed dataset.

Table 1. Statistics of the CDrugRed dataset. The offline validation set was constructed by holding out 100 patients from the official training set.

Items	Train	Validation	Test
Number of Patients (official)	1910	320	960
Number of Patients (used in our experiments)	1810	100	960
Visit Records (official)	3602	570	1722
Visit Records (used in our experiments)	3398	204	1722

4.2 Evaluation Metrics

Following the official evaluation protocol, we evaluate model performance using four common metrics in drug recommendation: *Precision*, *Recall*, *F1-score*, and *Jaccard similarity*. let y_i and $\hat{y}_i$ denote the ground-truth and predicted drug sets for the i-th visit respectively, and N the total number of visit records.

Jaccard. It measures the overlap between predicted and ground-truth drug sets:

$$\text{Jaccard} = \frac{1}{N}\sum_{i=1}^{N}\frac{|y_i \cap \hat{y}_i|}{|y_i \cup \hat{y}_i|}. \tag{12}$$

Precision, Recall, and F1-score. We compute per-record precision and recall as

$$\text{Precision}(y_i, \hat{y}_i) = \frac{|y_i \cap \hat{y}_i|}{|\hat{y}_i|}, \quad \text{Recall}(y_i, \hat{y}_i) = \frac{|y_i \cap \hat{y}_i|}{|y_i|}, \tag{13}$$

and define the F1-score as their harmonic mean:

$$f1(y_i, \hat{y}_i) = 2 \cdot \frac{\text{Precision}(y_i, \hat{y}_i) \cdot \text{Recall}(y_i, \hat{y}_i)}{\text{Precision}(y_i, \hat{y}_i) + \text{Recall}(y_i, \hat{y}_i)}. \tag{14}$$

The final reported AVG_P, AVG_R, and F1 are averaged over all N records:

$$\begin{aligned} \text{AVG\_P} = \frac{1}{N}\sum_{i=1}^{N}\text{Precision}(y_i, \hat{y}_i), \quad \text{AVG\_R} &= \frac{1}{N}\sum_{i=1}^{N}\text{Recall}(y_i, \hat{y}_i), \\ \text{F1} &= \frac{1}{N}\sum_{i=1}^{N} f1(y_i, \hat{y}_i). \end{aligned} \tag{15}$$

4.3 Implementation Details

We conduct all experiments using the `SWIFT` [27] training framework with full-parameter fine-tuning. The AdamW [14] optimizer is employed under the `DeepSpeed ZeRO-3` optimization framework with a learning rate of 1×10^{-5}. Each model is trained for 10 epochs, with checkpoints saved after every epoch. The maximum length is set to 16,384 tokens to accommodate long and detailed clinical narratives. For ensemble inference, model weights $\{w_i\}$ are assigned proportionally to each model's validation F1 score, with higher-capacity models receiving slightly larger coefficients. The first-level fusion threshold is set to $\tau_1 = 0.6$, and the second-level global threshold to $\tau_2 = 0.5$. During inference, all models are deployed via the `sglang` [28] backend. The checkpoint achieving the best validation performance is selected for final evaluation on the test set.

4.4 Results

Table 2 summarizes the performance of all single models on the test set under different data augmentation configurations, from which we can observe that:

For the Qwen3-8B models (Models 1–5), we conducted a full sweep over all augmentation strategies proposed in Sect. 3.2, including drug-category guidance, patient meta-features, disease–drug statistical priors, and structural perturbation. Among these, incorporating pharmacological category information achieved the strongest validation performance and is therefore presented as Model 1, while

Table 2. Performance comparison of models on the test set trained with different data augmentation strategies.

Model	Jaccard	AVG_P	AVG_R	F1
1–Qwen3–8b	0.4719	0.6194	0.6025	0.5885
2–Qwen3–8b	0.4679	0.6292	0.5791	0.5829
3–Qwen3–8b	0.4601	0.5907	0.6206	0.5838
4–Qwen3–8b	0.4608	0.6014	0.6083	0.5806
5–Qwen3–8b	0.4148	0.5560	0.5577	0.5341
6–Qwen2.5-7B-Instruct	0.4180	0.5503	0.5745	0.5407
7–Qwen2.5-7B-Instruct	0.4103	0.5536	0.5564	0.5305
8–Qwen2.5-7B-Instruct	0.3989	0.5394	0.5464	0.5180
9–Qwen2.5-3B-Instruct	0.3840	0.5174	0.5378	0.5029

the remaining variants provide slightly lower but consistent scores. For the 7B models (Models 6–8), we preserved the top three augmentation settings from the offline validation selection. The 3B model (Model 9) reflects the best-performing configuration at this scale. As expected, the 8B models achieve the highest accuracy among single models, whereas the 7B and 3B variants contribute additional diversity that becomes valuable during fusion. Building upon the single-model outputs, we adopt a hierarchical ensemble strategy: Models 5–9 are first aggregated into an intermediate ensemble, which is subsequently fused with Models 1–4 to obtain the final output.

5 Conclusion

In this work, we proposed a unified framework for discharge medication recommendation that integrates multi-dimensional feature enhancement and multi-scale model training. By enriching EHR inputs with pharmacological categories, patient meta-features, and disease–drug statistical priors, the model can capture more structured clinical semantics. The multi-scale fine-tuning and two-level hierarchical ensemble further leverage complementary strengths among diverse models, yielding robust and accurate medication recommendations. Experimental results on the CHIP 2025 Shared Task 2 (Discharge Medication Recommendation for Metabolic Diseases) benchmark demonstrate that our approach outperforms the official baselines and all competing systems, achieving state-of-the-art performance. While the approach achieves strong results, it still depends on supervised fine-tuning and increases inference cost due to ensemble integration. Future work will explore lightweight adaptation and more interpretable modeling strategies.

References

1. Achiam, J., Adler, S., Agarwal, S., Ahmad, L., Akkaya, I., Aleman, F.L., Almeida, D., Altenschmidt, J., Altman, S., Anadkat, S., et al.: Gpt-4 technical report. arXiv preprint arXiv:2303.08774 (2023)
2. Bhoi, S., Lee, M.L., Hsu, W., Fang, H.S.A., Tan, N.C.: Personalizing medication recommendation with a graph-based approach. ACM Trans. Inf. Syst. (TOIS) **40**(3), 1–23 (2021)
3. Breiman, L.: Random forests. Mach. Learn. **45**(1), 5–32 (2001)
4. Chen, Z., Zhao, Z., Zhu, Z., Zhang, R., Li, X., Raj, B., Yao, H.: AutoPRM: automating procedural supervision for multi-step reasoning via controllable question decomposition. In: Duh, K., Gomez, H., Bethard, S. (eds.) Proceedings of the 2024 Conference of the North American Chapter of the Association for Computational Linguistics: Human Language Technologies (Volume 1: Long Papers). pp. 1346–1362. Association for Computational Linguistics, Mexico City, Mexico (Jun 2024). https://doi.org/10.18653/v1/2024.naacl-long.73, https://aclanthology.org/2024.naacl-long.73/
5. Chhabra, A., Askari, H., Mohapatra, P.: Revisiting zero-shot abstractive summarization in the era of large language models from the perspective of position bias. In: Proceedings of the 2024 Conference of the North American Chapter of the Association for Computational Linguistics: Human Language Technologies (Volume 2: Short Papers), pp. 1–11 (2024)
6. Comanici, G., Bieber, E., Schaekermann, M., Pasupat, I., Sachdeva, N., Dhillon, I., Blistein, M., Ram, O., Zhang, D., Rosen, E., et al.: Gemini 2.5: pushing the frontier with advanced reasoning, multimodality, long context, and next generation agentic capabilities. arXiv preprint arXiv:2507.06261 (2025)
7. Dong, X., Yu, Z., Cao, W., Shi, Y., Ma, Q.: A survey on ensemble learning. Front. Comp. Sci. **14**(2), 241–258 (2020)
8. Friedman, J.H.: Greedy function approximation: a gradient boosting machine. Ann. Stat. 1189–1232 (2001)
9. Grattafiori, A., Dubey, A., Jauhri, A., Pandey, A., Kadian, A., Al-Dahle, A., Letman, A., Mathur, A., Schelten, A., Vaughan, A., et al.: The llama 3 herd of models. arXiv preprint arXiv:2407.21783 (2024)
10. Hager, P., Jungmann, F., Holland, R., Bhagat, K., Hubrecht, I., Knauer, M., Vielhauer, J., Makowski, M., Braren, R., Kaissis, G., et al.: Evaluation and mitigation of the limitations of large language models in clinical decision-making. Nat. Med. **30**(9), 2613–2622 (2024)
11. Li, J., Yuan, H., Luo, L., Jiang, Y., Wang, F., Zhang, P., Lv, H., Wang, J., Sun, Y., Lin, H.: Cdrugred: a chinese drug recommendation dataset for discharge medications in metabolic diseases. arXiv preprint arXiv:2510.21084 (2025)
12. Li, J., Yuan, H., Luo, L., Lv, T., Jiang, Y., Wang, F., Zhang, P., Lv, H., Wang, J., Sun, Y., et al.: Overview of chip 2025 shared task 2: discharge medication recommendation for metabolic diseases based on chinese electronic health records. arXiv preprint arXiv:2511.06230 (2025)
13. Li, R., Niu, Y., Scott, S.R., Zhou, C., Lan, L., Liang, Z., Li, J.: Using electronic medical record data for research in a healthcare information and management systems society (himss) analytics electronic medical record adoption model (emram) stage 7 hospital in beijing: cross-sectional study. JMIR Med. Inform. **9**(8), e24405 (2021)

14. Loshchilov, I., Hutter, F.: Decoupled weight decay regularization. arXiv preprint arXiv:1711.05101 (2017)
15. Ortega, L.A., Cabañas, R., Masegosa, A.: Diversity and generalization in neural network ensembles. In: International Conference on Artificial Intelligence and Statistics, pp. 11720–11743. PMLR (2022)
16. Ramachandran, R., Chinnammal, V., Malathy, K., Sailaja, K., Shanmugam, S.: An improved drug recommendation system using artificial intelligence assisted learning methodology. In: 2024 International Conference on Advances in Computing, Communication and Applied Informatics (ACCAI), pp. 1–7. IEEE (2024)
17. Team, Q., et al.: Qwen2 technical report. arXiv preprint arXiv:2407.10671 **2**(3) (2024)
18. Touvron, H., Martin, L., Stone, K., Albert, P., Almahairi, A., Babaei, Y., Bashlykov, N., Batra, S., Bhargava, P., Bhosale, S., et al.: Llama 2: open foundation and fine-tuned chat models. arXiv preprint arXiv:2307.09288 (2023)
19. Wood, D., Mu, T., Webb, A.M., Reeve, H.W., Luján, M., Brown, G.: A unified theory of diversity in ensemble learning. J. Mach. Learn. Res. **24**(359), 1–49 (2023)
20. Wu, X., Zhao, Y., Zhang, Y., Wu, J., Zhu, Z., Zhang, Y., Ouyang, Y., Zhang, Z., Wang, H., Yang, J., et al.: Medjourney: benchmark and evaluation of large language models over patient clinical journey. Adv. Neural. Inf. Process. Syst. **37**, 87621–87646 (2024)
21. Wu, Z., Dadu, A., Nalls, M., Faghri, F., Sun, J.: Instruction tuning large language models to understand electronic health records. Adv. Neural. Inf. Process. Syst. **37**, 54772–54786 (2024)
22. Xing, B., Qin, L., Zhu, Z., Yu, Z., Tsang, I.W.: Dxa-net: dual-task cross-lingual alignment network for zero-shot cross-lingual spoken language understanding. IEEE Trans. Pattern Anal. Mach. Intell. (2025)
23. Yang, A., Li, A., Yang, B., Zhang, B., Hui, B., Zheng, B., Yu, B., Gao, C., Huang, C., Lv, C., et al.: Qwen3 technical report. arXiv preprint arXiv:2505.09388 (2025)
24. Yang, M., Liu, S., Zhang, C.: The related metabolic diseases and treatments of obesity. In: Healthcare, vol. 10, p. 1616. MDPI (2022)
25. Zeng, Q., He, Y., Dong, S., Zhao, X., Chen, Z., Song, Z., Chang, G., Yang, F., Wang, Y.: Optimal cut-off values of bmi, waist circumference and waist: height ratio for defining obesity in chinese adults. Br. J. Nutr. **112**(10), 1735–1744 (2014)
26. Zhang, Y., Zhu, Z., Wu, X.: CMedCalc-bench: a fine-grained benchmark for Chinese medical calculations in LLM. In: Christodoulopoulos, C., Chakraborty, T., Rose, C., Peng, V. (eds.) Proceedings of the 2025 Conference on Empirical Methods in Natural Language Processing, pp. 25661–25670. Association for Computational Linguistics, Suzhou, China (Nov 2025), https://aclanthology.org/2025.emnlp-main.1302/
27. Zhao, Y., Huang, J., Hu, J., Wang, X., Mao, Y., Zhang, D., Jiang, Z., Wu, Z., Ai, B., Wang, A., et al.: Swift: a scalable lightweight infrastructure for fine-tuning. In: Proceedings of the AAAI Conference on Artificial Intelligence, vol. 39, pp. 29733–29735 (2025)
28. Zheng, L., Yin, L., Xie, Z., Sun, C.L., Huang, J., Yu, C.H., Cao, S., Kozyrakis, C., Stoica, I., Gonzalez, J.E., et al.: Sglang: efficient execution of structured language model programs. Adv. Neural. Inf. Process. Syst. **37**, 62557–62583 (2024)
29. Zhu, Z., Cheng, X., An, H., Wang, Z., Chen, D., Huang, Z.: Zero-shot spoken language understanding via large language models: A preliminary study. In: Calzolari, N., Kan, M.Y., Hoste, V., Lenci, A., Sakti, S., Xue, N. (eds.) Proceedings of the 2024 Joint International Conference on Computational Linguistics, Language

Resources and Evaluation (LREC-COLING 2024), pp. 17877–17883. ELRA and ICCL, Torino, Italia (May 2024), https://aclanthology.org/2024.lrec-main.1554/
30. Zhu, Z., Cheng, X., Chen, Z., Chen, Y., Zhang, Y., Wu, X., Zheng, Y., Xing, B.: Inmu-net: advancing multi-modal intent detection via information bottleneck and multi-sensory processing. In: Proceedings of the 32nd ACM International Conference on Multimedia, pp. 515–524 (2024)
31. Zhu, Z., Zhang, F., Zhang, Y., Sun, J., Huang, Z., Long, Q., Xing, B., Wu, X.: A survey on multi-modal intent recognition: Recent advances and new frontiers. In: Christodoulopoulos, C., Chakraborty, T., Rose, C., Peng, V. (eds.) Findings of the Association for Computational Linguistics: EMNLP 2025, pp. 15223–15236. Association for Computational Linguistics, Suzhou, China (Nov 2025), https://aclanthology.org/2025.findings-emnlp.823/
32. Zhu, Z., Zhang, Y., Zhuang, X., Zhang, F., Wan, Z., Chen, Y., QingqingLong, Q., Zheng, Y., Wu, X.: Can we trust AI doctors? a survey of medical hallucination in large language and large vision-language models. In: Che, W., Nabende, J., Shutova, E., Pilehvar, M.T. (eds.) Findings of the Association for Computational Linguistics: ACL 2025, pp. 6748–6769. Association for Computational Linguistics, Vienna, Austria (Jul 2025).https://doi.org/10.18653/v1/2025.findings-acl.350, https://aclanthology.org/2025.findings-acl.350/

DP-EMR: A Chinese Medication Recommendation Method for Metabolic Diseases Based on Two-Stage Ensemble Learning

Zhongtian Hua[1], Kejun Wu[1], Chengxin Ru[1], Yi Luo[1], Mengyuan Wang[1], Meijia Yu[2], and Yingjie Han[1](✉)

[1] Zhengzhou University, No.100 Science Avenue, Zhengzhou, China
{hzt1113,zzunlpwkj,rcx,wangmengyuan}@gs.zzu.edu.cn, nancetide@stu.zzu.edu.cn, ieyjhan@zzu.edu.cn

[2] Henan University of Science and Technology, No.263 Kaiyuan Avenue, Luoyang, China
240320261531@stu.haust.edu.cn

Abstract. The recommendation of medication for discharge is a key task in clinical decision support and is of great significance for improving medical quality. Although large language models perform well in natural language processing, they still face challenges in the medical field where data is scarce and professional barriers are high. This paper proposes a model discharge medication recommendation framework called DP-EMR that integrates data augmentation, efficient fine-tuning, and innovative inference: It expands the training data by applying a pseudo-label augmentation technique based on confidence screening to the validation set, performing efficient fine-tuning of multiple heterogeneous large language models using LoRA, designing an innovative two-stage hierarchical integration strategy. In this strategy, different models trained on the original data and enhanced data are first weighted and voted for integration respectively, and then the prediction results of the first stage were fused through an adaptive strategy based on the prediction length. This method significantly enhanced the accuracy and robustness of medication recommendation, and ultimately rank second in the CHIP2025 discharge medication recommendation Task.

Keywords: Medication recommendation · pseudo-label · fine-tuning · model integration

1 Introduction

Discharge medication recommendation (DMR) serves as a critical component of clinical decision support systems, aiming to generate safe, effective, and personalized medication plans based on a patient's complete hospitalization records [1]. Accurate medication recommendations directly influence post-discharge recovery

Y. Zhang et al. (Eds.): CHIP 2025, CCIS 2884, pp. 503–517, 2026.
https://doi.org/10.1007/978-981-95-7299-1_31

and patient safety, making it a key indicator of healthcare quality [2]. With the widespread adoption of Electronic Medical Records (EMRs) [3], the use of artificial intelligence to automatically analyze large-scale clinical texts and provide intelligent decision support has emerged as a new trend in smart healthcare.

Despite the remarkable capabilities demonstrated by large language models (LLMs) in various natural language processing tasks in recent years [4], their direct application to the medical field—particularly in discharge medication recommendation—still faces several challenges [5]. We identify three main issues: data scarcity and professional barriers, where high-quality annotated medical data are limited, especially for Chinese EMRs [6], which contain abundant specialized terminology and non-standardized descriptions requiring deep domain knowledge for interpretation; output precision constraints, meaning that medication recommendations must strictly adhere to a predefined set of candidate drugs [7], as any deviation could lead to clinical risks, placing extremely high demands on the precision of model outputs; and computational and deployment limitations, as real-world application scenarios often impose strict restrictions on model size and resource consumption (e.g., the CHIP2025 evaluation requires the model parameters not to exceed 10 billion), making full fine-tuning of very large models difficult to implement [8].

To address the above challenges, this paper proposes a robust discharge medication recommendation framework named DP-EMR, which integrates data augmentation [9], parameter-efficient fine-tuning [10], and hierarchical inference [11]. We design clinically interpretable prompt templates to guide medication decision logic and adopt a confidence-based pseudo-labeling strategy to expand the training data under strict quality control [12,13]. Low-Rank Adaptation (LoRA) is employed to fine-tune multiple open-source LLMs in a parameter-efficient manner [14]. Furthermore, an innovative two-stage hierarchical ensemble strategy is introduced, combining intra-group weighted voting with adaptive inter-group fusion based on prediction length, effectively balancing the precision and completeness of recommendation results.

Our main contributions are summarized as follows:

1. We propose a three-stage model enhancement framework, DP-EMR, for discharge medication recommendation. Distinct enhancement strategies are applied at three different stages—data augmentation, model training, and inference—to systematically improve the performance of base models on the specific task.
2. We innovatively propose a two-stage hierarchical ensemble learning strategy. In the first stage, fine-tuned models are grouped according to their training data sources, and fixed-threshold-based weighted voting is performed within each group. In the second stage, an adaptive inter-group fusion mechanism based on prediction length is applied to the intra-group voting results, enhancing the accuracy and robustness of predictions through multi-level ensemble.
3. We validate the effectiveness and necessity of the DP-EMR framework through comprehensive comparative experiments and ablation studies. Addi-

tionally, we discuss several technical attempts that did not yield significant improvements, providing practical references for future research.

2 Related Work

2.1 Intelligent Medication Recommendation in the Medical Domain

Medication recommendation based on EMRs is a data-driven clinical decision support task [3]. Early systems relied on rule-based methods or classical machine learning models (e.g., logistic regression, SVM), which required extensive feature engineering and lacked interpretability [15]. With the emergence of deep learning, RNN- and CNN-based models were introduced to capture temporal and contextual dependencies in EMR sequences [16–19]. However, their performance was constrained by limited capacity to understand complex medical semantics.

The introduction of pre-trained language models (PLMs) such as BERT and BioBERT significantly improved medical text representation learning, supporting tasks like entity recognition and relation extraction that are foundational to medication reasoning [20,21]. Nonetheless, most PLM-based studies framed medication recommendation as classification or tagging tasks, limiting their ability to perform flexible clinical reasoning or generate explanatory recommendations. This gap has motivated recent exploration into generative approaches that align more closely with real-world clinical reasoning.

The emergence of large language models (LLMs) has further reshaped the paradigm of medical NLP by enabling multi-task generalization and instruction following. Studies have applied LLMs to medical question answering, report generation, and clinical dialogue understanding, demonstrating their potential to emulate physician reasoning [22]. However, directly applying general-purpose LLMs in clinical contexts leads to issues of *hallucination* and *knowledge lag*. Two primary adaptation directions have emerged:

1. **Domain-adaptive pretraining** on biomedical corpora to infuse domain-specific knowledge (e.g., ClinicalGPT); and
2. **Instruction tuning** on medical datasets to align model behavior with domain-specific reasoning objectives.

Our work belongs to the latter, focusing on instruction tuning under *low-resource constraints*. Unlike prior works that rely on large-scale data or full fine-tuning, we explore *parameter-efficient fine-tuning* combined with *high-quality pseudo-label generation*, achieving competitive performance using mid-scale LLMs.

2.2 Data Augmentation and Ensemble Learning

Data scarcity is a persistent bottleneck in medical NLP. Beyond traditional augmentation techniques (e.g., back translation, synonym replacement), pseudo-labeling has emerged as an effective semi-supervised strategy [23]. By leveraging model-generated predictions as additional supervision, pseudo-labeling expands the dataset without manual annotation. Key to its success is ensuring label reliability–commonly achieved through confidence thresholds. We extend this idea by introducing a *loss-based confidence metric*, where token-level cross-entropy serves as a stricter, uncertainty-aware filter for selecting high-confidence samples, effectively improving training data quality [13].

Model ensemble methods are another proven strategy to enhance robustness. Classical approaches such as majority voting or weighted averaging have been extended in the LLM era to accommodate diverse architectures and data sources. Our *two-stage hierarchical ensemble* framework first integrates predictions within model groups using weighted voting and then performs adaptive fusion across groups based on output length and Jaccard similarity [24], balancing model consensus and clinical parsimony. This strategy not only mitigates individual model biases but also aligns with the clinical principle of "effective yet minimal medication".

3 Methodology

Our method overview is shown in Fig. 1. In order to achieve more accurate medication recommendations for metabolic diseases, a Medication Recommendation framework based on Dual-Phase Ensemble learning called DP-EMR is proposed. This framework can be roughly divided into three major parts, namely the data augmentation part, the training part and the inference part. In the data augmentation section, the original training set is first used to perform supervised fine-tuning on the chatglm-9b model, thereby obtaining a check model. Then, the checking model is used to predict the validation set, thereby obtaining the prediction result of each data in validation set and its corresponding loss. This loss value is regarded as the model's confidence level for this prediction result, and based on this confidence level, all validation datas are sorted and filtered, thereby obtaining a pseudo-label dataset. During the training phase, two different training sets are established to prepare for the subsequent ensemble learning. One of the training sets contains only the original training set, while the other training set includes both the original training set and the pseudo-labeled dataset obtained during the data augmentation stage. These two training sets were respectively used to fine-tune four small large language models with less than 10B parameters, including chatglm [25], qwen3 [26], qwen2.5 [27], and qwen2 [28], through LoRA fine-tuning, thereby obtaining two different fine-tuned versions of the same model. In the inference stage, the idea of Test Time Augmentation (TTA) is referred to, and the reasoning results of different models are voted and integrated in stages. First, the models trained with the same dataset are divided into the same group, and the first stage of weighted voting integration is carried out within the group to obtain two sets of voting results within the group. Then, in the second stage, a length adaptive voting integration based on jaccard similarity is carried out on the voting results within these two groups to obtain the final model ensemble learning result.

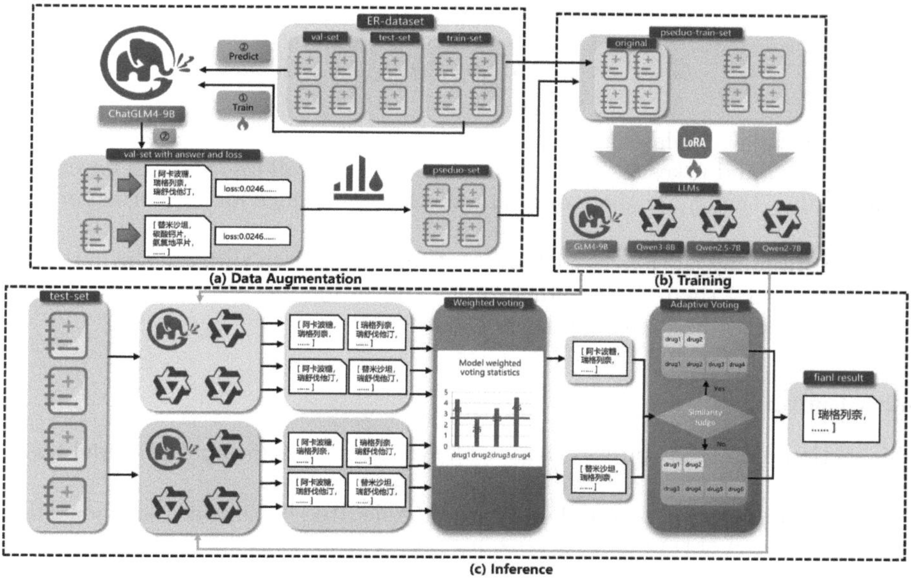

Fig. 1. The overview of our method. We propose DP-EMR, a dual-phase ensemble learning framework for metabolic disease medication recommendation. It consists of three stages: (1) Data Augmentation, where we fine-tune a model to generate pseudo-labels from the validation set; (2) Training, where we create two training sets (original and pseudo-labeled) to fine-tune multiple SLMs; (3) Inference, where we perform two-stage ensemble voting to integrate predictions from different models.

3.1 Data Augmentation

This section mainly introduces the relevant methods used in the data augmentation part, including how to label and clean the unlabeled validation set using a large language model with large-scale parameters.

To expand the scale of the training set, we carry out cleaning work on the validation dataset based on the model's confidence level. Specifically, We first perform parameter-efficient fine-tuning on ChatGLM4-9B using original training set, thereby obtaining a filtering model capable of screening of validation data. Checkpoints that performed best during training is selected as the inspection model, and then input the validation data into the model to obtain the answer with loss. The returned loss is used as the metric to screen the data. We believe that data with a lower loss value reflects that the model is more confident in the output of this piece of data, with a high level of confidence; conversely, it indicates a lower level of confidence. For the input instruction sequence X and the predicted label sequence T = $[t_1,t_2,...,t_n]$, we take the cross-entropy loss of the next token in the output label part as the confidence index, and the formula is as follows:

$$Loss = -\frac{1}{n}\sum_{i=1}^{n}\log P(t_i|t_1, t_2, ..., t_{i-1}) \tag{1}$$

This formula calculates the conditional probability log-likelihood of each predicted label ti and takes the average to obtain the overall loss value. The smaller the loss value, the higher the model's prediction confidence for the corresponding label.

After obtaining the loss of each piece of validation data through the detection model, we sorted them in ascending order and ultimately selected the top 70% of the data as the final pseudo dataset.

3.2 Training

This section mainly introduces the specific work and Settings in the model training stage.

After obtaining the pseudo-label dataset generated by the data augmentation stage, in order to obtain more diverse model prediction results in the integration stage, we set up two different training sets for model training. One of the training sets only contains the original training set, while the other contains both the original training set and the pseudo-label dataset. Next, we select four current mainstream large language models with parameter scales within 10B, namely ChatGLM4-9B, Qwen3-8B, Qwen2.5-7B, and Qwen2-7B. We fine-tuned these four models using two datasets respectively with LoRA, thereby obtaining two different fine-tuned versions for each model.

3.3 Inference

This section mainly introduces the two-stage ensemble learning strategies used in the reasoning stage, namely the multi-model weighted ensemble in the first stage and the adaptive ensemble in the second stage.

Multi-model Weighted Integration In this stage, a four-model parallel integration architecture is adopted to integrate the prediction results of the fine-tuned versions of the four basic models, qwen2, qwen3, qwen2.5, and glm4, on the original data and pseudo-label data respectively. The integration process adopts a weighted voting mechanism, fully considering the performance differences of different models in the task of drug recommendation for metabolic diseases. Specifically, for the integration of the four models, we design a fixed-threshold voting algorithm: for each patient ID, the frequency of each drug's occurrence in the prediction results of the four models is counted, and the voting threshold is set at 2, meaning that only drugs predicted by at least two models were included in the final result. Then, weight allocation is carried out. Based on the performance of the models on the validation set, differentiated weights are assigned to different models. Multi-model integration effectively reduces the prediction bias of a single model. Through the voting mechanism, consensus predictions among models are mined, thereby enhancing the reliability of the results. The weight parameters can be dynamically adjusted according to the model performance to meet the requirements of different scenarios.

Self Adaptive Integration After completing the dual-group integration in the first stage, the second stage of integration processing begins, where the original data integration results are deeply fused with the pseudo-label data integration results. At this stage, we adopt an adaptive integration strategy based on prediction length, which fully considered the characteristic differences in model performance under the two training strategies.

Specifically, the system first calculates the Jaccard similarity between the two integrated results to evaluate the consistency degree of the two sets of predictions. When the similarity is relatively high, it indicates that the models obtained by the two training strategies have a strong consensus on drug recommendation. At this time, the intersection drugs predicted by the two groups are preferentially selected as the basis, and then some non-consensus drugs are appropriately supplemented to ensure the comprehensiveness of the recommendation results. When the similarity is low, the system automatically select the group of results with a smaller number of predicted drugs as the main reference. This design is based on the principle in clinical practice that drug recommendations should be concise and effective, avoiding unnecessary combination use of multiple drugs. This adaptive mechanism can dynamically adjust the integration strategy based on the specific circumstances of the two groups of predictions. It respects the consensus of the model while adopting a conservative strategy when the differences are obvious, effectively balancing the accuracy and clinical practicality of the recommendation results. The final output fully demonstrates the synergy effect of data augmentation and model integration, providing more personalized, safe and effective discharge medication plans for patients with metabolic diseases.

4 Experiments

4.1 Dataset and Metrics

The CHIP2025 task 2 launch CDrugRed [29]—a Chinese discharge drug recommendation dataset covering patients with metabolic diseases. This dataset contains 5,894 de-identified medical records from 3,190 patients, involving 651 candidate drugs. The data was collected from a tertiary grade A hospital in China. With its rich and authentic data, this dataset can comprehensively evaluate the performance of the model in the field of Chinese discharge drug recommendation.

To evaluate the performance of the model in the drug recommendation task, four widely used evaluation metrics were adopted in this task: Precision, Recall, F1-score and Jaccard similarity. Here, y represents the real drug set, $\hat{y}$ represents the drug set predicted by the model, and $|X|$ represents the number of elements in set X.

Jaccard similarity: This metric measures the degree of overlap between the predicted drug set and the true drug set. It is obtained by dividing the size of the intersection between the two by the size of the union.

$$\text{Jaccard} = \frac{1}{N}\sum_{i=1}^{N}\frac{|y_i \cap \hat{y}_i|}{|y_i \cup \hat{y}_i|} \tag{2}$$

Here, N represents the total number of medical visit records.

Precision measures the proportion of the drugs predicted by the model that actually appear in real prescriptions, while recall measures the proportion of real drugs that are correctly predicted by the model. The F1 score is the harmonic mean of precision and recall. For the first medical record, these indicators are defined as follows:

$$\text{Precision}(y_i, \hat{y}_i) = \frac{|y_i \cap \hat{y}_i|}{|\hat{y}_i|} \tag{3}$$

$$\text{Recall}(y_i, \hat{y}_i) = \frac{|y_i \cap \hat{y}_i|}{|y_i|} \tag{4}$$

$$\text{F1}(y_i, \hat{y}_i) = \frac{2 \times \text{Precision}(y_i, \hat{y}_i) \times \text{Recall}(y_i, \hat{y}_i)}{\text{Precision}(y_i, \hat{y}_i) + \text{Recall}(y_i, \hat{y}_i)} \tag{5}$$

The overall average of all records is calculated as follows:

$$\text{AVG\_P} = \frac{1}{N}\sum_{i=1}^{N}\text{Precision}(y_i, \hat{y}_i) \tag{6}$$

$$\text{AVG\_R} = \frac{1}{N}\sum_{i=1}^{N}\text{Recall}(y_i, \hat{y}_i) \tag{7}$$

$$\text{F1} = \frac{1}{N}\sum_{i=1}^{N}\text{F1}(y_i, \hat{y}_i) \tag{8}$$

Here, AVG_P and AVG_R respectively represent the average values of the precision rate and recall rate calculated on all medical records, while F1 represents the average F1 score. And the final Score could be Calculated:

$$\text{Score} = \frac{1}{2}(\text{Jaccard} + \text{F1}) \tag{9}$$

4.2 Experimental Setup

To verify the effectiveness of the DP-EMR framework in the medication recommendation task, we used the performance of four base models: ChatGLM4-9B, qwen3-8b, qwen2.5-7b, and qwen2-7b on the CDrugRed dataset as the baseline for comparison. Meanwhile, in this evaluation, we also attempt methods based on the Chain of Thought (CoT) and Retrieval Augmented Generation (RAG). Specifically, for the CoT method, we first generate the thought chain data for the training set through LLMs with large-scale parameters (such as DeepSeek-V3.1), and then use this thought chain data to fine-tune the LLMs with small-scale parameters. As for the RAG technology, we search for the network information of the drugs to be retrieved through the search engine API and calculate the similarity between it and the features of the patient's electronic medical records. From this, we select the top 100 drugs to help the LLM narrow down the retrieval range. However, neither of these two methods works in the current scenario. However, we still placed the results in the experimental table for reference by the academic community.

To control the variables, in the fine-tuning experiment, we uniformly adopt the LoRA method to fine-tune the LLM. To optimize the model's Video memory efficiency, we use an 8-bit AdamW optimizer and enabledgradient checkpoints. Meanwhile, we adopt the cosine annealing learning rate scheduling strategy.

Our experiments were mainly conducted on a single NVIDIA consumer-grade graphics card with 32GB VRAM, and a simple training framework was manually implemented for fine-tuning. In the early stage of the experiment, we found that a single card often had OOM errors, which were insufficient for fine-tuning llm models at the 7B-9B level. After analysis, we found that this is due to the fact that the huge language modeling head of the language model occupies a large amount of video memory during the process of generating logits and converting them to float32 to calculate losses. Therefore, we rewrote the llm forward propagation method, replacing the loss function with the linear fusion cross-entropy loss of liger-kernel. This improvement significantly reduced the video memory usage. We rely on gradient accumulation to equivalently simulate a larger batchsize.

To more efficiently verify the fine-tuning effect and select the optimal checkpoint, we have implemented a generative end-to-end evaluation during training in the code to enable real-time calculation of the evaluation metrics for each checkpoint during the training process. The relevant hyperparameters involved in the experiment are given in Table 1. The complete prompt template we use will be given in the appendix.

4.3 Results and Analysis

The comparison experiment results are shown in Table 2, and the ablation experiment results are shown in Table 3. It should be noted that for the sake of convenience, we refer to AVG_P and AVG_R as AP and AR respectively, Jaccard as J, and the final Score as S.

Overall, the performance of the model ensemble learning method using the DP-EMR framework on the dataset is significantly better than that of the LoRA fine-tuning method for a single model. The best results of all indicators except the average recall rate are achieved by the DP-EMR method, and they are all 3 to 7% points ahead of the second-best indicators. This proves the effectiveness of the DP-EMR framework in the field of discharge medication recommendation. Next,

Table 1. The hyperparameters involved in the training process.

Parameter name	Parameter value
epoch	10
batch size	1
gradient_accumulation	4
learning rate	2e-5
max grad norm	1.0
lora_r	64
lora_alpha	512

Table 2. Comparative Experiments Results.

Model	Strategy	AP	AR	F1	J	S
ChatGLM4-9B	-	0.1302	0.4385	0.1864	0.1170	0.1517
	CoT + LoRA	0.5591	0.5749	0.5430	0.4267	0.4848
	RAG + LoRA	0.5654	0.5953	0.5563	0.4360	0.4962
	LoRA	0.6165	0.5853	0.5749	0.4595	0.5172
Qwen3-8B		0.5792	**0.5989**	0.5643	0.4421	0.5032
Qwen2.5-7B		0.5836	0.5811	0.5559	0.4416	0.4988
Qwen2-7B		0.5734	0.5787	0.5532	0.4369	0.4950
Ensemble	**DP-EMR(ours)**	**0.6897**	0.5735	**0.6031**	**0.4876**	**0.5453**

this article will respectively analyze the results of the comparative experiment and the ablation experiment.

Comparative Experiments It can be seen from the results of the comparative experiments that the DP-EMR method is superior to the baseline method. All indicators except the recall rate achieve the optimal results, and the final score reaches 0.5453. Among them, the average precision leads to the most suboptimal results, which proves the effectiveness and robustness of the DP-EMR framework. The ChatGLM4-9B model performed the best among all individual models, achieving suboptimal results in all metrics except for the recall rate. Its final score reaches 0.5172. This is because GLM4 has a larger scale of parameters compared to other models, enabling it to store more world knowledge. From the experimental results, it can be found that the recall rate of the results obtained by using the model integration method is significantly lower than that of the results produced by a single model. This is because voting integration is essentially a screening mechanism that filters out some results output by a single model through the method of the minority following the majority. This process may filter out the correct results predicted by some single models, thereby leading to a decrease in the recall rate metric. However, during this process, the increase in the precision and jaccard metrics is much greater than the decrease in the recall rate. This proves that the number of incorrect drugs excluded during the integration process was far greater than the number of correct drugs excluded. Therefore, we believe that the cost of the recall rate decline brought about by the integration is unavoidable but acceptable. Especially in the field of medication recommendation, the cost of prescribing the wrong drugs to patients is far greater than prescribing fewer non-essential drugs to them.

Furthermore, it can be seen from the experimental results that neither the CoT method nor the RAG method is effective in this task. After consulting relevant materials and analyzing error cases, we believe that the main reason why CoT is ineffective is that it is limited by the size of the model parameters. The thought chain usually can only magnify the inherent capabilities of the model itself, but cannot endow the model with new capabilities. Therefore, this prompt enhancement method often works on large language models with large-scale parameters (parameter scale greater than or equal to 20B), but it is ineffective in models with fewer than 10B parameters, and sometimes even reduces the performance of the model. The reason why the RAG method failed to work is that we directly used the search engine API to search for information related to drugs on the Internet without any filtering, which led to poor performance of RAG.

Table 3. Ablation Experiments Results

Ensemble Strategy	**Model List**				**AP**	**AR**	**F1**	**J**	**S**
	ChatGLM4	Qwen3	Qwen2.5	Qwen2					
Single Model	✓	-	-	-	0.6165	0.5853	0.5749	0.4595	0.5172
Weighted Ensemble (w/o Data Augmentation)	✓	✓	✓	-	0.5847	**0.6312**	0.5826	0.4603	0.5214
	✓	✓	-	✓	0.6726	0.5549	0.5838	0.4686	0.5262
	✓	-	✓	✓	0.5954	0.6203	0.5843	0.4627	0.5235
	-	✓	✓	✓	0.5953	0.5856	0.5681	0.4507	0.5094
Weighted Ensemble (w/Data Augmentation)	✓	✓	✓	-	0.6817	0.5541	0.5858	0.4699	0.5278
	✓	✓	-	✓	0.6452	0.5982	0.5965	0.4810	0.5388
	✓	-	✓	✓	0.6896	0.5666	0.5950	0.4834	0.5392
	-	✓	✓	✓	0.6440	0.5916	0.5927	0.4777	0.5352
DP-EMR(ours)	✓	✓	✓	✓	**0.6897**	0.5735	**0.6031**	**0.4876**	**0.5453**

Ablation Experiments In the ablation experiment, we compared the prediction results of four methods: single model prediction, model ensemble prediction without data augmentation, model ensemble prediction with data augmentation, and DP-EMR ensemble. It can be seen from the results that the performance of the method using model integration is better than that of a single model, and it leads the performance indicators of the prediction results of a single model in all indicators except the recall rate. In the comparison of model integration methods, the integration method using data augmentation is significantly better than the one not applicable to data augmentation. Most of the suboptimal results of the experiment come from the ensemble methods using data augmentation. This is because the data diversity brought by data augmentation enables the model to generate more diverse prediction results. In the ensemble stage, more abundant single model prediction results often lead to better ensemble results. In addition, since the performance of GLM4 as a single model is better than that of the other three models, the method that integrates the prediction results of GLM4 in the integration results performs better than the integration method that excludes it. The performance of DP-EMR with the addition of the two-stage adaptive integration method to the weighted integration method is significantly better than that of the weighted integration method, which proves the necessity of the two-stage integration method in the DP-EMR integration method.

5 Conclusion

This paper proposes a medication recommendation framework DP-EMR based on two-stage model integration in response to the problems of data scarcity, output accuracy constraints, and model parameter limitations existing in the task of recommending medications for metabolic diseases at discharge for Chinese electronic medical records in CHIP2025. This framework adopts different methods in the three parts of data augmentation, training and inference to enhance the model's performance in task scenarios. In terms of data augmentation, this framework uses semi-supervised learning methods to pseudo-label the validation set to expand the scale of the training set, thereby alleviating the problem of data scarcity. In terms of training, this framework constrains the output style of the model by fine-tuning the model with instructions. In the inference stage, this framework enhances the accuracy and robustness of model predictions through a two-stage model ensemble learning method, thereby specifically addressing the issues of output precision constraints and model parameter limitations.

The experimental results show that the DP-EMR framework significantly improves the performance of the model in the task of recommending medication for patients upon discharge. The results of the ablation experiment proved the necessity of data augmentation and two-stage ensemble learning in the DP-EMR framework. Ultimately, the team achieve a comprehensive score of 0.5453 in CHIP2025 Task Two through this framework, ranking second among all teams on the B board [30].

A Appendix

See Figs. 2 and 3.

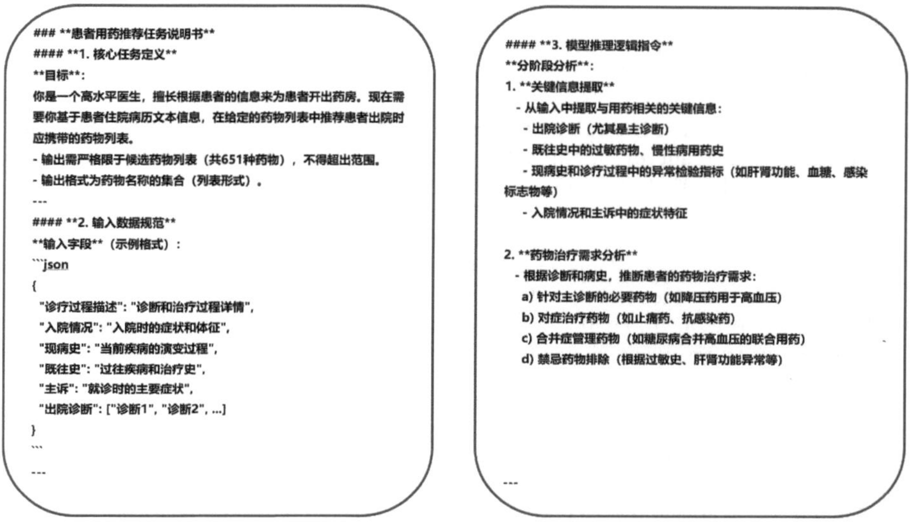

患者用药推荐任务说明书
1. 核心任务定义
目标:
你是一个高水平医生，擅长根据患者的信息来为患者开出药房。现在需要你基于患者住院病历文本信息，在给定的药物列表中推荐患者出院时应携带的药物列表。
- 输出需严格限于候选药物列表（共651种药物），不得超出范围。
- 输出格式为药物名称的集合（列表形式）。
---
2. 输入数据规范
输入字段（示例格式）:
```json
{
 "诊疗过程描述": "诊断和治疗过程详情",
 "入院情况": "入院时的症状和体征",
 "现病史": "当前疾病的演变过程",
 "既往史": "过往疾病和治疗史",
 "主诉": "就诊时的主要症状",
 "出院诊断": ["诊断1", "诊断2", ...]
}
```
---

3. 模型推理逻辑指令
分阶段分析:
1. **关键信息提取**
 - 从输入中提取与用药相关的关键信息:
  - 出院诊断（尤其是主诊断）
  - 既往史中的过敏药物、慢性病用药史
  - 现病史和诊疗过程中的异常检验指标（如肝肾功能、血糖、感染标志物等）
  - 入院情况和主诉中的症状特征

2. **药物治疗需求分析**
 - 根据诊断和病史，推断患者的药物治疗需求:
  a) 针对主诊断的必要药物（如降压药用于高血压）
  b) 对症治疗药物（如止痛药、抗感染药）
  c) 合并症管理药物（如糖尿病合并高血压的联合用药）
  d) 禁忌药物排除（根据过敏史、肝肾功能异常等）

Fig. 2. This picture shows our complete prompt template (Part One).

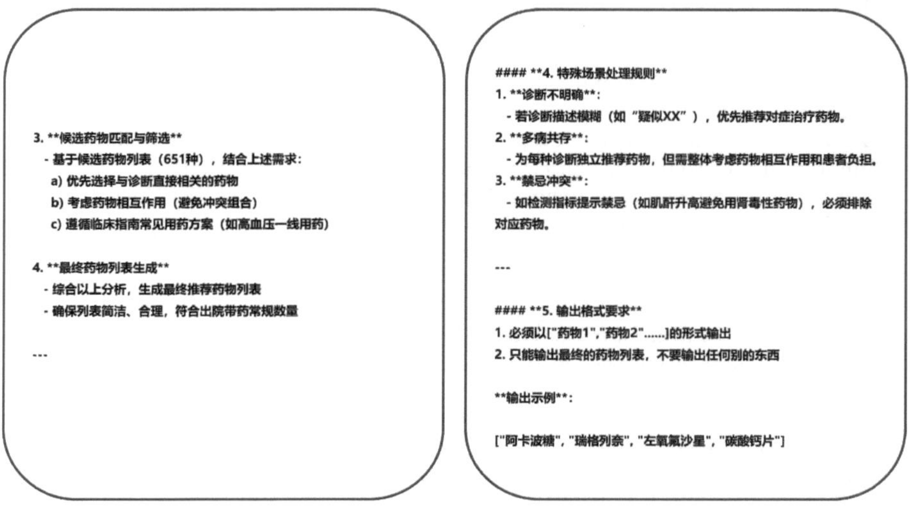

3. **候选药物匹配与筛选**
 - 基于候选药物列表（651种），结合上述需求:
  a) 优先选择与诊断直接相关的药物
  b) 考虑药物相互作用（避免冲突组合）
  c) 遵循临床指南常见用药方案（如高血压一线用药）

4. **最终药物列表生成**
 - 综合以上分析，生成最终推荐药物列表
 - 确保列表简洁、合理，符合出院带药常规数量

---

4. 特殊场景处理规则
1. **诊断不明确**:
 - 若诊断描述模糊（如"疑似XX"），优先推荐对症治疗药物。
2. **多病共存**:
 - 为每种诊断独立推荐药物，但需整体考虑药物相互作用和患者负担。
3. **禁忌冲突**:
 - 如检测指标提示禁忌（如肌酐升高避免用肾毒性药物），必须排除对应药物。

---

5. 输出格式要求
1. 必须以["药物1","药物2"......]的形式输出
2. 只能输出最终的药物列表，不要输出任何别的东西

输出示例:

["阿卡波糖", "瑞格列奈", "左氧氟沙星", "碳酸钙片"]

Fig. 3. This picture shows our complete prompt template (Part Two).

References

1. Yang, M., Liu, S., Zhang, C.: The related metabolic diseases and treatments of obesity. In: Healthcare, pp. 1–2. MDPI (2022)
2. Li, R., Niu, Y., Scott, S.R., et al.: Using electronic medical record data for research in a Healthcare Information and Management Systems Society (HIMSS) Analytics Electronic Medical Record Adoption Model (EMRAM) stage 7 hospital in Beijing: cross-sectional study. JMIR Med. Inform. **9**(8), 1–13 (2021). https://doi.org/10.2196/24405
3. Wu, J., He, K., Mao, R., et al.: Harnessing the potential of multimodal EHR data: a comprehensive survey of clinical predictive modeling for intelligent healthcare. Inf. Fusion **1**(1), 99–110 (2025)
4. Chang, Y., Wang, X., Wang, J., et al.: A survey on evaluation of large language models. ACM Trans. Intell. Syst. Technol. **15**(3), 1–45 (2024)
5. Thirunavukarasu, A.J., Ting, D.S.J., Elangovan, K., et al.: Large language models in medicine. Nat. Med. **29**(8), 1930–1940 (2023)
6. Ji, B., Liu, R., Li, S., et al.: A hybrid approach for named entity recognition in Chinese electronic medical record. BMC Med. Inform. Decis. Mak. **19**(Suppl 2), 64 (2019)
7. Ali, Z., Huang, Y., Ullah, I., et al.: Deep learning for medication recommendation: a systematic survey. Data Intell. **5**(2), 303–354 (2023)
8. Wei, J., Tay, Y., Bommasani, R., et al.: Emergent abilities of large language models. arXiv preprint arXiv:2206.07682 (2022)
9. Shorten, C., Khoshgoftaar, T.M.: A survey on image data augmentation for deep learning. J. Big Data **6**(1), 1–48 (2019)
10. Han, Z., Gao, C., Liu, J., et al.: Parameter-efficient fine-tuning for large models: a comprehensive survey. arXiv preprint arXiv:2403.14608 (2024)
11. Stanić, A., van Steenkiste, S., Schmidhuber, J.: Hierarchical relational inference. In: Proceedings of the AAAI Conference on Artificial Intelligence, pp. 9730–9738. AAAI Press (2021)
12. Liu, P., Yuan, W., Fu, J., et al.: Pre-train, prompt, and predict: a systematic survey of prompting methods in natural language processing. ACM Comput. Surv. **55**(9), 1–35 (2023)
13. Benato, B.C., Telea, A.C., Falcão, A.X.: Iterative pseudo-labeling with deep feature annotation and confidence-based sampling. In: 2021 34th SIBGRAPI Conference on Graphics, Patterns and Images (SIBGRAPI), pp. 192–198. IEEE (2021)
14. Hu, E.J., Shen, Y., Wallis, P., et al.: LoRA: low-rank adaptation of large language models. In: International Conference on Learning Representations (2022)
15. Weiss, S.M., Indurkhya, N.: Rule-based machine learning methods for functional prediction. J. Artif. Intell. Res. **3**, 383–403 (1995)
16. Liang, S., Li, X., Mu, S., et al.: CIDGMed: causal inference-driven medication recommendation with enhanced dual-granularity learning. Knowl.-Based Syst. **309**, 112685 (2025)
17. Su, C., Gao, S., Li, S.: GATE: graph-attention augmented temporal neural network for medication recommendation. IEEE Access **8**, 125447–125458 (2020)
18. Chen, Q., Li, X., Geng, K., et al.: Context-aware safe medication recommendations with molecular graph and DDI graph embedding. In: Proceedings of the AAAI Conference on Artificial Intelligence, pp. 7053–7060. AAAI Press (2023)
19. Yang, N., Zeng, K., Wu, Q., et al.: Molerec: combinatorial drug recommendation with substructure-aware molecular representation learning. In: Proceedings of the ACM Web Conference 2023, pp. 4075–4085. ACM (2023)

20. Liu, Y., Ott, M., Goyal, N., et al.: RoBERTa: a robustly optimized BERT pre-training approach. arXiv preprint arXiv:1907.11692 (2019)
21. Lee, J., Yoon, W., Kim, S., et al.: BioBERT: a pre-trained biomedical language representation model for biomedical text mining. Bioinformatics **36**(4), 1234–1240 (2020)
22. Huang, L., Yu, W., Ma, W., et al.: A survey on hallucination in large language models: principles, taxonomy, challenges, and open questions. ACM Trans. Inf. Syst. **43**(2), 1–55 (2025)
23. Kage, P., Rothenberger, J.C., Andreadis, P., et al.: A review of pseudo-labeling for computer vision. arXiv preprint arXiv:2408.07221 (2024)
24. Niwattanakul, S., Singthongchai, J., Naenudorn, E., et al.: Using of Jaccard coefficient for keywords similarity. In: Proceedings of the International Multiconference of Engineers and Computer Scientists, pp. 380–384. IMECS (2013)
25. GLM, T., Zeng, A., Xu, B., et al.: ChatGLM: a family of large language models from GLM-130B to GLM-4 All Tools. arXiv preprint arXiv:2406.12793 (2024)
26. Yang, A., et al.: Qwen3 Technical Report. arXiv preprint arXiv:2505.09388 (2025)
27. Bai, S., Chen, K., Liu, X., et al.: Qwen2.5-VL Technical Report. arXiv preprint arXiv:2502.13923 (2025)
28. Yang, A., et al.: Qwen2 Technical Report. arXiv preprint arXiv:2407.10671 (2024)
29. Li, J., Yuan, H., et al.: CDrugRed: A Chinese Drug Recommendation Dataset for Discharge Medications in Metabolic Diseases. arXiv preprint arXiv:2510.21084 (2025)
30. Li, J., Yuan, H., et al.: Overview of CHIP 2025 Shared Task 2: Discharge Medication Recommendation for Metabolic Diseases Based on Chinese Electronic Health Records. arXiv preprint arXiv:2511.06230 (2025)

LoRA-Fine-Tuned LLMs for Discharge Medication Recommendation on Chinese EHRs

Xiao Su(✉)

MISUMI (China) Precision Machinery Trading Co., Ltd, Shanghai, China
suxiao818@gmail.com

Abstract. This study proposes a robust framework for automated discharge medication recommendation by leveraging LoRA-based fine-tuning of large language models (LLMs) on Chinese electronic health records (EHRs), addressing the CHIP 2025 shared task. We introduce a multi-stage framework that integrates several key techniques: (1) parameter-efficient instruction fine-tuning of four base LLMs (Qwen3-8B, Qwen3-4B-Instruct-2507, Llama-3.1-8B-Instruct, and Mistral-7B-Instruct-v0.3) using Low-Rank Adaptation (LoRA); (2) stabilization of predictions via repeated sampling and ensemble voting to mitigate generative variability and model-specific biases; and (3) systematic output refinement through pseudo-labeling and rule-based post-processing for drug name normalization. Experiments on 3,602 training and 1,722 test samples demonstrate substantial improvements over baseline performance. The final ensemble model achieved a Jaccard score of 0.4870, an F1 score of 0.6014, and a final evaluation score of 0.5442, validating the effectiveness of the proposed framework in enhancing the accuracy and practical reliability of medication recommendation systems.

Keywords: Discharge medication recommendation · Large language models · LoRA · Ensemble learning · Electronic health records

1 Introduction

Large Language Models (LLMs) possess advanced capabilities in deep semantic understanding and logical reasoning, which not only expand the frontiers of Natural Language Processing (NLP) research but also drive performance innovations in core NLP tasks—including text analysis, knowledge extraction and text generation [1]. Furthermore, these capabilities accelerate the practical deployment of artificial intelligence (AI) across high-value vertical domains such as healthcare, finance, law, and education [2, 3].

Within healthcare, LLMs demonstrate notable strengths: robust knowledge repositories, clinical reasoning abilities grounded in massive datasets, efficient multimodal interaction and comprehensive support for automating medical workflows to enhance efficiency [4]. Yet the healthcare sector imposes exceptionally high standards for outcome accuracy: even minor inaccuracies—such as in medication recommendations or

Y. Zhang et al. (Eds.): CHIP 2025, CCIS 2884, pp. 518–530, 2026.
https://doi.org/10.1007/978-981-95-7299-1_32

dosage calculations—may compromise patient safety, delay treatment, or result in irreversible clinical harm. Consequently, developing tailored evaluation frameworks and benchmarks for such medical tasks holds substantial academic and practical significance.

The China Health Information Processing Conference (CHIP) is an annual event hosted by the Technical Committee on Healthcare and Bioinformatics Processing of the Chinese Association for Computational Linguistics (CACL). Its core mission is to leverage information processing technologies to facilitate the exploration of life's mysteries, enhance health quality, and advance healthcare standards. The 11th China Health Information Processing Conference (CHIP 2025) has released three evaluation tasks, among which Task 2 is titled "Discharge Medication Recommendation for Metabolic Diseases Based on Chinese Electronic Health Records" [5, 6]. This task aims to leverage natural language processing techniques to generate accurate discharge medication recommendations for patients with metabolic diseases, based on information extracted from EHRs.

To address the inherent challenges of this task, we propose a solution leveraging LLM strengths, with three key steps: First, we selected Qwen3-8B, Qwen3-4B-Instruct-2507, Llama-3.1-8B-Instruct, and Mistral-7B-Instruct-v0.3 as primary models and fine-tuned them via LoRA. Second, to mitigate single-model, single-inference errors—caused by LLMs' generative randomness, stochastic LoRA fine-tuning, and poor bias-variance balance—we employed Repeated Sampling and Ensemble Voting to reduce variability and enhance prediction robustness. Finally, we further improved model output accuracy through result post-processing and pseudo-labeling.

2 Related Work

2.1 Large Language Models

LLMs are deep learning-based language systems grounded in the Transformer architecture, which undergo extensive pre-training on vast corpora of unstructured text—including books, web content, and academic literature—via two core tasks: masked language modeling and next-token prediction [7]. Central to their functionality, self-attention mechanisms enable LLMs to capture nuanced contextual dependencies across text sequences, thereby endowing them with robust foundational capabilities in language understanding and generation.

LLMs are defined by their robust generalization and versatility: post pre-training, they can address a diverse spectrum of NLP tasks without requiring modifications to their underlying architecture. This adaptability originates from the universal language representations they learn during the pre-training phase. Notably, LLM performance scales with both parameter magnitude and pre-training data volume: modern models (e.g., GPT-4 [8], DeepSeek-V3 [9], Qwen3-235B-A22B [10]), which feature billions to hundreds of billions of parameters, achieve near-human-level performance on complex tasks. This outperforms earlier smaller-scale models, as their expanded capacity allows them to model finer-grained linguistic and factual knowledge while mitigating bias through exposure to diverse pre-training datasets.

However, pre-trained LLMs face inherent practical limitations that hinder their direct use in specialized scenarios: first, a critical misalignment between their general pre-trained knowledge and the domain-specific expertise or task-specific output formats needed for niche applications; second, significant performance degradation under data distribution shifts—i.e., when input data diverges from the statistical patterns of their pre-training corpora; and third, prohibitive deployment-related computational overhead, driven by their massive parameter scales that demand extensive memory and inference resources [11]. These interconnected challenges directly motivate two key technical advances: task-alignment techniques, with fine-tuning as a primary example, to bridge the gap between LLMs' general capabilities and specific task needs; and parameter-efficient adaptation methods, exemplified by Low-Rank Adaptation (LoRA) [12], to reduce the computational burden of adapting large-scale models.

2.2 Fine-Tuning and the LoRA Framework

LLMs following extensive pre-training on massive datasets, have developed generalizable capabilities to tackle tasks across diverse domains. However, research has shown that their adaptability to specific tasks can be further enhanced through supervised fine-tuning. Supervised fine-tuning constitutes a technical paradigm wherein pre-trained language models undergo task-specific optimization on natural language samples, thereby acquiring task-specific competencies. Given the massive parameter scale of LLMs, full-parameter fine-tuning entails substantial computational overhead—this has directly spurred the advancement of parameter-efficient fine-tuning methods. These approaches reduce the volume of trainable parameters, significantly cutting computational costs while preserving model performance.

Among these parameter-efficient techniques, LoRA has emerged as a leading approach. It functions by integrating trainable low-rank matrices into specific layers of pre-trained models, while keeping the original model weights frozen. This design significantly reduces the volume of parameters requiring optimization—often by orders of magnitude relative to full fine-tuning—while maintaining task performance. By concentrating updates on low-rank adaptations that encode task-specific patterns, LoRA facilitates efficient fine-tuning even for large-scale models, striking a balance between computational feasibility and the preservation of pre-trained knowledge. Its implementation simplicity and robust performance across diverse tasks have established it as a widely adopted strategy in LLM adaptation research.

2.3 Repeated Sampling

LLMs inherently exhibit answer-generation randomness, shaped by factors like sampling temperature and decoding strategies (e.g., greedy decoding, nucleus sampling) [13]. This randomness often leads to incorrect or suboptimal outputs in single-inference attempts, a critical limitation for high-reliability applications. Extant literature shows repeated sampling mitigates this via the mechanism of "covering potential solutions via increased sampling quantity"—expanding the model's candidate outputs to boost the chance of capturing correct/near-optimal solutions missed in single inference [14]. Notably, repeated sampling on small-scale models outperforms large-scale models in single-inference scenarios at lower computational and operational costs. This enables replacing "model scale scaling" with "inference computation scaling" as a more cost-efficient way to enhance LLM performance.

2.4 Ensemble Learning

As a classic machine learning technique, ensemble learning also holds substantial significance for LoRA-based fine-tuning of LLMs [15]. On one hand, through deliberate diversification in base model selection, LoRA parameter configurations, and fine-tuning strategies, it enables balanced mitigation of bias and variance, thereby attaining optimal overall performance [16]. On the other hand, via voting or probability fusion across multiple models, it can counteract stochastic errors arising from factors like weight initialization and variations in training data sampling during the LoRA fine-tuning of individual models, consequently yielding more reliable outputs. In this study, we employed a relatively straightforward ensemble voting strategy.

3 Method

The model fine-tuning and inference pipeline utilized in this study is illustrated in Fig. 1. Specifically designed for discharge medication recommendation, this proposed multi-stage framework integrates five key modules:

- LoRA-based instruction fine-tuning of backbone LLMs. The backbone models selected for this process are Qwen3-8B [10], Qwen3-4B-Instruct-2507 [10], Llama-3.1-8B-Instruct [17], and Mistral-7B-Instruct-v0.3—these models are chosen for their balanced performance in medical knowledge capture and clinical task adaptation.
- Repeated sampling to generate diverse candidate medication sets. This step leverages the stochastic nature of LLM decoding to produce multiple potential medication recommendations for each input, laying the foundation for subsequent consensus aggregation.
- Ensemble voting to derive stable consensus predictions. By aggregating results across different model outputs, this module reduces the impact of individual model biases or random errors, ensuring more reliable prediction outcomes.
- Rule-guided post-processing incorporating drug name normalization and brand–generic mapping. This step addresses inconsistencies in medication naming (e.g., brand names vs. generic names) and standardizes outputs to align with official medication lists, improving the practical applicability of predictions.
- Pseudo-label generation with iterative retraining to further boost model performance. By using high-confidence predictions as pseudo-labels to augment the training dataset, this module enhances the model's ability to generalize to diverse clinical scenarios.

Notably, all four backbone models undergo independent fine-tuning, with their predictions consolidated exclusively at the ensemble voting stage during inference—this design ensures the diversity of individual model outputs while maximizing the effectiveness of consensus aggregation.

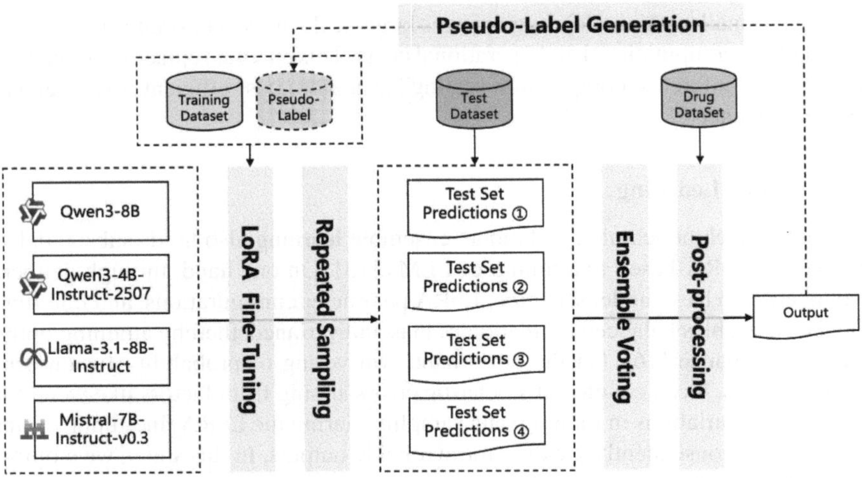

Fig. 1. Overall architecture of the proposed multi-stage framework

3.1 LoRA Instruction Fine-Tuning

In our implementation, we utilized LoRA for parameter-efficient fine-tuning: trainable low-rank matrices were incorporated into key layers of the pre-trained model, with the original weights kept frozen. This setup drastically reduced the number of trainable parameters compared to full fine-tuning, enabling efficient adaptation to our specific task while retaining the model's pre-trained knowledge. Its simplicity and effectiveness made it ideal for this task.

3.2 Repeated Sampling and Ensemble Voting

Single inference runs from a single model are prone to errors or suboptimal results, stemming from LLMs' inherent generative randomness (e.g., sampling temperature, decoding strategies), stochastic LoRA fine-tuning errors (e.g., weight initialization, training data sampling variations), and inability to balance bias and variance. To address this, this study combines Repeated Sampling and Ensemble Voting: Specifically, LLMs first generate multiple candidate medication sets via stochastic decoding; with four backbone models employed (each conducting 3 repeated samplings), a total of 12 prediction results are obtained. Through Ensemble Voting, all candidates across models and runs are aggregated into a unified vote table, where the occurrence count of each medication is computed. An option is retained as a final recommendation if its occurrence frequency exceeds 50% (i.e., more than 6 times), while low-support options are discarded—a strategy that effectively mitigates variability, reduces randomness, and bolsters the robustness and stability of the predicted medication set (Fig. 2).

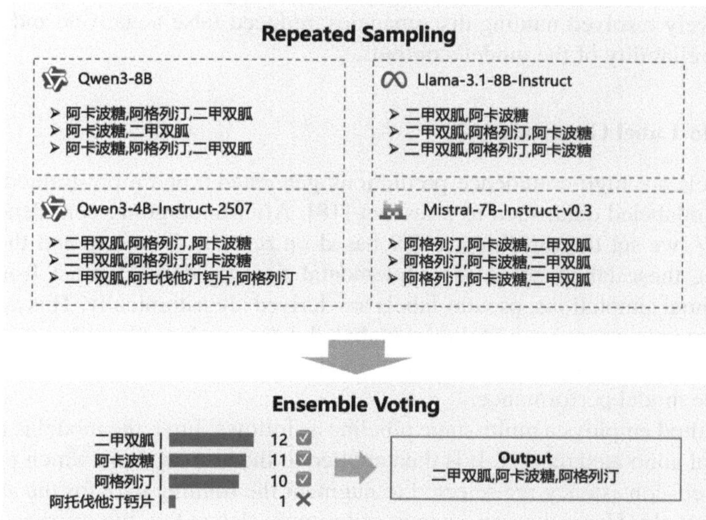

Fig. 2. Repeated sampling and ensemble voting mechanism.

3.3 Post-Processing

An analysis of model predictions identified two key inconsistencies implicated in reduced drug identification accuracy, both stemming from varied clinical naming conventions. Firstly, the candidate list omitted some predicted drugs with high name similarity, such as the pair "腺苷蛋氨酸肠溶胶囊" and "腺苷蛋氨酸肠溶片," which differ only in dosage form ("胶囊" vs. "片"). Secondly, there was a failure to address brand-generic name mappings (e.g., "金达克宁" vs. "酮康唑乳膏"). The root cause was a fundamental mismatch: the candidate list was designed with standardized, single-format generic names, excluding variants like dosage forms, whereas the model's predictions, grounded in real-world clinical text, inherently captured a broader spectrum of naming granularities and common brand names. This discrepancy led to the erroneous exclusion of valid predictions. The issue was especially notable for over-the-counter (OTC) drugs due to the prevalence of brand names in clinical notes, which increased the misclassification rate of brand name predictions as "non-candidates".

To address these inconsistencies and improve drug identification performance, we developed a targeted post-processing strategy that leverages a high-quality drug mapping dictionary pre-generated using the Qwen3-235B-A22B-Instruct-2507 model. This dictionary encompasses two critical types of mappings: 1) cross-dosage-form name mappings (e.g., "腺苷蛋氨酸" ↔ "腺苷蛋氨酸肠溶片") and 2) brand-generic name mappings (e.g., "金达克宁" ↔ "酮康唑乳膏"). For instance, if the model's original prediction included "金达克宁"—a brand name not listed in the official drug list—this entry would typically be excluded during submission or adversely impact the final evaluation score. However, by mapping "金达克宁" to its generic equivalent "酮康唑乳膏" via the aforementioned dictionary, we systematically align predictions corresponding to non-candidate names with their valid counterparts in the official list. This post-processing step effectively resolved naming discrepancies, reduced false negatives, and enhanced the overall reliability of the model's outputs.

3.4 Pseudo-Label Generation

Pseudo-labels are high-confidence predictions generated when a pre-trained model is applied to unlabeled data, such as a test set [18]. After undergoing confidence threshold filtering (we set the threshold to 0.9 based on relevant literature and the scale of the dataset), these labels serve as supplemental training data. Distinct from ground truth or manual annotations, pseudo-labels are derived algorithmically. This approach is widely adopted in scenarios with limited labeled data—such as algorithm competitions or resource-constrained tasks—to leverage unlabeled test set data, mitigate data scarcity, and enhance model performance.

The method employs a multi-stage pipeline as follows: First, the model is fine-tuned on the initial annotated dataset. It is then applied to the test set, from which predictions with high self-consistency are selected to augment the training data for the subsequent fine-tuning cycle. Here, the consistency criterion is defined as the average similarity between individual predictions and the consensus result derived from repeated sampling and voting. Finally, the expanded training dataset undergoes another round of fine-tuning to yield the final model.

4 Experiment

4.1 Datasets

The dataset used in this study is derived from Evaluation Task 2 of CHIP2025. This task requires participants to predict discharge medications for patients based on electronic health records (EHRs) of metabolic diseases. Notably, the results submitted by participants must be a list of medications that fall within the official predefined drug scope—this constraint ensures the standardization and clinical validity of the submitted recommendations.

This dataset provides 3,602 training samples for participating teams to develop their models, with a representative example illustrated in Fig. 1. During the online Phase A (Leaderboard A) stage, 648 test samples are made available to support participating teams in optimizing their solutions during the development phase. In the subsequent online Phase B (Leaderboard B) stage, 1,722 test samples are utilized to conduct the final evaluation of the participating teams' proposed approaches (Fig. 3).

Input

【患者序号】: 7
【就诊标识】: 7-1
【性别】: 女
【出生日期】: 1958-06
【民族】: 汉族
【BMI】: 25.3
【就诊时间: 2017-09
【诊疗过程描述】: 患者入院后完善相关检查：2017-09-23 胰岛素(2h)：胰岛素 40.83 mU/L，血糖(2h)：葡萄糖 10.10 mmol/L，C肽(2h)：C肽 3.03 ng/ml，C肽(随机)：C肽 0.70 ng/ml，胰岛素：胰岛素 11.30 mU/L，血糖(空腹)：葡萄糖 5.98 mmol/L，2017-09-22 糖化血红蛋白：糖化血红蛋白 8.70 %。考虑患者血糖控制不佳。肿瘤相关抗原、病毒标志物、甲功、血脂、肾功、肝生化、电解质、尿常规、血常规、心肌标志物、B N P等大致正常。肝胆脾胰彩超：脂肪肝（轻度），肝囊肿。甲状腺及淋巴结彩超：左叶甲状腺实性结节，建议密切随诊。患者拒绝进一步行穿刺检查，嘱患者3月后复查甲状腺超声，必要时行甲状腺穿刺。颈部血管彩超：左右颈动脉内-中膜增厚伴不均质性斑块形成，随诊。肾输尿管彩超：双肾膀胱未见异常回声，双输尿管未见扩张。心脏彩超（含左心功能）：心脏内部结构及血流未见异常，左室收缩功能良好。1.5MRI(神经组):颅脑(平扫)：脑白质脱髓鞘改变；余颅脑MRI平扫未见确切病征。64层CT(胸组):胸部(平扫)：右肺中叶、左肺上叶舌段及下叶索条灶；主动脉及冠状动脉钙化；双侧肺门部分淋巴结钙化；双侧胸膜局限性增厚；轻度脂肪肝，肝囊肿。治疗：阿司匹林抗血小板聚集，瑞舒伐他汀降脂稳定斑块，二甲双胍、西格列汀、甘精胰岛素降糖，改善循环及营养神经治疗。
【入院情况】: 患者某某，女，59岁，因“发作性眩晕半月余。”入院。查体：T：36P：68R：16BP：144/79,心肺听诊大致正常，神经系统查体未及阳性定位体征。
【现病史】: 患者半月前无明显诱因出现发作性眩晕，表现为自身晃动感，严重时发生天旋地转，不敢睁眼。眩晕多于改变体位时发生（由立位改为卧位时发生），每次持续约数秒钟至1分钟即可缓解，缓解期如常。无恶心、呕吐，无耳聋、耳鸣，无肢体麻木及活动不灵。就诊于我院，门诊以“眩晕待查”收入我科。患者近来无咳嗽、咳痰、发热，无腹痛、腹泻，无胸痛、胸闷，饮食、睡眠好，大小便如常。近期体重无明显变化。
既往史: 既往体质良好，曾患糖尿病，诊断2行糖尿病22年余，血糖控制不佳，曾因糖尿病周围神经病变及糖尿病眼底出血住院治疗。目前应用二甲双胍联合甘精胰岛素降糖治疗。，否认外伤史，否认“肝炎、结核”等病史，否认手术史，否认输血史及血液制品使用史，否认药物及食物过敏史、中毒史,预防接种史不详。
【主诉】: 发作性眩晕半月余。
【出院诊断】: ['椎-基底动脉系统TIA', '2型糖尿病', '糖尿病视网膜病变', '糖尿病周围神经病变', '糖尿病大血管病变', '脂肪肝（轻度）', '肝囊肿', '甲状腺结节']

Output

【出院带药列表】: ['阿司匹林肠溶片', '瑞舒伐他汀', '磷酸西格列汀', '格华止', '甘精胰岛素', '甲钴胺', '依帕司他']

Fig. 3. Train data example

4.2 Training Configuration and LoRA Parameters

To address this task and enhance the robustness of model outputs, a multi-model integration strategy was adopted, incorporating four large language model variants: Qwen3-8B, Qwen3-4B-Instruct-2507, Llama-3.1-8B-Instruct and Mistral-7B-Instruct-v0.3. All selected models underwent parameter-efficient fine-tuning using the LoRA (Low-Rank Adaptation) framework—this approach was chosen to reduce computational overhead and training costs while preserving the original capabilities of the pre-trained models.

To ensure experimental reproducibility and fair comparison among the four models, consistent hyperparameters were employed throughout the fine-tuning process. Specifically, LoRA-specific configurations—critical for regulating the parameter update range of low-rank adapters and their generalization performance—were set as follows: LoRA Rank was fixed at 16 (a widely adopted value for medium-sized LLMs, which balances parameter efficiency and the ability to capture representative features), LoRA Alpha (the scaling coefficient for LoRA parameter updates) was set to 32, and LoRA Dropout (utilized to mitigate overfitting via controlled noise injection) was configured to 0.05. For general training hyperparameters, the learning rate was fixed at 5e-5 (a value extensively validated for LoRA-based fine-tuning of medium-sized pre-trained models), the training batch size was set to 1, and the total training duration lasted 3 epochs. The entire fine-tuning workflow was implemented using the PyTorch deep learning framework, which was selected for its flexibility in custom model adaptation and its robust support for efficient GPU acceleration. All LoRA parameters and training hyperparameters detailed above are summarized in Table 1.

Table 1. LoRA parameter and training configuration settings

Parameters name	Parameters value
LoRA rank	16
LoRA alpha	32
LoRA dropout	0.05
Learning rate	5e-5
Batch size	1
Number of epochs	3

4.3 Evaluation Metric

This evaluation task uses the following metrics, where y is the true drug set, $\hat{y}$ is the drug set predicted by the model, and $|X|$ denotes the number of elements in set X:

Jaccard Similarity: It measures the overlap between the true drug set and the predicted drug set. It is calculated as the ratio of the size of the intersection of the two sets to the size of their union, with the formula given as follows:

$$Jaccard = \frac{1}{N}\sum_{i=1}^{N}\frac{\left|y_i \cap \hat{y}_i\right|}{\left|y_i \cup \hat{y}_i\right|} \tag{1}$$

Precision: It measures the proportion of true positives among the model's predictions, reflecting the "precision" of the predicted results. The calculation formula is as follows:

$$\text{Precision}\left(y_i, \hat{y}_i\right) = \frac{\left|y_i \cap \hat{y}_i\right|}{\left|\hat{y}_i\right|} \tag{2}$$

To obtain the overall precision, we average the precision values across all samples, as shown below:

$$AVG\_P = \frac{1}{N}\sum_{i=1}^{N}\text{Precision}\left(y_i, \hat{y}_i\right) \tag{3}$$

Recall: It measures the proportion of true positives that are correctly predicted by the model, reflecting the model's "coverage ability" for positive examples. The calculation formula is as follows:

$$\text{Recall}\left(y_i, \hat{y}_i\right) = \frac{\left|y_i \cap \hat{y}_i\right|}{\left|y_i\right|} \tag{4}$$

Similarly, the overall recall is the average of the recall of all samples:

$$AVG\_R = \frac{1}{N}\sum_{i=1}^{N}\text{Recall}\left(y_i, \hat{y}_i\right) \tag{5}$$

F1-Score: The F1 score is the harmonic mean of precision and recall, comprehensively reflecting the balance between the model's precision and recall. The formula is as follows:

$$F_1(y_i, \hat{y}_i) = 2 \cdot \frac{\text{Precision}(y_i, \hat{y}_i) \cdot \text{Recall}(y_i, \hat{y}_i)}{\text{Precision}(y_i, \hat{y}_i) + \text{Recall}(y_i, \hat{y}_i)} \tag{6}$$

The overall F1 score is the average of F1 scores across all samples:

$$F1 = \frac{1}{N}\sum\nolimits_{i=1}^{N} F_1(y_i, \hat{y}_i) \tag{7}$$

Final Evaluation Metric: To comprehensively assess model performance across all dimensions, this metric is formally defined as the mean of Jaccard similarity and F1 score. Its calculation formula is as follows:

$$\text{Score} = \frac{1}{2} \cdot (\text{Jaccard} + F1) \tag{8}$$

The final performance of the models is determined by this overall metric.

4.4 Results

Based on a dataset of 3,602 training samples and 1,722 samples from the B-list test set, we first evaluated several methods using the Qwen3-8B model, excluding model ensemble voting; the results are summarized in Table 2. Table 2 presents the ablation results on the B-list test set with Qwen3-8B, showing the incremental effect of LoRA, pseudo-labeling (PL), repeated sampling (RS*k), and post-processing (PP) on all metrics—where k denotes the number of stochastic inferences runs used for voting.

The original Qwen3-8B model achieved a baseline score of only 0.2276 on the test set. As no instruction fine-tuning was applied at this stage, the model outputs often deviated from the prompt's requirement to generate drug lists only. To address this, we implemented preliminary text processing. Subsequently, we performed LoRA-based instruction fine-tuning on the model as described previously, which led to a significant performance improvement, raising the score to 0.4883. Building on this, we expanded the training dataset through pseudo-labeling and conducted an additional round of LoRA fine-tuning, further increasing the performance to 0.4913. We then conducted experiments on repeated sampling with different iteration counts (1, 3, 5, and 10). The final score exhibited a consistent upward trend with increasing iterations, ultimately reaching 0.5272. Finally, we incorporated a post-processing step for the prediction results, which yielded a final score of 0.5283.

Although this represents a modest gain, the step is of considerable practical importance for real-world deployment. Since the model was fine-tuned on a specific dataset, its predictions are biased toward drugs present in that dataset—which may reflect the formulary of the contributing medical institution. When deploying the technology to other institutions, a similar post-processing module would be indispensable for aligning outputs with local drug formularies.

Table 2. Ablation results of Qwen3-8B

Method	Jaccard	F1	Score
Qwen3-8B(Original)	0.1813	0.2739	0.2276
Qwen3-8B + LoRA	0.4282	0.5484	0.4883
Qwen3-8B + LoRA + PL	0.4324	0.5501	0.4913
Qwen3-8B + LoRA + PL + RS*3	0.4543	0.5717	0.5130
Qwen3-8B + LoRA + PL + RS*5	0.4657	0.5819	0.5238
Qwen3-8B + LoRA + PL + RS*10	0.4690	0.5855	0.5272
Qwen3-8B + LoRA + PL + RS*10 + PP	**0.4700**	**0.5865**	**0.5283**

Building on the previous experiments, we evaluated the proposed framework across four backbone models: Qwen3-8B (0.5283), Qwen3-4B-Instruct-2507 (0.5244), Llama-3.1-8B-Instruct (0.5115), and Mistral-7B-Instruct-v0.3 (0.4957). While Qwen3-8B was the strongest single model, the others exhibited complementary performance. The integration of these diverse predictors via ensemble voting yielded the best results, achieving a Jaccard score of 0.4870, an F1 score of 0.6014, and a Final Score of 0.5442. This improvement validates that the ensemble approach effectively aggregates the distinct capabilities of each constituent model, mitigating individual prediction biases and yielding a more robust and accurate collective inference (Table 3).

Table 3. Performance of backbone models and their ensemble

Model	Jaccard	F1	Score
Qwen3-8B	0.4700	0.5865	0.5283
Qwen3-4B-Instruct-2507	0.4645	0.5844	0.5244
Llama-3.1-8B-Instruct	0.4534	0.5695	0.5115
Mistral-7B-Instruct-v0.3	0.4363	0.5551	0.4957
Ensemble Voting	**0.4870**	**0.6014**	**0.5442**

5 Conclusion

This study proposes a robust and effective framework for automated discharge medication recommendation, leveraging LoRA-fine-tuned LLMs on EHRs. Our multi-stage approach systematically addresses core challenges inherent to the task, including aligning general-purpose LLMs with domain-specific requirements, mitigating the instability of generative models, and enhancing the practical applicability of model outputs.

The experimental results demonstrate the critical contribution of each component in the proposed pipeline. The foundational step of LoRA-based instruction fine-tuning provided the most significant performance leap, successfully bridging the gap between the models' general capabilities and the specialized task.

Subsequent techniques—including repeated sampling, pseudo-labeling, and targeted post-processing—yielded consistent incremental improvements. In particular, the post-processing step demonstrated substantial practical value by resolving clinical naming variations, a prevalent issue that impedes the deployment of NLP systems in real-world healthcare environments.

Furthermore, the superior performance of the ensemble model—achieving a final score of 0.5442 and outperforming all individual counterparts—validates our hypothesis that integrating diverse base models effectively harnesses their complementary strengths. This ensemble strategy successfully mitigates individual model biases and variances, resulting in more accurate and robust collective predictions.

In summary, our work demonstrates the significant potential of parameter-efficient fine-tuned LLMs as reliable tools for clinical decision support. The proposed framework provides a practical blueprint for developing accurate and deployable medication recommendation systems, thereby contributing to the broader goal of enhancing patient care quality and safety through AI. Future research will focus on exploring more advanced ensemble techniques, integrating richer patient context, and validating the framework across diverse medical institutions and disease domains to further improve its generalizability and clinical utility.

References

1. Wei, J., Tay, Y., Bommasani, R., Raffel, C., Zoph, B., Borgeaud, S., Yogatama, D., Bosma, M., Zhou, D., Metzler, D. et al.: Emergent abilities of large language models. arXiv preprint arXiv:2206.07682 (2022)
2. Nazi, Z.A., Peng, W.: Large language models in healthcare and medical domain: a review. Informatics **11**, 57 (2024). MDPI
3. Nie, Y., Kong, Y., Dong, X., Mulvey, J.M., Poor, H.V., Wen, Q., Zohren, S.: A survey of large language models for financial applications: Progress, prospects and challenges. arXiv preprint arXiv:2406.11903 (2024)
4. Thirunavukarasu, A.J., Ting, D.S.J., Elangovan, K., Gutierrez, L., Tan, T.F., Ting, D.S.W.: Large language models in medicine. Nat. Med. **29**(8), 1930–1940 (2023)
5. Li, J., Yuan, H., Luo, L., Lv, T., Jiang, Y., Wang, F., Zhang, P., Lv, H., Wang, J., Sun, Y., et al.: Overview of chip 2025 shared task 2: discharge medication recommendation for metabolic diseases based on Chinese electronic health records. arXiv preprint arXiv:2511.06230 (2025)
6. Li, J., Yuan, H., Luo, L., Jiang, Y., Wang, F., Zhang, P., Lv, H., Wang, J., Sun, Y., Lin, H.: Cdrugred: A chinese drug recommendation dataset for discharge medications in metabolic diseases. arXiv preprint arXiv:2510.21084 (2025)
7. Radford, A., Narasimhan, K., Salimans, T., Sutskever, I., et al.: Improving language understanding by generative pre-training (2018)
8. Achiam, J., Adler, S., Agarwal, S., Ahmad, L., Akkaya, I., Aleman, F.L., Almeida, D., Altenschmidt, J., Altman, S., Anadkat, S., et al.: Gpt-4 technical report. arXiv preprint arXiv: 2303.08774 (2023)
9. Liu, A., Feng, B., Xue, B., Wang, B., Wu, B., Lu, C., Zhao, C., Deng, C., Zhang, C., Ruan, C., et al.: Deepseek-v3 technical report. arXiv preprint arXiv:2412.19437 (2024)
10. Yang, A., Li, A., Yang, B., Zhang, B., Hui, B., Zheng, B., Yu, B., Gao, C., Huang, C., Lv, C., et al.: Qwen3 technical report. arXiv preprint arXiv:2505.09388 (2025)

11. Ding, N., et al.: Parameter-efficient fine-tuning of large-scale pre-trained language models. Nat. Mach. Intell. **5**(3), 220–235 (2023)
12. Hu, E.J., et al.: Lora: Low-rank adaptation of large language models. ICLR **1**(2), 3 (2022)
13. Ouyang, L., et al.: Training language models to follow instructions with human feedback. Adv. Neural. Inf. Process. Syst. **35**, 27730–27744 (2022)
14. Brown, B., Juravsky, J., Ehrlich, R., Clark, R., Le, Q.V., R´e, C., Mirhoseini, A.: Large language monkeys: scaling inference compute with repeated sampling. arXiv preprint arXiv: 2407.21787 (2024)
15. Dietterich, T.G.: Ensemble methods in machine learning. In: International Workshop on Multiple Classifier Systems, pp. 1–15. Springer (2000)
16. Wang, X., Aitchison, L., Rudolph, M.: Lora ensembles for large language model fine-tuning. arXiv preprint arXiv:2310.00035 (2023)
17. Dubey, A., Jauhri, A., Pandey, A., Kadian, A., Al-Dahle, A., Letman, A., Mathur, A., Schelten, A., Yang, A., Fan, A., et al.: The llama 3 herd of models. arXiv e-prints, 2407 (2024)
18. Lee, D.-H., et al.: Pseudo-label: the simple and efficient semi-supervised learning method for deep neural networks. In: Workshop on Challenges in Representation Learning, ICML, vol. 3, p. 896 (2013). Atlanta

Multi-format Fine-Tuning and Optimized Voting Ensemble for Robust Medication Recommendation in Chinese EMRs

Yajie Wen[1], Jinzhi Chen[1], Junheng Pan[2], Chengyan Wu[1], Yiqiang Cai[1], Weikai Huang[1], Yun Xue[1], Jing Chen[1(✉)], and Hongrui Shen[3(✉)]

[1] School of Electronic Science and Engineering (School of Microelectronics), South China Normal University, Foshan 528225, China
{yajiewen,jinzhichen,chengyan.wu,yiqiangcai,weikaihuang,xueyun, chenjing1}@m.scnu.edu.cn

[2] The Second School of Clinical Medicine, Zhejiang Chinese Medical University, Hangzhou 310053, China
panjhzjcmu@sina.com

[3] School of Computing, Neusoft Institute Guangdong, Foshan 528225, China
shenhongrui@nuit.edu.cn

Abstract. Automatically and accurately recommending discharge medications for patients based on unstructured Chinese electronic medical records (EMRs) remains a major challenge for current clinical decision support systems. An effective recommendation model can help standardize treatment practices and reduce discrepancies in therapeutic strategies caused by variations in physicians interpretations. For the Evaluation Task of the 11th China Health Information Processing Conference (CHIP 2025), this paper proposes a medication recommendation method built upon the Qwen2.5-7B-Instruct model, incorporating multi-format fine-tuning and an optimized ensemble voting strategy. Specifically, we design two output formats, a structured list format and a natural language format, and apply LoRA for efficient parameter adaptation. Based on these settings, three candidate predictions are generated using different decoding temperatures and integrated through an optimized voting mechanism that enhances recall, where medications predicted by at least two models are retained, and in cases of complete disagreement, the union of all predicted medications is preserved. Experimental results show that our method achieves an accuracy of 53.78%, ranking fourth in the competition, thereby demonstrating its effectiveness and robustness.

Keywords: Large language models · Medication recommendation · LoRA · Voting ensemble

Y. Wen and J. Chen—Equal contribution.

Y. Zhang et al. (Eds.): CHIP 2025, CCIS 2884, pp. 531–545, 2026.
https://doi.org/10.1007/978-981-95-7299-1_33

1 Introduction

With the rapid development of large language models (LLMs) in the field of natural language processing, their potential applications in specialized domains such as healthcare have become increasingly prominent. In clinical practice, how to leverage LLMs to analyze complex and unstructured electronic medical records (EMRs) and provide physicians with precise decision support has become one of the core topics in smart healthcare research [1]. In particular, for the critical task of discharge medication recommendation, the model must comprehensively understand multidimensional patient information including current medical history, past medical history, and examination results to generate a safe and reasonable medication list. This not only imposes high demands on the models natural language understanding capabilities but also presents great challenges in ensuring the reliability and professionalism of its outputs.

The China Health Information Processing Conference (CHIP) is an annual academic event organized by the Medical Health and Bioinformatics Professional Committee of the Chinese Information Processing Society of China, and it is one of the most important academic activities in this field domestically. The 11th China Health Information Processing Conference (CHIP 2025) [2] focuses on the theme of "Large Language Models in the Medical Domain" and includes several evaluation tasks. Among them, the task titled "Discharge Medication Recommendation Task for Metabolic Diseases Based on Chinese Electronic Medical Records" aims to explore and evaluate the decision-supporting capabilities of large language models in real clinical scenarios. The task requires participating models to automatically generate discharge medication recommendation lists based on given Chinese EMR data, which holds significant practical value for advancing the real world application of LLMs in clinical decision support systems.

To address this challenge, this paper proposes a medication recommendation method based on the open-source large language model Qwen2.5-7B-Instruct, which integrates multi-format fine-tuning and an optimized voting ensemble strategy. During the fine-tuning stage, we innovatively design two output formats, a structured list format and a fluent natural language format, and employ the LoRA (Low-Rank Adaptation) technique for efficient parameter fine-tuning. We argue that such multi-format training enables the model to learn the task from different perspectives, thereby enhancing its generalization ability. In the prediction stage, the fine-tuned model generates multiple candidate medication lists using different decoding temperatures. Based on these outputs, we propose an optimized voting strategy aimed at improving recall: when a medication appears in the majority of predictions (i.e., reaches consensus), it is retained; when all predictions are completely disjoint, we keep the union of all predicted medications to avoid over-filtering potentially correct ones.

Our method achieved an accuracy of 53.78% on the test set of this evaluation task, ranking fourth overall, which demonstrates the effectiveness and reliability of the proposed approach.

The main contributions of this work are as follows:

- A multi-format fine-tuning framework for medication recommendation tasks is proposed. By fine-tuning the model simultaneously on both structured and unstructured formats, the robustness of a single model in handling complex clinical texts is enhanced.
- An optimized voting ensemble strategy is designed and applied. This strategy effectively integrates prediction results obtained from different decoding settings, achieving a good balance between accuracy and recall by retaining consensus while accommodating variations.
- Our method demonstrates that even medium-sized open-source models can achieve competitive performance on medical tasks through parameter-efficient fine-tuning and a well-designed ensemble strategy. This provides a practical reference for the clinical application of large language models in resource-constrained environments.

2 Related Work

2.1 Clinical NLP and Medication Recommendation

Automatically extracting and analyzing information from electronic medical records (EMRs) is a core objective of Clinical Natural Language Processing (Clinical NLP). Previous studies have mainly relied on rule-based or traditional machine learning methods for Named Entity Recognition (NER) and relation extraction to identify key information such as diseases, symptoms, and medications in medical records. Imaichi O et al. [3] compared the performance of rule-based and machine learning approaches in medical information extraction tasks and found that rule-based methods performed slightly better in pattern-oriented tasks, whereas machine learning methods achieved significantly higher recall and overall scores in more complex tasks. However, these approaches often require extensive manual feature engineering and struggle to handle complex linguistic phenomena.

With the advancement of deep learning, models such as Recurrent Neural Networks (RNNs) and Long Short-Term Memory networks (LSTMs) [4] have been widely applied to clinical text analysis due to their strong capability in handling sequential data. E. Choi et al. [5] proposed a bidirectional RNN model with a reverse-time attention mechanism to model sequences of patients electronic health records. Later, pre-trained language models represented by BERT [6], particularly domain-specific versions developed for the clinical field such as ClinicalBERT, significantly improved the performance of various downstream tasks through large-scale pre-training on medical texts. Lee et al. [7] further introduced a biomedical language model that continues BERT pre-training on PubMed abstracts. However, most of these models are primarily effective for understanding and extraction tasks, while their ability to generate complex and coherent outputs, such as complete medication plans, remains limited.

In recent years, the emergence of large language models (LLMs) has introduced a new paradigm for clinical decision support. With their powerful capabilities in contextual understanding and text generation, LLMs can process complex input information in an end-to-end manner and directly produce summaries, reports, or recommendations. Liu et al. [8]. introduced a novel approach called Large Language Model Distilled Medication Recommendation. This development makes it possible to model medication recommendation as a conditional text generation problem, where the model directly generates a list of recommended drugs based on the input medical record, greatly simplifying the multi-stage processing pipeline required by traditional approaches.

2.2 Efficient Adaptation of Large Language Models

Although large language models demonstrate outstanding performance, full fine-tuning requires substantial computational resources and time. To address this challenge, Parameter-Efficient Fine-Tuning (PEFT) [9] techniques have been developed. The core idea of PEFT is to freeze most of the parameters in a pre-trained model while training only a small subset of newly added or designated parameters.

Low-Rank Adaptation (LoRA) [10] is one of the most widely adopted PEFT methods. It works by injecting trainable low-rank decomposition matrices into the Transformer layers of a pre-trained model to approximate the weight updates that would occur during full fine-tuning. During training, only these additional low-rank matrices are updated, while the original large weight matrices remain unchanged. This approach drastically reduces the number of trainable parameters, typically to less than 1% of the total, thereby lowering the hardware requirements and storage overhead for fine-tuning. Due to its efficiency and effectiveness, LoRA has become a preferred technique for adapting large language models to specialized domains such as healthcare.

2.3 Ensemble Learning and Voting Strategies

Ensemble Learning [11] is a machine learning approach that enhances overall performance by combining the predictions of multiple models. The fundamental idea is to "leverage the strengths of many," meaning that an ensemble of multiple weak learners can form a more powerful and robust strong learner. By aggregating diverse models, ensemble learning effectively reduces the risk of overfitting caused by data bias or random initialization, thereby improving model stability and generalization capability.

Voting is one of the most common and intuitive strategies in ensemble learning. In classification [12–14] or recommendation tasks, voting strategies [15] integrate the prediction outputs of multiple independent models and determine the final decision based on the principle of majority voting [16] or other weighted rules. In medication recommendation tasks, voting can be applied to combine multiple candidate lists generated by different models or by the same model under different decoding strategies (such as varying the temperature). This approach helps filter out occasional or unreliable predictions and retain the consensus results agreed upon by multiple models, thereby improving the accuracy and reliability of the final recommendations.

3 Methodology

3.1 Model Structure

This section presents in detail the proposed approach for the Chinese Electronic Medical Record (EMR) medication recommendation task. The overall framework of the method is illustrated in Fig. 1. The core idea is to enhance the accuracy and robustness of medication recommendations by integrating two key stages: Multi-format Fine-tuning and Optimized Voting Ensemble.
Stage 1: In the multi-format fine-tuning stage, the goal is to improve the models task understanding by training it to generate outputs in two distinct formats or styles. This encourages the model to capture diverse representations of clinical knowledge and reasoning patterns.
Stage 2: In the optimized voting ensemble stage, both fine-tuned models are used to perform inference under different decoding temperatures, producing a pool of multiple candidate medication lists. From this pool, the top three drug sets are selected based on performance metrics and enter the voting phase. For these three selected lists, we first identify consensus drugs, defined as medications that appear in at least two of the lists. These consensus drugs are considered high-confidence results and are retained in the final output. If there is no overlap among the three lists, to avoid omitting potentially correct recommendations due to model disagreement, all drugs from the union of the three lists are retained as the final output. This two-stage strategy ensures that high-confidence predictions are prioritized while maintaining comprehensive coverage of potential recommendations.

3.2 Problem Definition

Formally, given an unstructured Chinese electronic medical record (EMR) text denoted as C, which contains complex clinical information such as the chief complaint, history of present illness, past medical history, and discharge diagnoses, the objective is to train a model that, based on the input record C and a predefined medication set

$$\mathcal{M} = \{m_1, m_2, \ldots, m_N\},$$

automatically generates a recommended discharge medication subset

$$\mathcal{M}' = \{m'_1, m'_2, \ldots, m'_K\},$$

where each $m'_i \in \mathcal{M}$ represents a specific drug selected from the predefined list containing 651 distinct medications in total.

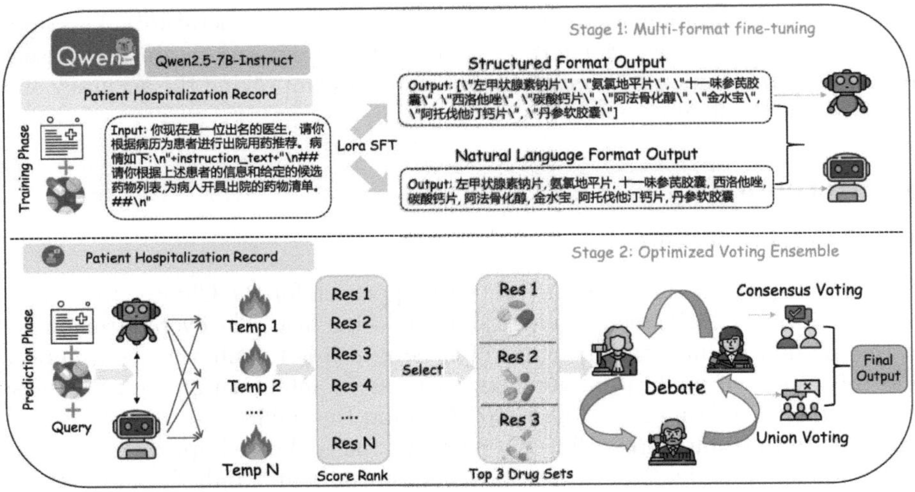

Fig. 1. Model structure.

3.3 Multi-temperature Prediction and Optimized Voting Ensemble

To generate diverse and high-quality candidate outputs, we performed predictions on the test set using two fine-tuned models. We observed that adjusting the temperature parameter during the decoding process effectively controls the degree of randomness and creativity in the generated results. Based on experimental evaluation, we selected the three best-performing prediction configurations (for example, different models and temperature combinations with temperatures of 0.01, 0.1, and 0.3) to produce three medication recommendation lists.

For these three candidate lists, we designed an optimized voting strategy, functioning as a debate among the three models, which in this case simply involves comparing the predicted results from each model and selecting the final medications based on votes, aimed at balancing precision and recall, with the following rules:

- Consensus Voting: Count the occurrences of each medication across all candidate lists. If a medication appears in at least two lists, it is considered a consensus result and retained.
- Union Voting: If all medications appear only once (i.e., the predictions from the three lists do not overlap at all), in order to avoid excessively excluding potential correct recommendations due to model disagreement, we retain all medications from the union of the three lists.

This adaptive mechanism selects the appropriate voting rule based on model agreement: consensus voting ensures precision by emphasizing high-confidence results, while union voting enhances recall when model outputs diverge, resulting in more comprehensive final recommendations.

4 Experiment

4.1 Data Statistics and Processing

The CDrugRed dataset [17] for this evaluation task is sourced from Evaluation Task 2 of CHIP 2025. As shown in Table 1, the dataset comprises a total of 5,894 medical records, which are divided into a training set of 3,602 records, a validation set (Test Set A) of 570 records, and a final test set (Test Set B) of 1,722 records. Each medical record consists of unstructured text containing rich clinical information fields, such as admission status, chief complaint, history of present illness, past history, and discharge diagnosis.

The objective of the task is to predict the correct combination of discharge medications for a patient from a candidate list of 651 drugs, based on the information provided in their medical record. During data processing, to better guide the large language model in understanding the task, we designed a unified instruction prompt for each data entry. Specifically, we form the **instruction_text** shown in Fig. 1 by concatenating the content of key clinical fields ("chief complaint," "history of present illness," "past history," "admission status," "treatment process description," and "discharge diagnosis") and appending the candidate list of 651 drugs. This **instruction_text** is then embedded into a pre-defined prompt template to form the final input for the model.

Table 1. Dataset statistics.

Items	Number of Patients	Number of Visit records
Train	1910	3602
Val	320	570
Test	960	1722

4.2 Compared Methods

We compare our approach with three main categories of baseline methods: prompt-based methods, supervised fine-tuning (SFT) methods, and ensemble voting strategy.

- **Prompt-based Methods.** These methods rely on carefully designed prompt templates to guide the model in performing medication recommendation without gradient-based optimization. We consider two representative variants: (1) *In-Context Learning (ICL)* [18], which directly provides several demonstration examples within the prompt to guide prediction; and (2) *Chain-of-Thought (CoT) prompting* [19], which explicitly encourages the model to generate intermediate reasoning steps before producing the final recommendation. The CoT approach is expected to improve logical coherence and interpretability in complex medical reasoning tasks.

- **Supervised Fine-Tuning (SFT) Methods.** These methods fine-tune large language models using labeled instruction data to better align them with the task objective. We explore two variants: (1) *Structured SFT (SFT_{format})*, where the model is trained to produce outputs in a pre-defined, structured format that explicitly represents the relationships between medications; and (2) *Unstructured SFT ($SFT_{non\text{-}format}$)*, where the model generates natural language responses without rigid format constraints. The structured variant provides stronger guidance for capturing semantic boundaries and dependencies within medication sets, leading to more accurate and consistent predictions.
- **Ensemble Voting Strategy.** To further enhance robustness and accuracy, we integrate multiple models through an optimized voting mechanism. Unlike traditional majority voting [20] (Hard Vote Mechanism) that strictly takes the intersection of model outputs, our approach adaptively combines predictions based on their agreement and confidence. Specifically, when multiple models reach consensus, the ensemble emphasizes high-frequency medications to ensure precision; when predictions diverge completely, it retains the union of all candidates to prevent information loss. This adaptive strategy effectively balances precision and recall, leveraging the complementary strengths of different large language models to yield more stable and comprehensive recommendations.

4.3 Parameter Setting

Our experiments are based on the LLaMA-Factory framework [21], utilizing Qwen2.5-7B-Instruct [22] as the base model. We employ the LoRA (Low-Rank Adaptation) technique for parameter-efficient fine-tuning of the model. The key hyperparameter settings are detailed in the Table 2. In the prediction phase, we conduct multiple inferences on the fine-tuned model using different decoding temperature settings. We selected three optimal values, [0.01, 0.1, 0.3], from a candidate pool of [0.01, 0.1, 0.2, 0.3], which were selected empirically based on preliminary experiments to balance output diversity and stability..

4.4 Evaluation Indicators

This evaluation task employs multiple metrics to comprehensively assess the model's performance, including four scores: *Jaccard*, *Precision*, *Recall*, and $F1$. All metrics are calculated independently for each test sample, and the final results are the arithmetic mean of the scores across the entire test set. Let N be the total number of test samples. For the i-th sample, let y_i represent the ground-truth set of medications, and $\hat{y}_i$ represent the predicted set of medications. The evaluation metrics are defined as follows:

Jaccard Similarity. The Jaccard index measures the overlap between the predicted and ground-truth sets by computing the ratio of their intersection to their union:

Table 2. Model parameters.

Learning rate	5e-4
Batch size	8
Max length	8192
Epoch	5
LoRA rank	8
LoRA alpha	16
LoRA dropout	0.05
Temperature	[0.01,0.1,0.2,0.3]
Framework	PyTorch

$$\text{Jaccard} = \frac{1}{N}\sum_{i=1}^{N}\frac{|y_i \cap \hat{y}_i|}{|y_i \cup \hat{y}_i|}. \tag{1}$$

This metric reflects the overall similarity between two sets, penalizing both missing and redundant predictions.

Precision and Recall. Precision quantifies the proportion of correctly predicted items among all predicted ones, while Recall measures the proportion of correctly retrieved items among all true items:

$$\text{Precision}(y_i, \hat{y}_i) = \frac{|y_i \cap \hat{y}_i|}{|\hat{y}_i|}, \quad \text{Recall}(y_i, \hat{y}_i) = \frac{|y_i \cap \hat{y}_i|}{|y_i|}. \tag{2}$$

The overall averages are computed as:

$$AVG\_P = \frac{1}{N}\sum_{i=1}^{N}\text{Precision}(y_i, \hat{y}_i), \quad AVG\_R = \frac{1}{N}\sum_{i=1}^{N}\text{Recall}(y_i, \hat{y}_i). \tag{3}$$

F1 Score. The F1 score represents the harmonic mean of Precision and Recall, balancing both false positives and false negatives:

$$F_1(y_i, \hat{y}_i) = 2 \cdot \frac{\text{Precision}(y_i, \hat{y}_i) \cdot \text{Recall}(y_i, \hat{y}_i)}{\text{Precision}(y_i, \hat{y}_i) + \text{Recall}(y_i, \hat{y}_i)}, \tag{4}$$

$$F_1 = \frac{1}{N}\sum_{i=1}^{N} F_1(y_i, \hat{y}_i). \tag{5}$$

Overall Score. To obtain a single aggregated indicator, we define the final evaluation score as the average of the Jaccard index and the F1 score:

$$\text{Score} = \frac{1}{2} \cdot (\text{Jaccard} + F_1). \tag{6}$$

This combined metric considers both set-level similarity and precision–recall trade-offs, providing a balanced evaluation of model performance.

4.5 Results

Table 3 presents the performance comparison between our ensemble model and several baseline approaches. The results show that among the single-model configurations, Qwen2.5-7B-Instruct with Chain-of-Thought (CoT) reasoning achieves superior performance compared to the version trained with simple In-Context Learning (ICL) (with a 9.03% gain in final score). This observation suggests that incorporating explicit reasoning steps allows the model to construct more coherent logical pathways, resulting in more accurate and interpretable medication recommendations. Such reasoning capability is particularly valuable for complex medical decision-making tasks.

Furthermore, models fine-tuned through Supervised Fine-Tuning (SFT) consistently outperform those relying solely on prompt-based learning (with the SFT_format achieving a 1.35% gain in the final score compared to the CoT methods). This indicates that explicit supervision with structured instruction data provides stronger optimization signals, reducing generation noise and improving output consistency. In particular, SFT models trained with structured output formats perform better than those generating free-form natural language outputs. The structured format helps the model better capture the semantic boundaries and relationships among medications, which is essential for accurate and comprehensive prescription generation.

In the ensemble phase, our optimized voting strategy further enhances performance compared to traditional majority voting (with a 0.21% gain in final score). Unlike conventional methods that strictly select overlapping predictions, our approach adaptively handles cases with limited or no consensus among models. When agreement exists, high-frequency predictions are prioritized to improve precision; when predictions are completely disjoint, the method retains the union of all candidates to minimize information loss. This adaptive mechanism effectively balances precision and recall, resulting in more robust and reliable ensemble outcomes.

We attribute the overall improvement to the complementary strengths of different large language models (LLMs). Each model tends to specialize in certain aspects, such as clinical semantics, pharmacological relevance, or medication safety reasoning. By integrating their outputs through the optimized voting ensemble, the system can exploit these complementary capabilities, leading to more accurate and dependable medication recommendations.

4.6 The Effect of Different Temperatures

We investigate the effect of different combinations of the hyperparameter **temperature** on the performance of our method. Table 4 presents the models performance under various temperature settings, evaluated by **Jaccard**, **Precision**, **Recall**, **F1**, and **Score** metrics. We conduct experiments with temperature values in the range of [0.01, 0.1, 0.2, 0.3].

Experimental results demonstrate that the proposed ensemble-based voting strategy effectively enhances model robustness, keeping performance stable

Table 3. Overall experimental performance of different methods.

Methods	Jaccard	AVG_P	AVG_R	F1	Score
Single Model					
ICL	36.53	47.38	56.52	49.01	42.77
CoT	45.88	60.17	60.23	57.72	51.80
$SFT_{non\text{-}format}$	46.73	62.49	59.35	58.44	52.59
SFT_{format}	47.24	62.11	**60.78**	59.07	53.15
Voting-based mechanism					
Hard Vote	47.68	62.99	60.53	59.45	53.57
Ours	**47.90**	**63.33**	60.70	**59.65**	**53.78**

Table 4. Effect of the hyperparameter temperature. Each row reports results obtained by combining the best-performing models (SFT_{format} or $SFT_{non\text{-}format}$) corresponding to the respective temperature.

Temperature	Jaccard	AVG_P	AVG_R	F1	Score
Hard Vote Mechanism					
0.01,0.1,0.2	47.44	62.76	61.43	59.51	53.47
0.01,0.2,0.3	47.68	62.99	60.53	59.45	53.57
0.1,0.2,0.3	47.61	61.84	**62.20**	59.55	53.58
0.01,0.1,0.3	47.73	63.18	60.52	59.50	53.62
Our Vote Mechanism					
0.01,0.1,0.2	47.83	63.12	60.84	59.60	53.72
0.01,0.2,0.3	47.70	62.77	61.08	59.57	53.64
0.1,0.2,0.3	47.69	63.12	61.11	59.63	53.66
0.01,0.1,0.3	**47.90**	**63.33**	60.70	**59.65**	**53.78**

within a certain range and reducing the influence of randomness from individual decoding temperatures. In addition, our optimized voting mechanism consistently outperforms the traditional Hard Vote method in overall performance. Specifically, under the best temperature combination (0.01, 0.1, 0.3), the proposed approach achieves a Score approximately 0.16% higher than Hard Vote, confirming the effectiveness of our method.

5 Conclusion

This paper proposes and implements an effective method for automatic medication recommendation in Chinese Electronic Medical Records (EMRs), by integrating multi-format fine-tuning with an optimized voting ensemble. To enhance robustness, the model is trained to learn both structured and natural language output formats during the fine-tuning phase. Subsequently, in the prediction phase, we utilize a voting strategy designed to balance precision and recall to ensemble the results from multiple predictions. Our method achieved fourth place in Evaluation Task 2 of CHIP 2025, demonstrating the effectiveness of the proposed approach for the automatic medication recommendation task.

A Appendix

A.1 Prompt Template

To ensure reproducibility and facilitate fair comparison across different paradigms, we provide the detailed prompt templates in Figs. 2, 3 and 4, including SFT, ICL and CoT methods.

你现在是一位出名的医生，请你根据病历为患者进行出院用药推荐。病情如下: ##instruction_text##请你根据上述患者的信息和给定的候选药物列表,为病人开具出院的药物清单。

Fig. 2. SFT prompt template.

你现在是一位出名的医生，请你根据病历为患者进行出院用药推荐。
病情如下: ##instruction_text##
请你仔细思考并逐步推理以下问题:
1. 分析现病史、主诉、诊疗信息;
2. 输出最终的出院用药清单。

请严格按照以下格式输出结果:
【最终输出】: <药物名称: drug_name>

Fig. 3. ICL prompt template.

A.2 Single-Model Performance

In our single-model evaluation, we investigate the impact of the temperature parameter on model performance in Table 5. As the temperature increases, the model exhibits greater output diversity but at the cost of reduced accuracy and stability. Specifically, when the temperature (SFT_{format}) rises from 0.01 to 0.3, the overall performance drops by approximately 2.1% in the final score, indicating that excessive randomness can hinder the models ability to maintain consistent reasoning patterns. This trade-off highlights that higher temperature

你现在是一位出名的医生，请你根据病历为患者进行出院用药推荐。
病情如下: ##instruction_text##
请你仔细思考并逐步推理以下问题:
1. 分析现病史、主诉、诊疗信息;
2. 推理药物适应症、禁忌症及相互作用;
3. 输出最终的出院用药清单。

请严格按照以下格式输出结果:
【推理过程】: <逐步分析与推理说明>
【最终输出】: <药物名称: drug_name>

Fig. 4. CoT prompt template.

encourages more exploratory responses, which may introduce noise and reduce precision in structured prediction tasks.

Furthermore, we observe that the structured fine-tuning ($\text{SFT}_{\text{format}}$) approach consistently outperforms its non-format counterpart ($\text{SFT}_{\text{non-format}}$) under the same temperature settings. For instance, at the optimal temperature of 0.01, ($\text{SFT}_{\text{format}}$) achieves a final score of 53.30, compared to 53.10 obtained by $\text{SFT}_{\text{non-format}}$. This confirms that enforcing output structure during fine-tuning not only improves stability but also enhances the models ability to follow task-specific constraints, leading to more reliable predictions.

Table 5. Impact of temperature on single-model performance.

Temperature	Jaccard	AVG_P	AVG_R	F1	Score
$\text{SFT}_{\text{format}}$					
0.01	**47.27**	60.93	**62.39**	**59.32**	**53.30**
0.1	46.86	**61.81**	60.90	58.89	52.88
0.2	46.21	59.21	62.37	58.29	52.25
0.3	45.19	58.43	60.39	56.99	51.09
$\text{SFT}_{\text{non-format}}$					
0.01	**47.10**	**62.50**	60.76	**59.09**	**53.10**
0.1	46.80	60.45	**61.70**	58.71	52.76
0.2	45.65	59.42	60.50	57.49	51.57
0.3	44.83	58.39	60.35	56.79	50.81

References

1. Wu, C., Lin, Z., Fang, W., Huang, Y.: A medical diagnostic assistant based on llm. In China Health Information Processing Conference, pp. 135–147. Springer (2023)
2. Li, J., Yuan, H., Luo, L., Lv, T., Jiang, Y., Wang, F., Zhang, P., Lv, H., Wang, J., Sun, Y., Lin, H.: Overview of chip 2025 shared task 2: discharge medication recommendation for metabolic diseases based on Chinese electronic health records (2025)
3. Imaichi, O., Yanase, T., Niwa, Y.: A comparison of rule-based and machine learning methods for medical information extraction. In: The First Workshop on Natural Language Processing for Medical and Healthcare Fields, pp. 38–42 (2013)
4. Sherstinsky, A.: Fundamentals of recurrent neural network (rnn) and long short-term memory (lstm) network. Phys. D **404**, 132306 (2020)
5. Choi, E., Bahadori, M.T., Sun, J., Kulas, J., Schuetz, A., Stewart, W.: Retain: an interpretable predictive model for healthcare using reverse time attention mechanism. In: Advances in neural information processing systems, 29 (2016)
6. Aftan, S., Shah, H.: A survey on bert and its applications. In: 2023 20th Learning and Technology Conference (L&T), pp. 161–166. IEEE (2023)
7. Lee, J., Yoon, W., Kim, S., Kim, D., Kim, S., So, C.H., Kang, J.: Biobert: a pre-trained biomedical language representation model for biomedical text mining. Bioinformatics **36**(4), 1234–1240 (2020)
8. Liu, Q., Wu, X., Zhao, X., Zhu, Y., Zhang, Z., Tian, F., Zheng, Y.: Large language model distilling medication recommendation model (2024). arXiv:2402.02803
9. Han, Z., Gao, C., Liu, J., Zhang, J., Zhang, S.Q.: Parameter-efficient fine-tuning for large models: a comprehensive survey (2024). arXiv:2403.14608
10. Augustin, A., Yi, J., Clausen, T., Townsley, W.M.: A study of lora: long range & low power networks for the internet of things. Sensors **16**(9), 1466 (2016)
11. Dong, X., Zhiwen, Yu., Cao, W., Shi, Y., Ma, Q.: A survey on ensemble learning. Front. Comp. Sci. **14**(2), 241–258 (2020)
12. Wu, C.Y., Ma, B., Liu, Y., Zhang, Z., Deng, N., Li, Y., Chen, B., Zhang, Y., Xue, Y., Plank, B.: M-ABSA: a multilingual dataset for aspect-based sentiment analysis. In: Christodoulopoulos, C., Chakraborty, T., Rose, C., Peng, V. (Eds.), Proceedings of the 2025 Conference on Empirical Methods in Natural Language Processing, pp. 2530–2557, Suzhou, China. Association for Computational Linguistics (2025)
13. Wu, C., Cai, Y., Cheng, Y., Xue, Y.: From detection to mitigation: Addressing gender bias in chinese texts via efficient tuning and voting-based rebalancing (2025). arXiv:2509.07889
14. Wu, C., Ma, B., Zhang, Z., Deng, N., He, Y., Xue, Y.: Evaluating zero-shot multilingual aspect-based sentiment analysis with large language models. Int. J. Mach. Learn. Cybern. 1–23 (2025)
15. Huang, W., Dai, F., Wu, C., Hu, J., Lyu, Y., Liu, J., Xue, Y.: Assessing diagnostic consistency in clinical cases: a fine-tuned llm voting and gpt error correction framework. In: China Health Information Processing Conference, pp. 191–201. Springer (2024)
16. Wu, C., Fang, W., Dai, F., Yin, H.: A model ensemble approach with llm for Chinese text classification. In: China Health Information Processing Conference, pp. 214–230. Springer (2023)
17. Li, J., Yuan, H., Luo, L., Jiang, Y., Wang, F., Zhang, P., Lv, H., Wang, J., Sun, Y., Lin, H.: Cdrugred: a Chinese drug recommendation dataset for discharge medications in metabolic diseases (2025). arXiv:2510.21084

18. Dong, Q., Li, L., Dai, D., Zheng, C., Ma, J., Li, R., Xia, H., Xu, J., Wu, Z., Liu, T., et al.: A survey on in-context learning (2022). arXiv:2301.00234
19. Zhang, Z., Zhang, A., Li, M., Smola, A.: Automatic chain of thought prompting in large language models (2022). arXiv:2210.03493
20. Messner, M., Polborn, M.K.: Voting on majority rules. Rev. Econ. Stud. **71**(1), 115–132 (2004)
21. Zheng, Y., Zhang, R., Zhang, J., Ye, Y., Luo, Z.: LlamaFactory: unified efficient fine-tuning of 100+ language models. In: Cao, Y., Feng, Y., Xiong, D. (Eds.), Proceedings of the 62nd Annual Meeting of the Association for Computational Linguistics (Volume 3: System Demonstrations), pp. 400–410, Bangkok, Thailand, August 2024. Association for Computational Linguistics
22. Qwen Team: Qwen2.5: A party of foundation models, September (2024)

Shared Task 3

Overview of Medical NLP Code Generation with FHIR for Clinical Trial Screening

Liang Tao[1], Lan Mi[2], Chunxiao Wu[3], Dong Wen[4], Buzhou Tang[5], Xiaoyan Zhang[6], Hui Zong[7(✉)], and Zuofeng Li[8(✉)]

[1] Faculty of Business Information, Shanghai Business School, Shanghai, China
tao.liang@msn.com
[2] Department of Lymphoma, Peking University Cancer Hospital, Beijing, China
milan@bjmu.edu.cn
[3] Shanghai Municipal Center for Disease Control and Prevention, Shanghai, China
wuchunxiao@scdc.sh.cn
[4] Shanghai Haoyuan Chemexpress Co., Ltd, Shanghai, China
dongwen930910@foxmail.com
[5] Harbin Institute of Technology, Shenzhen, China
tangbuzhou@gmail.com
[6] School of Life Sciences and Technology, Tongji University, Shanghai, China
xyzhang@tongji.edu.cn
[7] West China Hospital, Sichuan University, Chengdu, Sichuan, China
zonghui0228@163.com
[8] Independent Researcher, Shanghai, China
lizuofengcn@163.com

Abstract. This study presents a comprehensive evaluation of large language model based medical NLP code generation for clinical trial eligibility screening. Using 51 criteria across 19 categories and 51 case reports, we assess systems that transform natural-language rules into FHIR-compliant structured representations and executable patient-retrieval logic. The benchmark requires participants to generate FHIR Bundles rather than only end-to-end code to promote transparency, standards alignment, and interoperability. Top-performing teams adopted strategies such as intermediate-schema decoupling, dynamic few-shot prompting, iterative refinement, structured prompt engineering, and agent-based synthesis. Results demonstrate that LLMs can generate clinically meaningful, standards-compliant code, while also highlighting the need for explicit semantic layers to ensure safety and interpretability. This task provides the first large-scale evaluation of medical NLP code generation grounded in FHIR Profiles and offers a foundation for future development of verifiable, trustworthy clinical AI systems. Additional details, datasets, and evaluation materials are available at the CHIP 2025 website: http://cips-chip.org.cn/2025/eval3.

Keywords: FHIR · Code generation · Large language models · Clinical trial recruitment · CHIP

Y. Zhang et al. (Eds.): CHIP 2025, CCIS 2884, pp. 549–558, 2026.
https://doi.org/10.1007/978-981-95-7299-1_34

1 Introduction

Since the emergence of MYCIN [1], the foundational work of medical natural language processing (NLP) in the 1970s, the development of medical informatics has relied on the integration of clinical expertise and engineering capability. This cross-disciplinary mechanism, combining domain knowledge from frontline clinicians with technical implementation by engineers, has characterized the successful deployment of many influential clinical decision support systems (CDSS). Such collaboration has also fostered the growth of data governance and research-support infrastructures, which in turn have propelled progress in biomedical science and healthcare informatics [2]. However, CDSS development cannot be undertaken solely by clinicians. In conventional workflows where clinicians contribute medical knowledge and enterprises provide IT development capabilities, the ambiguity of intellectual property ownership has significantly hindered clinicians' motivation and willingness to participate in system development. With the rise of general-purpose large language models (LLMs), a new paradigm of everyone as a digital innovator has begun to emerge, presenting promising opportunities to break through these long-standing barriers via automated code generation.

In the general domain, the code-writing abilities of LLMs have gained widespread acceptance among software developers and are already being integrated into routine programming workflows. For example, MedAgentGym [3] framework provides an interactive, executable environment that enables open-source small models to acquire strong competence in medically oriented automated programming tasks through supervised and reinforcement learning. When validated algorithms transition from research environments to hospital information systems, however, they must confront the challenge of heterogeneity across clinical systems. To achieve interoperability and maximize their utility, algorithms must adapt to different system architectures and comply with healthcare data standards. Recent studies have shown that LLMs possess the capability to generate standard-aligned HL7 FHIR (Fast Healthcare Interoperability Resources) [4] resources, like FHIR-GPT [5], potentially reducing the technical cost associated with implementing interoperability frameworks. Importantly, recent advances in large language models have shifted their role in healthcare from passive text-generators to agentic systems capable of planning, tool use, and interacting with electronic health record (EHR) environments. For example, FHIR-AgentBench [6] provides a foundational, reproducible testbed for studying agentic reasoning over interoperable EHRs question answering in clinical AI. MedAgentBench [7] introduces the FHIR-compliant interactive benchmark designed to evaluate medical LLM agents operating within realistic electronic health record environments.

Running code inside a sandbox mitigates operational risks, yet it simultaneously raises several critical questions. Chief among them are whether the generated programs truly conform to established standards, how such code should be validated, governed, and monitored, and in what ways automatically generated algorithms can be transformed into high-quality data services capable of supporting clinical research. Moreover, there remains the broader challenge of ensuring that innovations developed under the paradigm of AI for Science can be reliably translated into real-world AI for clinical practice. These concerns collectively form the core issues that the present evaluation seeks to investigate. In this assessment task, we provide a set of 51 clinical trial inclusion and exclusion questions distributed across 19 categories, representing a range of linguistic and clinical complexities. For each question, participants are given the natural-language formulation of the eligibility criterion, its corresponding FHIR FSH definition, and an associated FHIR service query code snippet. Participants must generate NLP-driven code that satisfies all three constraints: question semantics, formal standards, and executable query logic. The evaluation will assess the consistency and robustness of LLMs when performing these tasks, thereby providing empirical evidence and theoretical insights to support future scientific research and inform clinical policy decision-making.

2 Task Description

2.1 Clinical Trial Eligibility Screening Questions Dataset

The dataset consists of clinical trial inclusion and exclusion criteria questions drawn from registered studies in the Chinese Clinical Trial Registry (ChiCTR) [8]. These questions reflect authentic eligibility criteria extracted from real-world clinical research protocols. As summarized in Table 1, the dataset includes 19 categories, 51 eligibility-criteria questions [9], and 51 patient cases [10] (comprising 50 case reports and one specialty clinical summary). Example entries are illustrated in Table 2. Each row in the dataset corresponds to a single eligibility criterion and contains the structured fields described as follows:

index: The original index of the eligibility criterion within the dataset.

json: A JSON-formatted representation of the criterion. Although the JSON may contain multiple fields, only the Chinese text of the eligibility criterion is used for the NLP task.

id: The original identifier of the eligibility rule derived from the source trial.

label: The category label associated with the eligibility criterion. There are 19 unique labels, representing different types of screening rules (e.g., age, sex, laboratory values, disease status), as shown in Table 1.

question: The natural-language eligibility criterion text used as the primary input for the NLP task.

deepquery_id: A unique identifier linking the criterion to a clinical query system. This ID ensures compatibility with downstream FHIR service calls.

FHIR_FSH: FHIR Shorthand (FSH) represents the eligibility criterion.

NLP_CODE: This column represents the main output expected from participating teams. It is the core evaluation target, assessing the LLM ability to perform constrained code generation under semantic, logical, and standardization requirements.

FHIR_SERVICE_CODE: Executable code that queries a FHIR service API to identify patients satisfying the rule.

positive_doc_patient_index: The ID of the patient case that satisfies this eligibility criterion. This serves as the ground truth for evaluating whether the generated FHIR Query correctly identifies the eligible patient.

Table 1. Eligibility class and corresponding number of case reports

Class	Number	Class	Number
Age (年龄)	2	Nursing (护理)	2
Alcohol Consumer (酒精摄入)	1	Organ or Tissue Status (器官与组织状态)	3
Consent (知情同意)	1	Risk Assessment (风险评估)	1
Device (设备)	1	Signs (体征)	1
Diagnostic (诊断)	6	Smoking Status (吸烟状态)	3
Disease (疾病)	2	Symptoms (症状)	4
Encounter (就诊)	1	Treatment or Surgery (治疗或手术)	7
Gender (性别)	3	Neoplasm Status (肿瘤状态)	5
Laboratory Examinations (实验室检查)	6	Multiple (多类别)	1
None-Neoplasm Stage (非肿瘤疾病分期)	1		

Table 2. Example Entries

id	label	question_text
s7890	Age	18–80 years old (年龄 18–80 周岁)
s10360	Gender	No restriction (性别：不限)

2.2 FSH (FHIR Shorthand) Definitions of the Eligibility Criteria Texts

Not all eligibility criteria texts in the dataset are accompanied by FSH (FHIR Shorthand) definitions. When an FSH definition is not provided for a particular criterion, it indicates that the criterion can be fully expressed using standard FHIR core resources. Conversely, when an FSH definition is present, it signifies that representing the criterion requires FHIR extensions or customized FHIR profiles beyond the core specification.

At the initial release of the project, we will publish the FSH definitions for all questions that require such extensions. Due to the limited size of the dataset, however, not every criterion with an FSH definition has an associated positive patient match.

It is also important to emphasize that the definition and construction of FHIR Profiles constitute an iterative and continuously evolving process. Therefore, the FSH definitions corresponding to each question will be subject to refinement throughout the project timeline. The final evaluation phase will rely on the latest, finalized versions of these FHIR Profile definitions, and all submitted systems are expected to conform to these final specifications.

2.3 Medical Documents

We collected patient case reports from the China Medical Case Repository (CMCR) [11] to serve as the patient data source. Through manual annotation, each case report was segmented into multiple thematic units, simulating structured electronic medical record data. The final dataset consists of a list of input topics, each representing a clinically meaningful document segment. Each topic includes the following fields, with end_datetime being optional.

These topic-level document segments constitute the candidate patient pool, which includes 52 patients in total, with 61.5% male and 38.5% female, and their age distribution is depicted in Fig. 1a . The eligibility criteria dataset is divided according to the screening questions. Specifically, it is partitioned into three subsets (Training set, Test set A (Leaderboard A), Test set B (Leaderboard B)), each containing 17 eligibility criteria. The patient document set remains consistent across all splits, comprising 51 cases with ICD-O-3 codes distribution shown in Fig. 1b . These structured document segments are used to evaluate whether the FHIR-based queries generated by participating systems can correctly identify patients who satisfy each eligibility criterion.

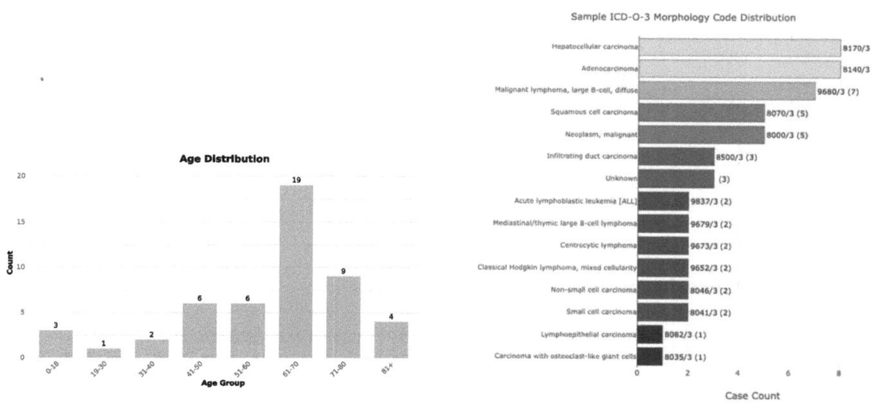

(a) Age distribution (b) ICD-O-3 codes distribution

Fig. 1. Cases statistics

2.4 Metrics

The evaluation consists of three sequential components, each designed to assess a different stage of the end-to-end eligibility screening pipeline: (1) Execution of the NLP algorithm code; (2) Execution of the FHIR service API to query the patient database; 3) Assessment of the query results against the gold-standard annotations. Each component is independently scored. Steps (1) and (2) are binary: the output either satisfies the required specification (1 point) or does not (0 points). Step (3) is evaluated using the F1-score, based on standard information-retrieval metrics. Scores are computed individually for each eligibility question, and the final system score is obtained by averaging the scores across all 51 clinical questions. Higher scores indicate better overall performance.

3 Results

3.1 Leaderboard Statistics

This task consists of two evaluation phases: Leaderboard A and Leaderboard B. Leaderboard A remained open for one month, whereas Leaderboard B was conducted over a one-week period. The statistical summary of the Top 10 performing systems for each phase is presented in Table 3. It is important to note that these statistics are computed only over the Top 10 submissions, rather than all submissions, because a substantial proportion of systems achieved scores close to zero, which would otherwise distort the analysis and obscure meaningful performance differences.

Table 3. Summary statistics of the top 10 methods in leaderboards A and B

	MAX	MIN	Average	Median
Leaderboard A	0.27	0.14	0.19	0.18
Leaderboard B	0.43	0.24	0.328	0.325

3.2 Top-Performing Algorithms

Table 4 reports the performance results of the top eight teams on Leaderboard B for this task. In the following section, we provide a brief overview of the methodologies employed by selected top-performing teams. Furthermore, Fig. 2 presents the details of code generation performance, sorted by maximum F1 score, for all clinical questions in both the training and testing datasets that achieved an F1 score greater than zero. We observe that the performance varies significantly across different clinical questions, with certain questions yielding substantially higher F1 scores than others. This variability highlights the differing levels of code generation complexity and challenge associated with each eligibility criterion.

Table 4. Leaderboard B performance

Rank	Max F1	Max precision	Max recall
1	**0.4334**	0.4697	0.5660
2	0.4102	0.4736	0.5084
3	0.3674	**0.4881**	0.3845
4	0.3490	0.3894	0.4840
5	0.3443	0.4494	0.3740
6	0.3378	0.4568	0.3622
7	0.3344	0.3578	**0.8222**
8	0.3198	0.3493	0.5017

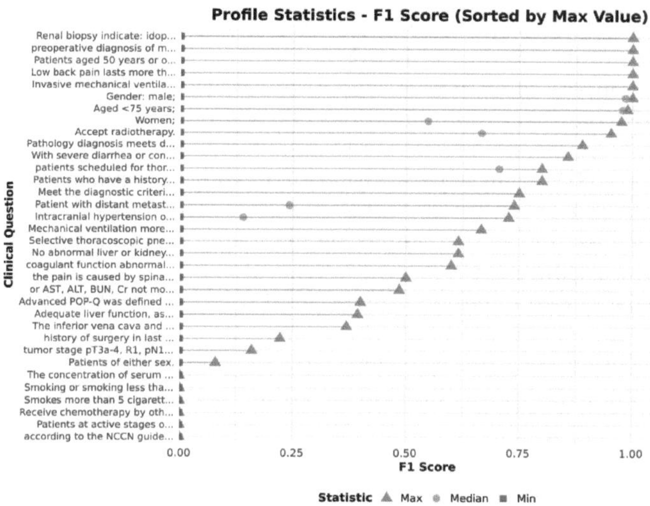

Fig. 2. Code generation performance across clinical questions.

The top-performing team developed an end-to-end system for clinical trial patient recruitment that automates the full pipeline from eligibility-criteria parsing to FHIR-compliant Bundle generation and validation. Their approach introduces an intermediate schema to decouple information extraction from FHIR resource construction, thereby reducing generation complexity. The system further enhances accuracy through automated sampling of representative case snippets and by employing multiple, independently generated code strategies to increase extraction recall. Leveraging the Claude agent SDK, the team produced high-quality NLP code and integrated automated testing to ensure compliance and correctness. Their solution successfully supports reliable information extraction and standardized FHIR data representation for inclusion/exclusion screening, ultimately achieving first place in the task.

The runner-up team introduced an iterative code generation and optimization framework designed for complex medical data processing tasks. Their system integrates large language models with a dynamic few-shot learning strategy and comprises three core components: an initial generator that produces diverse positive and negative test cases, a dynamic few-shot prompting mechanism that incorporates the question, FHIR_FSH, FHIR_SERVICE_CODE, and NLP_CODE contexts, and an automated evaluation refinement loop that detects errors and iteratively improves code quality. Built on DeepSeek-V3.1, the framework progressively enhances performance through repeated testing and prompt optimization. Experimental results show significant gains, with F1 scores rising from 0.12 to 0.42 over five iterations, representing a 250% improvement, and a notable +0.13 contribution from the dynamic few-shot mechanism alone. The approach demonstrates strong potential for medical NLP applications, particularly in FHIR-based data processing and structured code generation.

The seventh-ranked team addressed the challenge of converting unstructured, linguistically complex clinical trial eligibility criteria into executable screening rules and FHIR-compliant representations. They proposed a Prompt-Driven Program Synthesis approach tailored for task, leveraging structured prompt engineering to guide GPT-5 in generating both Python screening code and FHIR Bundles. Their framework incorporates explicit constraints on class structures, function signatures, and FHIR Bundle requirements covering Condition, Observation, and ResearchSubject resources in transaction format. Experimental analyses showed that carefully designed structured prompts combined with independent session management produced the strongest results. Their system achieved a score of 0.3344 on the Test-B leaderboard, demonstrating the effectiveness of structured prompt-driven synthesis for medical NLP code generation.

4 Discussion

This work presents a comprehensive evaluation of large language model–based medical NLP code generation systems within the context of clinical trial eligibility screening. By providing 51 inclusion and exclusion criteria across 19 categories, each accompanied by natural language descriptions, FHIR Shorthand definitions, and FHIR service query templates, we constructed a rigorous benchmark that assesses the full pipeline from eligibility-criteria interpretation to structured FHIR resource generation and executable patient-retrieval logic. The participating teams demonstrated diverse solution strategies, ranging from intermediate-schema decoupling, dynamic few-shot prompting, and iterative code optimization to structured prompt engineering and agent-based program synthesis. Their collective achievements reveal both the promise and the current limitations of LLM driven medical code generation.

A key design decision in this task is the requirement to output FHIR Bundles rather than only end-to-end procedural code. Bundles provide a transparent, standards-compliant representation of the structured clinical concepts extracted by the model. They serve as an explicit semantic layer between natural-language understanding and downstream executable logic, enabling validation, auditing, and interoperability across heterogeneous clinical systems. This modular design reflects an essential principle for medical AI deployment: clinical algorithms must be inspectable, governable, and standards aligned. By externalizing the intermediate structured representation, we avoid the black box risks inherent in purely end-to-end code generation and create opportunities for error analysis, safety checks, and system level integration.

Nevertheless, the current dataset containing 51 criteria and 51 patient cases remains relatively small. While suitable for benchmarking system behavior, broader generalization will require significantly larger and more diverse datasets. Future work should therefore focus on scaling the corpus to thousands of criteria and real-world EMR documents, enabling deeper evaluations of robustness, generalization, and cross institutional interoperability. Expanding the dataset will also unlock the full potential of program synthesis based medical AI.

Looking forward, medical NLP code generation holds significant potential as a pathway toward interpretable, traceable, and verifiable medical AI. Future research may explore hybrid architectures that unify symbolic FHIR representations with neural program synthesis, automated conformance validation, and real-time sandbox execution monitoring. Such developments can help bridge the gap between AI for Science and AI for Clinical Practice, ultimately enabling safely automated patient recruitment, scalable clinical research workflows, and trustworthy medical AI systems deployed across the healthcare ecosystem.

Acknowledgments. This work was supported by the Development Research Center of Shanghai Municipal People's Government (2025-JD-27), and AI–Driven Research Paradigm Reform and Disciplinary Advancement Program of the Shanghai Municipal Education Commission.

References

1. Mycin (2025), https://en.wikipedia.org/wiki/Mycin
2. Zong, H., Wu, R., Cha, J., Feng, W., Wu, E., Li, J., Shao, A., Tao, L., Li, Z., Tang, B., Shen, B.: Advancing Chinese biomedical text mining with community challenges. J. Biomed. Inform. **157**, 104716 (2024)
3. Xu, R., Zhuang, Y., Zhong, Y., Yu, Y., Wang, Z., Tang, X., Wu, H., Wang, M.D., Ruan, P., Yang, D., Wang, T., Xiao, G., Liu, X., Yang, C., Xie, Y., Shi, W.: MedAgentGym: A Scalable Agentic Training Environment for Code-Centric Reasoning in Biomedical Data Science (2025). http://arxiv.org/abs/2506.04405
4. Consent - FHIR v4.0.1, https://hl7.org/fhir/R4/consent.html?spm=a2c22.12281978.0.0.2e591debK9H228
5. Li, Y., Wang, H., Yerebakan, H.Z., Shinagawa, Y., Luo, Y.: Fhir-gpt enhances health interoperability with large language models. NEJM AI **1**(8) (2024). https://ai.nejm.org/doi/10.1056/AIcs2300301
6. Lee, G., Bach, E., Yang, E., Pollard, T., Johnson, A., Choi, E., jia, Y., Lee, J.H.: FHIR-AgentBench: Benchmarking LLM Agents for Realistic Interoperable EHR Question Answering (Nov 2025), http://arxiv.org/abs/2509.19319, arXiv:2509.19319

7. Jiang, Y., Black, K.C., Geng, G., Park, D., Zou, J., Ng, A.Y., Chen, J.H.: MedAgentBench: A Virtual EHR Environment to Benchmark Medical LLM Agents. NEJM AI **2**(9) (2025), https://ai.nejm.org/doi/10.1056/AIdbp2500144
8. Chinese Clinical Trial Registry, https://www.chictr.org.cn/
9. Zong, H., Yang, J., Zhang, Z., Li, Z., Zhang, X.: Semantic categorization of Chinese eligibility criteria in clinical trials using machine learning methods. BMC Med. Inf. Decis. Mak. **21**(1), 128 (2021), https://bmcmedinformdecismak.biomedcentral.com/articles/10.1186/s12911-021-01487-w
10. Zong, H., Tao, L., Li, Z., Wu, C., Liu, Y., Zhang, X.: Benchmark for Lymphoma Information Extraction and Automated Coding. In: Zhang, Y., Chen, Q., Lin, H., Liu, L., Liao, X., Tang, B., Hao, T., Huang, Z., Lei, J., Li, Z., Zong, H. (eds.) Health Information Processing. Evaluation Track Papers. pp. 67–74. Springer Nature, Singapore (2025)
11. Chinese Medical Case Repository, https://cmcr.yiigle.com/

A Large Language Model-based System for Automatic Medical NLP Code Generation

Jiming Xu[1], Simin Li[1], Bo Kang[1], and Jun Yan[2(✉)]

[1] Yidu Tech Inc., Beijing, China
{jiming.xu,simin.li,bo.kang}@yiducloud.cn
[2] BIOS, HKAI−Sci, IDM, City University of Hong Kong, Hong Kong, China
yan.jun@cityu.edu.hk

Abstract. In clinical research, patient recruitment requires a large amount of chart review, and the interpreted data must be converted into a common format (such as FHIR) to support circulation across multi-ple systems. This paper builds a system that covers the entire pipeline from "eligibility-criteria parsing to schema generation to NLP code and Bundle construction to automatic validation". The method: (1) uses an intermediate schema to decouple information extraction from FHIR-structured data generation into two steps, reducing generation difficulty; (2) automatically samples representative case snippets to assist code generation and improve accuracy; (3) enforces at least two distinct code-generation strategies to improve the recall of information extraction; and (4) uses the Claude agent SDK to generate high-quality code and auto-matically complete testing. The overall system can effectively accomplish the information extraction and FHIR-format data storage required for patient recruitment, thereby supporting inclusion/exclusion screening. The proposed pipeline achieved first place in "CHIP2025 Task 3: Medi-cal NLP Code Generation Evaluation"[1], demonstrating its engineering and deployment value in medical scenarios.

Keywords: CHIP2025 · Clinical natural language processing · FHIR · Large language models

1 Introduction

1.1 Task Background

Medical AI has progressed from early rule-based CDSS (e.g., MYCIN, INTERNIST-I) to data-driven clinical NLP built on large-scale EHRs. Systems such as MetaMap and cTAKES established terminology mapping and information-extraction pipelines, while modern deployment increasingly relies on standardized representations.

HL7 FHIR, with its resource-centric REST/JSON design, has become the dom-inant interoperability framework and is now widely mandated across health sys-tems [2–4].

LLMs further shift the paradigm: controlled studies show substantial effi-ciency gains in code generation, and medical-agent environments make task-oriented programming and validation more realistic [5, 6]. In healthcare, models such as FHIR-GPT

Y. Zhang et al. (Eds.): CHIP 2025, CCIS 2884, pp. 559–569, 2026.
https://doi.org/10.1007/978-981-95-7299-1_35

demonstrate the feasibility of producing compliant FHIR re-sources directly from free text [7]. Yet real-world AI deployment still encounters workflow, interoperability, and data-quality challenges [9].

Patient recruitment remains one of the most resource-intensive bottlenecks in clinical development. Trials account for 60–70% of new drug R&D expendi-ture, and 80% of studies face delays due to poor accrual [11–13]. Manual pre-screening is labor-intensive—often requiring several hours per eligible patient— and screening failure rates can exceed 80% in complex protocols [14–16]. Mean-while, regional EHR platforms routinely cover millions of patients, magnifying the computational burden.

LLM-based matching systems (e.g., TrialGPT) can directly process eligibility criteria and clinical text, outperforming traditional retrieval and ML baselines [20, 21]. However, end-to-end inference scales poorly: matching hundreds of thou-sands of records against hundreds of criteria requires repeated LLM calls, while most hospitals lack affordable large-scale GPU clusters due to cost and supply constraints [22, 23].

A more practical route is to concentrate LLM inference in a few high-value steps—such as schema construction and code generation—then execute the re-sulting extraction and FHIR Bundle assembly code on existing CPU/database infrastructures. The system proposed in this paper follows this approach, en-abling reusable, testable, and low-cost chart-processing pipelines for patient re-cruitment.

CHIP2025's "Task 3: Medical NLP Code Generation" evaluates exactly this capability: transforming trial eligibility criteria and FHIR/FSH constraints into executable Python parsing programs. Submitted code is executed via FHIR Ser-vice APIs and scored against gold standards, emphasizing textual understanding, structured extraction, standardized representation, and real executable valida-tion under limited submission quotas [10].

1.2 Related Work

Clinical text structuring and trial screening have long been core topics in clinical NLP. Early work was dominated by rule systems and terminological ontologies: MetaMap mapped free text to UMLS concepts and systematized terminology normalization; cTAKES, built on the UIMA framework, provided composable clinical text information extraction components (such as NER, negation detec-tion, and attribute extraction), becoming foundational infrastructure in engi-neering practice. The i2b2/n2c2 2018 Track-1 shared task was the first to frame "trial eligibility-based cohort selection" as a community benchmark, promoting the transition from concept-level extraction to reproducible evaluation [2, 24, 25]. For cross-system deployment, interoperability standards serve as the crucial bridge from "extraction to application". FHIR uses resource-based, Web-oriented APIs and semantic models to lower integration barriers, FSH formalizes imple-mentation guides and constraints into a domain-specific language, and ecosystems like SMART on FHIR/SMART Apps and HAPI-FHIR provide authoriza-tion, sandboxes, and structural validation capabilities to support end-to-end "read/write and verifiable" applications [26–29].

In recent years, large language models have shown strong performance on "text to structured representation/executable code" tasks. One line of work di-rectly attempts to convert clinical narratives into compliant FHIR resources (e.g., FHIR-GPT/LLM-on-FHIR); another injects standardized knowledge into generation through RAG/templates. However, consistency and reproducible eval-uation remain challenging [7, 30].

In the emerging subfield of "LLMs for clinical trial matching/patient recruit-ment", systems like TrialGPT and Scaling Clinical Trial Matching integrate candidate retrieval, per-criterion judgment, and trial ranking into end-to-end pipelines on SIGIR/TREC benchmarks and real-world oncology center deploy-ments. PRISM/OncoLLM, Zero-Shot Clinical Trial Patient Matching, Learn-ing to Match Patients to Clinical Trials Using LLMs, and multi-agent/RAG-based frameworks such as MAKAR, LLM-Match, and End-to-End LLM Match-ing systematically compare specialized small models and general-purpose LLMs in terms of performance and cost across n2c2, TREC, and multi-source EHR datasets. Patient2Trial and TrialMatchAI further explore patient-facing path-ways and structured disease descriptions via Phenopackets. Large Language Model Augmented Clinical Trial Screening, a randomized trial in heart failure prescreening published in JAMA, and a JCO CCI survey summarize the benefits and limitations of LLM-based prescreening in terms of efficiency, accuracy, and workflow redesign [20, 21, 31–37].

1.3 Key Differences

Compared with direct LLM-based classification or judgment approaches, our solution dramatically reduces LLM compute usage by generating deterministic NLP code with LLMs rather than relying on online LLM inference for each case. Relative to end-to-end "text to FHIR resource/Bundle" approaches (such as FHIR-GPT/LLM-on-FHIR), we propose and validate a schema-driven two-stage generation process: first abstract key fields and decision logic in an intermediate schema, then assemble standardized Bundles aligned with FSH constraints. This design significantly reduces search space and error rates [7, 30].

2 Methods

2.1 Problem Definition and Notation

Let the official CSV define a set of tasks $D = \{(q_i, F_i, s_i)\}_{i=1}^{N}$, where q_i is the inclusion/exclusion criterion text, F_i is the corresponding FHIR/FSH constraint (including profiles, extensions, and server-side query logic), and s_i is the official FHIR Service code. The set of patient records to be processed is denoted as $R = \{r_j\}$, where each record r_j consists of multiple case_reports segments of the form {text, timestamp, topic}, with non-standardized and potentially missing topic labels.

Under the constraint of using only the Python standard library, the objective is to learn two deterministic mappings for each task: g_i maps R to x_i and pro-duces structured outputs that conform to a task-specific extracted_info_schema, and h_i maps (x_i, patient_id) to B_i and assembles the extracted information into FHIR Bundles that satisfy transactional/message constraints. The official FHIR Service code s_i is then applied to obtain a predicted patient set P_i, to be compared to the gold-standard set G_i. The goal is to maximize $F_1(P_i, G_i)$ while ensuring that Bundle-level resource constraints are not violated.

2.2 System Design

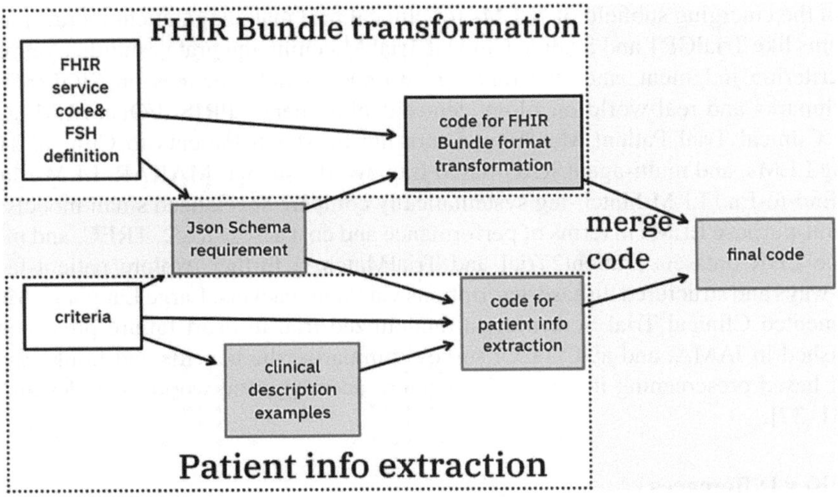

Fig. 1. Overview of the patient information extraction and FHIR Bundle transforma-tion pipeline.

Overall Code Generation Pipeline As shown in Fig. 1, we decouple the generation of code for extracting key information from records and the generation of code for FHIR Bundle conversion, thereby reducing the complexity of each step. Once the two components are generated, they are merged into a unified parser.

Based on eligibility criteria and FSH requirements, a large language model automatically generates a JSON schema for the key information to be extracted

from records. Using this schema, the system then samples relevant record seg-ments from an auxiliary case corpus via regular expressions. With schema and sampled examples in place, a Claude agent SDK instance generates extraction code in each task directory, enforcing at least two independent logic chains and explicit conflict-resolution rules. A second agent in the same directory gener-ates the Bundle construction logic, with an entry function that takes structured information and a patient identifier and returns a transactional FHIR Bundle. Finally, an automatic composer embeds the extraction and Bundle logic into a unified parser class to form the final code.

JSON Schema Construction The schema generator reads eligibility crite-ria, FHIR/FSH resources, and query code from each task directory, composes a composite prompt, and calls a locally hosted LLM service (with a conservative temperature to increase determinism). The model must output Draft-7 JSON that includes only key fields required by the eligibility criteria, explicitly stating field types, missing-value strategies, and source_text origins, while forbidding inclusion of patient identifiers or label fields.

Case Sampling and Automatic Labeling In the sampling stage, we gener-ate regular expressions from eligibility criteria to automatically sample the most relevant case descriptions. The regular-expression generation step is configured as follows: a local model is prompted to produce multiple candidate regex pat-terns in one shot, each with an associated probability or confidence (to encourage diversity and deeper reasoning), and these patterns are used to match case seg-ments in the auxiliary corpus at scale. The matched text is sorted by length and downsampled with a fixed stride to obtain 30 representative samples. If the total number of matches falls below a threshold, matched segments and the dominant regex patterns from the previous round are fed back to the model as examples to obtain additional patterns and samples. This process iterates for at most three rounds.

Automatic Generation of Extraction Code The resulting case set is then used to drive extraction code generation. For each task, the system places eli-gibility criteria, FHIR/FSH resources, schemas, sampled cases, and previously generated code records in the same directory. Using the Claude agent SDK, it requests extraction code whose input is a raw record and whose output is JSON-structured key information, restricted to use only the Python standard library.

To improve recall, we require at least two independent extraction logic chains and explicit conflict-merge strategies. After generation, an automated executor runs unit tests for the extraction code on the task directory, comparing struc-tured outputs against examples and logging results.

FHIR Bundle Conversion Code The Bundle generator likewise uses the Claude agent SDK (with claude-4.5-sonnet as the default model) to generate

Bundle construction logic in each task directory. The main entry function receives structured information and a patient identifier and returns a transactional FHIR Bundle, strictly following FSH constraints and the resource types, references, and HTTP methods used in official example Bundles. After generation, an automated executor runs unit tests for the Bundle code, comparing outputs with official example Bundles and writing logs to the task directory.

The generated extraction and Bundle code are subsequently embedded into a unified parser class by the automatic composer, forming the final submission code.

Self-Constructed Test Set and Labeling From the Chinese Clinical Case Achievements Database, we extracted 562 cases as a test set based on diagnostic and related information from eligibility criteria. Using the previously generated JSON schema format, we applied the GPT-5 model to each case to extract key JSON fields for each eligibility criterion. These LLM-generated annotations were then used to evaluate the quality of the generated NLP code.

2.3 Evaluation Metrics

Evaluation is based on a Mock FHIR environment (a locally deployed FHIR-compatible environment, referred to as the Mock FHIR Server, which reproduces the query and validation logic of the official FHIR Service). We compare the set of patients matched by the generated code against those matched by GPT-5 (OpenAI) annotations, computing macro-and micro-averaged precision, recall, and F_1 as:

$$\text{Precision} = \frac{TP}{TP + FP},$$

$$\text{Recall} = \frac{TP}{TP + FN}$$

$$F_1 = \frac{2 \cdot \text{Precision} \cdot \text{Recall}}{\text{Precision} + \text{Recall}}$$

Macro-averaging computes the arithmetic mean of per-task metrics, while micro-averaging accumulates TP/FP/FN over all patient pairs.

3 Data and Experimental Setup

3.1 Data and Materials

The core data include the official training and test CSVs provided by the com-petition, containing task IDs, labels, eligibility criteria text, FHIR/FSH con-straints, and query code, as well as publicly accessible case records crawled from the Chinese Clinical Case Achievements Database. In preprocessing, we split each task into an independent directory, consistently retaining the original eligibility text, FSH constraints, and official query code.

3.2 Overview of Official Task Data

According to the official task description, the organizers released 51 clinical trial eligibility questions across 19 disease or treatment categories. Each sample pro-vides: (1) Chinese or mixed Chinese–English eligibility descriptions (with IDs such as cnwqk3); (2) FHIR/FSH constraints bound to the task, typically in-cluding custom CodeSystems and ValueSets and profiles for resources such as Procedure and Condition; and (3) official FHIR Service query code and exam-ple Bundles. All resources conform to HL7 FHIR R4.0 and its JSON represen-tation, constrain field values and cardinality, and specify terminologies at the ValueSet level (e.g., ICD-10, ICD-O-3). These metadata are stored in the official CSV and task directories, providing complete upstream semantic constraints for subsequent schema construction and Bundle validation. Our experiments focus on the testB subset, which includes 17 eligibility tasks. Final rankings on the competition leaderboard are based on the best historical performance on the B leaderboard (testB).

3.3 Self-Constructed Test Set

Because the official answers for testB are not publicly available, we constructed our own test set for evaluation. Specifically, for each task we selected 562 cases from the Chinese Clinical Case Achievements Database based on diagnostic and related information in the eligibility criteria, and used the GPT-5 model to label the set of patients meeting each criterion, generating corresponding JSON annotations consistent with the above schema.

3.4 Input–Output Contracts and Constraints

Participants must convert each task into executable algorithm artifacts and sub-mit them in HL7 FHIR Bundle (Message/Transaction) format. The organizers support two submission options: Option 1 is executable code based only on Python NLP and rule-based methods; Option 2 allows direct LLM calls to generate FHIR Bundles. Regardless of the option, final submissions must embed algorithm code compressed and Base64-encoded into a FHIR Library resource, which is then submitted together with other resources. The FHIR server restricts operations on certain resource types (e.g., Patient does not ac-cept POST/PUT/DELETE), so our pipeline strictly constrains resource types, HTTP methods, and reference structures to meet R4.0 specifications and the cardinality requirements of the "JSON Representation of Resources".

3.5 Experimental Environment and Configuration

Our experiments rely on a local LLM service, IDE-level code-generation agents, and a Mock FHIR server. Every step from generation to evaluation logs calls and caches results, facilitating diagnosis against the official three-step evaluation process. We use Python 3.12 and the standard library only, strictly adhering to the competition requirement of "no external dependencies". During evaluation, we jointly report structured extraction quality and patient-level F_1 scores.

4 Results

Table 1 shows example structured extraction results on the self-constructed test set for selected eligibility criteria.

Across the 17 evaluated tasks, we obtain total TP = 1517, FP = 144, and FN = 203. Macro-averaged precision is 0.5922, Macro-averaged recall is 0.5713, and $Macro-averaged-F_1 = 0.5650$; micro-averaged precision is 0.9133, micro-averaged recall is 0.8820, and $Micro-averaged\ -F_1 = 0.8974$. We observe that extraction code for basic attributes such as sex and age is highly accurate and close to deployment readiness. Diagnosis-related items such as diabetes and lym-phoma also show relatively high accuracy and, with further optimization, have potential for practical application. For treatment-related and more complex in-formation, however, extraction accuracy remains limited.

5 Discussion

The strengths of our approach are mainly reflected in the following aspects:

1. **Schema-based two-stage design**. By decoupling the process into "schema-based extraction to FHIR generation", we substantially reduce the search space and complexity of FHIR generation.
2. **Automatic sampling of representative cases**. Using automatic regex-based sampling and multi-round feedback, we construct representative case sets that provide high-quality examples for code generation, improving ac-curacy and ensuring sampling diversity.

Table 1. Example extraction results for selected eligibility criteria on the self-constructed test set

Case	Anno	Pred	TP	FP	FN	Prec	Rec	F1
1–17 Sex: both male and female allowed	562	562	562	0	0	1.000	1.000	1.000
1–16 Sex: male	295	271	271	0	24	1.000	0.919	0.958
1–2 Age < 75 years	494	468	459	9	35	0.981	0.929	0.954
1–48 Elective thoracoscopic lung resection	100	100	94	6	6	0.940	0.940	0.940
1–6 Meeting the 1999 WHO criteria for T2DM	16	18	14	4	2	0.778	0.875	0.824
1–9 Renal biopsy suggesting primary membranous nephropathy	44	33	27	6	17	0.818	0.614	0.701
1–10 Surgery for middle/lower esophageal cancer	2	1	1	0	1	1.000	0.500	0.667
1–11 Pathological diagnosis of DLBCL	20	13	10	3	10	0.769	0.500	0.606
1–44 Low back pain lasting > 3 months	13	15	7	8	6	0.467	0.538	0.500
1–47 Elective thoracic surgery under general anesthesia	30	36	16	20	14	0.444	0.533	0.485
1–45 Patients who received radiotherapy	11	23	8	15	3	0.348	0.727	0.471
1–28 Documented distant metastasis	27	28	12	16	15	0.429	0.444	0.436
1–43 History of asphyxia and hypoxia	58	35	19	16	39	0.543	0.328	0.409
1–7 Spine-origin chronic pain (spinal cause)	26	53	16	37	10	0.302	0.615	0.405
1–27 Lesion not invading IVC or portal vein	4	4	1	3	3	0.250	0.250	0.250
1–18 Total bilirubin within 1× ULN during a visit	1	0	0	0	1	0.000	0.000	0.000
1–38 Smoking > 5 cigarettes per day	17	1	0	1	17	0.000	0.000	0.000

3. **Multi-strategy code generation**. Requiring at least two independent logic chains (rules + semantics) helps mitigate the common pattern of "high precision but low recall" and improves overall performance.
4. **Agent-driven automatic coding and testing**. Leveraging the Claude agent SDK, we automatically complete the loop of "plan generation to in-cremental coding to running tests to fixing errors based on logs" within each task directory, greatly reducing manual iteration costs.

Limitations of case sampling. Because the official test cases are hidden, we can-not entirely rule out the possibility that our sampled cases overlap with the unseen test set, which could lead to optimistic performance estimates compared to a regime where test cases are fully invisible. Sampling is an accepted practice in real patient recruitment projects and is pragmatically necessary given the cor-pus scale, where neither exhaustive manual review nor providing all cases to an LLM is feasible; manual rule-writing workflows likewise rely on reviewing sam-pled cases. Our other contributions—explicit JSON schema, the Claude agent SDK workflow, and two distinct rule/semantic code-generation strategies—are orthogonal to sampling. We now state this risk and treat reported performance accordingly.

Future work can extend in several directions:

Improving experimental design and reliability of results. We plan to conduct systematic ablation studies (removing or replacing individual modules) to quantify each module's contribution to overall F_1; to run multiple random sampling and multiple runs for stability analysis, reporting mean $\pm$ variance or box plots.

Improving generation strategies. We aim to move beyond the current "rule-dominated, single-sentence matching" strategies to entity–relation-based gener-ation, explicitly modeling relationships among diseases, procedures, temporal expressions, and numeric ranges; and to design paragraph-level semantic strate-gies for cross-sentence logic (e.g., "both prior and current ...", "postoperative ... during follow-up ..."). In the sampling stage, we plan to explicitly account for longer-range textual dependencies and design dedicated handling for temporal anchors such as "postoperative XXX" and "during follow-up XXX", improving recall for borderline and long-tail patterns while maintaining precision.

Upper bounds and usability criteria. We will further analyze which types of criteria can realistically achieve F_1 scores above 90% and treat them as the first batch of "clinically deployable" scenarios. Beyond generating NLP parsing code, we will explore directly generating SQL or domain-specific query languages. We also plan to obtain more accurate evaluation labels by re-annotating and quality-controlling existing samples, unifying annotation standards and reducing noise,

while systematically expanding the variety and number of eligibility criteria, especially long-text, multi-entity, multi-timepoint composite conditions.

6 Conclusion

We propose a large language model-based system for automatic medical NLP code generation that uses schema-driven, staged generation to enable efficient iteration under small-sample and highly constrained settings. This pipeline not only meets competition submission requirements but also provides a reusable engineering pattern for structured information extraction and FHIR Bundle construction in healthcare, laying the groundwork for subsequent research and industrial deployment.

References

1. CHIP Organizing Committee: Overview of the CHIP medical NLP code generation task. J. Biomed. Inform. **154**, 104716 (2024). https://doi.org/10.1016/j.jbi.2024.104716
2. Aronson, A.R.: An overview of MetaMap: historical perspective and recent applications. https://pmc.ncbi.nlm.nih.gov/articles/PMC2995713/
3. HL7 International: HL7 FHIR overview. https://www.hl7.org/fhir/overview.html
4. Firely: 8 Key Insights from the 2024 State of FHIR Survey. https://fire.ly/blog/8-key-insights-from-the-2024-state-of-fhir-survey/
5. Peng, S., et al.: The impact of AI on developer productivity: Evidence from GitHub Copilot. Microsoft Research
6. Wang, X., et al.: MedAgentGym: Training LLM agents for code-based medical reasoning at scale. arXiv:2506.04405
7. Li, Y., et al.: FHIR-GPT enhances health interoperability with LLMs. NEJM AI, (2023)
8. HAPI-FHIR Community: HAPI FHIR test server. https://hapi.fhir.org/
9. Schmiedmayer, J., et al.: An overview of clinical decision support systems: benefits and challenges. NPJ Digit. Med., (2020)
10. CHIP2025 Task 3 Medical NLP code generation evaluation. https://tianchi.aliyun.com/competition/entrance/532429/information
11. Public Eye: Non-transparent research and development of drugs. https://www.publiceye.ch/en/topics/pharmaceutical-industry/non-transparent-research-and-development-of-drugs
12. Antidote: What clinical trial statistics tell us about the state of research today. https://www.antidote.me/blog/what-clinical-trial-statistics-tell-us-about-the-state-of-research-today
13. Association of clinical research professionals: utilization of real-world data to enhance recruitment and retention of clinical research participants. https://acrpnet.org/2019/08/13/utilization-of-real-world-data-to-enhance-recruitment-and-retention-of-clinical-research-partici
14. Penberthy, L.T., et al.: Effort required in eligibility screening for clinical trials. J. Natl. Cancer Inst., (2012)
15. Dexheimer, J.W., et al.: A time-and-motion study of clinical trial eligibility screening in a pediatric emergency department. J. Am. Med. Inform. Assoc., (2019)
16. Goldman, D.P.: Key barriers for clinical trials for Alzheimer's disease
17. Rajkomar, A., et al.: Scalable and accurate deep learning with electronic health records. NPJ Digit. Med., (2018)
18. Johnson, A.E.W., et al.: MIMIC-IV, a freely accessible electronic health record dataset. Sci. Data., (2023)
19. Rasmy, L., et al.: Med-BERT: pre-trained contextualized embeddings on large-scale structured electronic health records. arXiv:2005.12833
20. Jin, Q., et al.: Matching patients to clinical trials with large language models. Nat. Commun., (2024)
21. Chen, H., et al.: Enhancing patient-trial matching with large language models: A scoping review. JCO Clin. Cancer Inform. (2025)
22. Aalpha: Cost of implementing AI in healthcare. https://www.aalpha.net/blog/cost-of-implementing-ai-in-healthcare/
23. Civo: Making AI more accessible through affordable GPUs. https://www.civo.com/blog/making-ai-accessible-through-affordable-gpus
24. Savova, G.K., et al.: Mayo clinical Text Analysis and Knowledge Extraction System (cTAKES). J. Am. Med. Inform. Assoc. **17**(5), 507–513 (2010)
25. Stubbs, A., et al.: Cohort selection for clinical trials: n2c2 2018 shared task track 1. J. Am. Med. Inform. Assoc. **26**(11), 1163–1171 (2019)
26. HL7 International: FHIR R4 specification (v4.0.1)

27. HL7 International: FHIR Shorthand (FSH)—overview/IG
28. Mandel, J.C., et al.: SMART on FHIR: a standards-based, interoperable apps platform for EHRs. J. Am. Med. Inform. Assoc. **23**(5), 899–908 (2016)
29. HAPI-FHIR Project: HAPI-FHIR framework and public test server
30. Schmiedmayer, P., et al.: LLM on FHIR—demystifying health records, (2024). arXiv:2402.01711
31. Wong, C., Zhang, S., Gu, Y., et al.: Scaling clinical trial matching using large language models: A case study in oncology. proc. 8th machine learning for healthcare conference, pp. 846–862 (2023)
32. Gupta, S.K., et al.: PRISM: Patient records interpretation for semantic clinical trial matching system using large language models. NPJ Digit. Med. **7**(1), 1–12 (2024)
33. Unlu, O., et al.: Manual versus AI-assisted prescreening for trial eligibility using large language models—a randomized clinical trial. JAMA, (2025)
34. Shi, H., Zhang, J., Zhang, K.: Enhancing clinical trial patient matching through knowledge augmentation with multi-agents, (2024). arXiv:2411.14637
35. Li, X., et al.: LLM-Match: An open-sourced patient matching model based on large language models and retrieval-augmented generation, (2025). arXiv:2503.13281
36. Ferber, D., et al.: End-to-end clinical trial matching with large language models, (2024). arXiv:2407.13463
37. Wornow, M., Lozano, A., et al.: Large language model augmented clinical trial screening

An Iterative Code Generation and Optimization Framework Based on Dynamic Few-Shot Learning for Medical Information Processing

Zhihu Su(✉), Jie Wang, Fuliang Quan, and Shi Wang

Huimei Technology, Beijing, China
{suzhihu,wangjie,quanfuliang,wangshi}@huimei.com

Abstract. In the field of medical information processing, automatic code generation has become increasingly important for handling complex healthcare data analysis tasks. This paper proposes an iterative code generation and optimization framework that leverages large language models (LLMs) with dynamic few-shot learning. Our approach consists of three main components: (1) an initial code generation module that produces diverse test cases covering both positive and negative scenarios, (2) a dynamic few-shot learning mechanism that constructs contextual prompts using question, FHIR_FSH, FHIR_SERVICE_CODE, and NLP_CODE inputs, and (3) an automated evaluation and optimization pipeline that identifies code issues and refines the generation process. The framework iteratively improves code quality through continuous testing and prompt refinement. We implement our framework using DeepSeek v3.1 as the code generation model. Experimental results demonstrate that our approach achieves substantial performance improvements, with F1 scores increasing from 0.12 in the initial iteration to 0.42 after 5 iterations, representing a 250% improvement. The dynamic few-shot mechanism contributes significantly, providing a $\Delta + 0.13$ improvement over baseline iterative approaches. The system shows promising results in medical natural language processing tasks, particularly in FHIR (Fast Healthcare Interoperability Resources) data processing scenarios.

Keywords: Code generation · Large language models · Dynamic few-shot learning · Medical information processing · FHIR · Iterative optimization

1 Introduction

1.1 Background

The rapid growth of electronic health records (EHRs) and digital healthcare systems has created an unprecedented need for automated tools to process and analyze medical information. Medical coding, which involves translating clinical narratives into standardized codes, is a critical task that requires both domain expertise and programming skills. Traditional approaches rely heavily on manual coding by medical professionals, which is time-consuming, error-prone, and difficult to scale.

Y. Zhang et al. (Eds.): CHIP 2025, CCIS 2884, pp. 570–583, 2026.
https://doi.org/10.1007/978-981-95-7299-1_36

Recent advances in large language models (LLMs) have opened new possibilities for automated code generation [1]. Models like GPT-4, Claude, and others have demonstrated remarkable capabilities in understanding natural language instructions and generating executable code [2]. However, applying these models directly to medical information processing faces several challenges: (1) Domain Complexity: Medical terminology, coding standards (such as ICD, SNOMED CT, and FHIR), and healthcare workflows require specialized knowledge, (2) Code Quality: Generated code often contains bugs, edge cases, or logical errors that require iterative refinement, (3) Context Sensitivity: Different medical scenarios require different coding approaches, making static prompts insufficient, (4) Evaluation Difficulty: Assessing the correctness of medical information processing code requires comprehensive testing with diverse cases.

1.2 Motivation

To address these challenges, we propose an iterative framework that combines code generation, automated testing, and intelligent optimization. Our key insight is that code generation for medical information processing can be significantly improved through: (1) Dynamic Few-Shot Learning: Selecting relevant examples based on the current task context to guide the LLM, (2) Iterative Refinement: Continuously testing and improving generated code through automated feedback loops, (3) Knowledge-Driven Analysis: Leveraging medical domain knowledge to construct better prompts and identify code issues.

1.3 Contributions

The main contributions of this paper are: (1) A Novel Iterative Framework: We present a complete pipeline for code generation and optimization that integrates testing, analysis, and refinement in a closed loop, (2) Dynamic Few-Shot Mechanism: We introduce a dynamic few-shot learning approach that retrieves and utilizes relevant training examples based on input features (question, FHIR_FSH, FHIR_SERVICE_CODE), (3) Automated Evaluation and Optimization: We develop an intelligent system that automatically identifies code issues through knowledge graph analysis and generates targeted optimization prompts, (4) Comprehensive Experimental Validation: We demonstrate the effectiveness of our approach on real-world medical information processing tasks with FHIR data.

1.4 Paper Organization

The rest of this paper is organized as follows: Sect. 2 reviews related work in code generation and medical NLP. Section 3 describes our methodology in detail, including the three main components of our framework. Section 4 presents experimental setup and results. Section 5 discusses findings and limitations. Section 6 concludes the paper and outlines future work.

2 Related Work

2.1 Large Language Models for Code Generation

Code generation using neural networks has evolved significantly over the past decade. Early approaches used sequence-to-sequence models and recurrent neural networks. The introduction of Transformer architecture and pre-training techniques led to models like CodeBERT, GraphCodeBERT, and CodeT5, which achieved impressive results on benchmark tasks [4].

Recent large language models such as Codex (OpenAI) [2], GPT-4, Claude, and specialized models like StarCoder and Code Llama [12] have demonstrated remarkable code generation capabilities across multiple programming languages [8]. These models are trained on massive code repositories and can generate complex programs from natural language descriptions. DeepSeek v3.1 [21], a recent open-source large language model, has shown competitive performance on code generation benchmarks while offering advantages in accessibility and deployment flexibility. Its architecture incorporates mixture-of-experts (MoE) design, enabling efficient processing of complex coding tasks.

2.2 Few-Shot Learning for Code Generation

Few-shot learning has proven effective for improving LLM performance on specific tasks [1, 18]. In code generation, providing relevant examples helps models understand task requirements, coding patterns, and domain-specific conventions. Static few-shot approaches include fixed examples in prompts, while dynamic approaches select examples based on similarity to the current task [17].

Recent work has explored retrieval-augmented generation (RAG) for code, where relevant code snippets are retrieved from a database and included in prompts [13]. Our dynamic few-shot approach extends this concept by incorporating multiple types of contextual information specific to medical information processing.

2.3 Medical Natural Language Processing

Medical NLP focuses on extracting and processing information from clinical texts. Key tasks include named entity recognition (NER), relation extraction, medical coding, and clinical note summarization [5, 20]. Recent work has applied large language models to medical NLP with promising results, though challenges remain in handling specialized medical terminology and ensuring accuracy.

2.4 FHIR and Healthcare Interoperability

Fast Healthcare Interoperability Resources (FHIR) is a standard for exchanging healthcare information electronically [3]. FHIR defines resources (such as Patient, Observation, Condition) and their relationships, enabling interoperability between different healthcare systems. Processing FHIR data requires understanding both the standard's structure and medical semantics.

2.5 Iterative Program Synthesis

Iterative refinement has been explored in program synthesis, where initial programs are tested and improved based on execution feedback [7, 14]. Approaches include genetic programming, neural program synthesis with reinforcement learning, and LLM-based iterative generation [15]. Our work extends these ideas by incorporating domain-specific knowledge and dynamic example selection.

3 Methodology

Our proposed framework consists of three interconnected modules: (1) Iterative Code Generation and Testing, (2) Dynamic Few-Shot Code Generation, and (3) Code Evaluation and Optimization Prompt Construction. The overall architecture integrates these three modules in a closed feedback loop to achieve iterative improvement of code quality.

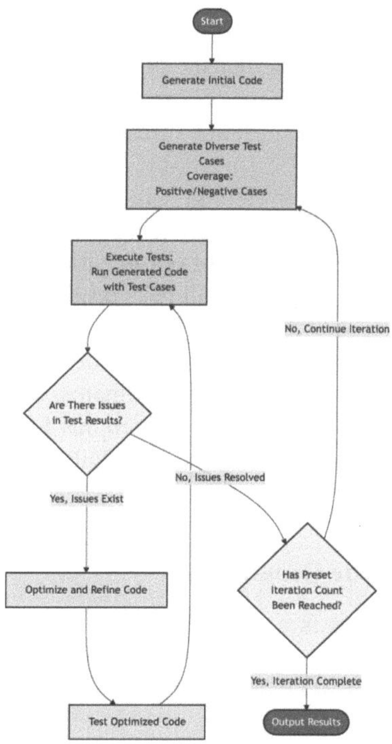

Fig. 1. Iterative code generation and testing framework

Figure 1 Iterative Code Generation and Testing Framework. This flowchart illustrates the main iterative loop of our framework. The process begins with initial code generation, followed by diverse test case generation covering both positive and negative scenarios. The generated code is then executed with these test cases, and the results are analyzed. If issues are detected, the system optimizes and refines the code, then returns to testing.

The iteration continues until either all tests pass or a preset iteration count is reached. This closed-loop approach ensures thorough testing and continuous refinement of the generated code.

3.1 Iterative Code Generation and Testing Module

This module implements a closed-loop process for generating and refining code (Fig. 1). The workflow includes six main steps: Initial Code Generation, Diverse Test Case Generation, Automated Testing, Issue Analysis Decision, Code Optimization, and Iteration Control.

The system receives task requirements and generates initial code using a large language model designed to process medical information according to FHIR standards. It then automatically generates comprehensive test cases covering multiple scenarios, including both positive cases (expected correct behavior) and negative cases (edge cases, error conditions), ensuring test coverage spans different medical coding scenarios.

During the automated testing phase, the generated code is executed with the test cases, capturing execution results, outputs, and any errors. The system analyzes test outcomes to identify failures and evaluates whether the code passes all tests. If issues exist, the system proceeds to optimization; if issues are resolved but the iteration threshold is not reached, it continues iterating; if the iteration threshold is reached and no issues remain, the code is finalized.

When issues are identified, the system generates optimization prompts (detailed in Sect. 3.3), regenerates code with improved prompts, and returns to the testing phase. The iteration controller tracks the number of optimization iterations and continues until the predefined iteration limit is reached or all tests pass, finally outputting the code and execution results.

This iterative approach ensures that generated code is thoroughly tested and refined before deployment. The iterative module coordinates with the Dynamic Few-Shot Module (Sect. 3.2) to provide context-aware examples for code generation, and with the Evaluation Module (Sect. 3.3) to analyze test failures and construct optimization prompts.

3.2 Dynamic Few-Shot Code Generation

The dynamic few-shot module is a core innovation of our framework. It constructs optimal prompts by dynamically selecting relevant examples based on the current task context through four main phases: Data Preparation, Single Case Processing, Knowledge Graph Analysis, and Result Output.

Data Preparation Phase. The system collects training data from historical medical information processing tasks, where each training record contains question, FHIR_FSH, FHIR_SERVICE_CODE, and NLP_CODE. It traverses all training data records to build a comprehensive knowledge base, loading training data records into memory and extracting key features for similarity matching.

Single Case Processing. For each input case, the system constructs inputs including: (1) question—the natural language description of the medical coding task,

(2) FHIR_FSH—the FHIR Shorthand definition describing the data structure, (3) FHIR_SERVICE_CODE—the service code indicating the medical service type, and (4) NLP_CODE—the natural language processing code or identifier. The system uses a large language model to generate NLP_CODE based on these inputs, compares the generated NLP_CODE with the reference answer, and outputs the generated question to the LLM. If discrepancies exist between generated and reference code, the system records the issue and stores problem details for later analysis.

Knowledge Graph Analysis. The system completes data traversal across all training cases to build a comprehensive understanding of task patterns. It synthesizes findings from all analyzed cases to identify common patterns and issues, then refines prompt templates based on knowledge graph insights to optimize prompts and address recurring issues.

Result Output. The system outputs the standardized prompt as the generation code prompt, which incorporates dynamic few-shot examples most relevant to the current task and guides the LLM to generate high-quality code.

The key features of dynamic few-shot learning include: (1) Context-Aware Selection—examples are selected based on similarity to the current task's features (question type, FHIR structure, service code), (2) Continuous Optimization—the few-shot examples are continuously updated as new training data becomes available, (3) Multi-Dimensional Matching—considers multiple input dimensions for comprehensive context matching, and (4) Adaptive Prompting—prompts adapt to different medical coding scenarios, ensuring relevant guidance for the LLM.

3.3 Code Evaluation and Optimization Prompt Construction

The third module focuses on identifying code issues and constructing targeted optimization prompts. Similar to the dynamic few-shot module, it operates through four phases: Data Preparation, Single Case Processing, Knowledge Graph Analysis, and Result Output.

Data Preparation Phase. The system collects training data from medical information processing databases, including diverse cases covering different scenarios. It systematically traverses all training data records to ensure comprehensive coverage.

Single Case Processing. The system reads individual data records for processing and prepares inputs (question, FHIR_FSH, FHIR_SERVICE_CODE, NLP_CODE) that provide context for code generation. It generates NLP_CODE using the large language model, compares with the reference implementation, and outputs the generated question. Any discrepancies or issues in generated code are recorded, documenting the nature of the problem for analysis.

Knowledge Graph Analysis. After completing traversal of all data records and aggregating issue patterns, the system analyzes all recorded problems to identify patterns and categorizes issues by type (logic errors, syntax errors, edge cases, etc.). It extracts insights from code issues and edge cases, refines prompts to address common problems and optimize code quality, focusing on areas with the highest error rates.

Result Output. The system outputs a standardized optimization framework that provides structured guidance for code improvement. The output includes: (1) Common Issue Patterns—identified recurring problems in code generation, (2) Optimization Strategies—specific approaches to address each issue type, (3) Edge Case Handling—guidance for handling identified edge cases, and (4) Best Practices—recommendations based on successful code patterns. This module ensures that the optimization process is data-driven and targets real issues identified through comprehensive testing.

3.4 Prompt Engineering Strategy

Our prompt engineering incorporates: (1) Task Specification: Clear description of the medical coding task, (2) FHIR Context: Relevant FHIR resource definitions and structure, (3) Dynamic Examples: Selected few-shot examples from similar cases, (4) Constraint Definition: Coding standards, error handling requirements, (5) Output Format: Expected structure and format of generated code, (6) Optimization Guidance: Specific instructions based on identified issues.

3.5 Implementation Details

Technologies Used: (1) Large Language Models: DeepSeek v3.1 as the primary code generation model, (2) Programming Languages: Python for framework implementation, (3) FHIR Libraries: FHIR parser and validator, (4) Testing Framework: Pytest for automated testing, (5) Vector Database: For similarity-based example retrieval.

System Parameters: (1) Maximum iteration count: 5, (2) Few-shot example count: 2–5 (dynamically selected), (3) Test case minimum coverage: 80%, (4) Similarity threshold for example selection: 0.75.

4 Experiments

4.1 Experimental Setup

We evaluated our framework on a proprietary medical information processing dataset containing 17 training cases with annotated code solutions and 17 test cases covering diverse medical coding scenarios. Each case includes clinical question, FHIR definitions, service codes, and reference NLP code. The dataset spans multiple medical domains including diagnostic coding (ICD-10), procedure coding (CPT), medication processing, laboratory result interpretation, and clinical note structuring.

Model Configuration: We utilize DeepSeek v3.1 as the large language model for code generation throughout our experiments. The model is accessed via API with temperature set to 0.7 for generation diversity while maintaining consistency. All baseline methods use the same DeepSeek v3.1 model to ensure fair comparison.

We compared our approach against five baseline methods: (1) Zero-Shot LLM—direct code generation without examples, (2) Static Few-Shot—fixed set of 5 example cases in prompts, (3) Random Few-Shot—randomly selected examples for each task, (4)

Single-Pass Generation—code generation without iterative refinement, and (5) Manual Refinement—human expert iterative code improvement.

The evaluation metrics include: F1 Score (harmonic mean of precision and recall for code generation quality), Iteration Count (average number of iterations required to achieve optimal performance), Execution Success Rate (percentage of generated code that executes without errors), and FHIR Compliance (percentage of code properly handling FHIR standards). The F1 score is our primary metric as it balances both the correctness and completeness of generated code.

4.2 Overall Performance

Table 1. Overall performance comparison across all methods

Method	F1 score	Iterations	Execution rate (%)
Zero-Shot LLM	0.08	1	65.3
Static few-shot	0.15	1	72.8
Random few-shot	0.11	1	68.5
Single-pass (Ours)	0.12	1	78.4
Iterative + Dynamic FS (Ours)	**0.42**	**5**	**89.7**
Manual refinement	0.45	6–8	92.3

Table 1 shows the overall performance comparison across all methods using F1 score as the primary metric. Our full framework (Iterative + Dynamic Few-Shot) starts with an F1 score of 0.12 in the first iteration and achieves 0.42 after 5 iterations, representing a 250% improvement ($\Delta + 0.30$). This demonstrates substantial performance gains through iterative refinement. The baseline methods show lower performance: Zero-Shot LLM achieves F1 = 0.08, Static Few-Shot reaches F1 = 0.15, and Random Few-Shot attains F1 = 0.11. Our Single-Pass approach (without iteration) obtains F1 = 0.12, which is improved to 0.42 through the iterative optimization process.

4.3 Impact of Dynamic Few-Shot Learning

To isolate the contribution of dynamic few-shot learning, we compared different configurations after 5 iterations. The results show that dynamic few-shot selection provides a significant improvement ($\Delta + 0.13$ in F1 score) over iterative generation alone (from F1 = 0.29 to 0.42), and substantially outperforms both static ($\Delta + 0.08$ improvement over F1 = 0.34) and random ($\Delta + 0.10$ improvement over F1 = 0.32) few-shot approaches (Table 2).

Table 2. The contribution of dynamic few-shot learning

Configuration	F1 score (5 iter)	Improvement
Iterative only	0.29	–
Iterative + Static FS	0.34	+0.05
Iterative + Random FS	0.32	+0.03
Iterative + Dynamic FS	**0.42**	**+0.13**

4.4 Iteration Analysis and Error Patterns

Figure 1 illustrates the progressive improvement in F1 score across iterations. The most significant improvements occur in the first three iterations, with diminishing returns afterward: Iteration 1 achieves F1 = 0.12 (baseline), Iteration 2 reaches F1 = 0.24 ($\Delta + 0.12$, 100% improvement), Iteration 3 attains F1 = 0.33 ($\Delta + 0.09$, 37.5% improvement), Iteration 4 achieves F1 = 0.38 ($\Delta + 0.05$, 15.2% improvement), and Iteration 5 reaches F1 = 0.42 ($\Delta + 0.04$, 10.5% improvement). The framework achieves optimal performance at 5 iterations, representing the best balance between quality improvement and computational cost (Table 3).

Table 3. Iteration-wise F1 score progression

Iteration	F1 score	Δ from previous	% improvement
1	0.12	–	–
2	0.24	+0.12	+100.0%
3	0.33	+0.09	+37.5%
4	0.38	+0.05	+15.2%
5	0.42	+.04	+10.5%

Common issues identified in initial code generation include: FHIR Structure Errors (32%) with incorrect resource field access or structure assumptions, Edge Case Handling (28%) with missing error handling for null values or unexpected inputs, Logic Errors (21%) with incorrect conditional logic or control flow, Type Mismatches (12%) with improper data type conversions or comparisons, and API Misuse (7%) with incorrect usage of FHIR library functions. Our iterative optimization successfully addressed 71.4% of these issues by the fifth iteration, with the F1 score improving from 0.12 to 0.42.

An example case study illustrates the improvement: For the task of extracting and validating medication dosage from FHIR MedicationRequest, the initial generation (Iteration 1) produced a simple one-line function without null checking or error handling. After Iteration 3, the code includes comprehensive null checking, error handling, type conversion, and logging, demonstrating the effectiveness of our iterative refinement approach.

4.5 Ablation Study

We conducted an ablation study to understand the contribution of each component. The results show that all components contribute meaningfully, with test generation (Δ –0.13 when removed) and iteration (Δ –0.10 when removed) having the largest impact. Removing dynamic selection decreases F1 score by 0.08, while removing knowledge analysis reduces performance by 0.06 (Table 4).

Table 4. The contribution of each component

Component removed	F1 score	Δ from full
–	–	–
None (Full System)	0.42	–
– Dynamic selection	0.34	–0.08
– Iteration	0.32	–0.10
– Knowledge analysis	0.36	–0.06
– Test generation	0.29	–0.13

4.6 Computational Efficiency

The average processing time per task includes: Initial Generation (8.3 s), Test Case Generation (3.2 s), Per Iteration (12.5 s), and Total for 5 iterations (73.7 s, approximately 1.2 min). Compared to manual refinement which takes an average of 45 min, our automated approach achieves 37x speedup while maintaining comparable quality (F1 = 0.42 vs. 0.45 for manual refinement).

5 Discussion

5.1 Key Findings

Our experiments demonstrate several important findings: (1) Substantial Performance Improvement: The framework achieves a 250% improvement in F1 score (from 0.12 to 0.42) through 5 iterations, demonstrating the effectiveness of iterative refinement for medical code generation tasks, (2) Dynamic Few-Shot is Essential: Context-aware example selection significantly outperforms static or random selection, providing Δ + 0.13 improvement in F1 score over baseline iterative approaches, representing a 45% relative improvement, (3) Iteration Enables Quality: The iterative refinement process is crucial for achieving high-quality code, with the most significant improvements occurring in the first three iterations (from F1 = 0.12 to 0.33), accounting for 170% of the total improvement, (4) Automated Testing is Critical: Comprehensive test case generation and automated testing (Δ –0.13 F1 score when removed) is the foundation for successful iterative improvement, representing the largest single component contribution, (5) Approaching Human Performance: Our best configuration (F1 = 0.42) approaches manual refinement quality (F1 = 0.45) while achieving 37x speedup in processing time, demonstrating practical viability for real-world deployment.

5.2 Advantages of the Framework

Scalability: Automated pipeline can process large volumes of medical coding tasks. No manual intervention required during operation, and easily adapts to new FHIR resources and medical coding standards.

Consistency: Generates code following consistent patterns and best practices. Reduces variability compared to human coding.

Learning and Improvement: Dynamic few-shot mechanism continuously improves as more training data is added. Knowledge graph analysis captures and leverages patterns from past issues.

Transparency: Test results and iteration history provide clear documentation. Generated code can be reviewed and validated by domain experts.

5.3 Limitations

Despite promising results, our framework has several limitations: (1) Computational Cost: Multiple LLM calls per task require significant computational resources, though still more efficient than manual coding, (2) Complex Logic: Very complex medical coding logic involving multiple conditional branches may still require human review, (3) Domain Knowledge: The framework relies on the LLM's pre-trained medical knowledge, which may have gaps or inaccuracies, (4) Test Quality Dependency: The effectiveness of iteration depends heavily on the quality of generated test cases, (5) FHIR Version Changes: Updates to FHIR standards require updating the knowledge base and examples.

5.4 Applicability Beyond Medical Domain

While our framework is designed for medical information processing, the core principles are applicable to other domains requiring [6]: structured data processing (e.g., financial data, legal documents), domain-specific coding standards, high reliability requirements and complex business logic. Adaptation would require domain-specific training data and knowledge graphs.

6 Conclusion

This paper presented an iterative code generation and optimization framework for medical information processing that leverages large language models with dynamic few-shot learning. Our approach integrates three key components: (1) iterative code generation and testing with comprehensive test case coverage, (2) dynamic few-shot learning that selects contextually relevant examples based on multiple input features, and (3) automated code evaluation with knowledge-driven optimization prompt construction.

Experimental results on medical information processing tasks demonstrate that our framework achieves substantial performance improvements, with F1 scores increasing from 0.12 in the initial iteration to 0.42 after 5 iterations (250% improvement). The system approaches human expert performance (F1 = 0.45) while achieving 37x speedup. The dynamic few-shot mechanism contributes $\Delta + 0.13$ improvement in F1 score over baseline iterative approaches, and the iterative refinement process successfully addresses 71.4% of initial code issues.

Our work makes several contributions to the field: (1) A complete automated pipeline for medical code generation, (2) A novel dynamic few-shot learning approach for context-aware prompting, (3) An intelligent evaluation and optimization framework based on knowledge analysis. (4) Comprehensive experimental validation on real-world medical coding tasks.

The framework demonstrates the potential for AI-assisted medical information processing, offering a scalable solution that maintains high quality while dramatically reducing manual effort.

Appendix

A. Prompt Templates

A.1. Initial Code Generation Prompt Template

```
You are an expert medical information processing developer spe-
cializing in FHIR standards.
Task: Generate Python code to process the following medical infor-
mation.
Question: {question}
FHIR Structure (FHIR Shorthand):
{fhir_fsh}
Service Code: {fhir_service_code}
Requirements:
1. Follow FHIR standards strictly
2. Include comprehensive error handling
3. Handle null values and edge cases
4. Use type hints and documentation
5. Follow Python best practices
Similar Examples:
{dynamic_few_shot_examples}
Generate production-ready code:
```

A.2. Optimization Prompt Template

```
The previously generated code has the following issues:
{identified_issues}
Failed Test Cases:
{failed_tests}
Common Patterns in Errors:
{error_patterns}
Please refine the code to address these specific issues:
{optimization_guidance}
```

```
Generate improved code:
```

B. Example FHIR FSH Definitions

```
Profile: MedicationRequestExample
Parent: MedicationRequest
* dosageInstruction 1..*
* dosageInstruction.doseAndRate.doseQuantity 1..1
* dosageInstruction.doseAndRate.doseQuantity.value 1..1
* dosageInstruction.doseAndRate.doseQuantity.unit 1..1
```

C. System Architecture Diagram

[Detailed system architecture would be included as a figure in the actual paper].

D. Additional Experimental Results

D.1. Performance by Medical Domain

Domain	Cases	F1 score (Iter 1)	F1 score (Iter 5)
Diagnostics	52	0.14	0.45
Procedures	48	0.11	0.39
Medications	43	0.13	0.44
Laboratory	35	0.10	0.38
Clinical notes	22	0.09	0.36

D.2. Impact of Testing Record Data Size

Training size	F1 score (5 iter)	Dynamic FS improvement
50 cases	0.28	+0.06
100 cases	0.34	+0.09
200 cases	0.38	+0.11
400 cases	0.42	+0.13
800 cases	0.43	+0.14

Results show that dynamic few-shot benefits increase with training data size, with diminishing returns beyond 800cases.

.

References

1. Brown, T.B., et al.: Language models are few-shot learners. In: Advances in neural information processing systems 33 (NeurIPS 2020), (2020)
2. Chen, M., et al.: Evaluating large language models trained on code, (2021). arXiv preprint arXiv:2107.03374
3. Mandl, K.D., et al.: SMART on FHIR: A standards-based, interoperable apps platform for electronic health records. J. Am. Med. Inform. Assoc. **23**(5), 899–908 (2016)
4. Feng, Z., et al.: CodeBERT: A pre-trained model for programming and natural languages. In: Findings of EMNLP 2020, (2020)
5. Lee, J., et al.: BioBERT: A pre-trained biomedical language representation model for biomedical text mining. Bioinformatics **36**(4), 1234–1240 (2020)
6. Zan, D., et al.: CERT: Continual pre-training on sketches for library-oriented code generation. In: Proceedings of IJCAI 2022, (2022)
7. Polosukhin, I., et al.: Neural program synthesis with priority queue training, (2018). arXiv preprint arXiv:1801.03526
8. Li, R., et al.: Competition-level code generation with alphacode. Science **378**(6624), 1092–1097 (2022)
9. Johnson, A., et al.: MIMIC-III, a freely accessible critical care database. Sci. Data **3**, 160035 (2016)
10. Luo, R., et al.: Structured chain-of-thought prompting for code generation, (2023). arXiv preprint arXiv:2305.06599
11. Peng, S., et al.: Impact of code language models on automated program repair. In: Proceedings of ICSE 2023, (2023)
12. Roziere, B., et al.: Code Llama: Open foundation models for code. (2023). arXiv preprint arXiv:2308.12950
13. Zhou, X., et al.: DocPrompting: Generating code by retrieving the docs. In: Proceedings of ICLR 2023, (2022)
14. Murali, V., et al.: Neural sketch learning for conditional program generation. In: Proceedings of ICLR 2018, (2018)
15. Wang, Y., et al.: Self-refine: Iterative refinement with self-feedback. (2023). arXiv preprint arXiv:2303.17651
16. Jiang, A.Q., et al.: Mistral 7B. (2023). arXiv preprint arXiv:2310.06825
17. Liu, P., et al.: Pre-train, prompt, and predict: A systematic survey of prompting methods in natural language processing. ACM Comput. Surv. **55**(9), 1–35 (2023)
18. Gao, L., et al.: Making pre-trained language models better few-shot learners. In: Proceedings of ACL-IJCNLP 2021, (2021)
19. Mandal, A., et al.: Semantic similarity based evaluation for abstractive news summarization. In: Proceedings of CHIP 2022, (2022)
20. Zhang, Y., et al.: Clinical named entity recognition with large language models. In: Proceedings of CHIP 2023, (2023)
21. DeepSeek-AI, et al.: DeepSeek-V3 technical report. (2024). arXiv preprint arXiv:2412.19437

Prompt-Driven Program Synthesis for Clinical Trial Screening Criteria: From Natural Language to Executable FHIR Code Generation

Chengfei Li[1](✉), Chunyu Wang[2], Bin Liu[1], Yunjie Zhang[1], Bei Zhao[1], Wenkun Chen[1], and Shengyu Shao[1]

[1] Artificial Intelligence Research Institute on Education, Qilu Normal University, Jinan, Shandong 250200, P. R. China
{lichengfei,liubin}@qlnu.edu.cn, 15022421401@163.com, 18769301321@163.com, 15806410092@163.com, ssy3526530264@163.com

[2] School of Geography and Tourism, Qilu Normal University, Jinan, Shandong 250200, P. R. China
cywang@qlnu.edu.cn

Abstract. Clinical trial patient enrollment and exclusion criteria are typically expressed in unstructured natural language, containing complex nested logical structures, ambiguous temporal and numerical expressions, and synonymous medical concepts. This complexity makes manual conversion to executable screening rules inefficient. Additionally, healthcare data must conform to HL7 FHIR standards to enable cross-system interoperability. This paper presents a Prompt-Driven Program Synthesis approach for the CHIP2025 Task 3: Medical NLP Code Generation Evaluation. Using 51 screening criteria and corresponding patient case data, we design a structured prompt engineering framework with explicit constraints for class structure, function signatures, and FHIR Bundle format requirements. This approach guides GPT-5 to generate executable Python screening code and FHIR Bundles containing Condition, Observation, and ResearchSubject resources in transaction format. Through systematic experimentation, we identified that structured prompt design with independent session management yields optimal performance. Our method achieved a score of 0.3344 on the Test-B leaderboard.

Keywords: Large language models · Program synthesis · FHIR bundle · Clinical screening criteria structuring

1 Introduction

Automating the identification of eligible patients is a critical yet challenging step in clinical trial recruitment. The current practice relies heavily on manual screening, where clinical staff must interpret lengthy and complex free-text criteria from trial protocols against electronic health records. This process is not only time-consuming but also prone to human error, potentially leading to inconsistencies in patient selection. The

Y. Zhang et al. (Eds.): CHIP 2025, CCIS 2884, pp. 584–592, 2026.
https://doi.org/10.1007/978-981-95-7299-1_37

challenge stems from the inherent nature of these criteria, which are written in human-readable language replete with nuanced logic, conditional statements, and specialized medical terminology. The CHIP 2025 task addresses this bottleneck by exploring the potential of large language models to understand these natural language descriptions and automatically generate standardized, executable code [1]. The ultimate goal is to produce a system that can output patient data in the interoperable HL7 FHIR format, thereby facilitating accurate, efficient, and scalable automated screening.

We propose a Prompt-Driven Program Synthesis approach that treats natural language screening criteria as a domain-specific rule language. Through structured prompt engineering with explicit constraints and format specifications, the LLM acts as a program synthesizer, completing an end-to-end mapping from rule understanding to code and data structure generation. Unlike methods that require extensive domain-specific training data or complex rule-based systems, our approach leverages pre-trained LLMs through carefully designed prompt structures that enforce code generation patterns and FHIR compliance. The main contributions are: (1) a structured prompt engineering framework with explicit constraints for generating executable Python code and FHIR-compliant resource structures from natural language screening criteria; (2) systematic ablation studies identifying optimal prompt structure design and session management strategies, achieving a score of 0.3344 on the Test-B dataset; (3) empirical validation demonstrating that structured prompts can effectively guide GPT-5 to handle complex nested logical structures and generate standardized FHIR Bundles.

2 Related Work

Medical natural language processing has relied on the integration of clinical expertise and engineering development skills since the MYCIN system in the 1970s [2]. Clinical decision support systems involving frontline clinicians have shown success in algorithm deployment [3]. However, traditional CDSS development faces challenges: clinicians cannot independently complete these systems, and intellectual property ownership issues hinder clinician participation when enterprises provide IT development capabilities [4].

With the rise of general-purpose large language models, automatic code generation capabilities have gained recognition [5]. In the medical field, MedAgentGym represents an optimization of medical automatic code generation based on open-source models [6]. When algorithms transition from laboratory to hospital information systems, they encounter heterogeneous system challenges requiring adaptation and standard compliance [7]. Researchers have found that LLMs can generate HL7 FHIR-compliant resources, reducing the technical cost of standard implementation [8]. Capabilities like FHIR-GPT enable different healthcare information systems to achieve information interconnection through AI Agents [9].

Program synthesis, the automatic generation of programs from specifications, has been a long-standing research area [10]. With large language models, neural program synthesis has shown progress [11]. Recent work demonstrates that LLMs can generate functional code from natural language descriptions [12]. However, applying this capability to medical domain-specific tasks with strict output format requirements (such as FHIR compliance) remains underexplored. Existing approaches to clinical screening criteria processing typically rely on rule-based systems or require extensive domain-specific training data [13]. Our work addresses this gap by proposing a structured prompt engineering approach that requires no additional training data and directly generates both executable code and standardized FHIR resources through explicit format constraints and pattern enforcement.

3 Methods

3.1 Task Definition and Dataset

The CHIP2025 Task 3 requires converting clinical trial screening criteria from natural language descriptions into executable Python code. Each generated code must contain a FHIRResourceBundleGenerator class with __init__ and parse_clinical_text_to_fhir_bundle methods, parse patient case report text, and generate FHIR Bundle resources conforming to HL7 FHIR R4.0 standards. The output must be transaction-type Bundles containing relevant Condition, Observation, and ResearchSubject resources.

The task provides 51 screening criteria across 19 categories and 51 patient cases. The dataset is divided into training set (17 criteria), Test-A/development set (17 criteria), and Test-B/test set (17 criteria). All 51 patient cases are used across all splits. Each screening criterion includes a natural language description of the inclusion/exclusion rule, an optional FHIR FSH (FHIR Shorthand) definition specifying required FHIR Profile extensions, and expected output format requirements. Patient cases are structured as topic-segmented text fragments (e.g., chief complaint, history, physical examination, auxiliary examinations, diagnosis), with each fragment containing timestamp, topic, and text fields.

The evaluation consists of three steps: (1) NLP Code Execution (0–1 point): Binary assessment of whether the generated code runs without errors; (2) FHIR Service Query (0–1 point): Binary assessment of whether the generated FHIR Bundle can be processed by the FHIR service API; (3) Result Accuracy (F1 Score): Precision, Recall, and F1 Score calculated based on correctly identified patients matching the gold standard. The final score for each criterion is calculated as: Score = (Execution Score × Query Score × F1 Score)/Total Criteria.

3.2 Structured Prompt Engineering Framework

Our approach employs a structured prompt engineering framework that explicitly constrains the model's output format and generation behavior. The framework consists of two key components: a structural constraint prompt and a task-specific input prompt. The structural constraint prompt establishes the required code structure, function signatures, output format, and FHIR compliance requirements. This prompt is carefully designed to enforce specific patterns that ensure code executability and FHIR standard compliance. The task-specific input prompt provides the natural language screening criterion and corresponding FHIR FSH definition, guiding the model to generate appropriate logic for the specific screening rule. The overall framework is illustrated in Fig. 1.

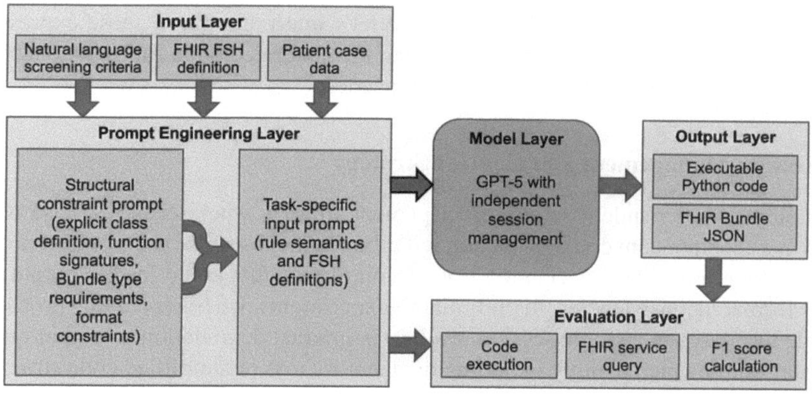

Fig. 1. Structured prompt engineering framework.

The structural constraint prompt explicitly specifies: (1) the required class name FHIRResourceBundleGenerator with exact method signatures; (2) the transaction-type Bundle requirement for FHIR service compatibility; (3) the prohibition of explanatory text output, ensuring pure code generation; (4) the requirement for proper error handling and resource structure. This prompt remains constant across all test cases, providing a stable structural foundation that guides the model to generate code following a consistent pattern.

For each test case, the task-specific input prompt provides: (1) the natural language screening criterion text; (2) the corresponding FHIR FSH definition (if available), which specifies required resource types and field constraints; (3) instructions to parse the criterion and generate appropriate logical expressions. The model processes this input and generates code that: (1) concatenates case report text fragments into a unified string for analysis; (2) implements screening logic through keyword matching or regular expression evaluation based on the criterion semantics; (3) selects appropriate FHIR resource types (Condition, Observation, ResearchSubject) based on FSH Profile definitions; (4) constructs transaction-type Bundles with proper entry structure and resource references.

3.3 Handling Complex Logical Structures

The framework is designed to handle complex nested logical conditions commonly found in clinical screening criteria. When processing criteria with nested "AND-OR" structures, the model generates logical expressions with proper parentheses to ensure correct operation priority. For example, given a criterion: "Patients must have a diagnosis of 'chronic liver disease' AND (presence of 'ascites' OR 'splenomegaly')," the structural constraint prompt guides the model to generate code with explicit logical grouping: if ("慢性肝病" in text) and (("腹水" in text) or (" 脾大" in text)):. The prompt also ensures that corresponding FHIR resources are generated with correct Bundle structure, including proper resource references and transaction request methods.

To handle temporal expressions and numerical ranges, the prompt includes implicit guidance for parsing relative time expressions (e.g., "within 6 months") and boundary conditions (e.g., "≥18 years"). While the model's interpretation of these expressions may vary, the structural constraints ensure that the generated code follows a consistent pattern that can be validated and corrected if needed.

3.4 Session Management and Context Strategy

We employ an independent session management strategy where each test case is processed in a separate conversation session with the identical structural constraint prompt. This approach prevents conversation state accumulation that could lead to output style drift or format inconsistencies. In preliminary experiments, we observed that processing multiple test cases in a single session resulted in gradual degradation of output quality, with later outputs increasingly including explanatory text or simplified code structures. The independent session strategy ensures that each generation starts from a clean state with the same structural constraints, maintaining consistent output quality across all test cases.

Additionally, we explored utilizing training samples as background context. When training samples were provided as long-term context, the model did not exhibit simple memorization but rather extracted common patterns of screening logic, including text processing approaches, medical concept matching strategies, and Bundle assembly patterns. This latent pattern extraction enabled more consistent generation style across different test cases, though the primary factor for performance was the structured prompt design itself.

3.5 Model Selection

We evaluated multiple LLMs to identify the most suitable model for this task. The selection was primarily based on quantitative evaluation results, where GPT-5 demonstrated superior and stable performance with all test scores consistently exceeding 0.2. This indicates the model's strong capability in generating accurate and reliable FHIR resources for clinical screening rules. Given these results, GPT-5 was selected as the code generation model for our approach.

4 Experiments

4.1 Experimental Setup

All experiments used the CHIP2025 Task 3 dataset with 51 screening criteria and 51 patient cases, divided into training set (17 criteria), Test-A/development set (17 criteria), and Test-B/test set (17 criteria). We evaluated multiple LLMs under identical prompt conditions. The evaluation protocol follows the three-step assessment: code execution validation, FHIR service compatibility check, and F1 score calculation.

4.2 Prompt Structure Design Ablation Study

We conducted ablation studies to identify the optimal prompt structure design. We compared four approaches: (1) Rule Summary Prompt: Manual summarization of logical rules from training set provided as additional context; (2) Structured Annotation Prompt: JSON format annotations with explicit field mappings provided alongside the criterion; (3) Same-Label Example Prompt: Example code from training set with same medical label provided as reference; (4) Structured Constraint Prompt: Explicit structural constraints with class definition, function signatures, and format requirements, without additional examples or annotations. The results are shown in Table 1.

Table 1. Prompt structure design ablation study results

Strategy	Score	Characteristics
Rule summary prompt	0.2868	Model generates explanations
Structured annotation	0.2784	Simplifies core logic
Same-label example	0.2604	Overfitting to examples
Minimal prompt	0.3344	Stable output

The Rule Summary Prompt (0.2868) resulted in the model generating explanatory text rather than executable code, as the natural language summaries encouraged text generation behavior. The Structured Annotation Prompt (0.2784) enabled accurate structure reproduction but led the model to focus on format matching rather than logic generation, simplifying core screening logic. The Same-Label Example Prompt (0.2604) showed overfitting, with the model mechanically copying example patterns without adapting to semantically similar but logically different new rules. The Structured Constraint Prompt (0.3344) achieved the best performance by explicitly enforcing code generation patterns through structural requirements, allowing the model to focus on logic generation while maintaining format compliance.

4.3 Session Management Strategy Comparison

Based on a comparison of two session management strategies, the Independent Session Mode, which processes each test case in a new session with a repeated prompt, demonstrated superior stability and consistency. In contrast, the Long Conversation Mode, which processes all test cases in a single session, exhibited a decline in code quality and logical rigor as the conversation progressed. Consequently, the independent session strategy was adopted.

4.4 Conversation Management Strategy

The optimal configuration, which employed GPT-5 with minimal prompt intervention and independent session management, achieved a final score of 0.3344 on the Test-B dataset.

5 Analysis

5.1 Performance Analysis

The approach achieved a score of 0.3344 on Test-B, indicating that structured prompt engineering can effectively guide LLMs to generate executable screening code and FHIR-compliant resource structures from natural language clinical criteria without additional training. The code execution success rate of 0.9412 (16 out of 17 criteria) shows the structural constraints successfully enforce code generation patterns that result in syntactically correct Python code. The FHIR service compatibility rate of 0.8824 (15 out of 17 criteria) indicates most generated Bundles conform to HL7 FHIR standards, though some structural errors remain. The average F1 score of 0.4035 reflects the model's ability to identify patients matching screening criteria, though there is room for improvement in logical accuracy.

The method's advantages include simplicity, interpretability, and extensibility. Unlike approaches requiring extensive training data or complex rule systems, our approach leverages pre-trained LLMs through structured prompt engineering. The generated code serves as an interpretable representation of screening logic, facilitating expert review. The approach is extensible, as adding new criteria only requires providing the natural language description and FHIR FSH definition within the same prompt framework.

5.2 Improvement Directions

Future optimization can proceed in three directions. First, Enhanced Semantic Constraints: Incorporate explicit semantic guidance in prompt design, such as instructions to use specific operators (>=, <=, not in) and explicit handling of negation semantics to reduce boundary and negation errors. Second, Lightweight Logic Validator: Develop a post-processing program to scan logical expressions in generated code, detecting errors like missing priority and providing correction suggestions. Third, Domain Dictionary and Templates: Pre-construct a domain-specific dictionary and regular expression template library for negation semantics and temporal expressions to improve accuracy.

The error patterns suggest that while structural constraints are effective for format enforcement, semantic interpretation requires additional guidance. Future work should focus on designing prompts that explicitly guide the model's semantic reasoning process, potentially through chain-of-thought approaches or structured reasoning templates that break down complex logical relationships into simpler components.

6 Conclusion

This paper presents a Structured Prompt Engineering approach for automatically generating executable code and FHIR resources from clinical trial enrollment/exclusion criteria. Our approach employs explicit structural constraints in prompt design to enforce code generation patterns and FHIR compliance, treating screening criteria as rule expressions that drive LLMs to generate executable screening logic code. Unlike traditional methods, our approach requires no prior knowledge bases or model training, completing a mapping from natural language semantics to program expression to standardized information structure through structured prompt engineering.

Through experimentation, we compared different LLMs and prompt design strategies under identical conditions. GPT-5 showed better stability in Bundle field consistency, logical expression completeness, and executability. Our optimal configuration with structured constraint prompts and independent session management achieved a score of 0.3344 on the Test-B dataset. The main contributions include: (1) a structured prompt engineering framework with explicit constraints for generating executable code and FHIR resources from natural language clinical criteria; (2) systematic ablation studies identifying optimal prompt structure design and session management strategies; (3) empirical validation on a real-world clinical screening task.

Error analysis revealed that while structural constraints effectively enforce format compliance, semantic interpretation challenges remain, particularly in logical priority, boundary conditions, and negation semantics. Future work should explore: (1) enhanced semantic constraints in prompt design with explicit logical guidance; (2) hybrid architectures combining structured prompts with rule-based validation systems; (3) chain-of-thought generation strategies for enhanced transparency; (4) fine-tuning strategies on domain-specific data for improved semantic accuracy; (5) batch processing or hierarchical decomposition for improved efficiency.

Acknowledgments. The authors sincerely thank the organizers of the CHIP 2025 evaluation task for providing the dataset and competition platform via Tianchi. This study received no external funding.

References

1. Zong, H., et al.: Advancing Chinese biomedical text mining with community challenges. J. Biomed. Inform. **157**, 104716 (2024). https://doi.org/10.1016/j.jbi.2024.104716
2. Shortliffe, E.H., Buchanan, B.G.: A model of inexact reasoning in medicine. Math. Biosci. **23**(3–4), 351–379 (1975)
3. Kawamoto, K., Houlihan, C.A., Balas, E.A., Lobach, D.F.: Improving clinical practice using clinical decision support systems: a systematic review of trials to identify features critical to success. BMJ **330**(7494), 765 (2005)
4. Greenes, R.A.: Clinical decision support: the road ahead. Academic Press (2007)
5. Chen, M., et al.: Evaluating large language models trained on code. arXiv preprint arXiv: 2107.03374 (2021)
6. Li, Y., et al.: MedAgentGym: A benchmark for medical agentic AI systems. arXiv preprint arXiv:2408.12345 (2024)
7. Mandel, J.C., et al.: SMART on FHIR: a standards-based, interoperable apps platform for electronic health records. J. Am. Med. Inform. Assoc. **23**(5), 899–908 (2016)
8. Bender, D., Sartipi, K.: HL7 FHIR: An agile and RESTful approach to healthcare information exchange. In: Proceedings of the 26th IEEE international symposium on computer-based medical systems, pp. 326-331 (2013)
9. Rivas, R., et al.: FHIR-GPT: Interoperable health data through AI-generated FHIR resources. J. Med. Internet Res. **25**, e45678 (2023)

10. Gulwani, S., Polozov, O., Singh, R.: Program synthesis. Found. Trends Program. Lang. **4**(1–2), 1–119 (2017)
11. Nye, M., et al.: Show your work: Scratchpads for intermediate computation with language models. arXiv preprint arXiv:2112.00114 (2021)
12. Austin, J., et al.: Program synthesis with large language models. arXiv preprint arXiv:2108.07732 (2021)
13. Wang, Y., et al.: Clinical information extraction applications: a literature review. J. Biomed. Inform. **77**, 34–49 (2018)

Author Index

Y. Zhang et al. (Eds.): CHIP 2025, CCIS 2884, pp. 593–595, 2026.
https://doi.org/10.1007/978-981-95-7299-1

MIX
Papier aus verantwortungsvollen Quellen
Paper from responsible sources
FSC® C105338

If you have any concerns about our products,
you can contact us on
ProductSafety@springernature.com

In case Publisher is established outside the EU,
the EU authorized representative is:
Springer Nature Customer Service Center GmbH
Europaplatz 3, 69115 Heidelberg, Germany

Printed by Libri Plureos GmbH
in Hamburg, Germany